NEW AMERICAN
Pocket Medical Dictionary
Second Edition

NEW AMERICAN
Pocket
Medical
Dictionary
Second Edition

EDITED BY

Nancy Roper MPhil, RSCN, RNT

Adapted from the fourteenth British Edition
by Jane Clark Jackson, BSN, RN, MSN,
CNM

Charles Scribner's Sons • New York

Second Edition copyright © 1988 by Churchill Livingstone Inc.

First Edition copyright © 1978 by Longman Inc.

Charles Scribner's Sons
Macmillan Publishing Company
866 Third Avenue, New York, NY 10022

ISBN 0-684-19031-1
Library of Congress Catalog Card Number 88-14973

10 9 8 7 6 5 4 3

Printed in the United States of America

Adapter's Preface

Nancy Roper's *Pocket Medical Dictionary* was first published more than fifty years ago. The fourteenth edition, recently published in Great Britain, continues to provide students and professionals in the allied health fields as well as lay readers with an accessible and transportable reference source. Once again, I have "Americanized" Ms. Roper's dictionary in order to make it more relevant for use in the United States. At the same time I have attempted to remain true to the original version wherever possible.

In the ten years since the *New American Pocket Medical Dictionary*, based on Ms. Roper's work, was first published there have been many innovations in the health care fields. This new edition has been revised and updated to reflect these changes. There are over one thousand new entries. The format has been redesigned to make the search task easier and faster. Wordbreaks have been indicated to aid in preparation of professional papers, and specialized information has been collected in seven appendices following the main dictionary.

Appendix 1 contains full page, 2-color line illustrations of the major body systems. At the appropriate anatomical term in the dictionary, the reader is directed to the relevant illustration.

Appendix 2 explains SI units and the metric system and provides useful conversion scales for certain chemical pathology tests and common units of measurement.

Appendix 3 details the range of normal human characteristics from blood and cerebrospinal fluid to vitamins and weights and heights.

Appendix 4, on poisons, combines an outline of substances commonly involved with the clinical features exhibited and a guide to treatment.

Appendix 5 contains the telephone numbers of State Poison Control Centers.

Appendix 6 lists familiar abbreviations covering professional degrees and organizations.

Appendix 7 lists commonly used abbreviations for recording nursing and medical records.

It is hoped that the second edition of the *New American Pocket Medical Dictionary* will be useful to nursing, medical, and other health care students and professionals as well as the growing numbers of lay people interested in increasing their medical knowledge and understanding.

I would like to extend my gratitude to Nancy Roper and to the publishers, both in Great Britain and in the United States, for help in this endeavor.

Jane Clark Jackson,
BSN, RN, MSN, CNM

Contents

How to use this dictionary

Main entries
These are listed in alphabetical order and appear in **bold** type. Derivative forms of the main entry also appear in **bold** type and along with their parts of speech are to be found at the end of the definition.

Wordbreaks
These are designed to provide guidance when preparing papers for publication, writing essays, and general correspondence. A centered bold dot · appears between letters of the main entry to indicate where the word(s) can be split at the end of a line. As far as possible the break has been limited to a single indication but because of the nature of many medical terms, alternative positions for the break have been included.

Separate meanings of main entry
Different meanings of the same word are separated by means of an arabic numeral before each meaning.

Subentries
Subentries relating to the defined headword are listed in alphabetical order and appear in *italic* type, following the main definition.

Parts of speech
The part of speech follows single word main entries and derivative forms of the main entry, and appears in *italic* type. For the parts of speech used in the dictionary, see the list of abbreviations on page x.

Cross-references
Cross-references alert you to related words and additional information elsewhere in the dictionary. Two symbols have been used for this purpose—an arrow ⇒ and an asterisk *. At the end of a definition, the arrow indicates the word you should then look up for related subject matter. In the case of a drug trade name, it will refer you to the approved name and main definition. For anatomical terms, the arrow will indicate an illustration in Appendix 1 to show the term's position in the body.
Within a definition an asterisk placed at the end of a word means that there is a separate entry in the dictionary which may be of use in providing further information.

Abbreviations

abbr abbreviation
adj adjective
adv adverb
e.g. for example
i.e. that is
i.m. intramuscular
i.v. intravenous
n noun
opp opposite
pl plural
sing singular
syn synonym
v verb
vi intransitive verb
vt transitive verb

Guide to pronunciation: consonants

ch (= tsh) as in cheese (chēz),
                 stitch (stich),
                 picture (pik′chėr).
   j (dzh)   judge (juj),
                 rigid (rij′id).
     sh   dish,
                 lotion (lō′-shun).
     zh   vision (vizh′-'n).
     ng   sing,
                 think (thingk).
      g Always hard as in good
      r This letter is often left unsounded or is slurred into the preceding vowel. In the combination 'er' (see Vowels) the 'r' is rarely trilled or marked. Where it receives its full consonantal value it is usually placed preceding a vowel; in most other cases its force is determined by individual taste and custom.
    th No attempt has been made to distinguish between the breathed sound as in 'think' and the voiced sound as in 'them.'
Accent: The accented syllable is indicated by a slanting stroke at its termination, e.g., fibrositis (fi-brė-sī′-tis).

Guide to pronunciation: vowels

a as in	fat, back, tap.
ā	lame, brain (brān), vein (vān).
à	far, calf (kàf), heart (hàrt), coma (kō'mà).
e	flesh, deaf (def), said (sed).
ē	he, tea (tē), knee (nē), anemia (an-ē'-mi-à).
ė	there, air (ėr), area (ėr'-i-à).*
i	sit, busy (biz'-i).
ī	spine, my, eye, tie
o	hot, cough (kof).
ō	bone, moan (mōn), dough (dō).
u	gum, love (luv), tough (tuf), color (kul'-ėr).
ū	mute, due, new, you, rupture (rup'-tūr).
aw	saw, gall (gawl), caul (kawl), water (waw'tėr).
oi	loin, boy.
oo	foot, womb (woom), wound (woond), rude (rood).
ow	cow, sound (sownd), gout (gowt).

* When followed by 'r', 'e'; is often sound as in 'her' or as 'u' in 'fur' (for example, 'ferment'); in '-er' as a final unaccented syllable, the 'e' is sometimes more or less elided (drawer, tower). See also consonant 'r' on page xi.

Prefixes which can be used as combining forms in compounded words

Prefix	Meaning	Prefix	Meaning
a-	without, not	brachy-	short
ab-	away from	brady-	slow
abdo- / abdomino-	abdominal	broncho-	bronchi
acro-	extremity	calc-	chalk
ad-	towards	carcin-	cancer
adeno-	glandular	cardio-	heart
aer-	air	carpo-	wrist
amb- / ambi-	both, on both sides	cata-	down
		cav-	hollow
amido-	NH₂ group united to an acid radical	centi-	a hundredth
		cephal-	head
amino-	NH₂ group united to a radical other than an acid radical	cerebro-	brain
		cervic-	neck, womb
		cheil-	lip
amphi-	on both sides, around	cheir-	hand
amyl-	starch	chemo-	chemical
an-	not, without	chlor-	green
ana-	up	chol-	bile
andro-	male	cholecysto-	gall bladder
angi-	vessel (blood)	choledocho-	common bile duct
aniso-	unequal	chondro-	cartilage
ant- / anti-	against, counteracting	chrom-	color
		cine-	film, motion
ante- / antero-	before	circum-	around
		co- / col- / com- / con-	together
antro-	antrum		
aorto-	aorta		
app-	away, from	coli-	bowel
arachn-	spider	colpo-	vagina
arthro-	joint	contra-	against
auto-	self	costo-	orib
		cox-	hip
bi-	twice, two	crani- / cranio-	skull
bili-	bile		
bio-	life	cryo-	cold
blenno-	mucus	crypt-	hidden, concealed
bleph-	eyelid	cyan-	blue
brachio-	arm		

Prefix	Meaning	Prefix	Meaning
cysto-	bladder	gala-	milk
cyto-	cell	gastro-	stomach
		genito-	genitals, reproductive
dacryo-	tear	ger-	old age
dactyl-	finger	glosso-	tongue
de-	away, from, reversing	glyco-	sugar
		gnatho	jaw
deca-	ten	gyne-	female
deci-	tenth		
demi-	half	hema-	blood
dent-	tooth	hemo-	
derma-	skin	hemi-	half
dermat-		hepa-	liver
dextro-	to the right	hepatico-	
dia-	through	hepato-	
dip-	double	hetgro-	unlikeness, dissimilarity
dis-	separation, against		
dorso-	dorsal	hexa-	six
dys-	difficult, painful, abnormal	histo-	tissue
		homeo-	like
		homo-	same
ecto-	outside, without, external	hydro-	water
		hygro-	moisture
electro-	electricity	hyper-	above
em-	in	hypo-	below
en-		hypno-	sleep
end-	in, into, within	hystero-	uterus
endo-			
ent-	within	iatro-	physician
entero-	intestine	idio-	peculiar to the individual
epi-	on, above, upon		
ery-	red	ileo-	ileum
eu-	well, normal	ilio-	ilium
ex-	away from, out, out of	immuno-	immunity
exo-		in-	not, in, into, within
extra-	outside	infra-	below
		inter-	between
		intra-	within
faci-	face	intro-	inward
ferri-	iron	ischio-	ischium
ferro-		iso-	equal
fibro-	fiber, fibrous tissue		
flav-	yellow	karyo-	nucleus
feto-	fetus	kerato-	horn, skin, cornea
fore-	before, in front of	kypho-	rounded, humped

Prefix	Meaning	Prefix	Meaning
lact-	milk	onc-	mass
laparo-	flank	onycho-	nail
laryngo-	larynx	oo-	egg, ovum
lepto-	thin, soft	oophor-	ovary
leuco-	} white	ophthalmo-	eye
leuko-		opisth-	backward
lympho-	lymphatic	orchido-	testis
		oro-	mouth
macro-	large	ortho-	straight
mal-	abnormal, poor	os-	bone, mouth
mamm-	} breast	osteo-	bone
mast-		oto-	ear
medi	middle	ova-	egg
mega-	large	ovari-	ovary
melano-	pigment, dark		
meso-	middle	pachy-	thick
meta-	between	pan-	all
metro-	uterus	para-	beside
micro-	small	patho-	disease
milli-	a thousandth	ped-	child, foot
mio-	smaller	penta-	} five
mono-	one, single	pento-	
muco-	mucus	per-	by, through
multi-	many	peri-	around
myc-	fungus	perineo-	perineum
myelo-	spinal cord, bone marrow	pharma-	drug
		pharyngo-	pharynx
myo-	muscle	phlebo-	vein
		phono-	voice
narco-	stupor	photo-	light
naso-	nose	phren-	diaphragm, mind
necro-	corpse	physio-	form, nature
neo-	new	pleuro-	pleura
nephro-	kidney	pluri-	many
neuro-	nerve	pneumo-	lung
noct-	night	podo-	foot
normo-	normal	polio	grey
nucleo-	nucleus	poly-	many, much
nyc-	night	post-	after
		pre-	} before
oculo-	eye	pro-	
odonto-	tooth	proct-	anus
oligo-	deficiency, diminution	proto-	first
		pseudo-	false

Prefix	Meaning	Prefix	Meaning
psycho-	mind	tabo-	tabes, wasting away
pyelo-	pelvis of the kidney	tachy-	fast
pyo-	pus	tarso-	foot, edge of eyelid
pyr-	fever	teno-	tendon
		tetra-	four
quadri-	four	thermo-	heat
quint	five	thoraco-	thorax
		thrombo-	blood clot
radi-	ray	thyro-	thyroid gland
radio-	radiation	tibio-	tibia
re-	again, back	tox-	poison
ren-	kidney	tracheo-	trachea
retro-	backward	trans-	across, through
rhin-	nose	tri-	three
rub-	red	trich-	hair
		tropho-	nourishment
sacchar-	sugar	ultra-	beyond
sacro-	sacrum	uni-	one
salpingo-	Fallopian tube	uretero-	ureter
sapro-	dead, decaying	urethro-	urethra
sarco-	flesh	uri-	urine
sclero-	hard	uro-	urine, urinary organs
scota	darkness	utero-	uterus
semi-	half		
sept-	seven	vaso-	vessel
sero-	serum	veno-	vein
socio-	sociology	ventro-	abdomen
sphygm-	pulse	vesico-	bladder
spleno-	spleen		
spondy-	vertebra	xanth-	yellow
steato-	fat	xero-	dry
sterno-	sternum	xiphi-	} ensiform cartilage of
sub-	below	xipho-	} sternum
supra-	above		
syn-	together, union, with	zoo-	animal

Suffixes which can be used as combining forms in compounded words

Suffix	Meaning	Suffix	Meaning
-able	able to, capable of	-gogue	increasing flow
-agra	attack, severe pain	-gram	a tracing
-al	characterized by, pertaining to	-graph	description, treatise, writing
-algia	pain		
-an	belonging to, pertaining to	-iasis	condition of, state
		-iatric	practice of healing
-ase	catalyst, enzyme, ferment	-itis	inflammation of
-asis	state of	-kinesis	
		-kinetic	motion
-blast	cell		
		-lith	calculus, stone
-caval	pertaining to venae cavae	-lithiasis	presence of stones
		-logy	science of, study of
-cele	tumor, swelling	-lysis lytic	breaking down,
-centesis	to puncture	-lytic	disintegration
-cide	destructive, killing		
-clysis	infusion, injection	-malacia	softening
-coccus	spherical cell	-megaly	enlargement
-cule	little	-meter	measure
-cyte	cell	-morph	form
-derm	skin	-ogen	precursor
-desis	to bind together	-odynia	pain
-dynia	pain	-oid	likeness, resemblance
		-ol	alcohol
-ectasis	dilation, extension	-ology	the study of
-ectomy	removal of	-oma	tumor
-emia	blood	-opia	eye
-esthesia	sensibility, sense-perception	-opsy	looking
		-ose	sugar
		-osis	condition, disease, excess
-facient	making		
-form	having the form of	-ostomy	to form an opening or outlet
-fuge	expelling		
-genesis		-otomy	incision of
-genetic	formation, origin	-ous	like, having the nature of
-genic	capable of causing		

xvii

Suffix	Meaning	Suffix	Meaning
-pathy	disease	-scope	instrument for visual examination
-penia	lack of		
-pexy	fixation	-scopy	to examine visually
-phage	ingesting	-somatic	pertaining to the body
-phagia	swallowing	-somy	pertaining to chromosomes
-phasia	speech		
-philia	affinity for, loving	-sonic	sound
-phobia	fear	-stasis	stagnation, cessation of movement
-phylaxis	protection		
-piesis	making	-sthenia	strength
-plasty	reconstructive surgery	-stomy	to form an opening or outlet
-plegia	paralysis		
-pnea	breathing		
-ptosis	falling	-taxis	arrangement, coordination, order
		-taxis	
-rhage	to burst forth	-taxy	
-rhaphy	suturing	-tome	cutting instrument
-rhea	excessive discharge	-tomy	incision of
-rhythmia	rhythm	-trophy	nourishment
		-trophy	turning
-saccharide	basic carbohydrate molecule	-urea	urine

A

A-200 Pyrinate *n* a pediculicide for control of head lice, pubic and body lice.

AA *abbr* Alcoholics* Anonymous.

abac·terial (ā-bak-tē′-ri-àl) *adj* without bacteria. A word used to describe a condition, for instance inflammation, which is not caused by bacteria.

abdo·men (ab′-dō-měn, ab-dō′-měn) *n* the largest body cavity, immediately below the thorax, from which it is separated by the diaphragm*. It is enclosed largely by muscle and fascia, and is therefore capable of change in size and shape. It is lined with a serous membrane, the peritoneum*, which is reflected as a covering over most of the organs. *acute abdomen* pathological condition within the abdomen requiring immediate surgical intervention. *pendulous abdomen* a relaxed condition of the anterior wall, allowing it to hang down over the pubis. *scaphoid abdomen* (navicular) concavity of the anterior wall.

abdomi·nal (ab-dom′-in-al) *adj* pertaining to the abdomen. *abdominal aoa* ⇒ Figures 10, 19. *abdominal breathing* more than usual use of the diaphragm and abdominal muscles to increase the input of air to and output from the lungs. It can be done voluntarily in the form of exercises. When it occurs in disease it is a compensatory mechanism for inadequate oxygenation. *abdominal excision of the rectum* usually performed by two surgeons working at the same time. The rectum is mobilized through an abdominal incision. The bowel is divided well proximal to the tumor. The proximal end is brought out as a permanent colostomy. Excision of the distal bowel containing the tumor together with the anal canal is completed through a perineal incision.

abdomino·centesis (ab-dom′-in-ō-sent-ē′-sis) *n* paracentesis* of the peritoneal cavity.

abdomino·pelvic (ab-dom-in-ō-pel′-vik) *adj* pertaining to the abdomen and pelvis* or pelvic cavity.

abdomino·perineal (ab-dom-in-ō-per-in-ē′-al) *adj* pertaining to the abdomen and perineum*.

ab·duct (ab-dukt′) *vt* to draw away from the median line of the body ⇒ adduct *opp*.

abduc·tion (ab-duk′-shun) *n* the act of abducting away from the midline ⇒ adduction *opp*.

abduc·tor (ab-duk′-tōr) *n* a muscle which, on contraction, draws a part away from the median line of the body. ⇒ adductor *opp*. *abductor policis longus* ⇒ Figure 3.

ab·errant (ab-er′-ant) *adj* abnormal; usually applied to a blood vessel or nerve which does not follow the normal course.

aber·ration (ab-er-rā′-shun) *n* a deviation from normal—aberrant *adj*. *chromosomal aberration* loss, gain or exchange of genetic material in the chromosomes of a cell resulting in deletion, duplication, inversion or translocation of genes. *mental aberration* ⇒ mental. *optical aberration* imperfect focus of light rays by a lens.

abio·trophy (ab-ē-ōt′-rō-fē) *n* premature loss of vitality or degeneration of certain cells or tissues, usually of genetic origin. ⇒ retinitis. chorea.

ab·lation (ab-lā′-shun) *n* removal. In surgery, the word means excision or amputation—**ablative** *adj*.

ablution (ab-lū′-shun) *n* act of cleaning or washing.

ABO incompatibility a blood group incompatibility between maternal and fetal blood based on Anti-A or Anti-B agglutinins in the maternal blood and the presence of A or B factors in the infant's blood. May cause hemolytic disease of newborn.

abort (ab-ōrt′) *vt* to terminate before full development.

aborti·facient (ab-ōr-ti-fā′-shi-ent) *adj* causing abortion. A drug or agent inducing expulsion of a nonviable fetus.

abort·ion (ab-ōr′-shun) *n* **1** abrupt termination of a process. **2** expulsion from a uterus of the product of conception before it is viable, i.e. before 20–24 weeks gestation or before the fetus weighs 500 g. ⇒ abortus—**abortive** *adj*. *complete abortion* the entire contents of the uterus are expelled. *criminal abortion* intentional evacuation of uterus by other than trained, licensed medical personnel, or when abortion is prohibited by law. *habitual abortion* (preferable syn.) *recurrent abortion* term used when abortion recurs in successive pregnancies. *incomplete abortion* part of the fetus or placenta is retained within the uterus. *induced abortion* (also called 'artificial') intentional evacuation of uterus. *inevitable abortion* one which has advanced to a stage where termination of pregnancy cannot be prevented. *missed*

1

abortion early signs and symptoms of pregnancy disappear and the fetus dies, but is not expelled for some time. ⇒ carneous mole. *septic abortion* one associated with uterine infection and rise in body temperature. *spontaneous abortion* one which occurs naturally without intervention. *therapeutic abortion* intentional termination of a pregnancy which is a hazard to the mother's life and health. *threatened abortion* slight blood loss per vagina while cervix remains closed. May be accompanied by abdominal pain. *tubal abortion* an ectopic* pregnancy that dies and is expelled from the fimbriated end of the Fallopian tube.

abor·tus (a-bōr´-tus) *n* an aborted fetus weighing less than 500 g. it is either dead or incapable of surviving.

abras·ion (ab-rā´-zhun) *n* **1** superficial injury to skin or mucous membrane from scraping or rubbing; excoriation. **2** can be used therapeutically for removal of scar tissue (dermabrasion).

abreac·tion (ab-rē-ak´-shun) *n* an emotional reaction resulting from recall of past painful experiences relived in speech and action during psychoanalysis or under the influence of light anesthesia, or drugs ⇒ narcoanalysis. catharsis.

ab·scess (ab´-ses) *n* localized collection of pus produced by pyogenic organisms. May be acute or chronic. ⇒ quinsy. *alveolar abscess* at the root of a tooth. *amoebic abscess* one caused by *Entamoeba hystolitica;* usual site is the liver, other sites are long brain and spleen ⇒ amoebiasis. *Brodie's abscess* chronic osteomyelitis* occurring without previous acute phase. *cold abscess* one occurring in the course of such chronic inflammation as may be due to *Mycobacterium tuberculosis. psoas abscess* ⇒ psoas.

abused child ⇒ battered baby syndrome.

acal·culia (a-kal-kūl´-ē-a) *n* inability to do simple arithmetic.

acapnia (ā-kap´-ni-à) *n* absence of CO_2 in the blood. Can be produced by hyperventilation—**acapnial,** *adj.*

acata·lasia (a-kat-al-āz´-i-a) *n* genetically determined absence of the enzyme catalase; predisposes to oral sepsis.

accessory nerve eleventh cranial nerve.

accommo·dation (ak-kom-mo-dā´-shun) *n* adjustment, e.g. the power of the eye to alter the convexity of the lens according to the nearness or distance of objects, so that a distinct image is always retained—**accommodative** *adj.*

accouche·ment (ak-koosh´-mong) *n* delivery in childbirth. Confinement.

accou·cheur (ak-koo-shėr´) *n* a man skilled in midwifery; an obstetrician.

accou·cheuse (ak-koo-shėrz´) *n* a midwife; a female obstetrician.

accre·tion (ak-krē´-shun) *n* an increase of substance or deposit round a central object; in dentistry, an accumulation of tartar or calculus round the teeth—**accrete** *adj. vt, vi,* **accretive** *adj.*

acebuto·lol (as-e-bū´-to-lol) *n* a β-adrenoceptor blocking agent used in cardiac dysrhythmias, angina pectoris and hypertension. (Sectral.)

acepha·lous (ā-sef´-a-lus) *adj* without a head.

acetabulo·plasty (as-et-ab´-ūl-ō-plas-ti) *n* an operation to improve the depth and shape of the hip socket (acetabulum); necessary in such conditions as congenital dislocation of the hip and osteoarthritis of the hip.

acetabu·lum (as-et-ab´-ūl-um) *n* a cuplike socket on the external lateral surface of the pelvis into which the head of the femur fits to form the hip joint—**acetabula** *pl.*

acetaminophen (a-sēt-a-min´-ō-fen) *n* a non-salicylate analgesic-antipyretic (Tylenol).

acet·ate (as´-e-tāt) *n* a salt of acetic* acid.

acetazol·amide (a-sē-ta-zol´-a-mīd) *n* oral diuretic of short duration. Carbonic anhydrase inhibitor. Used for treatment of glaucoma*. (Diamox.)

acetic acid (as-ēt´-ik-as´-id) *n* the acid present in vinegar. Three varieties are used medicinally: (a) glacial acetic acid, sometimes used as a caustic; (b) ordinary acetic acid, used in urine testing; (c) dilute acetic acid, used occasionally in cough mixtures.

aceto-acetic acid (as-ē´-tō-as-ē´-tik-as´-id) *n* (*syn* diacetic acid) a monobasic keto acid. Produced at an interim stage in the oxidation of fats in the human body. In some metabolic upsets, e.g. acidosis and diabetes mellitus, it is present in excess in the blood and escapes in the urine. (It changes to acetone if urine is left standing.) The excess acid in the blood can produce coma.

aceto-hexamide (as-ēt-ō-heks´-à-mīd) *n* an oral antidiabetic drug, one of the sulphonylureas*. (Dymelor.)

acet·one (as´-e-tōn) *n* inflammable liquid with characteristic odor; valuable as a solvent. *acetone bodies* ⇒ ketone.

aceton·emia (as-e-tōn-ēm′-i-a) *n* acetone bodies in the blood—**acetonemic** *adj*.

aceton·uria (as-e-tō-nū′-ri-a) *n* excess acetone bodies in the urine, causing a characteristic sweet smell—**acetonuric** *adj*.

acetyl·choline (as-et-il-kō′-lēn) *n* a chemical substance released from nerve endings to activate muscle, secretory glands and other nerve cells. The nerve fibers releasing this chemical are termed cholinergic. Hydrolyzed into choline and acetic acid by the enzyme acetylcholinesterase, which is present around the nerve endings and also in blood and other tissues.

acetyl·cysteine (as-et-il-sis′-tēn) *n* a mucolytic agent, invaluable in cystic* fibrosis. Also used in treatment of paracetamol overdose. (Mucomyst.)

acetyl·salicyclic acid (as-et-il-sal′-is-il-ik as′-id) *n* an extensively used mild analgesic. It forms the basis of a large number of proprietary analgesic tablets. Gastric irritant. Can cause hematemesis. Aspirin is the generic name.

acha·lasia (ak-a-lā′-zi-a) *n* failure to relax. *cardiac achalasia* ⇒ cardiac.

Achilles ten·don (ak-il′-ēz ten′-don) *n* the tendinous termination of the soleus* and gastrocnemius* muscles inserted into the heel bone (os calcis).

achlor·hydria (ā-klōr-hī′-dri-à) *n* the absence of free hydrochloric acid in the stomach. Found in pernicious anemia and gastric cancer—**achlorhydric** *adj*.

acholia (ā-kōl′-i-à) *n* the absence of bile*—**acholic** *adj*.

achol·uria (ā-kōl-ūr′-i-à) *n* the absence of bile* pigment from the urine. ⇒ jaundice—**acholuric** *adj*.

achondro·plasia (ā-kon-drō-plā′-zi-à) *n* an inherited condition characterized by arrested growth of the long bones resulting in short-limbed dwarfism with a big head. The intellect is not impaired. Inheritance is dominant—**achondroplastic** *adj*.

achroma·topsia (ā-krō-mat-op′-zi-à) *n* complete color blindness; only monochromatic grey is visible.

Achro·mycin (ak-rō-mī′-sin) *n* proprietary name for tetracycline*.

achylia (a-kī′-li-à) *n* absence of chylc*—**achylic** *adj*.

acid (as′-id) *n* any substance which in solution gives rise to an excess of hydrogen ions. Identified (a) by turning blue litmus

paper red; (b) by being neutralized by an alkali with the formation of a salt.

acid-alcohol-fast *adj* in bacteriology, describes an organism which, when stained, is resistant to decolorization by alcohol as well as acid, e.g. *Mycobacterium tuberculosis*.

acid-base balance equilibrium between the acid and base elements of the blood and body fluids.

acid·emia (as-id-ē′-mi-a) *n* abnormal acidity of the blood, giving increased hydrogen ions, and a below normal pH*. When it is caused by poor ventilation and increasing carbon dioxide it is termed *respiratory acidemia*. When it is caused by increased lactic acid production in muscles it is *metabolic acidemia* ⇒ acidosis.—**acidemic** *adj*.

acid-fast *adj* in bacteriology, describes an organism which, when stained, does not become decolorized when subjected to dilute acids.

acid·ity (as-id′-it-i) *n* the state of being acid or sour. The degree of acidity can be determined and interpreted on the pH* scale, pH 6.69 denoting a very weak acid and pH 1 a strong acid.

acidosis (as-id-ō′-sis) *n* depletion of the body's alkali reserve, with resulting disturbance of the acid-base balance. Acidemia*. ⇒ ketosis—**acidotic** *adj*.

acid phos·pha·tase (as-id fos′-fä-tāz) *n* an enzyme which synthesizes phosphate esters of carbohydrates in an acid medium. *acid phos·pha·tase test* an increase of this enzyme in the blood is indicative of carcinoma of the prostate gland.

acid·uria (as-id-ūr′-i-à) *n* excretion of an acid urine. Current work suggests there might be some association with mental subnormality.

acini (as′-in-ī) *n* minute saccules* or alveoli*, lined or filled with secreting cells. Several acini combine to form a lobule—**acinus** *sing*, **acinous, acinar** *adj*.

acme (ak′-mē) *n* 1 highest point. 2 crisis or critical state of a disease.

acne, acne vulgaris (ak′-nē vul-gār′-is) *n* a condition in which the pilosebaceous glands are overstimulated by circulating androgens and the excessive sebum* is trapped by a plug of keratin, one of the protein constituents of human hair. Skin bacteria then colonize the glands and convert the trapped sebum into irritant fatty acids responsible for the swelling and inflammation (pustules) which follow. Minocycline is the drug of choice.

3

acnei·form (ak-nē'-i-förm) *adj* resembling acne.

acous·tic nerve *n* eighth cranial nerve. ⇒ Figure 13.

ac·quired im·mune de·ficiency syn·drome (AIDS, *abbr.*) a reliably diagnosed disease that is at least moderately indicative of an underlying cellular immune deficiency, for example Kaposi's sarcoma in a patient aged less than 60 years or opportunistic infection where there is no known underlying cause of cellular immune deficiency nor any other cause of reduced resistance reported to be associated with the disease. Reported mainly in male homosexuals and bisexuals who have many sexual partners, a small number of intravenous drug abusers and a few hemophiliacs. Cause is unknown but it is thought to be due to a virus.

acri·flavine (ak-ri-flā'-vēn) *n* powerful antiseptic, used as a 1:1000 solution for wounds, and 1:4000 to 1:8000 for irrigation. Acriflavine emulsion is a bland, non-adherent wound dressing containing liquid paraffin. Proflavine and euflavine are similar compounds.

acro·cephalia; acro·cephaly (ak-rō-sef'-ä-li-a) *n* a congenital malformation whereby the top of the head is pointed and the eyes protrude, due to premature closure of sagittal and coronal skull sutures—**acrocephalic, acrocephalous** *adj.*

acro·cephalo·syndactyly (ak-rō-sef'-a-lō-sin-dak'-til-i) *n* a congenital malformation consisting of a pointed top of head, with webbed hands and feet. ⇒ Apert's syndrome.

acro·cyan·osis (ak-rō-sī-an-ō'-sis) *n* coldness and blueness of the extremities due to circulatory disorder—**acrocyanotic** *adj.*

acro·dynia (ak-rō-dīn'-i-a) *n* painful reddening of the extremities such as occurs in erythroedema* polyneuritis.

acro·megaly (ak-rō-meg'-a-li) *n* enlargement of the hands, face and feet, occurring in an adult due to excess growth hormone. In a child this causes gigantism. ⇒ growth hormone test—**acromegalic** *adj.*

acro·micria (ak-rō-mīk'-rē-a) *n* smallness of the hands, face and feet, probably due to deficiency of growth hormone from the pituitary gland.

acromio·clavicular (ak-rō-mi-ō-kla-vi'-kū-làr) *adj* pertaining to the acromion process (of scapula) and the clavicle.

acro·mion (ak-rō'-mi-on) *n* the point or summit of the shoulder; the triangular process at the extreme outer end of the spine of the scapula—**acromial** *adj.*

acronyx (ak'-rō-niks) *n* ingrowing of a nail.

acro·pares·thesia (ak-rō-pär-es-thē'-zi-a) *n* tingling and numbness of the hands.

acro·phobia (ak-rō-fō'-bē-à) *n* morbid fear of being at a height.

acry·lics (a-kril'-iks) *npl* a group of thermoplastic substances used in making prostheses—**acrylic** *adj.*

ACTH *abbr* adrenocorticotrophic hormone ⇒ corticotrophin.

Acthar gel (ak'-thar-jel) *n* a preparation of ACTH used for diagnostic testing of adrenocortical function and used therapeutically for lupus erythematosus, rheumatoid arthritis and allergies.

Acti-fed (ak'-ti-fed) *n* proprietary drug containing pseudoephedrine* and triprolidine*.

actin (ak'-tin) *n* one of the proteins in muscle cells; it reacts with myosin to cause contraction.

acting out *n* reduction of emotional distress by the release of disturbed or violent behavior, which is unconsciously determined and reflects previous unresolved conflicts and attitudes.

ac·tinic derma·toses *npl* skin conditions in which the integument is abnormally sensitive to ultraviolet light.

actin·ism (ak'-tin-izm) *n* the chemical action of radiant energy, especially in the ultraviolet spectrum—**actinic** *adj.*

actino·biology (ak-tin-ō-bī-ol'-ōj-i) *n* study of the effects of radiation on living organisms.

Actino·myces (ak-tin-ō-mī'-sēz) *n* a genus of parasitic fungus-like bacteria exhibiting a radiating mycelium. Also called 'ray fungus'. Many of the antibiotic drugs are produced from this genus.

actino·mycosis (ak-tin-ō-mī-kō'-sis) *n* a disease caused by the bacterium *Actinomyces israeli*, the sites most affected being the lung, jaw and intestine. Granulomatous tumors form which usually suppurate, discharging a thick, oily pus containing yellowish granules ('sulphur granules')—**actinomycotic** *adj.*

actino·therapy (ak-tin-ō-thè'-rap-i) *n* treatment by using infrared or ultraviolet radiation.

ac·tion (ak'-shun) *n* the activity or function of any part of the body. *antagonistic action* performed by those muscles which limit the movement of an opposing group. *compulsive action* performed by an individual at the supposed instigation of another's dominant will, but against his own. *impulsive action* resulting from a sudden urge rather than the will. *reflex action* ⇒ reflex. *sexual action* coitus, cohabitation, sexual intercourse. *specific action* that brought about by certain remedial agents in a particular disease, e.g. salicylates in acute rheumatism. *specific dynamic action* the stimulating effect upon the metabolism produced by the ingestion of food, especially proteins, causing the metabolic rate to rise above basal levels. *synergistic action* that brought about by the co-operation of two or more muscles, neither of which could bring about the action alone.

Acti·sorb (ak'-ti-sōrb) *n* activated charcoal pads for preventing odor from discharging wounds.

acti·vator (ak'-tiv-ā-tōr) *n* a substance which renders something else active, e.g. the hormone secretin*, the enzyme enterokinase*—**activate** *v*.

ac·tive (ak'-tiv) *adj* energetic. ⇒ passive* *opp. active hyperemia* ⇒ hyperemia. *active immunity* ⇒ immunity. *active movements* those produced by the patient using his neuromuscular mechanism. *active principle* an ingredient which gives a complex drug its chief therapeutic value, e.g. atropine is the active principle in belladonna.

acu·ity (ak-ū'-it-i) *n* sharpness, clearness, keenness, distinctness. *auditory acuity* ability to hear clearly and distinctly. Tests include the use of tuning fork, whispered voice and audiometer. In infants, simple sounds, e.g. bells, rattles, cup and spoon are utilized. *visual acuity* the extent of visual perception is dependent on the clarity of retinal focus, integrity of nervous elements and cerebral interpretation of the stimulus. Usually tested by Snellen's* test types at 6 meters.(20'.)

acu·punc·ture (ak'-ū-punk-tūr) *n* **1** the incision or introduction of fine, hollow tubes into edematous tissue for the purpose of withdrawing fluid. **2** a technique of insertion of special needles into particular parts of the body for the treatment of disease, relief of pain or production of anesthesia.

acute (a-kūt') *adj* short and severe; not long drawn out or chronic. *acute defibrination syndrome* (*syn* hypofibrinogenemia), excessive bleeding due to maternal absorption of thromboplastins from retained blood clot or damaged placenta within the uterus. A missed abortion, placental abruption, amniotic fluid embolus, prolonged retention in utero of a dead fetus and the intravenous administration of dextran can lead to ADS. *acute dilatation of the stomach* sudden enlargement of this organ due to paralysis of the muscular wall ⇒ paralytic ileus. *acute heart failure* cessation or impairment of heart action, in previously undiagnosed heart disease, or in the course of another disease. *acute yellow atrophy* acute diffuse necrosis of the liver; icterus gravis; malignant jaundice. *acute abdo·men* a pathological condition within the belly requiring immediate surgical intervention. *acute lympho·blastic leu·kemia* proliferation of circulating lymphoblasts (abnormal cells). The outlook is reasonably favorable in children and many can expect to be cured after a 2 year course of treatment. *acute myelblastic leu·kemia* proliferation of circulating myeloblasts. The condition is rapidly fatal if not treated: it requires intensive inpatient chemotherapy in a protected environment. The average duration of the first remission is 14 months.

acyan·osis (ā-sī-an-ō'-sis) *n* without cyanosis*.

acyan·otic (ā-sī-an-ot'-ik) *adj* without cyanosis*; a word used to differentiate congenital cardiovascular defects.

acyclo·vir (ā-sī'-clō-vīr) *n* an antiviral drug used to treat herpes simplex infections.

acyesis (ā-sī-ē'-sis) *n* absence of pregnancy—**acyetic** *adj*.

acys·tia (ā-sis'-ti-à) *n* congenital absence of the bladder—**acystic** *adj*.

Adam's apple *n* the laryngeal prominence in front of the neck, especially in the adult male, formed by the junction of the two wings of the thyroid cartilage.

adapta·bility (ad-apt-a-bil'-it-i) *n* the capacity to adjust mentally and physically to circumstances in a flexible way.

addic·tion (ad-dikt'-shŭn) *n* craving for chemical substances such as drugs, alcohol and tobacco which the addicted person finds difficult to control.

Addi·son's dis·ease (ad'-i-sonz) a condition due to deficient secretion of cortisol and aldosterone by the adrenal cortex. causing electrolytic upset, diminution of blood volume, lowered blood pressure, weight loss, hypoglycemia, great muscular weakness, gastrointestinal upsets and pigmentation of skin.

ad·duct (ad-dukt') *vt* to draw towards the midline of the body. ⇒ abduct *opp.*

adduc·tion (ad-dukt'-shun) *n* the act of adducting, drawing towards the midline. ⇒ abduction *opp.*

adduc·tor (ad-duk'-tŏr) *n* any muscle which moves a part toward the median axis of the body. ⇒ abductor *opp. adductor longus* ⇒ Figure 3. *adductor magnus* ⇒ Figure 3.

aden·ectomy (ad-en-ek'-to-mi) *n* surgical removal of a gland.

aden·itis (ad-en-īt'-is) *n* inflammation of a gland or lymph node. *hilar adenitis* inflammation of bronchial lymph nodes.

adeno·carcinoma (ad-en-ō-kàr-sin-ō'-mà) *n* a malignant growth of glandular tissue—**adenocarcinomata** *pl.* **adenocarcinomatous** *adj.*

adeno·fibroma (ad-en-ō-fī-brō'-mà) *n* ⇒ fibroadenoma.

aden·oid (ad'-en-oyd) *adj* resembling a gland. ⇒ adenoids.

adenoid·ectomy (ad-en-oyd-ek'-to-mi) *n* surgical removal from nasopharynx of adenoid tissue.

aden·oids (ad'-en-oydz) *npl* (pharyngeal tonsils) a mass of lymphoid tissue in the nasopharynx which can obstruct breathing and interfere with hearing.

aden·oma (ad-en-ō'-mà) *n* a non-malignant tumor of glandular tissue—**adenomata** *pl.* **adenomatous** *adj.*

adeno·myoma (ad-en-ō-mī-ō'-mà) *n* a non-malignant tumor composed of muscle and glandular elements, usually applied to benign growths of the uterus—**adenomyomata** *pl,* **adenomyomatous** *adj.*

aden·opathy (ad-en-op'-a-thi) *n* any disease of a gland, especially a lymphatic gland—**adenopathic** *adj.*

adeno·sclerosis (ad-en-ō-skle-rō'-sis) *n* hardening of a gland with or without swelling, usually due to replacement by fibrous tissue or calcification*—**adenosclerotic** *adj.*

adeno·sine diphosphate (ad-en'-ō-sēn dī-fos'-făt) **(ADP)** *n* an important cellular metabolite involved in energy exchange within the cell. Chemical energy is conserved in the cell, by the phosphorylation of ADP to ATP primarily in the mitochondrion, as a high energy phosphate bond.

aden·osine triphos·phate (ad-en'-ō-sēn trī-fos'-făt) **(ATP)** an intermediate high energy compound which on hydrolysis to ADP releases chemically useful energy. ATP is generated during catabolism and utilized during anabolism.

adeno·tonsil·lectomy (ad-en-ō-ton-sil-ek'-to-mi) *n* surgical removal of the adenoids and tonsils.

adeno·virus (ad-en-ō-vī'-rus) *n* a group of DNA-containing viruses composed of 47 serologically distinct types; 31 serotypes have been found in man, and many in various animal species. Some cause upper respiratory infection, others pneumonia, others epidemic keratoconjunctivitis.

ADH *abbr* antidiuretic hormone ⇒ vasopressin.

ad·hesion (ad-hē'-zhun) *n* abnormal union of two parts, occurring after inflammation; a band of fibrous tissue which joins such parts. In the abdomen such a band may cause intestinal obstruction; in joints it restricts movement; between two surfaces of pleura it prevents complete pneumothorax—**adherent** *adj,* **adherence** *n,* **adhere** *vi.*

adiaphoresis (ā-dī-a-fŏr-ē'-sis) *n* lack of perspiration or sweat—**adiaphoretic** *adj.*

adi·pose (ad'-ip-ōz) *n, adj* fat; of a fatty nature. The cells constituting adipose tissue contain either white or brown fat.

adi·posity (ad-i-pos'-it-i) *n* excessive accumulation of fat in the body.

adi·posuria (ad-i-pōs-ū'-ri-à) *n* ⇒ lipuria.

aditus (ad'-i-tus) *n* in anatomy, an entrance or opening.

adjust·ment (ad-just'-ment) *n* **1** the mechanism used in focusing a microscope. **2** stability within an individual and a satisfactory relationship between the individual and his environment.

adju·vant (ad'-joo-vant) *n* a substance included in a prescription to aid the action of other drugs. *adjuvant therapy* supportive measures in addition to main treatment.

ADL *abbr* activities of daily living; includes the usual hygiene and maintenance activities.

Adler's theory (ad'-lerz) the idea that neuroses arise from strong personal feelings of inferiority.

ad·nexa (ad-neks'-à) *n* structures which are in close proximity to a part—**adnexal** *adj. adnexa oculi* the lacrimal apparatus. *adnexa uteri* the ovaries and Fallopian tubes.

ado·lescence (ad-ō-les'-sens) *n* the period between the onset of puberty and full maturity; youth—**adolescent** *adj, n.*

adop·tion (ad-op'-shun) *n* the acquisition

of legal responsibility for a child who is not a biological offspring of the adopter.

adoral (ad-ōr′-ȧl) *adj* near the mouth.

ADP *abbr* adenosine diphosphate*.

adrenal (ad-rē′-nal) *adj* near the kidney, by custom referring to the adrenal glands, one lying above each kidney. (⇒ Figure 19). The *adrenal cortex* secretes mineral and glucocorticoids which control the chemical constitution of body fluids, metabolism and secondary sexual characteristics. Under the control of the pituitary gland via the secretion of corticotrophin*. The *adrenal medulla* secretes noradrenaline and adrenaline. ⇒ adrenalectomy.

adrenal function tests abnormal adrenalcortical function can be detected by measuring plasma cortisol. If hypoadrenalism is suspected the estimations can be repeated following the administration of synthetic ACTH (cortrosyn). Increased adrenal medullary function may be detected by measuring urinary vanyl* mandelic acid (VMA) excretion.

adren·alec·tomy (ad-rē′-nal-ek′-to-mi) *n* removal of an adrenal gland, usually for tumor. If both adrenal glands are removed, replacement administration of cortical hormones is required.

Adrena·lin (ad-ren′-ȧ-lin) *n* proprietary name for epinephrine.*

adren·ergic (ad-ren-ér′-jik) *adj* describes nerves which liberate either noradrenaline* or adrenaline* from their terminations. Most sympathetic nerves release noradrenaline. ⇒ cholinergic *opp*.

adreno·cortico·trophic hormone (ad-ren′-ō-kōr-ti-kō-trōf′-ik) ⇒ corticotrophin.

adreno·genital syn·drome (ad-ren-ō-jen′-it-al sin′-drōm) an endocrine disorder, usually congenital, resulting from abnormal activity of the adrenal cortex. A female child will show enlarged clitoris and possibly labial fusion, perhaps being confused with a male. The male child may show pubic hair and enlarged penis. In both male and female there is rapid growth, muscularity and advanced bone age.

adrenolytic (ad-re-nō-li′-tik) *adj.* that which antagonizes the action or secretion of adrenaline and nonadrenaline.

Adria·mycin (ād-ri-ȧ-mī′-sin) *n* proprietary name for doxorubicin*.

adsorb·ents (ad-sōrb′-ents) *npl* solids which bind gases or dissolved substances on their surfaces. Charcoal adsorbs gases and acts as a deodorant. Kaolin adsorbs bacterial and other toxins, hence used in cases of food poisoning.

adsorp·tion (ad-sōrp-shun) *n* the property of a substance to attract and to hold to its surface a gas, liquid or solid in solution or suspension—**adsorptive** *adj,* **adsorb** *vt.*

advance·ment *n* an operation to remedy squint. The muscle tendon opposite to the direction of the squint is detached and sutured to the sclera anteriorly.

adven·titia (ad-ven-tish′-i-ȧ) *n* the external coat, especially of an artery or vein—**adventitious** *adj.*

Aedes (á ē′-dēz) *n* a genus of mosquitoes which includes *Aedes aegypti,* the principal vector* of yellow* fever and dengue*.

AEG *abbr* air encelphalography or air encephalogram. ⇒ pneumoencephalography.

Aerobacter (ār-ō-bak′-ter) *n* generic name of bacteria made of short gram negative rods. Includes two species, *Aerobacter Aerogenes* and *Aerobacter Cloacae.*

aerobe (ā′ér-ōb) *n* a microorganism which requires O_2 to maintain life—**anaerobe***, *opp.*—**aerobic**, *adj,* **aerobic exercise** exercise which utilizes inspired O_2 for energy.

aero·genous (ā-ér-oj′-en-us) *adj* gas producing.

aero·phagia, aero·phagy (ā-ér-ō-fāj′-i-ȧ) *n* excessive air swallowing*.

aero·sol (ā′-ér-o-sol) *n* small particles finely dispersed in a gas phase. Commercial aerosol sprays may be used: (a) as inhalation therapy (b) to sterilize the air (c) in insect control (d) for skin application. Some aerosol sources (e.g. sneezing) are responsible for the spread of infection.

Aeros·porin (ā-ér-ō-spōr′-in) *n* proprietary name for polymyxin* B.

afeb·rile (ā-fēb′-rīl) *adj* without fever.

af·fect (af′-ekt) *n* emotion or mood.

affection (af-ek′-shun) the feeling or emotional aspect of mind making up one of the three aspects. ⇒ cognition, conation.

affect·ive (af-ek′-tiv) *adj* pertaining to emotions or moods. *affective psychosis* major mental illness in which there is grave disturbance of the emotions or mood. ⇒ psychosis.

affer·ent (af′-ér-ent) *adj* conducting inward to a part or organ; used to describe nerves, blood and lymphatic vessels ⇒

efferent *opp. afferent degeneration* that which spreads up sensory nerves.

affili·ation (af-il-ē-ā'-shun) *n* settling of the paternity of an illegitimate child on the putative father.

affin·ity (af-in'-it-i) *n* a chemical attraction between two substances, e.g. oxygen and hemoglobin.

afi·brino·gen·emia (ā-fī-brin'-ō-jen-ē'-mi-à) *n* inadequate fibrinogen-fibrin conversion; a serious disorder of blood coagulation—**afibrinogenemic** *adj.*

afla·toxin (af-la-toks'-in) *n* carcinogenic metabolites of certain strains of *Aspergillus flavus* which can infect peanuts and carbohydrate foods stored in warm humid climates. Four major aflatoxins: B_1, B_2, G_1 and G_2. Human liver cells contain the enzymes necessary to produce the metabolites of aflatoxins which predispose to liver cancer.

AFP *abbr* alphafetoprotein*.

after·birth *n* the placenta, cord and membranes which are expelled from the uterus after childbirth.

after·care *n* a term used to denote the care given during convalescence and rehabilitation. It need not be medical or nursing.

after·effect (af'-tėr-ē-fekt) *n* a response which occurs after the initial effect of a stimulus.

after·image *n* a visual impression of an object which persists after the object has been removed. This is called 'positive' when the image is seen in its natural bright colors; 'negative' when the bright parts become dark, while the dark parts become light.

after·pains *n* the pains felt after childbirth, due to contraction and retraction of the uterine muscle fibers.

agal·actia (a-gal-ak'-ti-à) *n* non-secretion or imperfect secretion of milk after childbirth—**agalactic,** *adj.*

agamma·globulin·emia (ā-gam-a-glōb'-ūl-in-ēm'-i-à) *n* absence of gammaglobulin in the blood, with consequent inability to produce immunity to infection—**agammaglobulinemic** *adj. Bruton's agammaglobulinemia* a congenital condition in boys, in which B-lymphocytes are absent but cellular immunity remains intact. ⇒dysgammaglobulinemia.

agang·lion·osis (a-gang-li-on-ō'-sis) *n* absence of ganglia, as those of the distant bowel ⇒ Hirschsprung's disease, megacolon.

agar (ā'gar) *n* a gelatinous substance obtained from certain seaweeds. It is used as a bulk-increasing laxative and as a solidifying agent in bacterial culture media.

age *n* ⇒ mental age, physiologic age.

age·ism *n* stereotyping people according to chronological age; overemphasizing negative aspects to the detriment of positive aspects.

agen·esis (ā-jen'-es-is) *n* incomplete and imperfect development—**agenetic** *adj.*

ag·gluti·nation (ag-gloo'-tin-ā'-shun) *n* the clumping of bacteria, red blood cells or antigen-coated particles by antibodies called 'agglutinins', developed in the blood serum of a previously infected or sensitized person or animal. Agglutination forms the basis of many laboratory tests—**agglutinable, agglutinative,** *adj,* **agglutinate** *vt, vi.*

ag·glutin·ins (ag-gloo'-tin-inz) *npl* antibodies which agglutinate or clump organisms or particles.

ag·glutin·ogen —ag-gloo'-tin-ō-jen) *n* an antigen which stimulates production of agglutinins*, used in the production of immunity, e.g. dead bacteria as in vaccine, particulate protein as in toxoid.

ag·gressin (a-gres'-in) *n* a metabolic substance, produced by certain bacteria to enhance their aggressive action against their host.

ag·gression (a-gre'-shun) *n* a feeling of anger or hostility—**aggressive** *adj.*

agi·tated de·pression (aj'-i-tā-ted dē-pre'-shun) persistent restlessness, with deep depression and apprehension. Occurs in affective psychoses.

aglos·sia (a-glos'-i-a) *n* absence of the tongue—**aglossic** *adj.*

aglut·ition (a-gloo-ti'-shun) *n* dysphagia*.

ag·nathia (ag-na'-thē-à) *n* absence or incomplete development of the jaw.

ag·nosia (ag-nō'-zē-à) *n* inability to appreciate sensory impressions—**agnosic** *adj. spatial agnosia* loss of spatial appreciation.

agon·ist (ag'-on-ist) *n* a muscle which shortens to perform a movement. ⇒ antagonist *opp.*

agora·phobia (ag-ōr-a-fō'-bi-à) *n* morbid fear of being alone in large open places—**agoraphobic** *adj.*

agran·ulo·cyte (ā-gran'-ū-lō-sīt) *n* a nongranular leukocyte.

agran·ulo·cytosis (ā-gran-ū-lō-sī-tō'-sis) *n* marked reduction in or complete absence of granulocytes* (polymorphonuclear leukocytes). Usually results from bone marrow depression caused by (a) hypersensitivity to drugs, (b) cytotoxic drugs or (c) irradiation. It is characterized by fever, ulceration of the mouth and throat and quickly leads to prostration and death. ⇒ neutropenia—**agranulocytic** *adj.*

agraphia (a-graf'-i-à) *n* loss of language facility. *motor agraphia* inability to express thoughts in writing, usually due to left precentral cerebral lesions. *sensory agraphia* inability to interpret the written word, due to lesions in the posterior part of the left parieto-occipital region—**agraphic** *adj.*

ague (ā'-gū) *n* malaria*.

AHG *abbr* Antihemophilic* globulin.

AID *abbr* artificial* insemination of a female with donor semen.

AIDS *abbr* acquired* immune deficiency syndrome.

AIDS-related complex a less severe condition than overt AIDS* (acquired immune deficiency syndrome) which occurs in some people who have contracted the AIDS virus. It may be asymptomatic or it may present as a febrile type of illness.

AJH *abbr* Artificial* insemination of a female with her husband's semen.

air *n* the gaseous mixture which makes up the atmosphere surrounding the earth. It consists of approximately 78% nitrogen, 20% oxygen, 0.04% carbon dioxide, 1% argon, and traces of ozone, neon, helium, etc. and a variable amount of water vapor. *air-bed* a rubber mattress inflated with air. *air hunger* a deep indrawing of breath which characterizes the late stages of uncontrolled hemorrhage. *air swallowing* swallowing of excessive air particularly when eating; it may result in belching or expulsion of gas via the anus.

akath·isia (ak'-ath-i'-zē-à) *n* a state of persistent motor restlessness; it can occur as a side-effect of neuroleptic drugs.

akin·etic (ā-kin-et'-ik) *adj* a word applied to states or conditions where there is lack of movement—**akinesia** *n.*

Akin·eton (ā-kin'-e-ton) *n* proprietary name for biperiden*.

alas·trim (al-as'-triṁ) *n* less virulent form of smallpox.

Albers-Schön·berg disease (al'-bārs-shern'-bärg) ⇒ osteopetrosis.

al'·bin·ism (al'-bin-izm) *n* congenital absence, either partial or complete, of normal pigmentation, so that the skin is fair,

the hair white and the eyes pink; due to a defect in melanin synthesis.

al·bino (al-bī'-nō) *n* a person affected with albinism—**albinotic** *adj*, **albiness** *female.*

albu·min (al-bū'-min) *n* a variety of protein found in animal and vegetable matter. It is soluble in water and coagulates on heating. *serum albumin* the chief protein of blood plasma and other serous fluids. ⇒ lactalbumin—**albuminous, albuminoid** *adj.*

al·bumi·nuria (al-bū-min-ūr'-i-à) *n* the presence of albumin in the urine. The condition may be temporary and clear up completely, as in many febrile states—**albuminuric** *adj.* ⇒ orthostatic albuminuria. *chronic albuminuria* leads to hypoproteinemia*.

albu·mose (al'-bū-mōz) *n* an early product of proteolysis. It resembles albumin, but is not coagulated by heat.

albumos·uria (al-bū-mōz-ū'-ri-à) *n* the presence of albumose in the urine—**albumosuric** *adj.*

albuterol (al-bū'-tèr-ol) *n* a bronchodilator derived from isoprenaline.* Does not produce cardiovascular side effects when inhaled in the recommended dosage. (Ventolin.)

al·cohol (al'-ko-hol) *n* (*syn* ethanol) a constituent of wines and spirits. Absolute alcohol is occasionally used by injection for the relief of trigeminal neuralgia and other intractable pain; rectified spirit (90% alcohol) is widely used in the preparation of tinctures; methylated spirit contains 95% alcohol with wood naphtha and is for external application only. Enhances the action of hypnotics and tranquilizers. *alcohol psychosis* Korsakoff's syndrome*.

al·cohol-fast *adj* in bacteriology, describes an organism which, when stained is resistant to decolorization by alcohol.

Al·coholics Anony·mous (AA) a fellowship of people who have had problems with alcohol addiction. Their aim is helping others with similar difficulties.

alcohol·ism (al'-ko-hol-izm) *n* poisoning resulting from alcoholic addiction. In its chronic form it causes severe disturbances of the nervous and digestive systems.

alcohol·uria (al-ko-hol-ū'-ri-à) *n* alcohol in the urine. It is the basis of one test for fitness to drive after drinking alcohol.

Aldac·tone (al-dak'-tōn) *n* proprietary name for spironolactone.

Aldoclor (al'-dō-klōr) *n* a proprietary drug

containing methyldopa* and chlorothia-zide*.

aldo·lase test an enzyme test; the serum enzyme aldolase is increased in diseases affecting muscle.

Aldo·met (al'-dō-met) *n* proprietary name for methyldopa*.

aldos·terone (al-dos'-tèr-ōn) *n* an adrenocortical steroid which, by its action on renal tubules regulates electrolyte metabolism; hence described as a 'mineralocorticoid'. Secretion is regulated by the renin*-angiotensin system. It increases excretion of potassium and conserves sodium and chloride.

aldosteron·ism (al-dos'-tèr-ōn-izm) *n* a condition resulting from tumors of the adrenal cortex in which the electrolyte imbalance is marked and alkalosis and tetany may ensue.

Aleppo boil (a-lep'-ō) ⇒ leishmaniasis.

alexia (a-leks'-i-à) *n* word blindness; an inability to interpret the significance of the printed or written word, but without loss of visual power. Can be due to a brain lesion or insufficient/inappropriate sensory experience during 'an initio' stage of learning—**alexic** *adj*.

ALG *abbr* antilymphocyte* globulin.

algae (al'-jē) *npl* lowest form of plant life, these plants contain chlorophyll and may be used for food or medicine.

algesia (al-jē'-zi-à) *n* excessive sensitiveness to pain; hyperesthesia ⇒ analgesia *opp*—**algesic** *adj*.

algesi·meter (al-jēz-im'-et-er) *n* an instrument which registers the degree of sensitivity to pain.

al·gid (al'-jid) *adj* used to describe severe attack of fever, especially malaria, with collapse, extreme coldness of the body, suggesting a fatal termination. During this stage the rectal temperature may be high.

algin·ates (al'-jin-ātz) *npl* seaweed derivatives which, when applied locally, encourage the clotting of blood. They are available in solution and in specially impregnated gauze.

alien·ation (ā-li-en-ā'-shun) *n* in psychology and sociology, estrangement from people.

ali·ment·ary (al-i-ment'-à-ri) *adj* pertaining to food.

ali·ment·ation (al-i-ment-ā'-shun) *n* the act of nourishing with food; feeding.

aliquot (al'-i-kwat) *n* part contained by the whole an integral number of times.

alka·lemia (al-kal-ēm'-i-à) *n*⇒ alkalosis—**alkalemic** *adj*.

alkali (al'-kal-ī) *n* soluble corrosive bases, including soda, potash and ammonia, which neutralize acids forming salts and combine with fats to form soaps. Alkaline solutions turn red litmus blue. *alkaline reserve* a biochemical term denoting the amount of buffered alkali (normally bicarbonate) available in the blood for the neutralization of acids (normally dissolved CO_2) formed in or introduced into the body.

alka·line (al'-kal-īn) *adj* **1** possessing the properties of or pertaining to an alkali. **2** containing an excess of hydroxyl over hydrogen ions. *alkaline phosphatase test* an increase in the enzyme alkaline phosphatase in the blood is indicative of such conditions as obstructive jaundice and various forms of bone disease.

alkalin·uria (al-kal-in-ūr'-i-à) *n* alkalinity of urine—**alkalinuric** *adj*.

alka·loid (al'-kal-oyd) *n* resembling an alkali. A name often applied to a large group of organic bases found in plants and which possess important physiological actions. Morphine, quinine, caffeine, atropine and strychnine are well-known examples of alkaloids—**alkaloidal** *adj*.

alka·losis (al-kal-ō'-sis) *n* (*syn* alkalemia) excess of alkali or reductions of acid in the body. Develops from a variety of causes such as overdosages with alkali, excessive vomiting or diarrhea and hyperventilation. Results in neuromuscular excitability expressed clinically as tetany*.

alkapton·uria (al-kap-tōn-ūr'-i-à) *n* the presence of alkaptone (homogentisic acid) in the urine, resulting from only partial oxidation of phenylalanine and tyrosine. Condition usually noticed because urine goes black in the diapers, or when left to stand. Apart from this, and a tendency to arthritis in later life, there are no ill-effects from alkaptonuria.

Alk·eran (al'-kėr-an) *n* proprietary name for melphalan*.

alkyl·ating agents (al'-kil-ā-ting ā'-jents) disrupt the process of cell division affecting DNA in the nucleus probably by adding to it alkyl groups—hence the name alkylating agents. Some are useful against malignant cell growth.

allelo·morphs (a-lē'-lō-mōrfz) *npl* originally used to denote inherited characteristics that are alternative and contrasting, such as normal color vision contrasting with color blindness, or the ability to taste or not to taste certain substances, or different blood groups. The basis of Mendelian inheritance of dominants and recessives. In modern usage allelomorph(s) is equivalent to allele(s), namely alternative forms of a gene at the same chromosomal location (locus)—**allelomorphic** *adj,* **allelomorphism** *n.*

aller·gen (al'-ėr-jen) *n* any antigen* capable of producing an altered state or manifestation of an immune response— **allergenic** *adj,* **allergenicity** *n.*

al·lergy (al'-ėr-jē) *n* an altered or exaggerated susceptibility to various foreign substances or physical agents. Colloquially, implies that an individual has become over-reactive to an antigen* which would not normally produce an adverse response (often difficult to prove). Sometimes caused by the interaction of an antigen with IgE antibody on the surface of mast cells. Scientifically, describes diseases due to an altered immune response, a state of altered reactivity. Some drug reactions, hay fever, insect bite reactions, urticarial reactions and asthma are classed as allergic diseases—**allergic** *adj.* ⇨ anaphylaxis, sensitization.

allo·cheiria (al-ō-chīr'-i-à) *n* an abnormality of tactile sensibility under test, wherein patient refers a given stimulus to the other side of the body.

allo·graft (al'-lō-graft) *n* grafting or transplanting an organ or tissue from one person to another who does not share the same transplantation antigens.

allopur·inal (al-lō-pū'-rin-ol) *n* a substance which prevents the formation of deposits of crystals from insoluble uric acid. Diminishes tophus* in gout and substantially reduces the frequency and severity of further attacks. Can cause skin rash. (Zyloprim.)

aloes (al'-ōz) *n* the dried juice from the cut leaves of a tropical plant. Powerful purgative with an intensely bitter taste.

alo·pecia (al-ō-pē'-shē-à) *n* baldness, which can be congenital, premature or senile. *alopecia areata* a patchy baldness, usually of a temporary nature. Cause unknown, probably autoimmune, but shock and anxiety are common precipitating factors. Exclamation mark hairs are diagnostic. *cicatrical alopecia* progressive alopecia of the scalp in which tufts of normal hair occur between many bald patches. Folliculitis decalvans is an alopecia of the scalp characterized by pustulation and scars.

Alo·phen (al'-ō-fen) *n* a proprietary compound containing phenolphthalin*.

alpha·chymo·trypsin (al-fa-kī-mō-trip'-sin) *n* a pancreatic enzyme used in ophthalmic surgery to dissolve the capsular ligament and allow the lens to be extracted through the pupil and out of the wound without undue physical manipulation. It is an anti-inflammatory agent when taken orally.

alpha·feto·protein (al-fa-fē'-tō-prō'-tēn) *n* present in maternal serum and amniotic fluid in cases of fetal abnormality.

alphaprodine hydrochloride (al-fa-prō'-dēn) *n* a synthetic narcotic analgesic, similar to meperidine. (Nisentil.)

alpha·toco·pherol (al-fa-tō-ko'-fėr-ol) *n* vitamin* E.

alprazolam (al-pra-zō'-lam) *n* an anti-anxiety drug, a benzodiazepine compound acting on the central nervous system. (Xanax.)

ALS *abbr* antilymphocyte* serum. Also advanced life support. Also amyotrophic* lateral sclerosis.

alterna·tive medi·cine the term currently in use for such diverse techniques as acupuncture, biofeedback, chiropractice, homeopathy, relaxation and yoga.

alum (al'-um) *n* potassium or ammonium aluminum sulfate. Used for its astringent properties as a mouthwash (1%) and as a douche (0.5%). Also used for precipitating toxoid. ⇨ APT.

alu·minum hydrox·ide (al-ūm'-in-um hī-droks'-īd) *n* an antacid with a prolonged action when used in the treatment of peptic ulcer. It is usually given as a thin cream or gel. There is no risk of alkalosis with long treatment, as the drug is not absorbed.

alu·minium paste (al-ūm'-in-um pāst) *n* a mixture of aluminium powder, zinc oxide and liquid paraffin, used as a skin protective in ileostomy. This paste is sometimes known as 'Baltimore paste'.

Alu·pent (al'-ū-pent) *n* proprietary name for metaproterenol sulfate*.

al·veolar abscess (al-vē'-ō-lar ab'-ses) ⇨ abscess.

al·veolar-capil·lary block syn·drome a rare syndrome of unknown etiology characterized by breathlessness, cyanosis* and right heart failure, due to thickening of the alveolar cells of the lungs, thus impairing diffusion of oxygen.

alveo·litis (al-vē-ōl-ī'-tis) *n* inflammation of alveoli, by custom usually referring to those in the lung; when caused by inhalation of an allergen such as pollen, it is termed *extrinsic allergic alveolitis.*

al·veolus (al-vē'-ōl-us) *n* **1** an air vesicle of the lung. **2** bone of the tooth socket, providing support for the tooth, partially absorbed when the teeth are lost. **3** a gland follicle or acinus—**alveoli** *pl*, **alveolar** *adj.*

Alz·heimer's dis·ease (alts'-hī-mèrz) *n* a dementing disease which is most commonly referred to as pre-senile dementia*; there are specific brain abnormalities.

amal·gam (à-mal'-gam) *n* any of a group of alloys containing mercury. *dental amalgam* an amalgam which is used for filling teeth; it contains mercury, silver and tin.

amant·adine (am-an'-ta-dēn) *n* an antiviral agent which reduces the length of illness in virus A_2 influenza (Hong Kong flu) and the frequency of respiratory complications. It evokes a response similar to but less powerful than that of dopa in relieving the tremor and rigidity in Parkinson's disease. (Symmetrel.)

amas·tia (a-maś-ti-à) *n* congenital absence of the breasts.

amaur·osis (am-aw-rō'-sis) *n* partial or total blindness—**amaurotic** *adj.*

ambi·dextrous (am-bi-deks'-trus) *adj* able to use both hands equally well—**ambidexter** *adj*, **ambidexterity** *n.*

ambiv·alence (am-biv'-al-ens) *n* coexistence at the same time in one person of opposite feelings, e.g. love and hate—**ambivalent** *adj.*

ambly·opia (am-bli-ōp'-i-à) *n* defective vision approaching blindness. ⇒ smoker's blindness—**amblyopic** *adj.*

ambu·lant (am'-bū-lant) *adj* able to walk.

ambu·latory (am'-bū-là-tōr-i) *adj* mobile, walking about. *ambulatory treatment* a term currently appearing in the literature to describe the monitoring of a patient at intermittent visits to the outpatients' department of a hospital. Also known as outpatient treatment.

ameba (àm-è'-bà) *n* ⇒ *amoeba.*

amebi·asis (am-ē-bī'-à-sis) *n* ⇒ *amoebiasis.*

amebi·cide (am-ē'-bis-īd) *n* ⇒ *amoebicide.*

ameb·oid (am-ē'-boyd) *n* ⇒ *amoeboid.*

ameb·oma (am-ē-bō'-mà) *n* amoeboma.

amelia (à-mē'-li-à) *n* congenital absence of a limb or limbs. *complete amelia* absence of both arms and legs.

amelior·ation (à-mē-li-ōr-ā'-shun) *n* reduction of the severity of symptoms.

amenor·rhea (ā-men-ō-rē'-à) *n* absence of the menses. When menstruation has not been established at the time when it should have been, it is *primary amenorrhea*; absence of the menses after they have once commenced is referred to as *secondary amenorrhea*—**amenorrheal** *adj.*

amentia (a-men'-shi-à) *n* mental subnormality from birth; to be distinguished from dementia which is acquired mental impairment.

amet·ria (ā-mēt'-ri-à) *n* congenital absence of the uterus.

amet·ropia (ā-mēt-rō'-pi-à) *n* defective sight due to imperfect retractive power of the eye—**ametropic** *adj*, **ametrope** *n.*

Ami·car (a'-mi-kar) proprietary name for aminocaproic acid*.

amik·acin (a-mi-kā'-sin) *n* an antibiotic for especial use in serious Gram-negative gentamicin-resistant infections; a semisynthetic derivative of kanamycin*, it has been altered structurally to resist degradation by bacterial enzymes. (Amikin.)

Amikin (á-mi-kin) *n* proprietary name for amikacin*.

amil·oride (am-il-ōr'-īd) *n* fairly mild diuretic, but has unusual potassium-conserving properties. When it is used, potassium supplements are rarely required, but continued use may lead to increased potassium in the blood. (Midamor.)

aminacrine (a-min'-à-krin) *n* nonstaining antiseptic similar to acriflavine, and used for similar purposes in the same strength.

amino·acid·opathy (àm-ēn'-ō-as-id-op'-ath-i) *n* disease caused by imbalance of amino acids.

amino acids (am-ēn'-ō-as'-idz) *n* organic acids in which one or more of the hydrogen atoms are replaced by the amino group, NH_2. They are the end product of protein hydrolysis and from them the body resynthesizes its own proteins. Ten cannot be elaborated in the body and are therefore essential in the diet—arginine, histidine, isoleucine; leucine, lysine, methionine, phenylalanine, threonine, tryptophan and valine. The remainder are designated non-essential amino acids.

amino·aciduria (am-ēn'-ō-às-id-ūr'-i-à) *n* the abnormal presence of amino acids in the urine; it usually indicates an inborn error of metabolism as in cystinosis* and

Fanconi's syndrome*—**aminoaciduric** *adj.*

amino·caproic acid (am-ēn'-ō-kap-rō'-ik-as'-id) *n* inhibits the plasminogen activators and has a direct hemostatic action by preventing the breakdown of fibrin. An antifibrinolytic agent. (Amicar.)

amino·gluteth·imide (am-ēn-ō-glooteth'-i-mīd) *n* a drug which is used to produce adrenal suppression in the hormone-dependent cancers. (Cytadren.)

amin·ophyl·line (am-in-of'-il-in) *n* theophylline with ethylene-diamine. A soluble derivative of theophylline*, widely used in the treatment of asthma, congestive heart failure and cardiac edema.

Amino·plex (a-min'-ō-pleks) *n* a proprietary synthetic preparation which is suitable for intravenous infusion: it contains those amino acids which are normally ingested as protein. It has been used to irrigate wounds with good results.

amino·salicylic acid (am-ēn-ō-sal-is-il'-ik) *n* an antibacterial drug, used orally as a tuberculostatic.

Aminosyn (a-min'-ō-sin) *n* a proprietary solution of amino acids which can be given orally or intravenously.

ami·tosis (a-mī-to'-sis) *n* division of a cell by direct fission—**amitotic** *adj.*

amitrip·tyline (am-i-trip'-til-in) *n* a tricyclic antidepressant similar to imipramine* but possessing a pronounced sedative effect which is of particular value in the agitated depressive. (Elavil, Endep.)

am·monia (am-ō'-ni-à) *n* a naturally occurring compound of nitrogen and hydrogen. In the human, several inborn errors of ammonia metabolism can cause mental retardation, neurological signs and seizures. *ammonia solution* (Liq. ammon) colorless liquid with a characteristic pungent odor. Used in urine testing—**ammoniated, ammoniacal** *adj.*

am·monium bicarb·onate (am-ō'-ni-um bī-kar'-bo-nāt) widely used in cough mixtures as a mild expectorant, and occasionally as a carminative in flatulent dyspepsia.

am·monium chlor·ide (am-ō'-ni-um klōr'-īd) used to increase the acidity of the urine in urinary infections. Occasionally given as a mild expectorant.

am·nesia (am-nē'-zē-à) *n* complete loss of memory; can occur after concussion, in dementia, hysteria and following ECT. The term *anterograde amnesia** is used when there is impairment of memory for recent events after an accident etc., and

retrograde amnesia when the impairment is for past events—**amnesic** *adj.*

amnio·centesis (am-nē-o-sen-tē'-sis) *n* piercing the amniotic cavity through the abdominal wall for the purpose of withdrawing a sample of fluid for examination to establish prenatal diagnosis of chromosomal abnormalities, spina bifida, metabolic errors, fetal hemolytic disease and so on.

amniog·raphy (am-nē-og'-ra-fē) *n* X-ray of the amniotic sac after injection of opaque medium into same: outlines the umbilical cord and placenta—**amniographical** *adj*, **amniographically** *adv.*

amnion (am'-nē-on) *n* the innermost membrane enclosing the fetus and containing the amniotic* fluid. It ensheaths the umbilical cord and is connected with the fetus at the umbilicus—**amnionic, amniotic** *adj.*

amnion·itis (am-nē-on-īt'-is) *n* inflammation of the amnion*.

amni·oscopy (am-nē-os'-ko-pē) *n* amnioscope passed through the abdominal wall enables viewing of the fetus and amniotic fluid. Clear, colorless fluid is normal; yellow or green staining is due to meconium and occurs in cases of fetal hypoxia—**amnioscopic** *adj*, **amnioscopically** *adv. cervical amnioscopy* can be performed late in pregnancy. A different instrument is inserted via the vagina and cervix for the same reasons.

amni·otic cav·ity (am-nē-ot'-ik) *n* the fluid-filled cavity between the embryo and the amnion.

amni·otic fluid *n* a liquid produced by the fetal membranes and the fetus which surrounds the fetus throughout pregnancy. As well as providing the fetus with physical protection, the amniotic fluid is a medium of active chemical exchange. It is secreted and reabsorbed by cells lining the amniotic cavity and is swallowed, metabolized and excreted as fetal urine. ⇒ amnioscopy. *amniotic fluid embolism* formation of an embolus in the amniotic sac and its transference in the blood circulation of mother to lung or brain. A rare complication of pregnancy. May occur at any time after rupture of the membranes. *amniotic fluid infusion* escape of amniotic fluid into the maternal circulation.

amni·otome (am'-nē-ot-ōm) *n* an instrument for rupturing the fetal membranes. Also called amnihook.

amni·otomy (am-nē-ot'-o-mē) *n* artificial rupture of the fetal membranes to induce or expedite labor.

amobarbital (am-ō-barb′-i-tol) *n* barbiturate of medium intensity and duration of action. (Amytal.) ⇒ barbiturates.

am·oeba (am-ē′-bà) *n* a protozoan. An elementary, unicellular form of life. The single cell is capable of ingestion and absorption, respiration, excretion, movement and reproduction by amitotic fission. One strain, *Entamoeba histolytica*, is the parasitic pathogen which produces amoebic dysentery* in man. ⇒ protozoon—**amoebae** *pl*, **amoebic** *adj*. Also spelled ameba.

amoebi·asis (am-ē-bī′-à-sis) *n* infestation of large intestine by the protozoon *Entamoeba histolytica*, where it causes ulceration by invasion of the mucosa. This results in passage per rectum of necrotic mucous membrane and blood, hence the term 'amoebic dysentery'. If the amoebae enter the portal circulation they may cause liver necrosis (hepatic abscess). Diagnosis is by isolating the amoeba in the stools. Regarded as a sexually transmitted disease among homosexual men.

amoebi·cide (am-ē′-bi-sīd) *n* an agent which kills amoebae—**amoebicidal** *adj*.

amoeb·oid (am-ē′-boyd) *adj* resembling an amoeba in shape or in mode of movement, e.g. white blood cells.

amoeb·oma (am-ē-bō′-mà) *n* a tumor in the caecum or rectum caused by *Entamoeba hystolytica*. Fibrosis may occur and obstruct the bowel.

amorph·ous (a-mōr′-fus) *adj* having no regular shape.

Am·oxil (a-moks′-il) *n* proprietary name for amoxycillin*.

amoxy·cillin (a-moks-i-sil′-lin) *n* antibiotic; penetrates bronchial secretions more readily than ampicillin* independent of the level of purulence, therefore preferable in chronic lower respiratory tract infections. In acute infections the sole advantage is its greater absorption and high blood levels for an equivalent dose. (Amoxil.)

amphet·amine (am-fet′-à-mēn) *n* a sympathomimetic agent (structurally related to adrenaline*) which is a potent CNS stimulant. It was formerly used as an appetite suppressant and in the treatment of depression but, because of its addictive potential and frequent abuse, its use is now restricted.

ampho·tericin B (am-fōt-ėr′-i-sēn-bē) anti-fungal agent given by i.v. infusion to treat serious systemic infections, e.g. histoplasmosis, candidiasis. It is taken as lozenges to eradicate *Candida* from the mouth; as cream or pessaries for the vagina and orally for treatment of bowel infections. (Fungizone.)

ampi·cillin (am-pi-sil′-lin) *n* an antibiotic active against many, but certainly not all, strains of *Esch. coli, Proteus, Salmonella* and *Shigella*; these are bacteria against which benzyl penicillin* is far less active. Ampicillin is also effective against benzyl penicillin-sensitive (but not resistant) staphylococci, streptococci and other Gram-positive bacteria. It has a wide range of activity and is a broad-spectrum antibiotic. Given orally and by injection. (Penbritin.)

am·pule (am′-pūl) *n* a hermetically sealed glass or plastic phial containing a single sterile dose of a drug.

am·pulla (am-pōol′-à) *n* any flask-like dilatation (Figure 17)—**ampullae** *pl*. **ampullar, ampullary, ampullate** *adj*. *ampulla of Vater* the enlargement formed by the union of the common bile duct with the pancreatic duct where they enter the duodenum.

ampu·tation (am-pū-tā′-shun) *n* removal of an appending part, e.g. breast, limb.

ampu·tee (am-pū-tē′) *n* a person who has had amputation of one or more limbs.

amygdalin (a-mig′-da-lin) *n* ⇒ Laetrile.

amyl·ase (am′-i-lāz) *n* any enzyme which converts starches into sugars. *pancreatic amylase* amylopsin*. *salivary amylase* ptyalin*. *amylase test* the urine is tested for starch to assess kidney function.

amyl nit·rite (am′il-nīt′-rīt) *n* volatile rapid-acting vasodilator, used by inhalation from crushed ampules. Its action is brief, and its main use is in the treatment of angina.

amy·loid (am′-i-loyd) *adj, n* resembling starch. An abnormal complex material which accumulates in certain disorders known as amyloidosis*.

amy·loid·osis (am-i-loyd-ō′-sis) *n* formation and deposit of amyloid* in any organ, notably the liver and kidney. *primary amyloidosis* has no apparent cause. *secondary amyloidosis* can occur in any prolonged toxic condition such as Hodgkin's disease, tuberculosis and leprosy. It is common in the genetic disease familial Mediterranean* fever.

amyl·olysis (am-il-ol′-is-is) *n* the digestion of starch—**amylolytic** *adj*.

amyl·opsin (am-il-op′-sin) *n* a pancreatic enzyme, which in an alkaline medium converts insoluble starch into soluble maltose.

amylum (am'-il-um) *n* starch*.

amyo·tonia con·genita (ā-mī-ō-tō'-nē-à con-jen'-it-à) (*syn* floppy baby syndrome) benign congenital hypotonia present at birth in the absence of demonstrable musculoneural pathology. Improvement occurs and the child's progress becomes normal.

amyotrophic lateral sclerosis (ā-mī-ō-trō'-fik la'ter-al sklêr-ō'-sis) (*abbr.*, ALS) a syndrome of progressive muscular weakness and atrophy with poor prognosis.

Amy·tal (am'-i-tal) proprietary name for amobarbital.*

ana·bolic com·pound (an-ab-ol'-ik) chemical substance which causes a synthesis of body protein. Useful in convalescence. Many of the androgens* come into this category.

anab·olism (an-ab'-ol-izm) *n* the series of chemical reactions in the living body requiring energy to change simple substances into complex ones. ⇒ adenosine diphosphate, adenosine triphosphate, metabolism.

anacid·ity (an-as-id'-it-ē) *n* lack of normal acidity, especially in the gastric juice. ⇒ achlorhydria.

anac·rotism (an-ak'-rot-izm) *n* an oscillation in the ascending curve of a sphygmographic pulse tracing, occurring in aortic stenosis—**anacrotic** *adj*.

anaer·obe (an'-ėr-ōb) *n* a microorganism which will not grow in the presence of molecular oxygen. When this is strictly so, it is termed an *obligatory anaerobe* the majority of pathogens are indifferent to atmospheric conditions and will grow in the presence or absence of oxygen and are therefore termed *facultative anaerobes*—**aerobe**, *opp*.—**anaerobic** *adj*.

anaero·bic respi·ration (an-ėr-ōb'-ik) *n* occurs when oxygen available to the fetus is limited, with the consequent production of lactic and pyruvic acids and a fall in the pH value of fetal blood. This can be measured in labor once the cervix has dilated—by taking a microsample of blood from the fetal scalp.

ana·leptic (an-à-lep'-tik) *adj*, *n* restorative. Analeptics in current use include caffeine, amphetamines, monoamine oxidase inhibitors and tricyclic antidepressants.

anal·gesia (an-al-jē'-zē-à) *n* loss of painful impressions without loss of tactile sense. ⇒ algesia *opp*—**analgesic** *adj*.

anal·gesic (an-al-je'-zik) *n* a drug which relieves pain.

anal·ogous (an-al'-a-gus) *adj* similar in function but not in origin.

analy·sis (an-al'-i-sis) *n* a term used in chemistry to denote the determination of the composition of a compound substance. ⇒ psychoanalysis—**analyses** *pl*, **analytic** *adj*, **analytically** *adv*.

analyst (an'-à-list) *n* a person experienced in performing analyses.

anaphia (an-af'-ē-à) *n* loss of or reduction in sense of touch.

ana·phyl·actic reac·tion (an-a-fil-ak'-tik) an adverse reaction due to the release of the constituents of acute inflammatory cells, generally as a result of antigens binding to IgE on mast cells and basophils. In hayfever* the reaction occurs mainly in the nose; in asthma* it occurs in the lower respiratory tract. In anaphylaxis* it occurs in many tissues throughout the body.

anaph·ylac·toid (an-a-fil-ak'-toyd) *adj* pertaining to or resembling anaphylaxis.

anaph·ylaxis (an-a-fil-aks'-is) *n* (*syn* serum sickness) a hypersensitive state of the body to a foreign protein (e.g. horse serum) so that the injection of a second dose after ten days brings about an acute reaction which may be fatal; in lesser degree it produces bronchospasm, pallor and collapse. ⇒ allergy, sensitization—**anaphylactic** *adj*.

ana·plasia (an-a-plāz'-ē-a) *n* loss of the distinctive characteristics of a cell, associated with proliferative activity as in cancer—**anaplastic** *adj*.

anar·thria (an-ar'-thrē-à) *n* a word restricted to those instances when a person does not produce any speech.

ana·sarca (an-a-sar'-kà) *n* serous infiltration of the cellular tissues and serous cavities; generalized edema—**anasarcous** *adj*.

anasto·mosis (an-as-to-mō'-sis) *n* **1** the intercommunication of the branches of two or more arteries or veins. **2** in surgery, the establishment of an intercommunication between two hollow organs, vessels or nerves—**anastomoses** *pl*, **anastomotic** *adj*, **anastomose** *vt*.

anat·omical pos·ition (an-a-tom'-ik-al) for the purpose of accurate description the anterior view is of the upright body facing forward, hands by the sides with palms facing forwards. The posterior view is of the back of the upright body in that position.

15

anat·omy (an-at′-ŏ-mē) *n* the science which deals with the structure of the body by means of dissection—**anatomical** *adj*, **anatomically** *adv*.

ancillary (an′-sil-ār-ē) *n* something that aids an action but is not necessary for the performance of the action.

Ancobon (an′-kŏ-bon) *n* proprietary name for flucytosine.*

Ancylos·toma (ang-ki-lō-stō′-mà) *n* (*syn* human hookworm). *Ancylostoma duodenale* is predominantly found in southern Europe and the Middle and Far East. *Necator americanus* is found in the Americas and tropical Africa. Mixed infections are not uncommon. Only clinically significant when infestation is moderate or heavy. Worm inhabits duodenum and upper jejunum, eggs are passed in stools, hatch in moist soil and produce larvae which can penetrate bare feet and reinfect people. Prevention is by wearing shoes and using latrines.

ancylosto·miasis (an-sī-lōs-tō-mī′-a-sis) *n* (*syn* hookworm disease) infestation of the human intestine with Ancylostoma giving rise to malnutrition and severe anemia.

andro·blastoma (an-drŏ-blas-tō′-mà) *n* (*syn* arrhenoblastoma) a tumor of the ovary; can produce male or female hormones and can cause masculinization in women or precocious puberty in girls.

andro·gens (an′-drŏ-jenz) *npl* hormones secreted by the testes and adrenal cortex, or synthetic substances, which control the building up of protein and the male secondary sex characteristics, e.g. distribution of hair and deepening of voice. When given to females they have a masculinizing effect. ⇒ testosterone—**androgenic, androgenous** *adj*.

android (an′-droyd) *adj*. resembling man. **android pelvis** a male type pelvis, funnel or heart shaped.

androphobia (an-drŏ-fō′-bi-à) *n* a morbid dislike or fear of men—**androphobic** *adj*.

anemia (an-ē′-mē-à) *n* a deficiency of hemoglobin in the blood due to lack of red blood cells and/or their hemoglobin content. Produces clinical manifestations arising from hypoxemia*, such as lassitude and breathlessness on exertion. Treatment is according to the cause and there are many—**anemic** *adj*. *aplastic anemia* is the result of complete bone marrow failure. *pernicious anemia* results from the inability of the bone marrow to produce normal red cells because of the deprivation of a protein released by gastric glands, called the intrinsic factor which is necessary for the absorption of vitamin B_{12} from food. An autoimmune mechanism may be responsible. *sickle-cell anemia* familial, hereditary hemolytic anemia peculiar to Blacks. The red cells are crescent-shaped. *splenic anemia* (*syn* Banti's disease) leukopenia, thrombocytopenia, alimentary bleeding, and splenomegaly which in turn is caused by portal hypertension. ⇒ Addison's disease *hemolytic* disease of the newborn *spherocytosis, thalassemia.*

anen·cephaly (an-en-sef′-a-lē) *n* congenital absence of the brain. The condition is incompatible with life; it can be detected by raised levels of alphafetoprotein in the amniotic fluid—**anencephalous, anencephalic** *adj*.

anes·thesia (an-es-thē′-zē-à) *n* loss of sensation. *general anesthesia* loss of sensation with loss of consciousness. In *local anesthesia* the nerve conduction is blocked directly and painful impulses fail to reach the brain. *spinal anesthesia* may be caused by (a) injection of a local anesthetic into the spinal sub-arachnoid space (b) a lesion of the spinal cord.

anes·thes·iology (an-es-thēz-ē-ol′-o-jē) *n* the science dealing with anesthetics, their administration and effect.

anes·thetic (an-es-thet′-ik) *n, adj* **1** a drug which produces anesthesia. **2** causing anesthesia. **3** insensible to stimuli—**anesthetize** *vt*. *general anesthetic* a drug which produces general anesthesia by inhalation or injection. *local anesthetic* a drug which injected into the issues or applied topically causes local insensibility to pain. *spinal anesthetic* ⇒ spinal.

anes·thetist (an-es′-thet-ist) *n* a person who is medically qualified to administer anesthetics.

aneur·ine (a-nū′-rin) *n* thiamine or vitamin B_1.

aneur·ysm (an′-ūr-izm) *n* dilation of a blood vessel, usually an artery, due to local fault in the wall through defect, disease or injury, producing a pulsating swelling over which a murmur may be heard. True aneurysms may be saccular, fusiform, or dissecting where the blood flows between the layers of the arterial wall—**aneurysmal** *adj*.

angi·ectasis (an-jē-ek′-tà-sis) *n* abnormal dilatation of blood vessels. ⇒ telangiectasis—**angiectatic** *adj*.

angi·itis (an-jē-ī′-tis) *n* inflammation of a blood or lymph vessel. ⇒ vasculitis—**angiitic** *adj*.

an·gina (an-jī'-nȧ) *n* sense of suffocation or constriction—**angina** *adj. angina pectoris* severe but temporary attack of cardiac pain which may radiate to the arms. Results from myocardial ischemia. Often the attack is induced by exercise (angina of effort).

angiocardio·graphy (an-jē-ō-kȧr-dē-og'-raf-i) *n* demonstration of the chambers of the heart and great vessels after injection of an opaque medium—**angiocardiographic** *adj*, **angiocardiogram** *n*, **angiocardiograph** *n*, **angiocardiographically** *adv*.

angioedema (an-jē-ō-e-dē'-mȧ) (*syn* angio-neurotic edema) *n* a severe form of urticaria* which may involve the skin of the face, hands or genitals and the mucous membrane of the mouth and throat; edema of the glottis may be fatal. Immediately there is an abrupt local increase in vascular permeability, as a result of which fluid escapes from blood vessels into surrounding tissues. Swelling may be due to an allergic hypersensitivity reaction to drugs, pollens or other known allergens, but in many cases no cause can be found.

angio·graphy (an-jē-og'-ra-fē) *n* demonstration of the arterial system after injection of an opaque medium—**angiographic** *adj*, **angiogram** *n*, **angiograph** *n*, **angiographically** *adv*.

angi·ology (an-jē-ol'-o-jē) *n* the science dealing with blood and lymphatic vessels—**angiological** *adj*, **angiologically** *adv*.

angioma (an-jē-ō'-mȧ) *n* a non-malignant tumor of blood vessels, usually capillaries.

angio·plasty (an'-jē-ō-plas-tē) *n* plastic surgery of blood vessels—**angioplastic** *adj. percutaneous transluminal coronary angioplasty* a balloon is passed into a stenosed coronary artery and inflated with contrast medium; it presses the atheroma against the vessel wall, thereby increasing the lumen.

angio·sarcoma (an-jē-ō-sȧr-kō'-mȧ) *n* a malignant tumor arising from blood vessels—**angiosarcomata** *pl*, **angiosarcomatous** *adj*.

angio·spasm (an'-jē-ō-spazm) *n* constricting spasm of blood vessels—**angiospastic** *adj*.

angio·tensin (an-jē-ō-ten'-sin) *n* an inactive substance formed by the action of renin* on a protein in the blood plasma. In the lungs angiotensin I is converted into angiotensin II, a highly active substance which constricts blood vessels

and causes release of aldosterone* from the adrenal cortex. (Hypertensin.)

angstrom unit (ang'-strom) *n* measure of wave length, especially of radiation.

ang·ular stomat·itis ⇒ stomatitis.

anhid·rosis (an-hī-drō'-sis) *n* deficient sweat secretion—**anhidrotic** *adj*.

anhid·rotics (an-hī-dro'-tiks) *n* any agent which reduces perspiration.

anhyd·remia (an-hīd-rēm'-ē-ȧ) *n* deficient fluid content of blood—**anhydremic** *adj*.

anhyd·rous (an-hīd'-rus) *adj* entirely without water, dry.

anict·eric (an-ik'-tėr-ik) *n* without jaundice.

aniline (an'-il-ēn) *n* an oily compound obtained from coal and used in the preparation of antiseptic dyes.

anir·idia (an-i-rid'-ē-ȧ) *n* lack or defect of the iris*; usually congenital.

aniso·coria (an-i-sō-kō'-rē-ȧ) *n* inequality in diameter of the pupils.

aniso·cytosis (an-i-sō-sī-tō'-sis) *n* inequality in size of red blood cells.

aniso·melia (an-i-sō-mē'-lē-ȧ) *n* unequal length of limbs—**anisomelous** *adj*.

aniso·metropia (an-i-sō-me-trō'-pē-ȧ) *n* a difference in the refraction* of the two eyes—**anisometropic** *adj*.

ankle clonus *n* a series of rapid muscular contractions of the calf muscle when the foot is dorsiflexed by pressure upon the sole.

ankylo·bleph·aron (ang-ki-lō-blef'-ȧ-ron) *n* adhesion of the ciliary edges of the eyelids.

anky·losing spond·ylitis (ang-ki-lō'-sing spon-dil-ī'-tis) ⇒ spondylitis.

anky·losis (ang-ki-lō'-sis) *n* stiffness or fixation of a joint as a result of disease. ⇒ spondylitis—**ankylosed** *adj*, **ankylose** *vt, vi*.

Anky·lostoma (ang-ki-lō-stō'-mȧ) *n* Ancylostoma*.

ankylosto·miasis (ang-ki-lō-stō-mī'-ȧ-sis) *n* Ancylostomiasis*.

an·nular (an'-ū-lȧr) *n* ring-shaped. *annular ligaments* hold in proximity two long bones, as in the wrist and ankle joints.

ano·dyne (an'-ō-dīn) *n* a remedy which relieves pain. ⇒ analgesic.

ano·genital (ā-nō-jen'-it-al) *adj* pertaining to the anus and the genital region.

anomaly (an-om'-a-lē) *n* that which is unusual or differs from the normal—**anomalous** *adj*.

anomia (an-ō'-mē-à) *n* inability to name objects or persons.

anomie (an'-ō-mē) *n* sociological term applied to a person who is lonely because he cannot relate with others and consequently no longer identifies with them.

anon·ychia (an-o-nik'-ē-à) *n* absence of nails.

ano·perin·eal (ā'-nō-pér-in-ē'-al) *adj* pertaining to the anus and perineum.

Anoph·eles (an-of'-i-lēz) *n* a genus of mosquito. The females of some species are the hosts of the malarial parasite, and their bite is the means of transmitting malaria* to man.

anoplasty (ān'-ō-plas-tē) *n* plastic surgery of the anus—**anoplastic** *adj*.

anor·chism (an-ōr'-kizm) *n* congenital absence of one or both testes—**anorchic** *adj*.

ano·rectal (ān-ō-rek'-tal) *adj* pertaining to the anus and rectum, e.g. a fissure.

anor·ectic (an-ōr-ek'-tik) *n* **1** appetite depressant. **2** one who suffers from anorexia nervosa.

anor·exia (an-ōr-eks'-ē-à) *n* loss of or impaired appetite for food. *anorexia nervosa* a complicated psychological illness, most common in female adolescents. There is minimal food intake leading to loss of weight and sometimes death from starvation—**anorexic, anorectic** *adj*.

anos·mia (an-oz'-mē-à) *n* absence of the sense of smell—**anosmic** *adj*.

anov·ular (an-ōv'-ū-làr) *adj* absence of ovulation. *anovular menstruation* is the result of taking contraceptive pills. *anovular bleeding* occurs in metropathia* hemorrhagica. An endometrial biopsy following an *anovular cycle* shows no progestational changes.

anox·emia (an-oks-ēm'-ē-a) *n* literally, no oxygen in the blood. Usually used to indicate hypoxemia—**anoxemic** *adj*.

an·oxia (an-oks'-ē-à) *n* literally, no oxygen in the tissues. Usually used to signify hypoxia—**anoxic** *adj*.

Antab·use (ant'-à-būs) *n* proprietary name for disulfiram*.

ant·acid (ant-as'-id) *n* a substance which neutralizes or counteracts acidity. Commonly used in alkaline stomach powders and mixtures.

antag·onism (ant-ag'-on-izm) *n* active opposition; a characteristic of some drugs. Antagonism also characterizes some muscles and organisms—**antagonistic** *adj*, **antagonist** *n*.

antag·onist (ant-ag'-on-ist) *n* a muscle that relaxes to allow the agonist to perform a movement. When applied to a drug it is one which blocks, nullifies or reverses the effects of another drug.

antagon·istic action ⇒ action.

antaphrodisiac (ant-af-rō-dēz'-ē-ak) *n* an agent that diminishes sexual desire; absence of sexual impulse. Also anaphrodisiac.

ante·flexion (an'-tē-flek'-shun) *n* the bending forward of an organ, commonly applied to the position of the uterus. ⇒ retroflexion *opp*.

ante·mortem (an-tē-mōr'-tem) *adj* before death. ⇒ postmortem *opp*.

ante·natal (an-tē-nā'-tal) *adj* prenatal*. ⇒ postnatal *opp*.—**antenatally** *adv*.

Ante·par (an'-te-pàr) *n* proprietary elixir and tablets containing piperazine.

ante·partum (an'-tē-pàr'-tum) *adj* before birth. ⇒ postpartum *opp. antepartum hemorrhage* ⇒ placental abruption.

an·terior (an-tē'-rē-ér) *adj* in front of; the front surface of; ventral ⇒ posterior *opp*.—**anteriorly** *adv*, *anterior chamber of the eye* the space between the posterior surface of the cornea and the anterior surface of the iris. ⇒ aqueous. *anterior tibial syndrome* severe pain and inflammation over anterior tibial muscle group, with inability to dorsiflex the foot.

antero·grade (an'-tér-ō-grād) *adj* proceeding forward. ⇒ retrograde *opp*. ⇒ amnesia.

ante·version (an'-tē-vėr'-shun) *n* the normal forward tilting, or displacement forward, of an organ or part. ⇒ retroversion *opp*—**anteverted** *adj*, **antevert** *vt*.

anthel·mintic (an-thel-min'-tik) *adj* describes any remedy for the destruction or elimination of intestinal worms.

anthracemia (an-thra-sēm'-ē-à) *n* anthrax septicemia—**anthracemic** *adj*.

anthra·cosis (an-thra-kō'-sis) *n* accumulation of carbon in the lungs due to inhalation of coal dust; may cause fibrotic reaction. A form of pneumoconiosis*—**anthracotic** *adj*.

Anthra-Derm *n* proprietary name for anthralin*.

anthralin (an'-thra-lin) *n* an ointment applied to the skin for the treatment of psoriasis. (Anthra-Derm.)

an·thrax (an'-thraks) *n* a contagious disease of cattle, which may be transmitted to man by inoculation, inhalation and ingestion, causing malignant pustule, woolsorter's disease and gastrointestinal anthrax respectively. Causative organism is *Bacillus* * *anthracis*. Preventive measures include prophylactic immunization of cattle and man.

anthro·poid (an'-thrō-poyd) *adj* resembling man. The word is also used to describe a pelvis that is narrow from side to side, a form of contracted pelvis*.

anthro·pology (an-thrō-pol'-o-jē) *n* the study of mankind. Subdivided into several specialities. ⇒ ethnology.

anthro·pometry (an-thrō-pom'-et-rē) *n* measurement of the human body and its parts for the purposes of comparison and establishing norms for sex, age, weight, race and so on—**anthropometric** *adj*.

anti·adrenergic (an'-tī-ad-ren-ér'-jik) *adj* neutralizing or lessening the effects of impulses produced by adrenergic postganglionic fibers of the sympathetic nervous system.

anti·aldosterone (an'-tī-al-dos'-tér-ōn) *n* any substance that acts as an aldosterone antagonist. Used in the treatment of edema and ascites of hepatic cirrhosis, edema of congestive heart failure and nephrotic syndrome ⇒ spironolactone.

anti·allergic (an'-tī-al-ér'-jik) *adj* preventing or lessening allergy.

anti·anabolic (an-tī-an-a-bol'-ik) *adj* preventing the synthesis of body protein.

anti·anemic (an-tī-an-ēm'-ik) *adj* used to prevent hemorrhage, e.g. vitamin* K.

anti·arrhyth·mic (an-tī-ā-rith'-mik) *adj* describes drugs and treatments used in a variety of cardiac rhythm disorders.

anti·bacterial (an-ti-bak-tēr'-ē-al) *adj* describes any agent which destroys bacteria or inhibits their growth.

anti·beri·beri (an-tī-bér'-ē-bér'-ē) *adj* against beri-beri*, e.g. the thiamine portion of vitamin B complex.

anti·bilharzial (an-tī-bil-hár'-zē-al) *adj* against *Bilharzia*. ⇒ *Schistosoma*.

anti·biosis (an-tī-bī-ōs'-is) *n* an association between organisms which is harmful to one of them. ⇒ symbiosis *opp*—**antibiotic** *adj*.

anti·biotics (an-tī-bī-ot'-iks) *npl* antibacterial substances derived from fungi and bacteria, exemplified by penicillin*. Later antibiotics such as tetracycline* are active against a wider range of pathogenic organisms, and are also effective orally. Others, such as neomycin* and bacitracin*, are rarely used internally owing to high toxicity, but are effective

when applied topically, and skin sensitization is uncommon.

anti·bodies (an'-ti-bod-ēz) *npl* ⇒ immunoglobulins.

anti·cholin·ergic (an-ti-kōl-in-érj'-ik) *adj* inhibitory to the action of a cholinergic nerve* by interfering with the action of acetylcholine*, a chemical by which such a nerve transmits its impulses at neural or myoneural junctions.

anti·cholin·esterase (an-ti-kōl-in-es'-tér-ās) *n* enzyme that destroys acetylcholine at nerve endings. Used for reversing the effects of muscle relaxant drugs.

anti·coag·ulant (an-ti-kō-ag'-ūl-ant) *n* an agent which prevents or retards clotting of blood, a small amount is made in the human body. Uses: (a) to obtain specimens suitable for pathological investigaton and chemical analyses where whole blood or plasma is required instead of serum; the anticoagulant is usually oxalate (b) to obtain blood suitable for transfusion, the anticoagulant usually being sodium citrate (c) as a therapeutic agent in the treatment of coronary thrombosis, phlebothrombosis (thrombophlebitis) etc. when aspirin should not be given.

anti·convul·sant (an-ti-kon-vul'-sant) *n* an agent which terminates a convulsion or prevents convulsions—**anticonvulsive** *adj*.

anti-D *n* anti-Rh_0, an immunoglobulin*, Rho Gam.

anti·depres·sants (an-ti-dē-pres'-ants) *npl* drugs which relieve depression. Those in the tricyclic group are the most widely prescribed: they are useful for endogenous depression. Another group is the monoamine* oxidase inhibitors whose widespread use is curtailed because of the need for users to take a strict diet to prevent toxic side-effects.

anti·diab·etic (an-tī-dī-ab-et'-ik) *adj* literally 'against diabetes'. Used to describe therapeutic measures in diabetes mellitus; the hormone insulin*, oral diabetic agents, e.g. tolbutamide*.

anti·diph·theritic (an-tī-dif-thér-it'-ik) *adj* against diphtheria. Describes preventive measures such as immunization to produce active immunity; therapeutic measures, for example, serum used to give passive immunity.

anti·diur·etic (an-tī-dī-ūr-et'-ik) *adj* reducing the volume of urine. *antidiuretic hormone* (*ADH*) vasopressin*.

anti·dote (an'-ti-dōt) *n* a remedy which

19

counteracts or neutralizes the action of a poison.

anti·embolic (an-ti-em'-bol-ik) *adj* against embolism*. Antiembolic stockings are worn to decrease the risk of deep vein thrombosis.

anti·emetic (an-tī-ē-met'-ik) *adj* against emesis*. Any agent which prevents nausea and vomiting.

anti·enzyme (an-tī-en'-zīm) *n* a substance which exerts a specific inhibiting action on an enzyme. Found in the digestive tract to prevent digestion of its lining, and in blood where they act as immunoglobulins*.

anti·epil·eptic (an-tī-ep-i-lep'-tik) *adj* describes drugs which reduce the frequency of epileptic attacks.

anti·feb·rile (an-ti-fēb'-ril) *adj* describes any agent which reduces or allays fever.

anti·fibrin·olytic (anti-fī-brin-ō-lit'-ik) *adj* describes any agent which prevents fibrinolysis*.

anti·fungal (an-ti-fun'-gal) *adj* describes any agent which destroys fungi.

anti·gen (an'-ti-jen) *n* any substance which, under favorable conditions, can stimulate the production of antibodies* (specific immune response*). ⇒ D-Vac antigens—**antigenic** *adj*.

anti·hemo·philic glob·ulin (AHG) factor VIII involved in blood* clotting, present in plasma; absent from serum; deficient in hemophilia*.

anti·hemor·rhagic (an-ti-hem-ōr-aj'-ik) *adj* describes any agent which prevents hemorrhage; used to describe vitamin* K.

anti·hista·mines (an-ti-hist'-à-mēnz) *npl* drugs which suppress some of the effects of released histamine*. They are widely used in the palliative treatment of hay fever, urticaria, angioneurotic edema and some forms of pruritis. They also have antiemetic* properties, and are effective in motion and radiation sickness. Side effects include drowsiness.

anti·hyper·tensive (an-ti-hī-pèr-ten'-siv) *adj* describes any agent which reduces high blood pressure.

anti·infect·ive (an-ti-in-fek'-tiv) *adj* describes any agent which prevents infection; used to describe vitamin* A.

anti·inflam·matory (an-ti-in-flam'-a-tōr-ē) *adj* tending to reduce or prevent inflammation.

antilep·rotic (an-ti-lep-rot'-ik) *adj* describing any agent which prevents or cures leprosy.

antiluetic (an-tī-lōō-et'-ik) *adj* any agent which prevents or cures syphilis (lues).

anti·lympho·cyte glob·ulin immunoglobulin* containing antibodies to lymphocyte membrane antigens, causing their inactivation or lysis and thus diminishing immune responses.

anti·lymph·ocyte serum (ALS) *n* serum containing antibodies which bind to lymphocytes inhibiting their function. Used to induce immunosuppression in a patient undergoing kidney transplant.

anti·malarial (an-tī-mal-ār'-ē-al) *adj* against malaria*.

anti·metab·olite (an-tī-met-ab'-ō-līt) *n* a compound which is sufficiently similar to the chemicals needed by a cell to be incorporated into the nucleoproteins of that cell, thereby preventing its development. Examples are methotrexate*, a folic acid antagonist, and mercaptopurine*, a purine antagonist. Antimetabolites are used in the treatment of cancer.

anti·microbial (an-ti-mī-krō'-bē-àl) *adj* against microbes.

anti·migraine (an-tī-mī'-grān) *adj* against migraine*.

anti·mitotic (an-tī-mī-tot'-ik) *adj* preventing reproduction of a cell by mitosis. Describes many of the drugs used to treat cancer.

anti·mutagen (an-tī-mū'-ta-jen) *n* a substance which nullifies the action of a mutagen*—**antimutagenic** *adj*.

antimycotic (an-tī-mī-kot'-ik) *adj* describes any agent which destroys fungi.

anti·neo·plastic (an-tī-nē-ō-plas'-tik) *adj* describes any substance or procedure which works against neoplasms*. ⇒ alkylating agents, cytotoxic, radiotherapy.

anti·neur·itic (an-tī-nū-rit'-ik) *adj* describes any agent which prevents neuritis. Specially applied to vitamin* B complex.

anti·oxid·ants (an-tī-oks'-id-ants) *npl* describes any substances which delay the process of oxidation.

anti·paras·itic (an-tī-pār-à-sit'-ik) *adj* describes any agent which prevents or destroys parasites.

anti·parkinson(ism) drugs (an-tī-pàr'-kin-son-izm) *npl* name given to the major transquilizing drugs such as the phenothiazines. They counter the side-effects of the neuroleptic or antipsychotic drugs.

anti·pellagra (an-tī-pel-ā'-grà) *adj* against

pellagra; a function of the nicotinic acid portion of vitamin* B complex.

anti·periodic (an-tī-pēr-ē-od′-ik) *n* an agent which prevents the periodic return of a disease, e.g. the use of quinine in malaria.

anti·peristal·sis (an-tī-per-i-stal′-sis) *n* reversal of the normal peristaltic action—**antiperistaltic** *adj.*

antiphlogistic (an-tī-flō-jis′-tik) *adj* an agent that helps relieve inflammation, e.g. Kaolin.

anti·prothr·ombin (an-tī-prō-throm′-bin) *n* arrests blood clotting by preventing conversion of prothrombin into thrombin. Anticoagulant.

anti·prur·itic (an-tī-proo-rit′-ik) *adj* describes any agent which relieves or prevents itching.

anti·pur·pura (an-tī-pur′-pū-rà) *adj* against purpura; a function of vitamin P (hesperidin).

anti·pyr·etic (an-tī-pī-ret′-ik) *adj* describes any agent which allays or reduces fever.

anti·rabic (an-tī-rā′-bik) *adj* describes any agent which prevents or cures rabies.

anti·rach·itic (an-tī-rak-it′-ik) *adj* describes any agent which prevents or cures rickets, a function of vitamin D*.

anti·reflux (an-tī-rē′-fluks) *adj* against backward flow. Usually refers to reimplantation of ureters into bladder in cases of chronic pyelonephritis* with associated vesicoureteric reflux. ⇒ Leadbetter-Politano operation.

anti·Rhesus (Rh) serum (an-tī-rē′-sus) given to Rh-negative women who have an Rh-positive baby in order to prevent the development of Rhesus antibodies which might cause erythroblastosis* fetalis in a subsequent pregnancy. Rho Gam.

anti·rheum·atic (an-tī-rōō-mat′-ik) *adj* describes any agent which prevents or lessens rheumatism.

anti·schisto·somal (an-ti-skis-tō-sō′-mal) *adj* describes any agent which works against *Schistosoma*.

anti·scorb·utic (an-tī-skōr-bū′-tik) *adj* describes any agent which prevents or cures scurvy, a function of vitamin* C.

anti·secret·ory (an-tī-sē′-kret-ōr-ē) *adj* describes any agent which inhibits secretion.

anti·sepsis (an-tī-sep′-sis) *n* prevention of sepsis (tissue infection); introduced into surgery in 1880 by Lord Lister, who used carbolic acid—**antiseptic** *adj.*

anti·sep·tics (an-ti-sep′-tiks) *npl* chemical substances which destroy or inhibit the growth of microorganisms. They can be applied to living tissues.

anti·sero·tonin (an-tī-sē′-rō-tōn′-in) *n* a substance which neutralizes or lessens the effect of serotonin*.

anti·serum (an-tī-sēr′-um) *n* a substance prepared from the blood of an animal which has been immunized by the requisite antigen; it contains a high concentration of antibodies.

anti·siala·gogue (an-tī-sī-al′-à-gog) *n* a substance which inhibits salivation.

anti·social (an-ti-sō′-shal) *adj* against society. A term used to denote a psychopathic state in which the individual cannot accept the obligations and restraints imposed on a community by its members—**antisocialism** *n.*

anti·spas·modic (an-tī-spaz-mod′-ik) *adj* describes any measure used to relieve spasm in muscle.

anti·static (an-ti-stat′-ik) *adj* preventing the accumulation of static electricity.

anti·steril·ity (an-tī-ster-il′-it-ē) *adj* against sterility; thought to be a function of vitamin* E.

anti·strepto·lysin (an-tī-strep-tō-lī′-sin) *adj* against streptolysins*. A raised antistreptolysin titer in the blood is indicative of recent streptococcal infection.

anti·syphil·itic (an-tī-sif-il-it′-ik) *adj* describes any measures taken to combat syphilis*.

anti·throm·bin (an-ti-throm′-bin) *n* antithrombin or antithrombins are substances occurring naturally in the blood, e.g. heparin*. ⇒ thrombin.

anti·thromb·otic (an-ti-throm-bot′-ik) *adj* describes any measures that prevent or cure thrombosis*.

anti·thymo·cyte glob·ulin (an-ti-thī′-mō-sīt glob′-ū-lin) **(ATG)** an immunoglobulin* which binds to antigens on thymic lymphocytes and inhibits lymphocyte-dependent immune responses.

anti·thyr·oid (an-tī-thī′-royd) *n* any agent used to decrease the activity of the thyroid gland.

anti·toxin an-ti-toks′-in) *n* an antibody which neutralizes a given toxin. Made in response to the invasion by toxin-producing bacteria, or the injection of toxoids—**antitoxic** *adj.*

anti·trepon·emal (an-tī-trep-ō-nēm′-àl) *adj* describes any measures used against infections caused by *Treponema*.

anti·tuber·cul·osis (an-tī-tū-ber-kū-lō'-sis) *adj* describes any measures used to prevent or cure tuberculosis—**antitubercular** *adj*.

anti·tum·or (an-ti-tū'-mor) *adj* against tumor formation; describes an agent which inhibits growth of tumor.

anti·tus·sive (an-ti-tus'-iv) *adj* describes any measures which suppress cough.

anti·venin (an-ti-ven'-in) *n* a serum prepared from animals injected with the venom of snakes; used as an antidote in cases of poisoning by snakebite.

anti·viral (an-tī-vī'-ràl) *adj* acting against viruses.

anti·vit·amin (an-tī-vīt'-à-min) *n* a substance interfering with the absorption or utilization of a vitamin.

antrect·omy (an-trek'-tō-mē) *n* excision of pyloric antrum* of stomach thus removing the source of the hormone gastrin in the treatment of duodenal ulcer.

Antrenyl (an'-tren-il) *n* proprietary name for oxyphenonium*.

antro·oral (an-trō-ōr'-àl) *adj* pertaining to the maxillary antrum and the mouth. *antrooral fistula* can occur after extraction of an upper molar tooth, the root of which has protruded into the floor of the antrum.

antros·tomy (an-tros'-tom-ē) *n* an artificial opening from nasal cavity to antrum* of Highmore (maxillary sinus) for the purpose of drainage.

ant·rum (ant'-rum) *n* a cavity, especially in bone—**antral** *adj. antrum of Highmore* in the superior maxillary bone.

Ant·rypol (an'-tri-pol) *n* proprietary name for suramin*.

Antuitrin (an-tū'-it-rin) *n* proprietary extract of the anterior pituitary gland.

Ant·urane (an-tūr-ān) *n* proprietary name for sulfinpyrazone*.

anuria (an-ū'-rē-à) *n* absence of secretion of urine by the kidneys. ⇒ suppression—**anuric** *adj*.

anus (ā'-nus) *n* the end of the alimentary canal, at the extreme termination of the rectum. It is formed of a sphincter muscle which relaxes to allow fecal matter to pass through—**anal** *adj. artificial anus* ⇒ colostomy. *imperforate anus* ⇒ imperforate.

Anusol (an'-ū-sol) *n* suppositories or ointment for the treatment of anorectal pain and itching.

anvil (an'-vil) *n* the incus, the middle of the three small bones of the middle ear. Shaped like an anvil.

anxiety (ang-zī'-et-ē) *n* feelings of fear, apprehension and dread. *anxiety neurosis state* a neurosis characterized by recurrent acute anxiety attacks (panics) or by chronic anxiety. The attacks consist of all the signs and symptoms of fear, leading up to fear of impending collapse and sometimes death. '*free floating anxiety*' a term used to indicate that the apprehension has external cause.

anxio·lytics (ang-zi-ō-lit'-iks) *npl* agents which reduce anxiety.

aorta (ā-ōr'-tà) *n* the main artery arising out of the left ventricle of the heart. ⇒ Figure 9.

aortic (ā-ōr'-tik) *adj* pertaining to the aorta. *aortic incompetence* regurgitation of blood from aorta back into the left ventricle. *aortic murmur* abnormal heart sound heard over aortic area; a systolic murmur alone is the murmur of aortic stenosis, a diastolic murmur denotes aortic incompetence. The combination of both systolic and diastolic murmurs causes the so-called 'to and fro' aortic murmur. *aortic stenosis* narrowing of aortic valve. This is usually due to rheumatic heart disease or a congenital bicuspid valve which predisposes to the deposit of calcium.

aort·itis (ā-ōr-tī'-tis) *n* inflammation of the aorta.

aort·og·raphy (ā-ōr-tog'-raf-ē) *n* demonstration of the aorta after introduction of an opaque medium, either via a catheter passed along the femoral or brachial artery or by direct translumbar injection—**aortographic** *adj*, **aortogram** *n*, **aortograph** *n*, **aortographically** *adv*.

apa·thy (a'-pà-thē) *n* 1 abnormal listlessness and lack of activity. 2 attitude of indifference—**apathetic** *adj*.

APC *n* tablets containing aspirin, phenacetin, and caffeine.

aperi·ents (a-pèr'-ē-ents) *npl* ⇒ laxatives.

aperi·stalsis (ā-pèr-is-tal'-sis) *n* absence of peristaltic movement in the bowel. Characterizes the condition of paralytic ileus—**aperistaltic** *adj*.

Apert's syn·drome (ā'-pèrts sin'-drōm) congenital craniosynostosis accompanied by deformities of the hands. ⇒ syndactyly, acrocephalosyndactyly.

apex (ā'-peks) *n* the summit or top of anything which is cone-shaped, e.g. the tip of the root of a tooth. ⇒ Figure 7—**ap-**

ices *pl.* **apical** *adj.* In a heart of normal size the *apical beat* (systolic impulse) can be seen or felt in the 5th left intercostal space in the mid-clavicular line. It is the lowest and most lateral point at which an impulse can be detected and provides a rough indication of the size of the heart.

Apgar score (ap′gàr) a measure used to evaluate the general condition of a newborn baby, developed by an American anesthetist, Dr. Virginia Apgar. A score of 0, 1, or 2 is given using the criteria of heart rate, respiratory effort, skin color, muscle tone and reflex response to a nasal catheter. A score of between 8 and 10 would indicate a baby in excellent condition, whereas a score of below 7 would cause concern.

aphagia (ā-fā′jē-à) *n* inability to swallow—**aphagic** *adj.*

aphakia (ā-fā′-kē-à) *n* absence of the crystalline lens. Describes the eye after removal of a cataract—**aphakic** *adj.*

aphasia (ā-fā′-zē-à) *n* often used interchangeably with dysphasia*. Disorder of the complex language function, in spite of normal hearing over the whole frequency range, which is thought to be due to brain lesion. There are several classifications but the most commonly used terms are *expressive* (*motor*) aphasia and *receptive* (*sensory*) aphasia although many patients exhibit deficiencies in both types—**aphasic** *adj.*

aphonia (a-fō′nē-à) *n* loss of voice from a cause other than a cerebral lesion—**aphonic** *adj.*

aphro·disiac (af-rō-dēz′-ē-ak) *n* an agent which stimulates sexual excitement.

aph·thae (af′-thē) *npl* small ulcers of the oral mucosa surrounded by a ring of erythema—**aphtha** *sing*, **aphthous** *adj.*

aph·thous stoma·titis (af′-thus stō-mà-tī′-tis) ⇒ stomatitis.

apic·ect·omy (āp-i-sek′-to-mē) *n* excision of the apex of the root of a tooth.

apicolysis (āp-ik-ol′-i-sis) *n* the parietal pleura is stripped from the upper chest wall to ensure collapse of the lung apex when it contains a tuberculous cavity.

aplasia (ā-plā′-zē-à) *n* incomplete development of tissue; absence of growth.

aplas·tic (ā-plas′tik) *adj* **1** without structure or form. **2** incapable of forming new tissue. *aplastic anemia* ⇒ anemia.

ap·nea (ap-nē′-à) *n* a transitory cessation of breathing as seen in Cheyne-Stokes

respiration*. It is due to lack of the necessary CO_2 tension in the blood for stimulation of the respiratory center—**apneic** *adj. apnea of the newborn* ⇒ periodic breathing *sleep apnea* failure of autonomic control of respiration which becomes more pronounced during sleep.

apo·crine glands (ap′-ō-krēn) modified sweat glands, especially in axiliac, genital and perineal regions. Responsible after puberty for body odor.

apo·dia (ā-pō′-dē-à) *n* congenital absence of the feet.

apo·mor·phine (a-pō-mōr′-fēn) *n* powerful emetic* when injected. Effective when gastric irritant emetics are useless, as in phenol poisoning.

apo·neurosis (ap-ō-nū-rō′-sis) *n* a broad glistening sheet of tendon-like tissue which serves to invest and attach muscles to each other, and also to the parts which they move—**aponeuroses** *pl*, **aponeurotic** *adj.*

apon·euros·itis (ap-ō-nū-rō-sī′-tis) *n* inflammation of an aponeurosis.

apo·physis (ap-of′-is-is) *n* a projection, protuberance or outgrowth. Usually used in connection with bone.

apo·plexy (ap′-ō-pleks-ē) *n* condition more commonly referred to as cerebro-.vascular* accident (stroke)—**apoplectic**, **apoplectiform** *adj.*

appen·dectomy (ap-pen·dek′-to-mē) *n* appendicectomy*.

appendi·cectomy (ap-pen-dis-ek′-to-mē) *n* excision of the appendix* vermiformis.

appen·dicitis (ap-pen-dis-ī′-tis) *n* inflammation of the appendix* vermiformis.

appen·dix (ap-pen′-diks) *n* an appendage. *appendix vermiformis* a worm-like appendage of the cecum about the thickness of a pencil and usually measuring from 50.8 to 152.4 mm in length (⇒ Figure 18). Its position is variable and it is apparently functionless—**appendices** *pl*. **appendicular** *adj.*

apper·cep·tion (ap-pèr-sep′-shun) *n* clear perception of a sensory stimulus, in particular where there is identification or recognition—**apperceptive** *adj.*

appli·cator (ap′-li-kā-tor) *n* an instrument for local application of remedies.

appo·sition (ap-o-zish′-un) *n* the approximation or bringing together of two surfaces or edges.

apraxia (ā-praks′-e-à) *n* inability to deal effectively with or manipulate objects as a result of a brain lesion—**apraxic, apractic** adj. constructional apraxia inability to arrange objects to a plan.

Apresoline (ă-pres'-ō-lēn) n proprietary name for hydralazine*.

APT abbr alum precipitated diphtheria toxoid. A diphtheria prophylactic used mainly for children.

apti·tude (ap'-ti-tūd) n natural ability and facility in performing tasks, either mental or physical.

apyr·exia (ā-pī-reks'-ē-à) n absence of fever—**apyrexial** adj.

Apyr·ogen (ā-pī'-rō-jen) n a proprietary brand of sterile distilled water in hermetically sealed ampules. It is free from pyrogen*. Used to make up drugs supplied in powder form, when they are to be given by injection.

apyrogenic (ā-pī-rō-jen'-ik) adj not fever producing.

aqua (ak'-wà) n water. aqua destillata distilled water. aqua fortis nitric acid. aqua menthae piperitae peppermint water.

Aqua·mephy·ton (ak-wa-mef-i'-ton) proprietary name for phytonadione, Vitamin K.

aque·duct (ak'-wi-dukt) a canal. aqueduct of Sylvius the canal connecting the 3rd and 4th ventricles of the brain; aqueductus cerebri.

aque·ous (ā'-kwi-us) adj watery. aqueous humor the fluid contained in the anterior and posterior chambers of the eye. ⇒ Figure 15.

arachi·donic acid (ar-ak'-id-on-ik) one of the essential fatty acids. Found in small amounts in human and animal liver and organ fats. A growth factor.

arachis oil (ar'-ak-is) oil expressed from groundnuts. Similar to olive oil.

arach·nodac·tyly (ar-ak-nō-dak'-til-ē) n congenital abnormality resulting in spider fingers.

arach·noid (ar-ak'-noyd) adj resembling a spider's web. arachnoid membrane a delicate membrane enveloping the brain and spinal cord, lying between the pia mater internally and the dura mater externally; the middle serous membrane of the meninges—**arachnoidal** adj.

Aralen (ār'-à-len) n proprietary name for chloroquine*.

Ara·mine (ār'-à-mēn) n proprietary name for metaraminol*.

arboriz·ation (ar-bor-ī-zā'-shun) n an arrangement resembling the branching of a tree. Characterizes both ends of a neurone, i.e. the dendrons and the axon as it supplies each muscle fiber.

arbo·viruses (ar-bō-vī'-rus-es) npl an abbreviation for RNA viruses transmitted by arthropods. Members of the mosquito-borne group include those causing yellow fever, dengue and viruses causing infections of the CNS. Sandflies transmit the virus causing sandfly fever. The tickborne viruses can cause hemorrhagic fevers.

ARC abbr AIDS*-related complex.

arch of aorta ⇒ Figure 10.

arc·us sen·ilis (ar'-kus sen-il'-is) an opaque ring round the edge of the cornea, seen in old people.

are·ola (ār-ē'-o-là) n The pigmented area round the nipple of the breast. A secondary areola surrounds the primary areola in pregnancy—**areolar** adj.

ARF abbr 1 acute renal failure ⇒ renal. 2 acute respiratory failure. ⇒ respiratory failure.

Arf·onad (ar'-fo-nad) proprietary name for trimetaphan*.

argin·ase (ar'-jin-āz) n an enzyme found in the liver, kidney and spleen. It splits arginine into ornithine and urea.

argin·ine (ar'-jin-ēn) n one of the essential amino acids. Used in treatment of acute liver failure to tide patient over acute ammonia intoxication.

arginino·succin·uria (ar-jin-ēn'-ō-suks-in-ū'-rē-à) n the presence of arginine and succinic acid in urine. Currently associated with mental subnormality.

argon (ar'-gon) n a rare insert gas used in measurement. Less than 0.1% in atmospheric air.

Argyll Robert·son pupil (ar-gil' rob'-ertson pū'-pil) one which reacts to accommodation, but not to light. Diagnostic sign in neurosyphilis*, but not all examples are syphilitic. Other important causes include disseminated sclerosis and diabetes mellitus. In the non-syphilitic group the pupil is not small, but often dilated and unequal and is called atypical.

aribo·flavin·osis (ā-rī-bō-flāv-in-ōs'-is) n a deficiency state caused by lack of riboflavine* and other members of the vitamin B complex. Characterized by cheilosis, seborrhea, angular stomatitis, glossitis and photophobia.

Aristocort (ar-is'-to-kōrt) n proprietary name for triamcinalone*.

Arnold·Chiari mal·formation (ar'-nōlt kē'-a-rē) n a group of disorders affecting the base of the brain. Commonly occurs in hydrocephalus associated with meningocele and myelomeningocele. There are degrees of severity but usually there is some 'kinking' or 'buckling' of the brain stem with cerebellar tissue herniating through the foramen magnum at the base of the skull.

AROM *abbr* active range of motion; artificial rupture of membranes.

arrec·tores pit·orum (àr-ek-tōr'-ēz pi-lōr'-um) internal, plain, involuntary muscles (⇒ Figure 12) attached to hair follicles, which, by contraction, erect the follicles, causing 'gooseflesh'—arrector pili *sing*.

ar·rheno·blast·oma (ā-rēn-ō-blas-tō'-mà) *n* ⇒ androblastoma.

ar·rhyth·mia (ā-rith'-mē-à) *n* any deviation from the normal rhythm, usually referring to the heart beat. ⇒ sinus extrasystole, fibrillation, heart, Stokes-Adams syndrome, tachycardia.

Arruga suture (à-rū'-gà) purse-string suture placed around eye in the treatment of detached retina.

ar·senic (àr'-sen-ik) *n* a metal which, in some forms, is a potent toxin, causing malaise, anemia, gastrointestinal and nervous symptoms.

Ar·tane (àr'-tān) proprietary name for trihexyphenidyl*.

arte·fact (àr'-te-fakt) *n* any artificial product resulting from a physical or chemical agency; an unnatural change in a structure or tissue.

arter·algia (àr'-ter-al'-jē-à) *n* pain in an artery.

arterectomy (àr-tèr-ek'-to-mē) *n* excision of an artery or part of an artery.

arteri·ography (ar-tēr-ē-o'-gra-fē) *n* demonstration of the arterial system after injection of an opaque medium—**arteriographic** *adj*, **arteriogram** *n*, **arteriograph** *n*, **arteriographically** *adv*.

arteri·ole (àr-tēr'-ē-ōl) *n* a small artery, joining an artery to a capillary.

arteri·opathy (àr-tēr-ē-op'-à-thē) *n* disease of any artery—**arteriopathic** *adj*.

arterio·plasty (àr-tēr'-ē-ō-plas-tē) *n* plastic surgery applied to an artery—**arterioplastic** *adj*.

arteriorrhaphy (àr-tē-rē-ōr'-raf-ē) *n* a plastic procedure or suturing of an artery, as in obliteration of an aneurysm.

arterio·sclerosis (àr-tēr-ē-ō-sklèr-ō'-sis) *n* degenerative arterial change associated with advancing age. Primarily a thickening of the media and usually associated with some degree of atheroma*—**arteriosclerotic** *adj*. *cerebral arteriosclerosis* a syndrome characterized by progressive memory loss, confusion and childlike behavior.

arteri·otomy (àr-tēr-ē-ot'-ō-mē) *n* incision or needle puncture of an artery.

arterio·venous (àr-tēr-ē-ō-vēn'-us) *adj* pertaining to an artery and a vein, e.g. an arteriovenous aneurysm, fistula, or shunt for hemodialysis. *arteriovenous filtration* hemofiltration*.

arter·itis (àr-tèr-ī'-tis) *n* an inflammatory disease affecting the middle walls of the arteries. It may be due to an infection such as syphilis or it may be part of a collagen disease. The arteries may become swollen and tender and the blood may clot in them. *Giani cell arteritis* occurs in the elderly and mainly in the scalp arteries. Blindness can ensue if there is thrombosis of the ophthalmic vessels. Treatment with cortisone is effective—**arteritic** *adj*.

ar·tery (àr'-tèr-ē) *n* a vessel carrying blood from the heart to the various tissues. The internal endothelial lining provides a smooth surface to prevent clotting of blood. The middle layer of plain muscle and elastic fibers allows for distension as blood is pumped from the heart. The outer, mainly connective tissue layer prevents overdistension. The lumen is largest nearest to the heart; it gradually decreases in size—**arterial** *adj*. *artery forceps* forceps used to produce hemostasis*.

ar·thral·gia (àrth-ral'-jē-à) *n* (*syn* articular neuralgia, arthrodynia) pain in a joint, used especially when there is no inflammation—**arthralgic** *adj*. *intermittent* or *periodic arthralgia* is the term used when there is pain, usually accompanied by swelling of the knee at regular intervals.

arthrectomy (àrth-rek'-to-mē) *n* excision of a joint.

ar·thritis (àrth-rī'-tis) *n* inflammation of one or more joints which swell, become warm to touch, are painful and are restricted in movement. There are many causes and the treatment varies according to the cause. ⇒ arthropathy—**arthritic** *adj*. *arthritis deformans juvenilis* ⇒ Still's disease. *arthritis nodosa* gout*.

arthro·clasis (àrth-rō-klā'sis) *n* breaking down of adhesions within the joint cavity to produce a wider range of movement.

arthro·desis (àrth-rō-dē'-sis) *n* the stiffening of a joint by operative means.

arthro·dynia (àrth-rō-dī'-nē-à) *n* ⇒ arthralgia—**arthrodynic** *adj*.

arthroendoscopy (àrth-rō-en-dos'-kop-ē) *n* visualization of the interior of a joint using an endoscope*—**arthroendoscopic** *adj*, **arthroendoscopically** *adv*.

arthro·graphy (àrth-rog'-raf-ē) *n* a radiography examination to determine the internal structure of a joint, outlined by contrast media—either a gas or an opaque medium or both—**arthrographic** *adj*, **arthrogram** *n*, **arthrograph** *n*, **arthrographically** *adv*.

arthro·logy (àrth-rol'-oj-ē) *n* the science which studies the structure and function of joints, their diseases and treatment.

arthro·pathy (àrth-rop'-ath-ē) *n* any joint disease—**arthropathies** *pl*, **arthropathic** *adj*. The condition is currently classified as: *enteropathic arthropathies* resulting from chronic diarrheal diseases; *psoriatic arthropathies* psoriasis; *seronegative arthropathies* include all other instances of inflammatory arthritis other than rheumatoid arthritis; *seropositive arthropathies* include all instances of rheumatoid arthritis.

arthro·plasty (àrth'-rō-plas-tē) *n* surgical remodelling of a joint—**arthroplastic** *adj*. *cup arthroplasty* articular surface is reconstructed and covered with a vitallium cup. *excision arthroplasty* gap is filled with fibrous tissue as in Keller's* operation. *Girdlestone arthroplasty* excision arthroplasty of the hip. *replacement arthroplasty* insertion of an inert prosthesis of similar shape. *total replacement arthroplasty* replacement of the head of femur and the acetabulum, both being cemented into the bone.

arthro·scope (àrth'-rō-skōp) *n* an instrument used for the visualization of the interior of a joint cavity. ⇒ endoscope—**arthroscopic** *adj*.

arthros·copy (àrth-ros'-kop-ē) *n* the act of visualizing the interior of a joint—**arthroscopic** *adj*.

arth·rosis (àr-thrō'-sis) *n* degeneration in a joint.

arth·rotomy (àrth-rot'-o-mē) *n* incision into a joint.

artic·ular (àr-tik'-ū-làr) *adj* pertaining to a joint or articulation. Applied to cartilage, surface, capsule, etc. *articular neuralgia* ⇒ arthralgia.

articul·ation (àr-tik-ū-lā'-shun) *n* **1** the junction of two or more bones; a joint. **2** enunciation of speech—**articular** *adj*.

artifact (àrt'-i-fakt) *n* any artificial product; an unnatural change in a structure or tissue. Also spelled artefact.

arti·ficial anus *n* ⇒ colostomy.

arti·ficial blood *n* a fluid able to transport O_2 which has been used successfully in the USA and Japan. Jehovah's Witnesses acted as subjects for clinical trials.

arti·ficial feeding ⇒ enteral.

arti·ficial insemin·ation ⇒ insemination.

arti·ficial kid·ney ⇒ dialyser.

arti·ficial limb ⇒ prosthesis, orthosis.

arti·ficial lung ⇒ respirator.

arti·ficial pace·maker cardiac pacemaker. ⇒ cardiac.

arti·ficial pneumo·thorax ⇒ pneumothorax.

arti·ficial respir·ation ⇒ resuscitation.

asbes·tos (as-bes'-tos) *n* a fibrous, mineral substance which does not conduct heat and is incombustible. It has many uses, including brake linings, asbestos textiles and asbestos-cement sheeting.

asbest·osis (as-bes-tōs'-is) *n* a form of pneumoconiosis* from inhalation of asbestos dust and fiber. ⇒ mesothelioma.

ascar·iasis (as-kàr-ī'-a-sis) *n* infestation by the ascarides*. The bowel is most commonly affected but, in the case of roundworm, infestation may spread to the stomach, liver and lungs.

ascari·cide (as-kar'-is-īd) *n* a substance lethal to ascarides*—**ascaricidal** *adj*.

ascar·ides (as-kar'-i-dēz) *npl* nematode worms of the family Ascaridae, to which belong the roundworm (*Ascaris lumbricoides*) and the threadworm (*Oxyuris vermicularis*).

ascend·ing colon ⇒ Figure 18.

Aschoff's nod·ules (ash'-hofs) nodules in the myocardium in rheumatism.

as·cites (a-sī'-tēz) *n* (*syn* hydroperitoneum) free fluid in the peritoneal cavity—**ascitic** *adj*.

ascor·bic acid (a-skōr'-bik) vitamin* C. A water-soluble vitamin which is necessary for healthy connective tissue, particularly the collagen fibers and cell walls. It is present in fresh fruits and vegetables. It is destroyed by cooking in the presence of air and by plant enzymes released when cutting and grating food; it is also lost by storage. Deficiency causes scurvy. Used as nutritional supplement in anemia and to promote wound healing.

asep·sis (ā-sep'-sis) *n* the state of being

free from living pathogenic microorganisms—**aseptic** *adj*.

asep·tic tech·nique a precautionary method used in any procedure where there is a possibility of introducing organisms into the patient's body. Every article used must have been sterilized.

ASLO *abbr* antistreptolysin* O.

aspara·ginase (as-par'-a-jin-ās) *n* an enzyme derived from micro-organisms. Rarely useful in the treatment of asparagine-requiring acute lymphoblastic leukemias.

aspartame (a-spàr'-tām) *n* artificial sweetener made from the amino acids phenylalanine and aspartic acid. (Equal and Nutrasweet.)

asper·gill·osis (as-pèr-ji-lō'-sis) *n* opportunist infection, mainly of lungs, caused by any species of *Aspergillus*. ⇒ bronchomycosis.

Asper·gillus (as-pèr-jil'-us) *n* a genus of fungi, found in soil, manure and on various grains. Some species are pathogenic.

asper·mia (ā-sperm'-ē-à) *n* lack of secretion or expulsion of semen—**aspermic** *adj*.

as·phyxia (as-fiks'-ē-à) *n* suffocation; cessation of breathing. The O_2 content of the air in the lungs falls while the CO_2 rises and similar changes follow rapidly in the arterial blood. *blue asphyxia, asphyxia livida* deep blue appearance of a newborn baby; good muscle tone, responsive to stimuli. *white (pale) asphyxia, asphyxia pallida* more severe condition of newborn; pale, flaccid, unresponsive to stimuli. ⇒ respiratory distress syndrome.

aspir·ation (as-pi-rā'-shun) *n* (*syn* paracentesis, tapping) the withdrawal of fluids from a body cavity by means of a suction or siphonage apparatus—**aspirate** *vt*. *aspiration pneumonia* inflammation of lung from inhalation of foreign body, usually fluid or food particles.

aspir·ator (as'-pi-rā-tor) *n* a negative pressure apparatus for withdrawing fluids from cavities.

as·pirin (as'-pir-in) *n* acetylsalicylic* acid.

as·sertive·ness train·ing aims at developing self-confidence in personal relationships. It focuses on the honest expression of feelings, both negative and positive; the technique is learned by role playing in a therapeutic setting followed by practice in actual situations.

as·simi·lation (as-sim-i-lā'-shun) *n* the process whereby the already digested foodstuffs are absorbed and utilized by the tissues—**assimilable** *adj*, **assimilate** *vt, vi*.

assis·ted venti·lation mechanical assistance with breathing. Babies requiring extended periods of assisted ventilation are at great risk of developing bronchopulmonary dysplasia, which can result in repeated chest infections.

associ·ation (as-sō-si-ā'-shun) *n* a word used in psychology. *association of ideas* the principle by which ideas, emotions and movements are connected so that their succession in the mind occurs. *controlled association* ideas called up in consciousness in response to words spoken by the examiner. *free association* ideas arising spontaneously when censorship is removed; an important feature of psychoanalysis*.

astereo·gnosis (as-stèr-ē-og-nō'-sis) *n* loss of power to recognize the shape and consistency of objects.

as·thenia (as-thē'-nē-à) *n* lack of strength; weakness, debility—**asthenic** *adj*.

asthen·opia (as-thē-nō'-pē-à) *n* poor vision—**asthenopic** *adj*, **asthenope** *n*.

asthma (az'-mà) *n* paroxysmal dyspnea* characterized by wheezing and difficulty in expiration because of muscular spasm in the bronchi. Recent advances in immunology reveal that mast cells in bronchial walls produce immunoglobulin on encountering pollen grains; when another grain is inhaled, the alveolar mast cells burst producing an asthmatic attack. New anti-asthmatic drugs can prevent this. ⇒ bronchial asthma, renal asthma—**asthmatic** *adj*.

astig·matism (as-tig'-màt-izm) *n* defective vision caused by inequality of one or more refractive surfaces, usually the corneal, so that the light rays do not converge to a point on the retina. May be congenital or acquired—**astigmatic, astigmic** *adj*.

astrin·gent (as-trin'-jent) *adj* describes an agent which contracts organic tissue, thus lessening secretion—**astringency, astringent** *n*.

astro·cytoma (as-trō-sī-tō'-mà) *n* a slowly growing tumor of the glial tissue of brain and spinal cord.

AST test aspartate transferase is an enzyme normally present in liver, heart, muscles and kidneys. Values greater than 400 units per milliliter of serum are abnormal and are the commonest indication of liver disease.

Astrup test (as′-trup) estimates the degree of acidosis by measuring the pressures of oxygen and carbon dioxide in arterial blood.

asym·metry (ā-sim′-et-rē) *n* lack of similarity of the organs or parts on each side.

asymptom·atic (ā-simp-tom-at′-ik) *adj* symptomless.

asynclitism (ā-sin′-klit-izm) *n* anterior or posterior deflection of the saggital suture in presentation of the fetal head.

Atabrine (a′-tà-brēn) *n* proprietary name for quinacrine*.

atarac·tic (at-a-rak′-tik) *adj* describes drugs that, without drowsiness, help to relieve anxiety, thus providing emotional equilibrium thereby reducing the incidence of leukotomy. ⇒ tranquilizers.

Ata·rax (at′-à-raks) *n* proprietary name for hydroxyzine*.

atav·ism (at′-à-vizm) *n* the reappearance of a hereditary trait which has skipped one or more generations—**atavic, atavistic** *adj*.

ataxia, ataxy (ā-taks′-ē-à, ā-taks′-ē) *n* defective muscular control resulting in irregular and jerky movements; staggering—**ataxic** *adj*. *ataxic gait* ⇒ gait. *Friedreich's ataxia* ⇒ Friedreich's.

atel·ectasis (at-el-ek′-ta-sis) *n* numbers of pulmonary alveoli do not contain air due to failure of expansion (congenital atelectasis) or resorption of air from the alveoli (collapse*)—**atelectatic** *adj*.

aten·olol (at-en′-ol-ol) *n* cardioselective beta adrenoceptor antagonist; an effective hypotensive. (Tenormin.)

ATG *abbr* antithymocyte* globulin.

athero·genic (ath-e-rō-jen′-ik) *adj* capable of producing atheroma*—**atherogenesis** *n*.

ather·oma (ath-e-rō′-mà) *n* deposition of hard yellow plaques of lipoid material in the intimal layer of the arteries. May be related to high level of cholesterol in the blood or excessive consumption of refined sugar. Of great importance in the coronary arteries in predisposing to coronary thrombosis—**atheromatous** *adj*.

athero·scler·osis (ath-e-rō-skle-rō′-sis) *n* co-existing atheroma and arteriosclerosis—**atherosclerotic** *adj*.

atheto·sis (ath-e-tō′-sis) *n* a condition marked by purposeless movements of the hands and feet and generally due to a brain lesion—**athetoid, athetotic** *adj*.

ath·lete's foot tinea pedis. ⇒ tinea.

Ativan (at′-i-van) *n* proprietary name for lorazepam*.

atom (at′-om) *n* the smallest particle of an element capable of existing individually, or in combination with one or more atoms of the same or another element—**atomic** *adj*. *atomic weight* the weight of an atom compared with that of an atom of hydrogen, more recently with that of an atom of the carbon isotope ^{12}C.

atomization (at-om-īz-ā′-shun) *n* a mechanical process whereby a liquid is divided into a fine spray.

atom·izer (at′-om-īz-èr) *n* nebulizer*.

atonic (ā-ton′-ik) *adj* without tone; weak—**atonia, atony, atonicity** *n*.

atopic syn·drome (ā-top′-ik sin′-drōm) a constitutional tendency to develop infantile eczema, asthma, hay fever or all three when there is a positive family history.

ATP *abbr* adenosine* triphosphate.

atra·curium (at-rà-cū′-rē-um) *n* a non-depolarizing relaxant drug which is destroyed spontaneously in the body by the Hofmann* reaction. (Tracrium.)

atresia (ā′-trē′-zē-à) *n* imperforation or closure of a normal body opening, duct or canal—**atresic, atretic** *adj*.

atrial fibril·lation (ā′-trē-al fib-ril-ā′-shun) chaotic irregularity of artrial rhythm without any semblance of order. The ventricular rhythm, depending on conduction through the atrioventricular node, is irregular. Commonly associated with mitral stenosis or thyrotoxicosis.

atrial flut·ter (ā′-trē-al flu′-tèr) rapid regular cardiac rhythm caused by irritable focus in atrial muscle and usually associated with organic heart disease. Speed of atrial beats between 260 and 340 per minute. Ventricles usually respond to every second beat, but may be slowed by carotid sinus pressure.

atrial sep·tal de·fect (ā′-trē-al sep′-tal) non-closure of foramen ovale at birth resulting in congenital heart defect.

atrio·ventricular (ā′-trē-ō-ven-trik′-ū-làr) *adj* pertaining to the atria and the ventricles of the heart. Applied to a node, tract and valves.

atrium (ā′-trē-um) *n* cavity, entrance or passage. One of the two upper cavities of the heart (⇒ Figure 9)—**atria** *pl*, **atrial** *adj*.

Atro·mid-S (a′-trō-mid es) *n* proprietary name for clofibrate*.

atrophic rhin·itis (ā-trō′-fik-rhīn-ī′-tis) (*syn* ozena) an atrophic condition of the nasal mucous membrane with associated crusting and fetor.

atrophy (a'-trō-fē) *n* wasting, emaciation, diminution in size and function—**atrophied, atrophic** *adj. acute yellow atrophy* massive necrosis of liver associated with severe infection, toxemia of pregnancy or ingested poisons. *progressive muscular atrophy* (*syn* motor neuron disease) disease of the motor neurons of unknown cause, characterized by loss of power and wasting in the upper limbs. May also have upper motor neuron involvement (spasticity) in lower limbs.

atro·pine (at'-rō-pēn) *n* principal alkaloid of belladonna. Has spasmolytic, mydriatic and central nervous system depressant properties. Given before anesthetic to decrease secretion in bronchial and salivary systems and to prevent cardiac depression by depressing the vagus nerve, thus quickening the heart beat. *atropine methonitrate* is used in pylorospasm and in spray preparations for asthma and bronchospasm.

ATS *abbr* antitetanus serum. Contains tetanus antibodies. Produces artificial passive immunity. A test dose is given to ensure that the patient will not develop an anaphylactic* reaction.

ATT *abbr* antitetanus toxoid. Contains inactivated but antigenically intact tetanus toxins. Produces active immunity.

attenu·ation (at-ten-ū-ā'-shun) *n* the process by which pathogenic microorganisms are induced to develop or show less virulent characteristics. They can then be used in the preparation of vaccines—**attenuant, attenuated** *adj,* **attenuate** *vt, vi.*

atti·tude (at'-ti-tūd) *n* **1** a settled mode of thinking. **2** body posture or position. **fetal attitude** a characteristic posture of the fetus indicating the relations of the fetal parts to each other.

at·trition (at-tri'-shun) *n* wear of the occlusal* surfaces of the teeth by use.

atypi·cal (ā-tip'-ik-al) *adj* not typical; unusual, irregular; not conforming to type, e.g. atypical pneumonia.

audio·gram (aw'-dē-ō-gram) *n* a visual record of the acuity of hearing tested with an audiometer.

audi·ology (aw-dē-ol'-o-jē) *n* the scientific study of hearing—**audiological** *adj,* **audiologically** *adv.*

audio·meter (aw-dē-om'-et-ėr) *n* an apparatus for the clinical testing of hearing. It generates pure tones over a wide range of pitch and intensity—**audiometric** *adj,* **audiometry** *n.*

audio·metrist (aw-dē-om'-et-rist) *n* a person who is qualified to carry out audiometry*.

audi·tory (aw'-dit-ō-rē) *adj* pertaining to the sense of hearing *auditory acuity* ⇒ acuity. *auditory area* that portion of the temporal lobe of the cerebral cortex which interprets sound. *auditory canal* ⇒ Figure 13. *auditory meatus* the canal between the pinna and eardrum. *auditory nerves* the eighth pair of cranial nerves. *auditory ossicles* the three small bones—malleus, incus and stapes—stretching across the cavity of the middle ear.

aura (aw'-rà) *n* a premonition; a peculiar sensation or warning of an impending attack, such as occurs in epilepsy*.

aural (awr'-àl) *adj* pertaining to the ear.

Aureo·mycin (aw-rē-ō-mī'-sin) *n* proprietary name for chlortetracycline*. ⇒ tetracycline.

aur·icle (aw'-rik-l) *n* **1** the pinna of the external ear. ⇒ Figure 13. **2** an appendage to the cardiac atrium*. **3** commonly used mistakenly for atrium*—**auricular** *adj.*

auricu·lar fibrill·ation (aw-rik'-ū-lar fíb-ril-ā'-shun) atrial* fibrillation.

auricu·lar flut·ter (aw-rik'-ū-lar flut'-ėr) atrial* flutter.

auriculo·ventricular (aw-rik'-ū-lō-ven-trik'-ū-lar) *adj* atrioventricular*.

auri·scope (aw'-ris-kōp) *n* an instrument for examining the ear, usually incorporating both magnification and illumination.

auro·thiomalate (aw-rō-thī'-ō-màl-āt) *n* gold injection useful in chronic discoid lupus erythematosus and rheumatoid arthritis. Urine should be tested for albumen before each injection. (Myochrysine.)

auscul·tation (aws-kul-tā'-shun) *n* a method of listening to the body sounds, particularly the heart, lungs and fetal circulation for diagnostic purposes. It may be: (a) immediate, by placing the ear directly against the body (b) mediate, by the use of a stethoscope—**auscultatory** *adj,* **auscult, auscultate** *v.*

Austral·ian anti·gen an antigen* which is associated with hepatitis* B virus. Found in blood of 0.1 percent of Americans without manifestations of disease. Rates are higher in tropical areas. This blood may induce hepatitis in other people, so must not be used for transfusion.

Austral·ian lift better described as shoulder lift. A method of lifting a heavy patient, whereby his weight is taken by the upper shoulder muscles of the two lifters, and the lift is achieved by straightening the lifters' flexed hips.

autism (aw'-tizm) *n* a condition of self-absorption. There is retreat from reality into a private world of thought, fantasies and in extreme cases hallucinations.

autistic person (aw-tis'-tik) a person, usually a child, who has lost or never achieved normal contact with other people and is totally withdrawn and preoccupied with his own fantasies, thoughts and stereotyped behavior such as rocking.

autoagglutin·ation (aw-tō-a-gloo-ti-nā'-shun) *n* the clumping together of the body's own red blood cells caused by autoantibodies; this occurs in acquired hemolytic anemia, an autoimmune disease.

auto·antibody (aw-tō-an'-ti-bod-ē) *n* an antibody which can bind to normal constituents of the body, such as DNA, smooth muscle and parietal cells.

auto·antigen (aw-tō-an'-ti-jen) *n* antigens in normal tissues which can bind to autoantibodies.

auto·clave (aw'-tō-klāv) **1** *n* an apparatus for high-pressure steam sterilization. **2** *vt* sterilize in an autoclave.

auto·digestion (aw-tō-di-jest'-chun) *n* self-digestion of tissues within the living body. ⇒ autolysis.

auto·eroticism (aw-tō-e-rot'-is-izm) *n* self-gratification of the sex instinct. ⇒ masturbation—**autoerotic** *adj*.

auto·graft (aw'-tō-graft) *n* tissue grafted from one part of the body to another.

auto·immune dis·ease (aw-tō-im-mūn') an illness caused by, or associated with, the development of an immune response to normal body tissues. Hashimoto's disease, myxedema, Graves' disease and pernicious anemia are examples.

auto·immunization (aw-to-im-mūn-īz-ā'-shun) *n* the process which leads to an autoimmune disease.

auto·infection (aw-tō-in-fek'-shun) *n* ⇒ infection.

auto·intoxication (aw-tō-in-toks-i-kā'-shun) *n* poisoning from faulty or excessive metabolic products elaborated within the body. Such products may be derived from infected or dead tissue.

aut·olysis (aw-tol'-is-is) *n* autodigestion* which occurs if digestive enzymes escape into surrounding tissues—**autolytic** *adj*.

auto·matic (aw-tō-mat'-ik) *adj* performed without the influence of the will; spontaneous; nonvolitional acts; involuntary acts.

automa·tism (aw-tom'-at-izm) *n* organized behavior which occurs without subsequent awareness of it; somnambulism, hysterical and epileptic states.

auto·nomic (aw-tō-nom'-ik) *adj* independent, self-governing. *autonomic nervous system (ANS)* is divided into parasympathetic and sympathetic portions. They are made up of nerve cells and fibers which cannot be controlled at will. They are concerned with reflex control of bodily functions.

autoplasty (aw'-tō-plas-tē) *n* replacement of tissue by a graft of tissue from the same body—**autoplastic** *adj*, **autoplast** *n*.

aut·opsy (aw'-top-sē) *n* the examination of a dead body (cadaver) for diagnostic purposes.

auto·some (aw'-tō-sōm) *n* a chromosome other than a sex chromosome (gonosome).

auto·sug·gestion (aw-tō-su-jest'-yun) *n* self-suggestion; uncritical acceptance of ideas arising in the individual's own mind. Occurs in hysteria*.

auto·trans·fusion (aw-tō-trans-fū'-zhun) *n* the infusion into a patient of the actual blood lost by hemorrhage, especially when hemorrhage occurs into the abdominal cavity.

avas·cular (ā-vas'-kū-lar) *adj* bloodless; not vascular, i.e. without blood supply. *avascular necrosis* death of bone from deficient blood supply following injury or possibly through disease, often a precursor of osteoarthritis—**avascularity** *n*, **avascularize** *vt*, *vi*.

Avazyme (a'-va-zīm) *n* proprietary name for chymotrypsin.

Aven·tyl (a'-ven-tl) *n* proprietary name for nortriptyline*.

aver·sion ther·apy (a-vėr'-zhun) a method of treatment by deconditioning. Effective in some forms of addiction and abnormal behavior.

avian (ā'-vi-an) *adj* pertaining to birds. *avian tubercle bacillus (Myobacterium avium)* resembles the other types of tubercle bacilli in its cultural requirements. Avian tuberculosis is also caused by *M. tuberculosis* and *M. xenopi*; both cause disease in man.

avi·din (av'-i-din) *n* a high molecular weight protein with a high affinity for biotin* which can interfere with the absorption of biotin. Found in raw egg white.

avir·ulent (ā-vīr′-ū-lent) *adj* without virulence*.

avitamin·osis (ā-vīt-a-min-ōs′-is) *n* any disease resulting from a deficiency of vitamins.

avul·sion (a-vul′-shun) *n* a forcible wrenching away, as of a limb, nerve or polypus.

ax·illa (aks-il′-à) *n* the armpit.

axil·lary (aks′-il-ār-ē) *adj* applied to nerves, blood and lymphatic vessels, of the armpit. *axillary artery* ⇒ Figure 10. *axillary vein* ⇒ Figure 11.

axis (aks′-is) *n* 1 the second cervical vertebra. 2 an imaginary line passing through the center; the median line of the body—**axial** *adj*.

axon (aks′on) *n* that process of a nerve cell conveying impulses away from the cell; the essential part of the nerve fiber and a direct prolongation of the nerve cell—**axonal** *adj*.

axono·tmesis (aks-on-ot-mēs′-is) *n* (*syn* neuronotmesis, neurotmesis) peripheral degeneration as a result of damage to the axons of a nerve. The internal architecture is preserved and recovery depends upon regeneration of the axons, and may take many months (about 25.4 mm a month is the usual speed of regeneration). Such a lesion may result from pinching, crushing or prolonged pressure.

azacytidine (ā-zà-sī′-ti-dēn) *n* an antimetabolite used in the treatment of leukemia.

aza-thio·prine (az-à-thī′-ō-prēn) *n* immunosuppressive drug. Works by competing against purine, an essential metabolite for cell division. (Imuran.)

azlo·cillin (az-lō-sil′-in) *n* a pencillin antibiotic which is particularly active against *Pseudomonas* infections. (Azlin.)

azoo·spermia (ā-zō-ō-spėrm′-ē-à) *n* sterility of the male through non-production of spermatozoa.

azo·temia (az-ōt-ēm′-ē-à) *n* uremia.

azo·turia (az-ōt-ūr′-ē-a) *n* pathological excretion of urea in the urine—**azoturic** *adj*.

AZT *abbr.* azidothymidine. Experimental drug used for AIDS.*

Azulfidine (ā-zul′-fi-dēn) *n* proprietary name for sulfasalazine.*

azygos (az′-i-gos) *adj* occurring singly, not paired. *azygos veins* three unpaired veins of the abdomen and thorax which empty into the inferior vena cave—**azygous** *adj*.

B

Bab·inski's re·flex (bab-in′-skēz) or sign. Movement of the great toe upwards (dorsiflexion) instead of downwards (plantar flexion) on stroking the sole of the foot. It is indicative of disease or injury to upper motor neurons and is present in organic but not hysterical hemiplegia. Babies exhibit dorsiflexion, but after learning to walk they show the normal plantar flexion response.

bacil·lemia (bas-il-ēm′-ē-à) *n* the presence of bacilli in the blood—**bacillemic** *adj*.

Bacille-Calmette-Gueria (ba-sēl′-kalmet′-gār′-ē-à) *n* ⇒ BCG.

bacil·luria (bas-il-ū′-rē-à) *n* the presence of bacilli in the urine—**bacilluric** *adj*.

Bacil·lus (bas-il′-us) *n* a genus of bacteria consisting of aerobic. Gram-positive, rod-shaped cells which produce endospores. The majority are motile by means of peritrichate flagella. These organisms are saprophytes and their spores are common in soil and dust of the air. Colloquially, the word is still used to describe any rod-shaped microorganism. *Bacillus anthracis* causes anthrax in man and in animals.

baci·tracin (bas-i-trā′-sin) *n* an antibiotic used mainly for external application in conditions resistant to other forms of treatment. It does not cause sensitivity reactions.

bac·lofen (bak′-lō-fen) *n* a drug which reduces spasticity of voluntary muscle; mode uncertain. Side effects include nausea, vomiting, diarrhea, gastric discomfort, muscular incoördination, hypotonia, mental confusion, vertigo and drowsiness. Particularly useful for multiple sclerosis. (Lioresal.)

bacter·emia (bak-te-rēm′-ē-à) *n* the presence of bacteria in the blood—**bacteremic** *adj*.

bac·teria (bak-tē′-rē-à) *n* a group of microorganisms, also called the 'schizomycetes'. They are typically small cells of about 1 micron in transverse diameter. Structurally there is a protoplast, containing cytoplasmic and nuclear material (not seen by ordinary methods of microscopy) within a limiting cytoplasmic membrane, and a supporting cell wall. Other structures such as flagella, fimbriae and capsules may also be present. Individual cells may be spherical, straight or curved rods or spirals; they may form chains or masses and some show branching with mycelium formation. They may produce various pigments including chlorophyll. Some form endospores. Reproduction is chiefly by simple binary fission. They may be free living, saprophytic or parasitic; some are pathogenic to man, animals and plants—**bacterium** *sing.* **bacterial** *adj.*

bacteri·cide (bak-tēr′-i-sīd) *n* any agent which destroys bacteria—**bactericidal** *adj.* **bactericidally** adv.

bacteri·cidin (bak-tēr-i-sīd′-in) *n* an antibody which kills bacteria.

bacteri·ologist (bak-tēr-ē-ol′-oj-ist) *n* a person who is an expert in bacteriology.

bacteri·ology (bak-tēr-ē-ol′-oj-ē) *n* the scientific study of bacteria—**bacteriological** *adj.* **bacteriologically** *adv.*

bacteri·olysin (bak-tē-rē-ō-lī′-sin) *n* a specific antibody formed in the blood which causes dissolution of bacteria.

bacteri·olysis (bak-tēr-ē-ol′-is-is) *n* the disintegration and dissolution of bacteria—**bacteriolytic** *adj.*

bacterio·phage (bak-tēr′-ē-ō-fāj) *n* a virus parasitic on bacteria. Some of these are used in phagetyping staphylococci etc.

bacterio·stasis (bak-tēr-ē-ō-stā′-sis) *n* arrest or hindrance of bacterial growth—**bacteriostatic** *adj.*

bacteri·uria (bak-tē-rē-ū′-rē-à) *n* the presence of bacteria in the urine (100,000 or more pathogenic microorganisms per ml). Acute urinary tract infection may be preceded by, and active pyelonephritis may be associated with asymptomatic bacteriuria.

Bact·rim (bak′-trim) *n* proprietary name for co-trimoxazole*.

baker's itch 1 contact dermatitis* resulting from flour or sugar. **2** itchy papules from the bite of the flour mite *Pyemotes*.

BAL *abbr* British anti-lewisite. ⇒ dimercaprol.

balan·itis (bal-an-ī′-tis) *n* inflammation of the glans penis.

balano·posthitis (bal-an-ō-pos-thī′-tis) *n* inflammation of the glans penis and prepuce.

bal·anus (bal′-an-us) *n* the glans of the penis or clitoris.

bald·ness *n* ⇒ alopecia.

Bal·kan beam (bal′-kan bēm) wooden beam attached to a hospital bed whereby a Thomas' bed splint can be slung up, with pulleys and weights attached, to allow movement and provide counterbalance to the weight of the splint and leg.

bal·lotte·ment (bal-lot′-mon(g)) *n* testing for a floating object, especially used to diagnose pregnancy. A finger is inserted into the vagina and the uterus is pushed forward; if a fetus is present it will fall back again, bouncing in its bath of fluid—**ballottable** *adj.*

bal·sam of Peru (bawl′-sam of pė-rū′) a viscous aromatic liquid from the trunks of South American trees. Mild antiseptic used with zinc ointment for sores.

bal·sam of Tolu (bawl′-sam of tō-loo′) brown aromatic resin. Constituent of Friar's* balsam. Used as syrup of Tolu in cough syrups.

Balti·more paste (bal′-ti-mōr) ⇒ aluminium paste.

band·age (band′-aj) *n* traditionally a piece of cloth, calico, cotton, flannel etc. of varying size and shape applied to some part of the body: (a) to retain a dressing or a splint (b) to support, compress, immobilize (c) to prevent or correct deformity. There are now several proprietary circular bandages that are applied with an applicator to almost any part of the body.

Bank·art's oper·ation (bank′-harts) for recurrent dislocation of shoulder joint; the defect of the glenoid cavity is repaired.

Banthine (ban′-thēn) *n* proprietary name for methantheline.*

Ban·ti's dis·ease (ban′-tēz) ⇒ anemia.

Barbad·os leg (bar-bā′-dōs) (*syn* elephant leg) ⇒ elephantiasis.

bar·ber's itch ⇒ sycosis barbae.

bar·bitu·rates (bàr-bit′-ū-rātz) *npl* a widely used group of sedative drugs derived from barbituric acid (a combination of malonic acid and urea). Small changes in the basic structure result in the formation of rapid-acting, medium or long-acting barbiturates and a wide range is now available. Continual use may result in addiction. Action potentiated in presence of alcohol. As barbiturates produce tolerance and psychological and physical dependence, have serious toxic side-effects and can be fatal following large overdose, they have been replaced in clinical use by safer drugs e.g. benzodiazepines.

barbi·turism (bàr-bit′-ū-rizm) *n* addiction to any of the barbiturates. Characterized by confusion, slurring of speech, yawning, sleepiness, depressed respiration, cyanosis and even coma.

bar·botage (bàr-bot-àzh′) *n* a method of extending the spread of spinal anesthesia whereby local anesthetic is directly mixed with aspirated cerebrospinal fluid and reinjected into the subarachnoid space.

bar·ium enema (bår'-ē-um) the retrograde introduction of barium sulfate suspension, plus a quantity of air, into the large bowel via a rectal catheter, during fluoroscopy.

bar·ium sul·fate (bår'-ē-um sul'-fāt) a heavy insoluble powder used, in an aqueous suspension, as a contrast agent in X-ray visualization of the alimentary tract.

bar·ium sul·fide (bår'-ē-um sul'-fid) the chief constituent of depilatory creams. ⇒ depilatories.

Bar·low's dis·ease (bàr'-lōz) infantile scurvy*.

baro·trauma (bår-ō-traw'-mà) n injury due to a change in atmospheric or water pressure, e.g. ruptured eardrum.

bar·rier nurs·ing (bår'-ē-èr) a method of preventing the spread of infection from an infectious patient to others. It is achieved by isolation technique. *reverse barrier nursing* every attempt is made to prevent carrying infection to the patient.

barthol·initis (bàr-tol-in-ī'-tis) n inflammation of Bartholin's* glands.

Bar·tholin's glands (bàr'-to-linz) two small glands situated at each side of the external orifice of the vagina. Their ducts open just outside the hymen.

bartonellosis (bàr-to-nel-ō'-sis) n nonprotozoal hemolytic anemia. Syn. oroya fever.

basal gan·glia (bå'-sal gan'-glē-à) grey cells at the cerebral base concerned with modifying and coordinating voluntary muscle movement. Site of degeneration in Parkinson's disease.

basal meta·bolic rate BMR. the oxygen consumption is measured when the energy output has been reduced to a basal minimum, that is the patient is fasting and is physically and mentally at rest. The result is expresssed in kilocalories as a percentage of the norm for a subject of the same age, sex and surface area.

basal nar·cosis (nàr-kō'-sis) the pre-anesthetic administration of narcotic drugs which reduce fear and anxiety, induce sleep and thereby minimize postoperative shock.

base (bās) n 1 the lowest part. ⇒ Figure 7. 2 the main part of a compound. 3 in chemistry, the substance which combines with an acid to form a salt—**basal, basic** *adj*.

basic life support a term which describes maintenance of a clear airway and cardiopulmonary function.

basi·lar·ver·tebral insuf·ficiency (bå'-si-lar vèr-tē'-bral in-suf-ish'-ens-ē) vertebrobasilar* insufficiency.

ba·silic (bas-il'-ik) *adj* prominent. *basilic vein* on the inner side of the arm (⇒ Figure 10). *median basilic* a vein at the bend of the elbow which is generally chosen for venepuncture.

baso·phil (bå'-zō-fil) n 1 a cell which has an affinity for basic dyes. 2 a basophilic granulocyte (white blood cell) which takes up a particular dye; its function appears to be phagocytic and it contains heparin and histamine.

baso·philia (bå-zō-fil'-ē-à) n 1 increase of basophils in the blood. 2 basophilic staining of red blood corpuscles.

Batch·elor plas·ter (bach'-e-lor plas'-ter) a type of double abduction plaster, with the legs encased from groins to ankles, in full abduction and medial rotation. The feet are then attached to a wooden pole or 'broomstick'. Alternative to frog plaster, but the hips are free.

bath n 1 the apparatus used for bathing. 2 the immersion of the body or any part of it in water or any fluid; or the application of spray, jet or vapor of such a fluid to the body. The term is modified according to (a) temperature, e.g. cold, contrast, hot, tepid (b) medium used, e.g. mud, sand, water, wax (c) medicament added, e.g. Milton, potassium permanganate, saline, sulfur (d) function of medicament, e.g. astringent, disinfectant (c) part bathed, e.g. arm bath, sitz bath (f) environment, e.g. bed bath. ⇒ hydrotherapy.

bat·tered baby syn·drome the manifestations in an infant of the results of inflicted injury. Described by Caffey in 1957. Widened to battered *child* syndrome by Kempe in 1961; also known as 'child abuse' and 'non-accidental injury'. All these terms reflect the physical injuries done to the child to the exclusion of the emotional problems of the parents. 'Child abuse' is therefore preferred by many people. ⇒ battering.

bat·tering n striking another person repeatedly so causing injury; the lesions are frequently multiple involving mainly the head, soft tissues, long bones and the thoracic cage. Clinically, the resulting injuries cannot be unequivocally explained by natural disease or simple accident. Usually there is accompanying psychological damage. Three groups of people are particularly vulnerable—babies, wives (women) and the elderly. ⇒ battered baby syndrome, wife/woman battering, elderly abuse.

Bazin's dis·ease (ba-zaz') (*syn* erythema induratum). a chronic recurrent disorder, involving the skin of the legs of women. There are deep-seated nodules which later ulcerate.

BCG *abbr* Bacille-Calmette-Guerin. An attenuated form of tubercle bacilli; it has lost its power to cause tuberculosis, but retains its antigenic function; it is the base of a vaccine used for immunization against tuberculosis.

bear·ing down *n* 1 a pseudonym for the expulsive pains in the second stage of labor. 2 a feeling of weight and descent in the pelvis associated with uterine prolapse or pelvic tumors.

beat (bēt) *n* pulsation of the blood in the heart and blood vessels. *apical beat* ⇒ apex. *dropped beat* refers to the loss of an occasional ventricular beat as occurs in extrasystoles* *premature beat* an extrasystole*.

beclo·methasone (bek-lō-meth'-à-zōn) *n* anti-asthmatic corticosteroid drug prepared in inhaler or spin-haler* (Beclovent, Vanceril).

Beclovent (bek'-lō-vent) *n* proprietary name for beclomethasone.*

bed·bug *n* a blood-sucking insect belonging to the genus *Cimex*. *Cimex lecturlarius* is the most common species in temperate zones and *C. hemipterus* in tropical zones. They live and lay eggs in cracks and crevices of furniture and walls. They are nocturnal in habit and their bites leave a route for secondary infection.

bed·sore ⇒ pressure sore.

bed·wetting *n* ⇒ enuresis.

behav·ior (bē-hā'-vūr) *n* the observable behavioral response of a person to an internal or external stimulus. *behavior modification* in a general sense, an inevitable part of living, resulting from the consistent rewarding or punishing of response to a stimulus, whether that response is negative or positive. Some education systems deliberately employ a behavior modification approach to maximize learning. *behavior therapy* a kind of psychotherapy to modify observable, maladjusted patterns of behavior by the substitution of a learned response or set of responses to a stimulus. The treatment is designed for a particular patient and not for the particular diagnostic label which has been attached to him. Such treatment includes assertiveness training, aversion therapy, conditioning and desensitization.

be·havior·ism (bē-hā'-vūr-izm) *n* a word used in psychology to describe an approach which studies and interprets behavior by objective observation of that behavior without reference to the underlying subjective mental phenomena such as ideas, emotions and will. Behavior is a series of conditioned reflexes.

Beh·çet syn·drome (bā'-sets) described by Behçet in 1937. Starts with ulceration of mouth and/or genitalia with eye changes such as conjunctivitis, keratitis or hypopyon iritis. One site may be affected months or years before the others. There may also be skin nodules, thrombophlebitis and arthritis of one or more of the large joints. Pulmonary, gastrointestinal and neurological complications are being increasingly reported. Cause unknown; some favor virus, others an allergic vasculitis. No effective treatment apart from attempts to suppress worst phases with steroids. Blindness may result from ocular complications.

bejel (bej'-el) *n* a long-lasting, non-venereal form of syphilis* mainly affecting children in the Middle East and Africa. It usually starts in the mouth and then affects the skin, so that it is easily transmitted. It is rarely fatal and is treated with penicillin.

belch·ing (bel'-ching) *n* noisy oral emission of gas, mainly swallowed air, from the gullet and the stomach.

bella·donna (bel-à-don'-à) *n* deadly nightshade (*Atropa belladonna*). Powerful antispasmodic. The alkaloid from deadly nightshade is poisonous but from it, atropine* and hyoscyamine* are extracted.

'belle indifference' (bel in-dif-ér-ons') the incongruous lack of appropriate emotion in the presence of incapacitating symptoms commonly shown by patients with hysteria. First noted by Janet in 1893.

Beller·gal (bel'-er-gal) *n* proprietary combination of phenobarbital*, belladonna* alkaloids and ergotamine*. Useful for menopausal syndrome, premenstrual tension and migraine.

Bellocq's sound or cannula (bel-oks') *n* a curved tube used for plugging the posterior nares.

Bell's palsy facial hemiparesis* from edema of the seventh (facial) cranial nerve. Cause unknown.

beme·gride (bem'-i-grīd) *n* a respiratory stimulant; can be given intravenously.

ben·actyzine (ben-ak'-ti-zēn) *n* tranquilizing drug with selective action, producing sense of detachment from environment. Used in anxiety and tension neuroses. (Deprol.)

Bena·dryl (ben'-à-dril) *n* proprietary name for diphenhydramine*.

Bence-Jones pro·tein (bens-jōnz' prō'-tēn) protein bodies appearing in the urine of some patients with myclomatosis*. On heating the urine they are precipitated out of solution at 50°–60° C; they redissolve on further heating to boiling point and reprecipitate on cooling.

bendro·flumethiazide (bend-rō-flū-meth-ī'-à-zīd) *n* an oral diuretic of the thiazide group: it decreases the reabsorption of sodium and chloride in the kidney tubules: its duration of action is about 20–24 hours. Used with caution in renal or hepatic failure. ⇒ diuretics, thiazides. (Corzide, Naturetin, Rauzide.)

bends *npl* ⇒ caisson disease.

Benedict's solution (ben'-e-dikts sol-ū'-shun) a solution of copper sulfate which is easily reduced, producing color changes. Used to detect the presence of glucose.

Ben·emid (ben'-i-mid) *n* proprietary name for probenecid*.

benign (bē-nīn') *adj* 1 non-invasive, non-cancerous (of a growth). 2 describes a condition or illness which is not serious and does not usually have harmful consequences. *benign myalgic encephalomyelitis* (*BME*) a flu-like illness with symptoms including dizziness, muscle fatigue and spasm, headaches and other neurological pain. A high percentage of BME sufferers have a higher level of Coxsackie B antibodies in their blood than the rest of the population.

Bennett's fracture (ben'-ets) fracture of proximal end of first metacarpal involving the articular surface.

Bentyl (ben'-tl) *n* proprietary name for dicyclomine* hydrochloride.

benzal·konium (ben-zal-kō'-nē-um) *n* antiseptic with detergent action. Used as 1% solution for skin preparation, 1 : 20,000–1 : 40,000 for irrigation of wounds. Incompatible with soap, with loss of activity.

ben·zathine peni·cillin (ben'-zà-thēn) a slowly absorbed, long-acting antibiotic which can be given by mouth or intramuscularly. It is effective against most Gram-positive microorganisms—streptococci, staphylococci and pneumococci. (Bicillin, Penidural.) ⇒ penicillin.

ben·zene (ben'-zĕn) *n* a colorless inflammable liquid obtained from coal tar. Extensively used as a solvent. Its chief importance in the medical sphere is in industrial toxicology. Continued exposure to it results in leukopenia, anemia, purpura and, rarely, leukemia.

benzo·caine (ben'-zō-kān) *n* relatively non-toxic surface anesthetic for skin and mucous membranes. Used as dusting powder (10%), ointment (10%), suppositories (5 g), and lozenges (1½ g). Occasionally given orally in gastric carcinoma.

benzo·diaze·pines (ben-zō-dī-az'-e-pēns) *npl* a group of minor transquilizers which have similar pharmacological activities such as reducing anxiety, relaxing muscles, sedating and having hypnotic effects. Includes Ativan, Librium, Valium, Xanax.

ben·zoic acid (ben-zō'-ik) an antiseptic* and antifungal* agent used as a food preservative and in pharmaceutical preparations; also in keratolytic* ointments. Rarely given orally owing to irritant effects. Saccharin* is a derivative of this acid.

ben·zoin (ben'-zō-in) *n* a resin of balsam used as a topical protective and as an expectorant. ⇒ Friar's balsam.

benz·phetamine (benz-fet'-à-mēn) *n* a drug similar to amphetamine*; it can be used orally in the treatment of obesity. (Didrex.)

benz·thiazide (benz-thī'-à-zīd) *n* thiazide diuretic. (Exna.) ⇒ diuretics.

benz·tropine (benz-trō'-pēn) *n* a drug similar to atropine* but also has antihistaminic, local anesthetic and sedative functions. It reduces the muscle rigidity and cramp of parkinsonism. (Cogentin.)

ben·zyl ben·zoate (ben'-zil ben'-zō-āt) aromatic liquid; has ascaricidal properties and is used mainly in the treatment of scabies.

ben·zyl peni·cillin ⇒ penicillin.

bephen·ium hydroxy·naphthoate (befen'-ē-um hī-droks-i-naf'-thō-āt) an anthelmintic which is effective against hookworm and roundworm. It is given on an empty stomach at least 1 hour before food.

beri·beri (ber'-ē-ber'-ē) *n* a deficiency disease caused by lack of vitamin B_1. It occurs mainly in those countries where the staple diet is polished rice. The symptoms are pain from neuritis, paralysis, muscular wasting, progressive edema, mental deterioration and, finally, heart failure.

beryl·liosis (ber-il-i-ō'-sis) *n* an industrial disease; there is impaired lung function because of interstitial fibrosis from inhalation of beryllium. Steroids are used in treatment.

Besnier's pru·rigo (bez'-nē-az proo-rī'-gō) an inherited flexural neurodermatitis with impaired peripheral circulation giving rise to dry thickened epidermis and outbreaks of eczema in childhood. Old term for atopic* syndrome. ⇒ eczema.

beta blocker (bā'-tà blok'-ėr) a drug which prevents stimulation of the beta-adrenergic receptors, thus decreasing the heart's activity.

Beta·dine (bā'-tà-dēn) *n* a proprietary brand of povidone* iodine, available as aerosol spray, surgical scrub, scalp lotion and ointment.

beta·methasone (bā-ta-meth'-à-sōn) *n* synthetic corticosteroid drug which is effective on low dosage. It is similar to prednisolone*. (Betnelan, Celestone.)

bethan·echol (beth-an'-e-kol) *n* a compound resembling carbachol* in activity, but relatively nontoxic. Used in urinary retention, abdominal distension and myasthenia gravis. (Myotonachol.)

Betnelan (bet'-ne-lan) *n* proprietary name for betamethasone*.

Bet·novate (bet'-nō-vàt) *n* proprietary brand of cream or ointment containing betamethasone*. More effective than those containing hydrocortisone, but it can be absorbed through the skin and can produce local or systemic side effects.

bib·lio·therapy (bib'-lē-ō-ther'-a-pē) *n* literally means book therapy; it is being used to tap elderly patients' capacity to experience joy in life, and to help them meet their need for self fulfillment.

bicar·bonate (bī-kàr'-bon-āt) *n* a salt of carbonic acid. *blood bicarbonate* that in the blood indicating the alkali reserve. Also called 'plasma bicarbonate'.

bicel·lular (bī-sel'-ū-làr) *adj* composed of two cells.

biceps (bī'-seps) *n* a muscle possessing two heads or points of origin. ⇒ Figure 4. *biceps femoris* ⇒ Figure 5.

Bicil·lin (bī-sil'-in) *n* proprietary name for benzathine penicillin*.

bi·concave (bī-kon'-kāv) *adj* concave or hollow on both surfaces.

bi·convex (bī-kon'-veks) *adj* convex on both surfaces.

bi·cornuate (bī-kõrn'-ù-āt) *adj* having two horns, generally applied to a double uterus or a single uterus possessing two horns.

bi·cuspid (bī-kus'-pid) *adj* having two cusps or points. *biscuspid teeth* the premolars. *biscuspid valve* the mitral valve between the left antrium and ventricle of the heart.

bidet (bē-dā') *n* low-set, trough-like basin in which the perineum can be immersed, whilst the legs are outside and the feet on the floor. Can have attachments for douching the vagina or rectum.

bifid (bī'-fid) *n* divided into two parts. Cleft or forked.

bifur·cation (bī-fur-kā'-shun) *n* division into two branches—**bifurcate** *adj, vt, vi.*

biguan·ides (bī'-gwan-īdz) *npl* (*syn* diguanides) oral antidiabetic agents. They do not act on the islets of Langerhans but appear to stimulate the uptake of glucose by muscle tissue in diabetic subjects. Unwanted side-effects include lactic acidosis.

bi·lateral (bī-lat'-ėr-al) *adj* pertaining to both sides—**bilaterally** *adv.*

bile (bīl) *n* a bitter, alkaline, viscid, greenish-yellow fluid secreted by the liver and stored in the gall-bladder. It contains water, mucin, lecithin, cholesterol, bile salts and the pigments bilirubin and biliverdin. *bile ducts* the hepatic and cystic, which join to form the common bile duct (⇒ Figure 18). *bile salts* emulsifying agents, sodium glycocholate and taurocholate—**bilious, bilary** *adj.*

Bil·harzia (bil-hàr'-zē-à) *n* ⇒ Schistosoma.

bilhar·ziasis (bil-hàr-zī'-à-sis) *n* ⇒ schistosomiasis.

bili·ary (bil'-ē-àr-ē) *adj* pertaining to bile. *biliary colic* pain in the right upper quadrant of abdomen, due to obstruction of the gallbladder or common bile duct, usually by a stone; it is severe and often occurs about an hour after a meal; it may last several hours and is usually steady which differentiates it from other forms of colic. Vomiting may occur. *biliary fistula* an abnormal track conveying bile to the surface or to some other organ.

bil·ious (bil'-yus) *adj* **1** a word usually used to signify vomit containing bile. **2** a non-medical term, usually meaning 'suffering from indigestion'.

bili·rubin (bil-ē-roo'-bin) *n* a pigment largely derived from the breakdown of hemoglobin from red blood cells destroyed in the spleen. When it is released it is fat-soluble, gives an indirect reaction with Van* den Bergh's test and is potentially harmful to metabolically active tissues in the body, particularly the basal nuclei of the immature brain. *indirect bilirubin* is transported to the blood attached to albumen to make it less likely to enter and damage brain cells. In the liver the enzyme glucuronyl transferase conjugates indirect fat-soluble bilirubin with glucuronic acid to make it water-soluble, in which state it is relatively non-toxic, reacts directly with Van den Bergh's test and can be excreted in stools and urine. ⇒ phototherapy.

bili·rubin·emia (bil-ē-rū-bin-ēm'-ē-à) *n* the presence of bilirubin in the blood. Some times used (incorrectly) for an excess of bilirubin in the blood. ⇒ hyperbilirubinemia.

bili·uria (bil-ē-ū'-rē-à) *n* (choluria) the presence of bile pigments in the urine—**biliuric** *adj*.

bili·verdin (bil-ē-vėr'-din) *n* the green pigment of bile formed by oxidation of bilirubin.

Bill·roth's oper·ation (bil'-rōts) partial gastrectomy. Type 1: excision of the lower part of the stomach with anastomosis of the remaining part to the duodenum. Type II: resection of the distal end of the stomach with closure of the lines of section and gastrojejunostomy.

bi·lobate (bī-lō'-bāt) *adj* having two lobes.

bi·lobular (bī-lōb'-ū-làr) *adj* having two little lobes or lobules.

bi·manual (bī-man'-ū-àl) *adj* performed with both hands. A method of examination used in gynecology whereby the internal genital organs are examined between one hand on the abdomen and the other hand or finger within the vagina.

bin·aural (bīn-aw'-ràl) *adj* pertaining to, or having two ears. Applied to a type of stethoscope*.

bind·er (bīn'-dėr) *n* type of many-tailed bandage which can be applied to the abdomen to provide external pressure while the internal pressure is decreasing, e.g. in childbirth, paracentesis of the abdomen.

Binet's test (be-nāz') properly Binet-Simon scale. First used in 1905. A series of graded intelligence tests in which an individual's intelligence level (mental age) is compared with his chronological age. A forerunner of IQ tests.

binge-purge syn·drome (binj-pėrj) ⇒ bulimia*.

bin·ocular vis·ion (bīn-ok'-ū-làr) the focusing of both eyes on one object at the same time, in such a way that only one image of the object is seen. It is not an inborn ability but is acquired in the first few months of life.

bi·novular (bīn-ov'-ū-làr) *adj* derived from two separate ova. Binovular twins may be of different sexes. ⇒ uniovular *opp*.

bio·chemistry (bī-ō-kem'-is-trē) *n* the chemistry of life—**bio-chemical** *adj*.

bio·engi·neering (bī-ō-en-jin-ēr'-ing) *n* designing sophisticated microelectronic or mechanical equipment for external use by patients; for attachment to patients, or placement inside patients.

bio·ethics (bī-ō-eth'-iks) *n* the application of ethics* to biological problems.

bio·feedback (bī-ō-fēd'-bak) *n* presentation of immediate visual or auditory information about usually unconscious body functions such as blood pressure, heart rate and muscle tension. Either by trial and error or by operant conditioning a person can learn to repeat behavior which results in a satisfactory level of body functions.

bio·hazard (bī'-ō-haz-àrd) *n* anything which presents a hazard to life. Some specimens for the pathological laboratory are so labelled.

bio·logical age (bī-ō-loj'-ik-àl) *n* the term applied to age as assessed from appearance and behavior, thus some people are old at 40 while others are young at 60.

bi·ology (bī-ol'-o-jē) *n* the science of life, dealing with the structure, function and organization of all living things—**biological** *adj*. **biologically** *adv*.

bi·opsy (bī'-op-sē) *n* excision of tissue from a living body for microscopic examination to establish diagnosis.

bio·rhythm (bī-ō-rith'-um) *n* any of the recurring cycles of physical, emotional and intellectual activity which affect people's lives—**biorhythmic** *adj*.

bio·sensors (bī-ō-sens'-ors) *npl* non-invasive instruments which measure the result of biological processes, for example local skin temperature and humidity; or biological response to, for example, external pressure.

bio·technology (bī-ō-tek-nol'-o-jē) *n* the use of biological knowledge in the scientific study of technology and vice versa—**biotechnical** *adj.* **biotechnically** *adv.*

bi·otin (bī'-ō-tin) *n* a member of vitamin B complex; also known as vitamin H and as coenzyme R. Probably synthesized by intestinal flora. Lack of it may cause dermatitis in human beings.

bi·parous (bip'-ār-us) *adj* producing two offspring at one birth.

biperi·den (bī-per'-i-den) *n* a drug which acts on the autonomic nervous system: useful for drug-induced parkinsonism. (Akinaton.)

bi·polar (bī-pō'-làr) *adj* having two poles.

BIPP *n* a pasty mixture of bismuth subnitrate, iodoform, and liquid paraffin. Used as antiseptic dressing in acute osteitis.

birth (bèrth) *n* the act of expelling the young from the mother's body; delivery; being born. *birth canal* the cavity or canal of the pelvis through which the baby passes during labor. *birth certificate* a legal document given on registration, within 42 days of a birth. *birth control* prevention or regulation of conception by any means; contraception. *birth injury* any injury occurring during parturition, e.g. fracture of a bone, subluxation of a joint, injury to peripheral nerve, intracranial hemorrhage. *birth mark* naevus*. *premature birth* one occurring after the infant is viable, but before term. *birth rate* the number of live births per 1000 people in a given year.

bisa·codyl (bī-sà-kō'-dil) *n* a synthetic laxative which is not absorbed when taken orally but has a contact stimulant action on the bowel lining. It is also available as suppositories. (Dulcolax.)

bi·sexual (bī-seks'-ū-àl) *adj* 1 having some of the physical genital characteristics of both sexes; a hermaphrodite. When there is gonadal tissue of both sexes in the same person, that person is a true hermaphrodite. 2 describes a person who is sexually attracted to both men and women.

bismuth (biz'-muth) *n* a greyish metal. *bismuth carbonate* a mild antacid, used with other alkalis in dyspepsia and peptic ulcer. *bismuth salicylate* gastric sedative used in gastroenteritis. *bismuth sodium tartrate* a soluble compound used occasionally by intramuscular injection in infective arthritis. *bismuth subgallate* yellow, insoluble powder. Used as dusting powder in eczema and in suppositories for hemorrhoids. Occasionally given orally as an astringent.

bis·toury (bis'-tū-rē) *n* a long narrow knife, straight or curved, used for cutting from within outwards in the opening of a hernial sac, an abscess, sinus or fistula.

Bitot's spots (bē'-tōz) (*syn* xerosis conjunctivae) collections of dried epithelium, flaky masses and microorganisms at the sides of the cornea. A manifestation of vitamin A deficiency.

bit·ters (bit'-terz) *npl* substances, the extracts of which are used as tonics.

bi·valve (bī'-valv) *adj* having two blades such as in the vaginal speculum. In orthopedic work, the division of a plaster of Paris splint into two portions—an anterior and posterior half.

black·head (blak'-hed) *n* ⇒ comedo.

black lung disease a form of pneumoconiosis arising from exposure to coal dust; an industrial disease of coal miners.

black·water fever a malignant form of malaria* occurring in the tropics, especially Africa. There is great destruction of red blood cells, and this causes a very dark colored urine.

blad·der (blad'-àr) *n* a membranous sac containing fluid or gas.

Blalock-Hanlon oper·ation (bla'-lok han'-lon) a surgical opening between the right and left atrium of the heart in patients with complete transposition.

Blalock's oper·ation (bla'-loks) anastomosis of the pulmonary artery (distal to obstruction to the right ventricular outflow) to a branch of the aorta to increase pulmonary blood flow. Most often performed for Fallot's* tetralogy.

bland *adj* mild, non-irritating, soothing.

blastocyst (blas'-tō-sist) *n* a stage in mammalian embryo development consisting of the inner cell mass and a trophoblast layer enclosing the blastocele. Also called blastodermic vesicle.

Blasto·myces (blas-tō-mī'-sēz) *n* a genus of pathogenic yeast-like organisms—**blastomycetic** *adj.*

blasto·mycosis (blas-tō-mī-kō'-sis) *n* granulomatous condition caused by budding, yeast-like organisms called Blastomyces. May affect skin, viscera and bones—**blastomycotic** *adj.*

blas·tula (blas'-tū-là) *n* an early stage in development of the fertilized ovum when the morula* becomes cystic and infolds to become the gastrula.

bleb (bleb) *n* a large blister*. ⇒ bulla, vesicle.

bleeder (blēd'-ėr) *n* one who is subject to frequent loss of blood, as one suffering from hemophilia*.

'bleed·ing time' (blēd'-ing tīm) the time required for the spontaneous arrest of bleeding from a skin puncture; under controlled conditions this forms a clinical test.

blennor·rhagia (blen-ō-rāj'-ē-à) *n* **1** a copious mucous discharge particularly from the vagina or male urethra, **2** Gonorrhea.

blennor·rhea (blen-ōr-ē'-à) *n* blennorrhagia*.

bleo·mycin (blē-ō-mī'-sin) *n* an antibiotic. (Blenoxane.)

bleph·aritis (blef-ȧr-īt'-is) *n* inflammation of the eyelids, particularly the edges—**blepharitic** *adj*.

bleph·aron (blef'-ȧr-on) *n* the eyelid; palpebra—**blephara** *pl*.

blepharo·plasty (blef-ȧr-ō-plast'-ē) *n* tarsoplasty—**blepharoplastic** *adj*.

bleph·aroptosis (blef-ȧr-op'-to-sis) *n* ⇒ ptosis—**blepharoptotic** *adj*.

blepharo-spasm (blef'-ȧr-ō-spazm) *n* spasm of the muscles in the eyelid. Excessive winking—**blepharospastic** *adj*.

blind loop syn·drome (blīnd loop) resulting from intestinal obstruction of surgical anastomosis; there is stasis in the small intestine which encourages bacterial growth thus producing diarrhea and malabsorption.

blind sight (blīnd sīt) following damage to the visual cortex, some patients have been diagnosed blind after traditional testing. However, they may be trained to use functional residual vision.

blind spot (blīnd spot) the spot at which the optic nerve leaves the retina. It is insensitive to light.

blis·ter (blis'-tėr) *n* separation of the epidermis from the dermis by a collection of fluid, usually serum or blood.

blister·ing fluid (blis'-tėr-ing floo'-id) liquor* epispasticus, a counterirritant.

Blocad·ren (blok'-à-dren) *n* proprietary name for timolol* maleate.

blood (blud) *n* the red viscid fluid filling the heart and blood vessels. It consists of a colorless fluid, plasma, in which are suspended the red blood corpuscles, or erthrocytes, the white corpuscles, or leukocytes, and the platelets, or thrombocytes. The plasma contains a great many substances in solution including factors which enable the blood to clot. *defibrinated blood* that in which the fibrin is removed by agitation. *laked blood* that in which the red cells are hemolysed. *occult blood* blood which is not visible to the naked eye but whose presence can be detected by chemical tests.

blood bank a special refrigerator in which blood is kept after withdrawal from donors until required for transfusion.

blood-brain bar·rier the membranes between the circulating blood and the brain. Some drugs can pass from the blood through this barrier to the cerebrospinal fluid, others cannot, e.g. streptomycin.

blood casts casts of coagulated red blood corpuscles, formed in the renal tubules and found in the urine.

blood clot·ting primary phase: the vessel closes itself off from circulation and a plug of tiny particles (platelets) collects to fill the gap, attracted by collagen present in the blood vessel walls. Collagen is normally separated from flowing blood by a thin layer of cells which line the vessel wall: blood only comes into contact with collagen when a break occurs in this lining and the first platelets stick to it. These first two steps—contraction, plug—are normal in hemophilia A and B. Secondary phase: involves coagulation over and through the platelet mass. Plasma coagulation factors are as follows:

Factor No	Synonyms
I	Fibrinogen
II	Prothrombin
III	Tissue thromboplastin
IV	Calcium ions
V	Proaccelerin
VII	Factor VII
VIII	Antihemophilic factor (AHF)
IX	Christmas factor
X	Stuart factor (Power factor)
XI	Plasma thromboplastin antecedent (PTA)
XII	Hageman factor
XIII	Fibrin-stabilizing factor

Factor VIII is affected in hemophilia A; Factor IX is affected in hemophilia B (Christmas disease). In von Willebrand's disease there is a deficiency in both Factor VIII and in platelet function.

blood count calculation of the number of red or white cells per cubic millimeter of blood, using a hemocytometer. *differential blood count* the estimation of the relative proportions of the different leukocyte cells in the blood. The normal differential count is: polymorphs, 65%–70%, lymphocytes, 20%–25%, monocytes, 5%, eosinophils, 0%–3%, basophils, 0%–0.5%. In childhood the proportion of lymphocytes is higher.

blood crossmatching a method of mixing a sample of a blood donor's red blood cells with the recipient's blood (major crossmatching), and mixing a sample of the recipient's blood with the donor's blood (minor crossmatching). Done before a blood transfusion to determine compatibility of the blood.

blood culture after withdrawal of blood from a vessel, it is incubated in a suitable medium at an optimum temperature, so that any contained organisms can multiply and so be isolated and identified under the microscope. ⇒ septicemia.

blood forma·tion hemopoiesis*.

blood gas tension ⇒ tension.

blood glu·cose pro·files used to make rational adjustments to treatment of individual diabetic patients. They can show the peaks and troughs and the duration of action of a given insulin preparation, which can vary from patient to patient. Blood samples are taken on fasting, 2 h after breakfast, before lunch, 2 h after lunch, before the evening meal, at bedtime and possibly during the night. Some patients are independent for collecting these profiles and do so at home.

blood groups ABO system. There are four groups, A, B, AB and O. The cells of these groups contain the corresponding antigens, A, B, A and B, except group O cells, which contain neither antigen A nor B. For this reason group O blood can be given to any of the other groups and it is known as the 'universal donor'. In the plasma there are agglutinins* which will cause agglutination of any cell carrying the corresponding antigen, e.g. group A plasma contains anti-B agglutinins; group AB plasma contains no agglutinins. Group AB is therefore known as the 'universal recipient' and can receive A, B and O blood. This grouping is determined by (a) testing a suspension of red cells with anti-A and anti-B serum or (b) testing serum with known cells. Transfusion with an incompatible ABO group will cause a severe hemolytic reaction and death may occur unless the transfusion is promptly stopped. High titer agglutinins: in some

persons the anti-A or anti-B content of the plasma is unusually high and their agglutinating and hemolytic effect must be neutralized by dilution in a recipient's blood stream. Such blood can be transfused only to a recipient of the same ABO group as the donor. Blood containers are usually labelled to show the presence of high titer agglutinins. *Rhesus blood group* the red cells contain four pairs of antigens which are known by the letters Cc, Dd, Ee and Ff. The letters denote allelomorphic genes which are present in all cells except the sex cells where a chromosome can carry C or c, but not both. In this way the Rhesus genes and blood groups are derived equally from each parent. When the cells contain only the cde groups, then the blood is said to be Rhesus negative (Rh−); when the cells contain C, D or E singly or in combination with cde, then the blood is Rhesus positive (RH+). These groups are antigenic and can, under suitable conditions, produce the corresponding antibody in the serum. These antibodies are then used to detect the presence of Rh groups in cells. Antibodies to the Rh group are produced by (a) transfusion with Rh incompatible blood (b) immunization during pregnancy by fetal cells containing the antigen entering the mother's circulation. This can cause erythroblastosis* fetalis. ⇒ rhesus incompatibility.

blood-let·ting venesection*.

blood plasma ⇒ plasma.

blood press·ure the pressure exerted by the blood on the blood vessel walls. Usually refers to the pressure within the arteries which may be measured in millimeters of mercury using a sphygmomanometer. The arterial blood pressure fluctuates with each heart beat, having a maximum value (the systolic pressure) which is related to the ejection of blood from the heart into the arteries and a minimum value (diastolic pressure) when the aortic and pulmonary valves are closed and the heart is relaxed. Usually valves for both systolic and diastolic pressures are recorded (e.g. 120/70). ⇒ hypertension, hypotension.

blood sedi·men·tation rate (BSR) ⇒ erythrocyte sedimentation rate.

blood serum the fluid which exudes when blood clots; it is plasma minus the clotting agents.

blood sugar the amount of glucose in the circulating blood; varies within the normal limits. This level is controlled by various enzymes and hormones, the most important single factor being insulin*. ⇒ hyperglycemia, hypoglycemia.

blood trans·fusion ⇒ transfusion.

blood urea the amount of urea* (the end product of protein metabolism) in the blood; varies within the normal range. This is virtually unaffected by the amount of protein in the diet, when the kidneys which are the main organs of urea excretion are normal. When they are diseased the blood urea quickly rises. ⇒ uremia.

BLS *abbr* basic* life support.

'blue baby' the appearance produced by some congenital heart defects. The appearance, by contrast, of a newborn child suffering from temporary anoxia is described as 'blue asphyxia'.

blue pus bluish discharge from a wound infected with *Pseudomonas aeruginosa* (*pyocyanea*).

blux·ism (bluks'-izm) *n* teeth clenching; it can cause headache from muscle fatigue.

BME *abbr* benign* myalgic encephalomyelitis.

BMR *abbr* basal* metabolic rate.

BM stix chemically impregnated 'stick' for estimating the capillary blood sugar by color change.

BMT *abbr* bone marrow transplant/transplantation. ⇒ transplantation.

BNF *abbr* British National Formulary. ⇒ formulary.

body im·age the image in an individual's mind of his own body. Distortions of this occur in anorexia* nervosa, parietal lobe tumors and trauma. ⇒ mutilation.

body language non-verbal symbols that express a person's current physical and mental state. They include body movements, postures, gestures, facial expressions, spatial positions, clothes and other bodily adornments.

Boeck's dis·ease (beks) a form of sarcoidosis*.

Bohn's nod·ules (bōns no'-dūls) tiny white nodules on the palate of the newly born.

boil (boil) *n* (*syn* furuncle) an acute inflammatory condition surrounding a hair follicle; caused by *Staphylococcus aureus*. Usually attended by suppuration; it has one opening for drainage in contrast to a carbuncle*.

bolus (bō'-lus) *n* **1** a soft, pulpy mass of masticated food. **2** a large dose of a drug

given at the beginning of a treatment program to raise the blood concentration rapidly to a therapeutic level.

bond·ing (bond'-ing) *n* the emotional tie one person forms with another, making an enduring and special emotional relationship. There is a fundamental biological need for this to occur between an infant and its parents. When newborn babies have to be nursed in an intensive care unit, special arrangements have to be made to encourage bonding between the parents and their new baby.

bone (bōn) *n* connective tissue in which salts, such as calcium carbonate and calcium phosphate, are deposited to make it hard and dense. The separate bones make up the skeleton*.

bone graft the transplantation of a piece of bone from one part of the body to another, or from one person to another. Used to repair bone defects or to supply osteogenic tissue.

bone mar·row the substance contained within bone cavities. At birth the cavities are filled with blood-forming *red marrow* but in later life, deposition of fat in the long bones converts the red into *yellow bone marrow*. *bone marrow puncture* an investigatory procedure whereby a sample of marrow is obtained by aspiration after piercing the sternum or iliac crest. *bone marrow transplant* ⇒ transplantation.

Bonne·vie-Ull·rich syn·drome (bun-vē' ul'-rik) ⇒ Noonan syndrome.

bor·acic acid (bōr-as'-ik) ⇒ boric acid.

bor·ax (bōr'-aks) *n* mild antiseptic similar to boric* acid. Used in alkaline mouthwashes. Glycerin of borax, and borax with honey are used as throat paints, but should be applied sparingly.

bor·borygmi (bor-bor-ig'-mē) *n* rumbling noises caused by the movement of gas in the intestines.

Bordetella (bor-de-tel'-à) *n* a genus of Brucellaceae bacteria. *B. pertussis* causes whooping cough.

boric acid (bōr'-ik-as'-id) (*syn* boracic acid) mild antiseptic used mainly as eye lotions and ear drops. Dusting powders and lotions should not be applied to large raw areas, as there is a danger of boric poisoning.

Born·holm dis·ease (bōrn'-hŏm) (*syn* epidemic myalgia) a viral disease due to B group of coxsackieviruses named after the Danish island where it was described by Sylvest in 1934. 2–14 days incubation. Symptoms include sudden onset of severe pain in lower chest or abdominal or lumbar muscles. Breathing may be difficult, because of the pain, and fever is common. May last up to one week. There is no specific treatment.

botul·ism (bot'-ŭ-lĭzm) *n* an intoxication with the preformed exotoxin of *Clostridium botulinum*. Vomiting, constipation, ocular and pharyngeal paralysis and sometimes aphonia manifest witihin 24–72 h of eating food contaminated with the spores, which require anaerobic conditions to produce the toxin. Hence the danger of home–canned vegetables and meat.

bou·gie (boo'-zhē) *n* a cylindrical instrument made of gum elastic, metal or other material. Used in varying sizes for dilating strictures, e.g. esophageal or urethral.

bov·ine (bō'-vīn) *adj* pertaining to the cow or ox. *bovine tuberculosis* ⇒ tuberculosis.

bowel (bow'-el) *n* the large intestine. ⇒ intestine.

bowleg (bō'-leg) *n* varum genu*.

Boyle's anes·thetic mach·ine (boilz) apparatus by which chloroform, ether, nitrous oxide gas and oxygen may be administered. Adapted for use with cyclopropane*.

brach·ial (brā'-kē-al) *adj* pertaining to the arm. Applied to vessels in this region and a nerve plexus at the root of the neck. *brachial artery* ⇒ Figure 9. *brachial vein* ⇒ Figure 10.

brach·ialis (brā-kē-al'-is) *n* ⇒ Figure 4.

brachio·cephalic artery (brā-kē-ō-sef-al'-ik) ⇒ Figure 9.

brachio·cephalic vein ⇒ Figure 10.

brachio·adialis (brā'-kē-ō-ad-ē-al'-is) ⇒ Figure 4.

brach·ium (brā'-kē-um) *n* the arm (especially from shoulder to elbow), or any arm-like appendage—**brachia** *pl*. **brachial** *adj*.

Bradford frame (brad'-ford) a stretcher type of bed used for: (a) immobilizing spine; (b) resting trunk and back muscles; (c) preventing deformity. It is a tubular steel frame fitted with two canvas slings allowing a 100–150 mm gap to facilitate the use of a bedpan.

Bradley method of childbirth (brad'-lē) preparation of mother and father for childbirth, utilizing relaxation techniques. Also called husband-coached childbirth.

brady·cardia (brā-di-kàr'-dē-à) *n* slow rate of heart contraction, resulting in a slow pulse rate. In febrile states, for each degree rise in body temperature the expected increase in pulse rate is ten beats per minute. When the latter does not occur, the term 'relative bradycardia' is used.

bra·in (brān) *n* the encephalon; the largest part of the central nervous system: it is contained in the cranial cavity and is surrounded by three membranes called meninges. The fluid inside the brain contained in the ventricles, and outside in the subarachnoid space acts as a shock absorber to the delicate nerve tissue. ⇒ Figure 1. *brain death* a condition described over the last few decades. Stringent criteria are essential in many organ transplant programs. ⇒ death.

bran *n* the husk of grain. The coarse outer part of cereals, especially wheat, high in dietary* fiber and the vitamin* B complex.

bran·chial (brang'-kē-al) *adj* pertaining to the fissures or clefts which occur on each side of the neck of the human embryo and which enter into the development of the nose, ears and mouth. *branchial cyst* a cyst* in the neck arising from abnormal development of the branchial* cleft/s.

brand name the trade mark or proprietary name of a drug.

Brandt Andrews tech·nique (brant-an'-drōoz) an obstetric maneuver involving elevation of the uterus abdominally while holding the cord just taut—no traction. When the uterus is lifted the placenta will be in the cervix or upper vagina and is then expelled by suprapubic pressure directed below the fundus of the elevated uterus.

Braun's frame (brounz frām) a metal frame, bandaged for use, and equally useful for drying a lower leg plaster and for applying skeletal traction (Steinmann's* pin or Kirschner* wire inserted through the calcaneus) to a fractured tibia, after reduction.

Braxton Hicks sign (braks'-ton-hiks) intermittent painless contractions of the uterus observed throughout pregnancy.

break-bone fever (brāk'-bōn fē'-vèr) ⇒ dengue.

breast (brest) *n* **1** the anterior upper part of the thorax. **2** the mammary gland. *breast bone* the sternum.

breath-H₂ (hydrogen) test for disaccharide intolerance. An indirect method for detecting lactase deficiency.

breech (brēch) *n* the buttocks. ⇒ buttock.

breech/birth presentation refers to the position of a baby in the womb such that the buttocks would be born first: the normal position is head first.

bregma (breg'-mà) *n* the anterior fontanel. ⇒ fontanel.

bretylium tosylate (bre-til'-ē-um to'-sil-āt) antihypertensive drug. (Bretylol.)

bretylol (bre'-til-ol) *n* proprietary name for bretylium* tosylate.

Brevital (brev'-i-tol) *n* proprietary name for methohexital*.

Bri·canyl (brik'-a-nil) *n* proprietary name for terbutaline*.

Bright's dis·ease (brīts) inflammation of the kidneys. ⇒ nephritis.

bril·liant green antiseptic aniline dye. Used as lotion (1:1000), paint (1%) and ointment (2%).

Broad·bent's sign (brod'-bents sīn) visible retraction of the left side and back, in the region of the 11th and 12th ribs, synchronous with each heart beat and due to adhesions between the pericardium and diaphragm. ⇒ pericarditis.

broad liga·ments lateral ligaments; double fold of parietal peritoneum which hangs over the uterus and outstretched Fallopian tubes, forming a lateral partition across the pelvic cavity.

broad thumb syn·drome Rubenstein-Taybi* syndrome.

Broca's ar·ea (brōk'-às) often described as the motor center for speech; situated at the commencement of the sylvian fissure in the left hemisphere of the cerebrum. Injury to this center can result in language deficiency, including inability to speak.

Brodie's ab·scess (brō'-dēz) chronic abscess* in bone.

brom·ides (brō'-mīdz) *npl* a small group of drugs, exemplified by potassium bromide, which have a mild depressant action on the central nervous system. Used extensively in epilepsy before phenobarbital was introduced; now rarely used in nervous insomnia and restlessness, sometimes in association with chloral* hydrate.

bromi·drosis (brom-i-drō'-sis) *n* a profuse, fetid perspiration, especially associated with the feet—**bromidrotic** *adj*.

brom·ism (brō'-mizm) *n* chronic poisoning due to continued or excessive use of bromides*.

bromo·criptine (brō-mō-krip'-tēn) *n* a dopamine receptor agonist useful in parkinsonism and hyperprolactinemia. (Parlodel.)

bromo·sulph·thalein test (brō-mō-sulf'-tha-lēn) used to assess liver function; 5 mg per kg of body weight of the blue dye are injected intravenously. If more than 5% of the dye is circulating in the blood 45 min after injection, there is impaired hepatic function.

brompheniramine maleate (brom-fen-ir'-à-mēn mal'-ē-āt) an antihistamine used for rhinitis and allergy symptoms. (Dimetane.)

Brompton cocktail (bromp'-ton kok'-tāl) a mixture containing alcohol, morphine and cocaine for relieving pain in terminally-ill patients. Name is applied to different mixtures.

bron·chi (brong'-kī) *npl* the two tubes into which the trachea* divides at its lower end. ⇒ Figures 6, 7—**bronchus** *sing*. **bronchial** *adj*.

bron·chial asthma (brong'-kē-àl-az'-mà) reversible airflow obstruction precipitated in different patients by intake of allergens, infection, vigorous exercise or emotional stress. There is often a family history of asthma* and/or other allergic conditions.

bron·chial tubes (brong'-kē-àl-tūbz) *npl* subdivisions of the bronchi* after they enter the lungs.

bronchi·ectasis (brong-kē-ek'-ta-sis) *n* dilatation of the bronchial tubes which, when localized, is usually the result of pneumonia or lobar collapse in childhood, but when more generalized is due to some inherent disorder of the bronchial mucous membrane as in cystic fibrosis. Associated with profuse, fetid, purulent expectoration. Characterized by recurrent respiratory infections and digital clubbing. Leads to eventual respiratory failure—**bronchiectatic** *adj*.

bronchi·ole (brong'-kē-ōl) *n* one of the minute subdivisions of the bronchi* which terminate in the alveoli or air sacs of the lungs—**bronchiolar** *adj*.

bronchiolectasis (brong-kē-ō-lek'-ta-sis) *n* dilatation of the bronchioles.

bronchio·litis (brong-kē-ōl-īt'-is) *n* inflammation of the bronchioles*, usually in children in the first year of life—**bronchiolitic** *adj*.

bron·chitis (brong-kī'-tis) *n* inflammation of the bronchi *acute bronchitis* as an isolated incident is usually a primary viral infection occurring in children as a complication of the common cold, influenza, whooping cough, measles or rubella. Secondary infection occurs with bacteria, commonly *Streptococcus pneumoniae* or *Haemophilus influenzae*. Acute bronchitis in adults is usually an acute exacerbation of chronic bronchitis precipitated by a viral infection but sometimes by a sudden increase in atmospheric pollution. In *simple chronic bronchitis* the bronchial mucous glands are hypertrophied and the patient's only complaint is of cough productive of mucoid sputum. In *chronic obstructive bronchitis* the bronchial mucous membrane has so hypertrophied that the bronchial lumen is narrowed, causing airflow obstruction resulting in wheezing and leading to respiratory insufficiency and sometimes eventual respiratory failure—**bronchitic** *adj*.

broncho·constrictor (brong-kō-con-strik'-tor) *n* any agent which constricts the bronchi.

broncho·dilator (brong-kō-dī'-lā-tor) *n* any agent which dilates the bronchi.

broncho·genic (brong-kō-jen'-ik) *adj* arising from one of the bronchi.

bron·chography (brong-kog'-raf-ē) *n* radiological demonstration of the bronchial tree after introduction of a small amount of a liquid contrast medium—**bronchographic** *adj*. **bronchogram** *n*. **bronchograph** *n*. **bronchographically** *adv*.

broncho·mycosis (brong-kō-mī-kō'-sis) *n* general term used to cover a variety of fungal infections of the bronchi and lungs, e.g. pulmonary candidiasis*, aspergillosis*—**bronchomycotic** *adj*.

bron·chophony (brong-kof'-ō-nē) *n* abnormal transmission of voice sounds heard over consolidated lung or over a thin layer of pleural fluid.

broncho·pleural fis·tula (brong-kō-ploo'-ràl fis'-tūl-à) pathological communication between the pleural cavity and one of the bronchi.

broncho·pneumonia (brong'-kō-nū-mō'-nē-à) *n* a term used to describe a form of pneumonia in which areas of consolidation are distributed widely around bronchi and not in a lobar pattern—**bronchopneumonic** *adj*.

broncho·pulmonary (brong'-kō-pul'-mon-är-ē) *adj* pertaining to the bronchi and the lungs—**bronchopulmonic** *adj*.

bronchorrhea (brong-kō-rē'-à) *n* an ex-

cessive discharge of mucus from the bronchial mucous membrane—**bronchorrhoeal** *adj*.

broncho·scope (brong'-kō-skōp) *n* an endoscope* used for examining and taking biopsies from the interior of the bronchi. Also used for removal of inhaled foreign bodies. Traditional bronchoscopes are rigid tubes; modern bronchoscopes are flexible fiberoptic instruments—**bronchoscopic** *adj*. **bronchoscopy** *n*. **bronchoscopically** *adv*.

broncho·spasm (brong'-kō-spazm) *n* sudden constriction of the bronchial tubes due to contraction of involuntary plain muscle in their walls—**bronchospastic** *adj*.

bronchospirometer (bron-kō-spī-rom'-et-êr) *n* an instrument for measuring the capacity of one lung—**bronchospirometric** *adj*; **bronchospirometry** *n*.

bronchostaxis (brong-kō-stak'-sis) *n* hemorrhage from a bronchial wall.

broncho·stenosis (brong-kō-sten-ōs'-is) *n* narrowing of one of the bronchi—**bronchostenotic** *adj*.

broncho·tracheal (brong-kō-trāk'-ē-àl) *adj* pertaining to the bronchi and trachea.

bron·chus (brong'-kus) ⇒ bronchi.

Bronkaid Mist (Brong'-kād) proprietary name for epinephrine*.

Bronkephrine (brong-kef'-rin) *n* proprietary name for ethylnorepinephrine*.

Bronkosol (brong'-ko-sol) *n* proprietary name for isoetharine*.

brow (brow) *n* the forehead; the region above the supraorbital ridge.

Broxil (broks'-il) proprietary name for phenethicillin*.

Bru·cella (broo-sel'-là) *n* a genus of bacteria causing brucellosis* (undulant fever in man; contagious abortion in cattle). *Brucella abortus* is the bovine strain. *Brucella melitensis* the goat strain, both transmissible to man via infected milk.

brucel·losis (broo-sel-lō'-sis) *n* (*syn* melitensis) an infective reticulosis. A generalized infection in man resulting from one of the species of *Brucella*. There are recurrent attacks of fever and mental depression. The condition may last for months. An industrial disease in relation to occupations involving contact with bovine animals infected by *Brucella abortus*, their carcasses or untreated products; or with laboratory specimens containing *Brucella abortus*, by reason of employment as a farmworker, veterinary worker, slaughterhouse worker, laboratory worker or in any other work relating to the care, treatment, examination or handling of such animals, carcasses or products. The condition is also called 'Malta fever', 'abortus fever'. 'Mediterranean fever'' and 'undulant fever'.

Brudzin·ski's sign (brood-zin'-skēz) immediate flexion of knees and hips on raising head from pillow. Seen in meningitis.

bruise (brooz) *n* (*syn* contusion) a discoloration of the skin due to an extravasation of blood into the underlying tissues; there is no abrasion of the skin. ⇒ ecchymosis.

bruit (broo'-ē) *n* ⇒ murmur.

bruxism (bruk'-sizm) *n* abnormal grinding of teeth. Often producing excessive wear or attrition.

Bryant's gal·lows' trac·tion (brī'-ants) skin traction* is applied to the lower limbs, the legs are then suspended vertically (from an overhead beam), so that the buttocks are lifted just clear of the bed. Used for fractures of the femur in children up to 4 years.

BSE *abbr* breast self-examination.

BSP *abbr* bromosulphthalein*.

BSR *abbr* blood sedimentation rate. ⇒ erythrocyte sedimentation rate.

BTS *abbr* blood transfusion service.

bubo (bū'-bō) *n* enlargement of lymphatic glands, especially in the groin. A feature of soft sore (chancroid), lymphogranuloma inguinale and plague—**bubonic** *adj*.

buc·cal (buk'-ål) *adj* pertaining to the cheek or mouth.

Buck's extension a traction apparatus composed of a weight and a pulley to apply extension to a limb.

Buerger's disease (bėr'-gėrz) (*syn* Thromboangiitis obliterans) a chronic obliterative vascular disease of peripheral vessels which results in intermittent claudication*. In an investigation, the incidence of HLA-A9 and HLA-B5 was significantly greater in those with Buerger's disease than in the controls. *Buerger's exercises* were designed to treat this condition. The legs are placed alternately in elevation and dependence to assist perfusion of the extremities with blood.

buffer (buf'-ėr) *n* **1** generally, a mixture of substances in solution with the ability to bind both hydrogen and hydroxyl ions and the property of resistance to pH change when acids or alkalis are added. **2** anything used to reduce shock or jarring due to contact.

bulbar (bul'-bår) *adj* pertaining to the medulla* oblongata. *bulbar palsy or paralysis* paralysis* which involves the labioglossopharyngeal (lips, tongue and pharynx) region and results form degeneration of the motor nuclei in the medulla oblongata. The patient is deprived of the safety reflexes and is in danger of choking and aspiration pneumonia. Associated with feeding difficulties in profoundly handicapped children.

bulbo·urethral (bul-bō-ūr-ēth'-rål) *adj* applied to two racemose* glands (Cowper's) which open into the bulb of the male urethra. Their secretion is part of seminal fluid.

bulimar·exia (bū-lēm-å-reks'-ē-å) *n* bulimia*.

bu·limia (bū-lēm'-ē-å) *n* an eating disorder involving repeated episodes of uncontrolled consumption of large quantities of food in a short time. Many anorectics have a history of such episodes *bulimia nervosa* (*syn* binge-purge syndrome) self-induced vomiting after meals.

bulla (bool'-là) *n* a large watery blister. In dermatology, bulla formation is characteristic of the pemphigus group of dermatoses, but occurs sometimes in other diseases of the skin, e.g. in impetigo, in dermatitis herpetiformis etc.—**bullae** *pl*, **bullate, bullous** *adj*.

bumet·anide (bū-met'-an-īd) *n* potent loop diuretic. ⇒ diuretics. (Bumex.)

Bumex (bū'-meks) *n* proprietary name for bumetanide*.

BUN *abbr* blood urea nitrogen*.

bundle (bun'-dl) *n* a group of fibers. *Bundle of His* atrioventricular bundle. A bundle of fibers in the heart for conducting impulses.

bunion (bun'-yun) *n* (*syn* hallux valgus) a deformity on the head of the metatarsal bone at its junction with the great toe. Friction and pressure of shoes at this point cause a bursa to develop. The prominent bone, with its bursa, is known as a bunion.

Bunsen burner (bun'-sen) a gas burner with side openings that admit so much air that the carbon is completely burned so that the flame is only slightly luminous but very hot.

buph·thalmos (buf-thal'-mos) *n* (*syn* oxeye) congenital glaucoma.

bupi·vacaine (bū-piv'-à-kān) *n* one of the longer acting local anesthetics suitable for regional nerve block. Synthetic; less toxic than cocaine*. (Marcaine.)

buprenor·phine (bū-pre'-nŏr-fēn) *n* an analgesic which has a longer action than morphine and is of low dependence. (Buprenex.)

Burch colpo·suspension oper·ation (burch) the vagina is suspended from the ileopectineal ligament. Carried out for severe stress incontinence of urine.

Bur·kitt's lym·phoma (bur'-kits lim-fŏ'-mà) a malignant lymphoma frequently of the jaw but other sites as well. Affects principally children. Occurs almost exclusively in areas of Africa and New Guinea where malaria is endemic.

burn *n* a lesion of the tissues due to chemicals, dry heat, electricity, flame, friction or radiation; classified as partial or full thickness according to the depth of skin destroyed; the latter requiring skin grafts. The prevention of shock, infection and malnutrition are important aspects of treatment.

burn·out syn·drome *n* a controversial term currently used to denote depletion of energy experienced by a person who feels overwhelmed by other people's problems. Such a person becomes an inoperative member of the group and he opts out.

Burow's solution (bur'-ōwz) aluminum acetate, an antiseptic solution.

burr *n* an attachment for a surgical drill which is used for cutting into tooth or bone.

bursa (bur'-sà) *n* fibrous sac lined with synovial membrane and containing a small quantity of synovial fluid. Bursae are found between (a) tendon and bone (b) skin and bone (c) muscle and muscle. Their function is to facilitate movement without friction between these surfaces—**bursae** *pl*.

bur·sitis (bur-sī'-tis) *n* inflammation of a bursa. *olecranon bursitis* inflammation of the bursa over the point of the elbow. *prepatellar bursitis* (*syn* housemaid's knee) a fluid-filled swelling of the bursa in front of the knee cap (patella). It is frequently associated with excessive kneeling. A blow can result in bleeding into the bursa and there can be infection with pyogenic pathogens.

Bus·copan (būs-kō'-pan) *n* proprietary name for a derivative of hyoscine (hyoscine-N-butyl bromide), an antispasmodic which relaxes smooth muscle in peptic ulcer, colic and related conditions, however it is most effective if given by injection.

bu·sulphan (bū-sul'-fan) *n* a cytotoxic, alkylating drug used in chronic myeloid leukemia and polycythemia. Regular blood counts are essential, as the compound is a powerful depressant of bone marrow. (Myleran.)

buta·caine (bū'-tà-kān) *n* a synthetic local anesthetic similar to cocaine*. Used in ophthalmology as 2% solution which, unlike cocaine, does not dilate the pupil. (Butyn.)

Butazolidin (bū-tà-zol'-i-din) *n* proprietary name for phenylbutazone*.

but·tock (but'-ok) *n* one of the two projections posterior to the hip joints. Formed mainly of the gluteal* muscles.

butylamino·benzoate (bū-til-am-in-ō-ben'-zō-āt) *n* local anesthetic used as ointment (1%), suppositories (1 g), or dusting powder.

Butyn (bū'-tin) *n* proprietary name for butacaine*.

butyro·phenones (bū-ti-rō-fē'-nonz) *npl* substances which are dopamine blockers; they produce extrapyramidal side-effects.

BWS *abbr* battered woman (wife) syndrome. ⇒ battering.

bypass surgery ⇒ cardiac* bypass operation.

byssi·nosis (bis-in-ō'-sis) *n* a form of pneumoconiosis* caused by inhalation of cotton or linen dust.

C

cacao (kà-kā'-ō) *n* the seeds of *Theobroma cacao* from which chocolate, cocoa and cocoa butter are prepared.

ca·chet (kash-ā') *n* a flat capsule formed of rice paper, enclosing any bitter powdered drug which is to be taken orally.

ca·chexia (ka-keks'-ē-à) *n* a term denoting a state of constitutional disorder, malnutrition and general ill-health. The chief signs of this condition are bodily emaciation, sallow unhealthy skin and heavy lusterless eyes—**cachectic** *adj*.

ca·daver (ka-dav'-èr) *n* a corpse. In a medical context it implies a dead body which is dissected in a medical school, or in a mortuary at a postmortem.

cad·mium (kad'-mē-um) *n* a metallic element present in zinc ores and used in several industries. Inhalation of fumes over time can cause serious lung damage. Food can be contaminated, for example by contact with cadmium containing industrial waste.

CaEDTA *abbr* calcium disodium edetate, a chelating agent. Used in lead poisoning and as eyedrops in the treatment of lime burns.

caes·ium 137 (sē′-se-um) (^{137}Cs) a radioactive substance which, when sealed in a container, can be used for beam therapy instead of cobalt; when sealed in needles or tubes it can be used for local application instead of radium.

caf·feine (kaf-ē′-in) *n* the central nervous system stimulant which is present in tea and coffee. It has been given as a diuretic, but its main use is in analgesic preparations.

caisson disease (kā′-son) (*syn* the bends; decompression sickness) results from sudden reduction in atmospheric pressure, as experienced by divers on return to surface, airmen ascending to great heights. Caused by bubbles of nitrogen which are released from solution in the blood; symptoms vary according to the site of these. The condition is largely preventable by proper and gradual decompression technique.

Cala·dryl (kal′-à-dril) *n* proprietary lotion and cream containing calamine* and diphenhydramine*.

cala·mine (kal′-à-mīn) *n* zinc carbonate tinted pink with ferric oxide. Widely employed in lotions and creams for its mild astringent action on the skin. *calamine lotion* calamine dissolved in a weak solution of carbolic acid (phenol) for its anesthetic effect in relieving itch.

Calan (ka′-lan) *n* proprietary name for verapamil*.

calcaneus (kal-kā′-nē-us) *n* the heel bone; the os calcis, largest of the tarsal bones.

calcar·eous (kal-kā′-rē-us) *adj* pertaining to or containing lime or calcium; of a chalky nature.

calcif·erol (kal-sif′-e-rol) *n* one of a group of fat-soluble compounds which have antirachitic properties and can be produced artificially. This, or natural vitamin D, is essential for the uptake and utilization of calcium. Given in rickets and to prevent hypocalcemia in celiac disease, in parathyroid deficiency and lupus vulgaris. (Sterogyl 15.)

calcifi·cation (kal-sif-i-kā′-shun) *n* the hardening of an organic substance by a deposit of calcium salts within it. May

be normal, as in bone, or pathological, as in arteries.

calci·tonin (kal-si-tōn′-in) *n* (*syn* thyrocalcitonin) hormone produced in the thyroid parafollicular or 'C' cells. It may play a role in regulating the blood calcium level. In therapeutic doses it lowers serum calcium and inhibits resorption of bone. It may be of benefit in Paget's* disease.

calcium (kal′-sē-um) *n* a metallic element. Taken into the body as a constituent of certain foods its functions include: aiding in coagulation of blood and in formation of bones and teeth, preventing rickets, producing milk in lactation and activating enzymes.

cal·cium chlor·ide (kal′-sē-um klōr′-īd) a salt of calcium occurring as deliquescent granules, very soluble in water. Occasionally given by injection in calcium defiency, but, owing to is irritant properties, other calcium salts are preferred. Can be given by i.v. injection for cardiac resuscitation.

cal·cium glucon·ate (kal′-sē-um glū′-kon-āt) a well tolerated and widely used salt of calcium. Indicated in all calcium deficiency states, in allergic conditions and in lead poisoning.

cal·cium lac·tate (kal′-sē-um lak′-tāt) a soluble salt of calcium, less irritating than calcium chloride. Used orally like calcium gluconate in all calcium deficiency states.

cal·cium oxalate (kal′-sē-um oks′-à-lāt) *n* a salt which, if it occurs in high concentrations in the urine, may lead to the formation of urinary calculi.

cal·culus (kal′-kū-lus) *n* an abnormal concretion composed chiefly of mineral substances and formed in the passages which transmit secretions, or in the cavities which act as reservoirs for them. *dental calculus* mineralized dental plaque deposited on the tooth surface— **calculi** *pl,* **calculous** *adj*.

Cald·well-Luc operat·ion (kold′-wel-look) (*syn* radical antrostomy*) an opening is made above the upper canine tooth into the anterior wall of the maxillary antrum and an antrostomy for dependent drainage.

cali·per (kal′-ip-ėr) *n* **1** a two-pronged instrument for measuring the diameter of a round body. Used chiefly in pelvimetry. **2** a two-pronged instrument with sharp points which are inserted into the lower end of a fractured long bone. A weight is attached to the other end of the caliper, which maintains a steady pull on the distal end of the bone. **3** *Thomas' walking caliper* is similar to the Thomas' splint, but the W-shaped junction at the lower end is replaced by two small iron rods which slot into holes made in the heel of the boot. The ring should fit the groin perfectly, and all weight is then born by the ischial tuberosity.

cal·losity (kal-os′-it-ē) *n* (*syn* keratoma) a local hardening of the skin caused by pressure or friction. The epidermis becomes hypertrophied. Most commonly seen on the feet and palms of the hands.

cal·lus (kal′-us) *n* **1** a callosity. **2** the partly calcified tissue which forms about the ends of a broken bone and ultimately accomplishes repair of the fracture. When this is complete the bony thickening is known as *permanent callus*—**callous** *adj.*

calor (kal′-or) *n* heat; one of the four classic local signs of inflammation—the others are dolor*, rubor*, tumor*.

ca·loric test (kal-ōr′-ik) irrigation of the external ear canal with warm and/or cold fluid to assess vistibular disease; if the ear is normal there is nystagmus*; a diseased ear may not produce nystagmus.

cal·orie (kal′-ō-rē) *n* a unit of heat. In practice the calorie is too small a unit to be useful and the kilocalorie is the preferred unit in studies in metabolism. A kilocalorie (kcal. Cal) is the amount of heat required to raise the temperature of 1 kg of water by 1° C. In science generally, the calorie has been replaced by the joule as a unit of energy, work and heat; a joule is approximately 1/4 calorie.

calor·ific (kal-or-if′-ik) *adj* describes any phenomena which pertain to the production of heat.

calvarium (kal-vā′-rē-um) *n* the vault of the skull; the skull cap.

cam·phor (kam′-for) *n* carminative and expectorant internally, and used as a camphorated tincture of opium in cough mixtures. Applied externally in the form of camphorated oil as an analgesic and as a rubefacient—**camphorated** *adj.*

Campylo·bacter (kam′-pil-ō-bak′-ter) *n* a Gram-negative motile rod bacterium. It causes an acute diarrheal illness lasting several days.

canal (kan-al′) *n* a duct or channel. *canal of Schlemm* ⇒ Figure 15.

canali·culotomy (kan-a-lik-ūl-ot′-o-mē) *n* excision of the posterior wall of the ophthalmic canaliculus* and conversion of drainage 'tube' into a bony channel.

cana·licu·lus (kan-a-lik′-ū-lus) *n* a minute capillary passage. Any small canal, such as the passage leading from the edge of the eyelid to the lacrimal sac or one of the numerous small canals leading from the Haversian canals and terminating in the lacunae of bond—**canaliculi** *pl.* **canalicular** *adj.* **canaliculization** *n.*

cancel·lous (kan′-sel-lus) *n* resembling latticework; light and spongy; like a honeycomb.

can·cer (kan′-sèr) *n* a general term which covers any malignant growth in any part of the body. The growth is purposeless, parasitic, and flourishes at the expense of the human host. Characteristics are the tendency to cause local destruction, to invade adjacent tissues and to spread by metastasis. Frequently recurs after removal. Carcinoma refers to malignant tumors of epithelial tissue, sarcoma to malignant tumors of connective tissue—**cancerous** *adj.*

cancero·cidal (kan-sèr-ō-sīd′-àl) *adj* lethal to cancer.

cancero·phobia (kan-sèr-ō-fō′-bē-à) *n* obsessive fear of cancer–**cancerophobic** *adj.*

can·crum oris (kan′-krum ōr′-is) *n* gangrenous stomatitis of cheek in debilitated children. Often called 'noma'. Associated with measles in malnourished African children.

Can·dida (kan′-di-dà) *n* (*syn* Monilia) a genus of dimorphic fungi. Yeast-like cells which form some filaments. They are widespread in nature. *Candida (Monilia) albicans* is a commensal of the gastro-intestinal tract of man. It causes infections such as thrush, vulvovaginitis, balanoprosthitis and systemic disease in some physiological and pathological states. Disease can result from disturbed flora due to use of wide-spectrum antibiotics, steroids, immunosuppressive and/or cytotoxic drugs. Infection can also occur during pregnancy or secondary to debilitating general disease such as diabetes mellitus or Cushing's syndrome. Oral infection can be due to poor oral hygiene, including carious teeth and ill-fitting dentures.

candidi·asis (kan-did-ī′-à-sis) *n* (*syn* candidosis, moniliasis thrush) disease caused by infection with a species of *Candida.*

cani·cola fever (kan-i-kō′-là) leptospirosis*.

can·ine (kān′-īn) *adj* of or resembling a dog. *canine teeth* four in all, two in each jaw, situated between the incisors and the premolars. Those in the upper jaw are popularly known as the 'eye teeth'.

canker (kang'-kėr) *n* white spots on mucous membrane of the mouth.

canna·bis indica (kan'-ab-is in'-dik-à) (*syn* marijuana, pot, hashish) Indian hemp, a narcotic drug once used as a cerebral sedative in nervous disorders. Possession and use of cannabis is illegal in many countries.

can·nula (kan'-ū-là) *n* a hollow tube for the introduction or withdrawal of fluid from the body. In some patterns the lumen is fitted with a sharp-pointed trocar to facilitate insertion which is withdrawn when the cannula is *in situ*—**cannulae** *pl.*

cannu·lation (kan-ū-lā'-shun) *n* insertion of a cannula*.

canthar·ides (kan-thar'-i-dēz) *n* a blistering agent prepared from the dried Spanish beetle *Cantharides*.

can·thus (kan'-thus) *n* the angle formed by the junction of the eyelids. The inner one is known as the *nasal canthus* and the outer as the *temporal canthus*—**canthi** *pl*, **canthal** *adj*.

Capas·tat (kap'-a-stat) proprietary name for capreomycin*.

CAPD *abbr* continuous* ambulatory peritoneal dialysis.

capel·ine ban·dage (*syn* divergent spica) a bandage applied in a circular fashion to the head or an amputated limb.

capil·lary (kap'-il-ā-rē) *n* (literally, hairlike) any tiny thin-walled vessel forming part of a network which facilitates rapid exchange of substances between the contained fluid and the surrounding tissues. *bile capillary* begins in a space in the liver and joins others, eventually forming a bile duct. *blood capillary* unites an arteriole and a venule. *capillary fragility* an expression of the case with which blood capillaries may rupture. *lymph capillary* begins in the tissue spaces throughout the body and joins others, eventually forming a lymphatic vessel.

Capoten (kap'-o-ten) *n* proprietary name for captopril.

capreo·mycin (kap-rē-ō-mī'-sin) *n* peptide antibiotic derived from *Streptomyces capreolus*. Its main indication is as a secondary drug in treating drug resistant tuberculosis. (Capastat.)

capsicum (kap'-si-kum) *n* African pepper (cayenne), used as a carminative and rubefacient.

cap·sule (kap'-sūl) *n* **1** the ligaments which surround a joint. **2** a gelatinous or rice paper container for noxious drugs. **3** the outer membranous covering of certain organs, such as the kidney, liver, spleen, adrenals—**capsular** *adj*.

capsul·ectomy (kap-sūl-ek'-to-mē) *n* the surgical excision of a capsule. Refers to a joint or lens; less often to the kidney.

capsul·itis (kap-sūl-ī'-tis) *n* inflammation of a capsule. Sometimes used as a synonym for frozen* shoulder.

capsul·otomy (kap-sūl-ot'-om-ē) *n* incision of a capsule usually referring to that surrounding the crystalline lens of the eye.

capto·pril (kap'-tō-pril) *n* a drug which inhibits angiotensin-converting enzyme (ACE), thus preventing the formation of active angiotensin II $\Rightarrow$ angiotensin. (Capoten.)

caput succed·aneum (kap'-ut suk-sē-dā'-nē-um) *n* an edematous swelling of the baby's soft scalp tissue which is apparent at or shortly after birth. The swelling is diffuse, not delineated by scalp suture lines and usually disappears rapidly.

carbacel (kär'-bà-sel) *n* proprietary name for carbachol*.

car·bachol (kär'-ba-kol) *n* parasympathetic nervous system stimulant similar to acetylcholine* but active orally and has a sustained action by injection. Given in postoperative retention of urine and intestinal atony, and as eye drops for glaucoma. (Carbacel, Miostat.)

car·bamaze·pine (kär-bam-az'-e-pēn) *n* an anticonvulsant which also relieves pain; especially useful in trigeminal neuralgia. (Tegretol.)

carbamino·hemoglobin (kär-bam-in'-ō-hē-mo-glō'-bin) *n* a compound formed between carbon dioxide and hemoglobin. Part of the carbon dioxide in the blood is carried in this form.

carbarsone (kar'-bar-sōn) *n* arsenic compound used in amoebiasis, sometimes in association with emetine.

carbeni·cillin (kär-ben-i-sil'-in) *n* the only semisynthetic penicillin to show any reasonable activity against the antibiotic-resistant *Pseudomonas aeruginosa*. Unfortunately, even carbenicillin is not highly active against this organism. High concentrations can be achieved in the urine to destroy *Pseudomonas* there, but much larger doses of the order of 30–40 g a day are required to achieve sufficient concentration in the tissues. Such large doses can only be given by intravenous infusion. (Pyopen.)

carbi·dopa (kȧr-bi-dō′-pȧ) *n* when added to levodopa* allows reduction of dose, decreases frequency of adverse reactions and improves control of symptoms.

carbinoxamine maleate (kȧr-bin-oks′-ȧ-mĕn mal′-ē-āt) *n* an antihistamine used for rhinitis and symptoms of allergy. (Clistin.)

Carbocaine (kȧr′-bō-kān) *n* proprietary name for mepivacaine*.

carbo·hydrate (kȧr-bō-hī′-drāt) *n* an organic compound containing carbon, hydrogen and oxygen. Formed in nature by photosynthesis in plants. Carbohydrates are heat producing; they include starches, sugars and cellulose, and are classified in three groups—monosaccharides, disaccharides and polysaccharides.

car·bolic acid (kȧr-bol′-ik as′-id) ⇒ phenol.

carbol·uria (kȧr-bol-ū′-rē-ȧ) *n* green or dark-colored urine due to excretion of carbolic acid, as occurs in carbolic acid poisoning—**carboluric** *adj.*

car·bon (kȧr′-bon) *n* a non-metallic tetrad element occurring in all living matter. *carbon dioxide* a gas; a waste product of many forms of combustion and metabolism, excreted via the lungs. Accumulates in respiratory insufficiency or respiratory failure and carbon dioxide tension* in arterial blood (P_2CO_2) increases above the reference range of 36–44 mmHg (c 5.0 kPa). *carbon monoxide* a poisonous gas which forms a stable compound with hemoglobin, thus blocking its normal reversible oxygen-carrying function and causing signs and symptoms of hypoxia to ensue. *carbon tetrachloride* colorless volatile liquid with an odor similar to chloroform. Used as an anthelmintic against hookworm and tapeworm, sometimes in combination with chenopodium oil. Previous fasting and subsequent purging is necessary. Inhalation of the vapors can depress central nervous system activity and cause liver and kidney damage.

car·bonic anhydrase (kȧr-bon′-ik an-hī′-drās) a zinc-containing enzyme which facilitates the transfer of carbon dioxide from tissues to blood and to alveolar air by catalyzing the decomposition of carbonic acid into carbon dioxide and water.

carboxy·hemoglobin (kȧr-boks′-i-hēm-ō-glō′-bin) *n* a stable compound formed by the union of carbon monoxide and hemoglobin; the red blood cells thus lose their respiratory function.

carboxy·hemoglobin·emia (kȧr-boks′-i-hēm-ō-glō′-bin-ē′-mē-ȧ) *n* carboxyhemoglobin* in the blood—**carboxyhemoglobinemic** *adj.*

carboxy·hemoglobin·uria (kȧr-boks′-i-hēm-ō-glō′-bin-ūr′-ē-ȧ) *n* carboxyhemoglobin* in the urine—**carboxyhemoglobinuric** *adj.*

car·buncle (kȧr′-bung-kl) *n* an acute inflammation (usually caused by *Staphylococcus*) involving several hair follicles and surrounding subcutaneous tissue, forming an extensive slough with several discharging sinuses.

carcino·gen (kȧr-sin′-ō-jen) *n* any cancer-producing substance or agent—**carcinogenic** *adj,* **carcinogenicity** *n.*

carcino·genesis (kȧr-sin-ō-jen′-e-sis) *n* the production of cancer—**carcinogenetic** *adj.*

carcin·oid syn·drome (kȧr′-sin-oyd sin′-drōm) the name given to a histologically malignant but clinically mostly benign tumor of the appendix that may secrete serotonin*, which stimulates smooth muscle causing diarrhea, asthmatic spasm, flushing and other miserable symptoms. Methysergide may give prompt relief of the diarrhea.

carcin·oma (kȧr-sin-ō′-mȧ) *n* a cancerous growth of epithelial tissue (e.g. mucous membrane) and derivatives such as glands, *carcinoma-in-situ* asymptomatic condition with cells closely resembling cancer cells. A very early cancer. Well described in uterus and prostate. Previously called pre-invasive carcinoma—**carcinomata** *pl,* **carcinomatous** *adj.*

car·cinoma·tosis (kȧr-sin-ō-mȧ-tō′-sis) *n* a condition in which cancer is widespread throughout the body.

car·dia (kȧr′-dē-ȧ) *n* the esophageal opening into the stomach.

car·diac (kȧr′-dē-ak) *adj* 1 pertaining to the heart 2 pertaining to the cardia. *cardiac achalasia* food fails to pass normally into the stomach, though there is no obvious obstruction. The esophagus does not demonstrate normal waves of contraction after swallowing; this prevents the normal relaxation of the cardiac sphincter. Associated with loss of ganglion cells within muscle layers of at least some areas of the affected esophagus. *cardiac arrest* complete cessation of the heart's activity. Failure of the heart action to maintain an adequate cerebral circulation in the absence of a causative and irreversible disease. The clinical picture of cessation of circulation in a patient who was not expected to die at the time. This naturally rules out the seriously ill patient who is dying slowly with an incurable disease. *cardiac asthma* nocturnal paroxysmal dyspnea precipitated by pulmonary congestion resulting from left-sided heart failure. ⇒ asthma. *cardiac bed* one which can be manipulated so that the patient is supported in a sitting position. *cardiac bypass operation* the bypassing of sclerosed vessels supplying heart muscle by grafting a vein from the leg. *cardiac catheterization* ⇒ catheterization. *cardiac cycle* the series of movements through which the heart passes in performing one heart beat which corresponds to one pulse beat and takes about one second ⇒ diastole, systolic. *cardiac edema* gravitational edema. Such patients excrete excessive aldosterone which increases excretion of potassium and conserves sodium and chloride. Anti-aldosterone drugs useful, e.g. spironalactone, triamterine. Both act as diuretics. ⇒ edema. *cardiac pacemaker* an electrical apparatus for maintaining myocardial contraction by stimulating the heart muscle. A pacemaker may be permanent, emitting the stimulus at a constant and fixed rate, or it may fire only on demand when the heart does not spontaneously contract at a minimum rate. *cardiac tamponade* compression of heart. Can occur in surgery and penetrating wounds or rupture of the heart—from hemopericardium.

cardi·algia (kàr-dē-al′-jē-à) *n* literally, pain in the heart. Often used to mean heartburn (pyrosis*).

cardio·genic (kàr-dē-ō-jen′-ik) *adj* of cardiac origin, such as the shock in coronary thrombosis.

cardio·graph (kàr′-dē-ō-graf) *n* an instrument for recording graphically the force and form of the heart beat—**cardiographic** *adj*, **cardiogram** *n*, **cardiographically** *adv*.

cardi·ologist (kàr-dē-ol′-oj-ist) *n* a person who specializes in diagnosing and treating diseases of the heart.

cardi·ology (kàr-dē-ol′-o-jē) *n* study of the structure, function and diseases of the heart.

cardio·megaly (kàr-dē-ō-meg′-a-lē) *n* enlargement of the heart.

cardi·omyopathy (kàr-dē-ō-mī-op′-ath-ē) *n* an acute, subacute, or chronic disorder of heart muscle, of unknown etiology or association, often with associated endocardial or sometimes with pericardial involvement (WHO definition)—**cardiomyopathic** *adj*.

cardiopathy (kàr-dē-op′-ath-ē) heart disease—**cardiopathic,** *adj*.

cardio·phone (kàr′-dē-ō-fōn) *n* a microphone strapped to patient which allows audible and visual signal of heart sounds. By channelling pulse through an electrocardiograph, a graphic record can be made. Can be used for the fetus.

cardioplasty (kàr-dē-ō-plas′-tē) plastic operation to the cardiac sphincter of the stomach.

cardio·plegia (kàr-dē-ō-plē′-jē-à) *n* the induction of electromechanical cardiac arrest. *cold cardioplegia* cardioplegia combined with hypothermia to reduce the oxygen consumption of the myocardium during open heart surgery.

cardio·pulmonary (kàr-dē-ō-pul′-mon-ā-rē) *adj* pertaining to the heart and lungs. *cardiopulmonary bypass* used in open heart surgery. The heart and lungs are excluded from the circulation and replaced by a pump oxygenator—**cardiopulmonic** *adj*, *cardiopulmonary resuscitation (CPR)* ⇒ resuscitation.

Cardioquin (kàr′-dē-ō-kwin) *n* proprietary name for quinidine.

cardio·rator (kàr-dē-ō-rā′-tor) *n* apparatus for visual recording of the heart beat.

cardio·renal (kàr-dē-ō-rēn′-al) *adj* pertaining to the heart and kidney.

cardio·respiratory (kàr-dē-ō-resp′-ir-à-tōr-ē) *adj* pertaining to the heart and the respiratory system.

cardi·orraphy (kàr-dē-ōr′-af-ē) *n* stitching of the heart wall; usually reserved for traumatic surgery.

cardio·scope (kàr′-dē-ō-skōp) *n* an instrument fitted with a lens and illumination, for examining the inside of the heart—**cardioscopic** *adj*, cardioscopically *adv*.

cardiospasm (kàr′-dē-ō-spazm) *n* spasm of the cardiac sphincter between the esophagus and the stomach, causing retention within the esophagus. Usually no local pathological change is found.

cardio·thoracic (kàr-dē-ō-thōr-as′-ik) *adj* pertaining to the heart and thoracic cavity. A specialized branch of surgery.

cardio·tocograph (kàr-dē-ō-tó-kō-graf) *n* the instrument used in cardiotocography*.

cardio·tocography (kàr-dē-ō-to-kog′-raf-ē) *n* a procedure whereby the fetal heart rate is measured either by an external microphone or by the application of an electrode to the fetal scalp, recording the fetal ECG and from it the fetal heart rate. Using either an internal catheter which is passed into the amniotic cavity, or an external transducer placed on the mother's abdomen, the maternal contractions can also be measured. Both measurements are fed through a monitor in such a way that extraneous sounds are excluded and both measurements are recorded on heat-sensitive paper.

cardi·otomy syn·drome (kȧr-dē-ot'-o-mē) pyrexia, pericarditis and pleural effusion following heart surgery. It may develop weeks or months after the operation and is thought to be an autoimmune reaction.

cardio·toxic (kȧr-dē-ō-toks'-ik) adj describes any agent which has injurious effect on the heart.

cardio·vascular (kȧr-dē-ō-vas'-kū-lȧr) adj pertaining to the heart and blood vessels.

cardio·version (kȧr-dē-ō-vėr'-shun) n use of electrical countershock for restoring the heart rhythm to normal.

car·ditis (kȧr-dī'-tis) n inflammation of the heart. A word seldom used without the appropriate prefix, e.g. endo-, myo-, pan-, peri-.

car·ies (kār'-ēz) n 1 inflammatory decay of bone, usually associated with pus formation 2 a microbial disease of the calcified tissue of the teeth characterized by demineralization of the inorganic portion and destruction of the organic substance of the tooth—**carious** adj.

ca·rina (kȧ-rī'-nȧ) n a keel-like structure exemplified by the keel-shaped cartilage at the bifurcation of the trachea into two bronchi—**carinal** adj.

cario·genic (kā-rē-ō-jen'-ik) adj any agent causing caries*, by custom referring to dental caries.

carmin·ative (kȧr-min'-a-tiv) adj. n having the power to relieve flatulence and associated colic. The chief carminatives administered orally are aromatics, e.g. cinnamon, cloves, ginger, nutmeg and peppermint.

carmus·tine (kȧr-mus'-tēn) n an alkylating cytotoxic agent.

car·neous mole (kȧr'-nē-us mōl) a fleshy mass in the uterus comprising blood clot and a dead fetus or parts thereof which have not been expelled with abortion.

caro·tenes (kār'-ō-tēns) npl a group of naturally occurring pigments within the larger group of carotenoids*. Carotene occurs in three forms—alpha (α), beta (β) and gamma (γ). The β form is converted in the body to vitamin A; it is therefore a provitamin.

caroten·oids (ka-rot'-e-noyds) npl a group of about 100 naturally occurring yellow to red pigments found mostly in plants, some of which are carotenes*.

ca·rotid (kȧr-ot'-id) n the principal artery on each side of the neck. At the bifurcation of the common carotid into the internal and external carotids there are: (a) the *carotid bodies* a collection of chemoreceptors which, being sensitive to chemical changes in the blood, protect the body against lack of O_2 (b) the *carotid sinus* a collection of receptors sensitive to pressure changes; increased pressure causes slowing of the heart beat and lowering of blood pressure.

car·pal tun·nel syn·drome (kar'-pal tun'-nel) nocturnal pain, numbness and tingling in the area of distribution of the median nerve in the hand. Due to compression as the nerve passes under the fascial band. Most common in middle-aged women.

car·phology (kȧr-fol'-o-jē) n involuntary picking at the bedclothes, as seen in exhaustive or febrile delirium. syn. floccillation.

carpo·metacarpal (kȧr'-pō-met-ȧ-kȧr'-pal) adj pertaining to the carpal and metacarpal bones, the joints between them and the ligaments joining them.

carpo·pedal (kȧr-pō-pē'-dal) adj pertaining to the hands and feet. *carpopedal spasm* (*syn* Trousseau's sign) spasm of hands and feet in tetany*, provoked by constriction of the limb.

carpus (kȧr'-pus) n the wrist, consisting of eight small bones arranged in two rows—**carpal**, adj. $\Rightarrow$ Figure 3.

car·rier (kār'-ē-ėr) n 1 a person who, without manifesting an infection, harbors the microorganism which can cause the overt infection, and who can transmit infection to others. 2 a person who carries a recessive (i.e. a non-manifesting) gene at a specific chromosome location (locus).

car·tilage (kȧr'-til-aj) n a dense connective tissue capable of withstanding pressure. There are several types according to the function it has to fulfill. There is relatively more cartilage in a child's skeleton but much of it has been converted into bone by adulthood—**cartilaginous** adj.

car·uncle (ka-rung'-kl) n a red fleshy projection. Hymenal caruncles surround the entrance to the vagina after rupture of the hymen. The lacrimal caruncle is the fleshy prominence at the inner angle of the eye.

cas·cara (kas-kar'-a) *n* purgative bark, used as the dry extract in tablets and as liquid extract and elixir for chronic constipation.

caseat·ion (kā-zē-ā'-shun) *n* the formation of a soft, cheese-like mass, as occurs in tuberculosis—**caseous** *adj*.

casein (kā'-sē-in) *n* a protein produced when milk enters the stomach, the result of the precipitation of caseinogen. Coagulation occurs and is due to the action of rennin* upon the caseinogen* in the milk, splitting it into two proteins, one being casein. The casein combines with calcium and a clot is formed. *casein hydrolysate* predigested protein food derived from casein, easily added to other foods to increase the protein content. *syn* paracasein.

casein·ogen (kā-sē-in'-o-jen) *n* the principal protein in milk. It is not soluble in water but is kept in solution in milk by inorganic salts. The proportion to lactalbumin* is much higher in cows' milk than in human milk. In the presence of rennin* it is converted into insoluble casein.

case·ous degener·ation (kā'-sē-us dē-jen-er-ā'-shun) cheese-like tissue resulting from atrophy in a tuberculoma or gumma.

Casoni test (ka-sō'-nē) intradermal injection of 0·2 ml of fresh, sterile hydatid fluid. A white papule indicates a hydatid* cyst.

cast *n* 1 fibrous material and exudate which has been molded to the form of the cavity or tube in which it has collected; this can be identified under the microscope. 2 a rigid casing made with plaster of Paris and applied to immobilize a part of the body.

cas·tor oil (kas'-tor) a vegetable oil which has a purgative action when taken orally. Also used with zinc ointment for diaper rash and pressure sores.

cas·tration (kas-trā'-shun) *n* surgical removal of the testicles in the male, or of the ovaries in the female. Castration can be part of the treatment for a hormone-dependent cancer—**castrated** *adj*, **castrate** *n*, *vt*.

CAT *abbr* computed* axial tomography.

cata·bolism (kat-á-bol-izm) *n* the series of chemical reactions in the living body in which complex substances, taken in as food, are broken down into simpler ones accompanied by the release of energy. This energy is needed for anabolism and the other activities of the body $\Rightarrow$ adenosine triphosphate, metabolism—**catabolic** *adj*.

cata·lase (kat'-a-lāz) *n* an enzyme present in most human cells to catalyze the breakdown of hydrogen peroxide.

ca·taly·sis (kat-al'-i-sis) *n* an increase in the rate at which a chemical action proceeds to equilibrium through the medium of a catalyst or catalyser. If there is retardation it is negative catalysis—**catalytic** *adj*.

cata·lyst (kat'-a-list) *n* (*syn* catalyser, enzyme, ferment) an agent which produces catalysis*. It does not undero any change during the process.

cata·plexy (kat'-a-pleks-ē) *n* a condition of muscular rigidity induced by severe mental shock or fear. The patient remains conscious—**cataplectic** *adj*.

Cat·apres (kat'-a-pres) proprietary name for clonidine*.

cat·aract (kat'-à-rakt) *n* an opacity of the crystalline lens or its capsule. It may be congenital, senile, traumatic or due to metabolic defects, in particular diabetes mellitus. *hard cataract* contains a hard nucleus, tends to be dark in color and occurs in older people. *soft cataract*. one without a hard nucleus, occurs at any age, but particularly in the young. Cataract usually develops slowly and when mature is called a *ripe cataract*—**cataractous** *adj*.

ca·tarrh (ka-tàr') *n* chronic inflammation of a mucous membrane with constant flow of a thick sticky mucus—**catarrhal** *adj*.

cata·tonic schizo·phrenia (kat-a-ton'-ik skiz-ō-frēn'-ē-a) $\Rightarrow$ schizophrenia.

cat cry syn·drome cri* du chat' syndrome.

cat·echol·amines (kat-e-kōl'-a-mēns) *npl* any of a group of amines which are secreted in the human body to act as neurotransmitters; epinephrine, norepinephrine and dopamine are examples. Some of them have been synthesized and they can be prescribed as treatment.

cat·gut (kat'-gut) *n* a form of ligature and suture of varying thickness, strength and absorbability, prepared from sheep's intestines. After sterilization it is hermetically sealed in a container. The 'plain' variety is usually absorbed in 5–10 days. 'Chromicized' catgut and 'iodized' catgut will hold for 20–40 days.

cath·arsis (kà-thàr'-sis) *n* in psychology, the outpouring from the patient's mind—**cathartic** *adj.*

cath·eter (kath'-e-tèr) *n* a hollow tube of variable length and bore, usually having one fluted end and a tip of varying size and shape according to function. Catheters are made of many substances including soft and hard rubber, gum elastic, glass, silver, other metals and plastic materials, some of which are now radioopaque. They have many uses, from insufflation of hollow tubes to introduction and withdrawal of fluid from body cavities. A recent innovation is the fiberoptic cardiac catheter which, when in situ, picks up pulses of light from which the oxygen saturation of the blood can be determined.

cath·eter·ization (kath-e-ter-īz-ā'-shun) *n* insertion of a catheter, most usually into the urinary bladder. *cardiac catheterization* a long plastic catheter or tubing is inserted into an arm vein and passed along to the right atrium, ventricle and pulmonary artery for (a) recording pressure in these areas (b) introducing contrast medium prior to X-ray and high speed photography. Especially useful in the diagnosis of congenital heart defects—**catheterize** *vt.*

cath·etron (kath'-e-tron) *n* a high rate dose, remotely controlled, afterloading device for radiotherapy. Hollow steel catheters are placed in the desired position. They are then connected to a protective safe by hollow cables. The radioactive cobalt moves from the safe into the catheters. After delivery of the required dose, the cobalt returns to the safe, thus avoiding radiation hazard to staff.

cat scratch fever a virus infection resulting from a scratch by a cat. There is fever and glandular swelling about a week after the incident. Recovery is usually complete, although there may be some abscesses.

cau·da (kaw'-dà) *n* a tail or tail-like appendage—**caudal, caudate** *adj.*

cau·dal anesthetic (kaw'-dal an-es-thet'-ik) an anesthetic administered by means of an approach to the epidural space through the caudal canal in the sacrum.

caul (kawl) *n* the amnion, instead of rupturing as is usual to allow the baby through, persists and covers the baby's head at birth.

cauli·flower growth (kaul'-i-flour grōth) a proliferative free-growing type of cancer which forms an excrescence on the affected surface.

causal·gia (kaws-al'-jē-à) *n* excruciating neuralgic pain, resulting from physical trauma to a cutaneous nerve. Also known as reflex sympathetic dystrophy.

caus·tic (kaws'-tik) *adj, n* corrosive or destructive to organic tissue; the agents which produce such results. Used to destroy over-growths of granulation tissue, warts or polypi. Carbolic acid, carbon dioxide snow and silver nitrate (lunar caustic) are most commonly employed.

cauter·ize (kaw'-tèr-īz) *vt* to cause the destruction of tissue by applying a heated instrument, a cautery*—**cauterization** *n.*

cautery (kaw'-tèr-ē) *n* ⇒ cauterize.

cavern·ous (kav'-èr-nus) *adj* having hollow spaces, *cavernous sinus* a channel for venous blood, on either side of the sphenoid bone. It drains blood from the lips, nose and orbits. Sepsis in these areas can cause cavernous sinus thrombosis.

cavi·tation (kav-it-ā'-shun) *n* the formation of a cavity, as in pulmonary tuberculosis.

cav·ity (kav'-it-ē) *n* a hollow; an enclosed area. *abdominal cavity* that below the diaphragm; the abdomen. *buccal cavity* the mouth. *cerebral cavity* the ventricles of the brain. *cranial cavity* the brain box formed by the bones of the cranium. *medullary cavity* the hollow center of a long bone, containing yellow bone marrow or medulla. *nasal cavity* that in the nose, separated into right and left halves by the nasal septum. *oral cavity* buccal cavity. *pelvic cavity* that formed by the pelvic bones, more particularly the part below the iliopectineal line. *peritoneal cavity* a potential space between the parietal and visceral layers of the peritoneum. Similarly, the *pleural cavity* is the potential space between the pulmonary and parietal pleurae which in health are in contact in all phases of respiration. *synovial cavity* the potential space in a synovial joint. *uterine cavity* that of the uterus, the base extending between the orifices of the uterine tubes.

CCU *abbr* coronary care unit. ⇒ intensive care/therapy unit.

CDH *abbr* congenital* dislocation of the hip.

ce·costomy (sē-kos'-to-mē) *n* a surgically established fistula between the cecum* and anterior abdominal wall, usually to achieve drainage and/or decompression of the cecum. It is usually created by inserting a widebore tube into the cecum at operation.

ce·cum *n* the blind, pouch-like commencement of the colon* in the right iliac fossa. To it is attached the vermiform appendix; it is separated from the ileum by the ileocecal valve—**cecal** *adj*.

Cedil·anid (sē-de-lan′-id) *n* proprietary name for deslanoside*.

cef·triaxone (sef-tri-aks′-ōn) *n* a semisynthetic cephalosporin with a half-life of 8 h, a single i.m. dose of which is claimed to be extremely effective against gonorrhea. (Rocephin.)

cefurox·ime (sef-ūr-oks′-ēm) *n* a useful drug for penicillin resistant strains of microorganisms. (Zinacef.)

Celestone (sel′-es-tōn) *n* proprietary name for betamethasone*.

celiac (sē′-lē-ak) *adj* relating to the abdominal cavity; applied to arteries, veins, nerves and a plexus. *celiac disease (syn gluten-induced enteropathy)* due to intolerance to the protein gluten* in wheat and rye, it being the gliadin fraction that is the harmful substance. Sensitivity occurs in the villi of the small intestine, and produces the malabsorption syndrome. Symptoms become apparent at 3–6 months, soon after the child is weaned on to cereals, as up to this time the digestion is not interfered with. On weaning the absorption of fats is impaired, and large amounts of split fats may be excreted in the stools (steatorrhca*).

celioscopy (sē-lē-oś-ko-pē) *n* laparoscopy*.

cell (sel) *n* a histological term for a minute mass of protoplasm containing a nucleus. Some cells, e.g. the erythrocytes, are non-nucleated and others may be multinucleated—**cellular** *adj*.

Cello·phane (sel′-ō-fān) *n* the trade name for a brand of a transparent, impermeable derivative of cellulose. Used in face masks: to protect, and prevent evaporation from surgical dressings.

cell medi·ated immunity ⇒ immunity.

cellu·litis (sel-ū-lī′-tis) *n* a diffuse inflammation of connective tissue, especially the loose subcutaneous tissue. When it involves the pelvic tissues in the female it is called parametritis. When it occurs in the floor of the mouth it is called Ludwig's angina.

cellu·lose (sel′-ū-lōs) *n* a carbohydrate forming the outer walls of plant and vegetable cells. A polysaccharide which cannot be digested by man but supplies fiber for stimulation of peristalsis.

Celontin (sel-on′-tin) *n* proprietary name for methsuximide*.

Cel·sius (sel′-sē-us) having one hundred divisions or degrees. Usually applied to the thermometric scale in which the freezing point of water is fixed at 0° and the boiling point at 100°. The centigrade thermometer was first constructed by Celsius (1701–1744).

cemen·tum (sem-en′-tum) *n* the layer of calcified tissue covering the surface of the root of the tooth.

cen·sor (sen′-sor) *n* term employed by Freud to define the resistance which prevents repressed material from readily reentering the conscious mind from the subconscious (unconscious) mind.

centi·grade (sen′-ti-grād) *n* ⇒ Celsius.

cen·tral cyanosis (sen′-tral sī-an-ōs′-is) ⇒ cyanosis.

cen·tral intra-epitheal neo·plasia (sen′-tral in-tra-ep-i′-thē-al ne-o-plā′-zē-a) **(CIN)** a grading system.
CIN 1 mild dysplasia
CIN 2 moderate dysplasia
CIN 3 severe dysplasia, carcinoma in situ.

central nervous system (CNS) the brain and spinal cord and their nerves and end organs. Controls voluntary acts.

cen·tral ven·ous pres·sure *n* the pressure of the blood within the right atrium. It is measured by an indwelling catheter and a pressure manometer.

centri·fugal (sen-trif′-ū-gàl) *adj* efferent. Having a tendency to move outwards from the center, as the rash in smallpox.

centri·fuge (sen′-tri-fūj) *n* an apparatus which subjects solutions to centrifugal forces by high-speed rotation, thereby separating substances of different densities into discrete bands within the liquid phase. It is usually used to separate ('spin down') particulate material (e.g. subcellular particles) from a suspending liquid.

centri·petal (sen-trip′-et-al) *adj* afferent. Having a tendency to move towards the center, as the rash in chickenpox.

centrosome (sen′-trō-sōm) *n* a minute spot in the cytoplasm of animal cells supposed to be concerned with division of the nucleus.

cephal·algia (sef-al-al′-jē-à) *n* pain in the head; headache.

cephal·exin (sef-al-eks′-in) cephalosporin* an antibiotic which, unlike cephaloridine*, is well absorbed when given orally. Useful for urinary infections. (Keflex.)

cephal·hematoma (sef-al-hēm-a-tō'-mà) *n* a collection of blood in the subperiosteal tissues of the scalp.

ceph·alic (sef-al'-ik) *adj* pertaining to the head; near the head. *cephalic vein* ⇒ Figure 10. *cephalic version* ⇒ version.

cephalo·cele (sef-al'-ō-sēl) *n* hernia of the brain; protrusion of part of the brain through the skull.

cephalo·hematoma (sef-al-ō-hēm-a-tō'-ma) cephalhematoma*.

cephal·ometry (sef-al-om'-et-rē) *n* measurement of the living human head.

cephalopelvic disproportion (CPD) inability of the fetus to pass safely through the pelvis in labor, due to contraction of the pelvis, unfavorable attitude, position or presentation of the fetus, or large size of fetus in relation to pelvic size. May be associated with inefficient uterine contractions, lack of moldability of fetal head, or rigidity of perineum.

cephal·osporin (sef-al-ō-spōr'-in) *n* a large group of antibiotics produced by a mold obtained from sewage in Sardinia in 1948.

cephalothin (sef'-al-ō-thin) *n* a semi-synthetic broad spectrum cephalosporin antibiotic. (Keflin.)

ceph·radine (sef'-ra-dīn) *n* a mixed antibiotic used mainly for urinary tract infections. It is usually given orally but an injectable form is also available. (Velosef.)

Cephulac (sef'-ū-lak) *n* proprietary preparation of lactulose.

cere·bellar gait ⇒ gait.

cerebel·lum (sèr-i-bel'-um) *n* that part of the brain which lies behind and below the cerebrum (⇒ Figures 1, 11). Its chief functions are the co-ordination of fine voluntary movements and the control of posture—**cerebellar** *adj*.

cer·ebral (sèr'-e-bral; sèr-ē'-bral) *adj* pertaining to the cerebrum. *cerebral compression* arises from any space-occupying intracranial lesion. *cerebral palsy* non-progressive brain damage before the completion of brain development resulting in a range of mainly motor conditions ranging from clumsiness to severe spasticity.

cer·ebration (sèr-e-brā'-shun) *n* mental activity.

cerebro·spinal (sèr-i-brō-spī'-nal) *adj* pertaining to the brain and spinal cord. *cerebrospinal fluid* the clear fluid filling the ventricles of the brain and central canal of the spinal cord. Also found beneath the cranial and spinal meninges in the pia-arachnoid space.

cerebro·vascular (sèr-i-brō-vas'-kū-lar) *adj* pertaining to the blood vessels of the brain. *cerebrovascular accident (CVA)* interference with the cerebral blood flow due to embolism, hemorrhage or thrombosis. Signs and symptoms vary according to the duration, extent and site of tissue damage; there may only be a passing, even momentary inability to move a hand or foot; weakness or tingling in a limb; stertorous breathing, incontinence of urine and feces, coma; paralysis of a limb or limbs and speech deficiency (aphasia). *syn* stroke.

cer·ebrum (sèr'-e-brum; sèr-ē'-brum) *n* the largest and uppermost part of the brain (⇒ Figure 11); it does not include the cerebellum, pons and medulla. The longitudinal fissure divides it into two hemispheres, each containing a lateral ventricle. The internal substance is white, the outer convoluted cortex is grey—**cerebral** *adj*.

ce·rumen (se-roo'-men) *n* a wax-like, brown secretion from special glands in the external auditory canal—**ceruminous** *adj*.

cer·vical (sèr'-vi-kal) *adj* **1** pertaining to the neck **2** pertaining to the cervix (neck) of an organ. *cervical amnioscopy* ⇒ amnioscopy. *cervical canal* the lumen of the cervix uteri, from the internal to the external os. *cervical nerve roots* ⇒ Figure 11. *cervical rib* (*syn* thoracic inlet syndrome) a supernumerary rib in the cervical region, which may present no symptoms or it may press on nerves of the brachial plexus. *cervical smear* ⇒ Pap test. *cervical vertebrae* ⇒ Figure 3.

cervi·cectomy (sèr-vi-sek'-to-mē) *n* amputation of the uterine cervix.

cervi·citis (sèr-vis-ī'-tis) *n* inflammation of the uterine cervix.

cer·vix (sèr'-viks) *n* a neck. *cervix uteri, uterine cervix* the neck of the uterus (⇒ Figure 17)—**cervical** *adj*.

ces·arean sec·tion (ses-ār'-ē-an) *n* delivery of the fetus through an abdominal incision. It is said to be named after Caesar, who is supposed to have been born in this way. When delivery is accomplished extra-peritoneally, the term 'low cervical cesarian section' is used.

ces·tod (ses'-tōd) *n* tapeworm ⇒ Taenia.

Cetav·lon (set'-av-lon) *n* proprietary name for cetrimide*.

Cetri·hex (set'-ri-heks) *n* a proprietary mixture of cetrimide* and pHisoHex*.

cetr·imide (set'-ri-mīd) *n* an antiseptic with detergent properties, however, during storage it can become contaminated with *Pseudomonas aeruginosa*. Used as 1% solution for wound, burns and skin sterilization. (Cetavlon.)

CF *abbr* cystic* fibrosis.

CFT *abbr* complement* fixation test.

Chadwick's sign (chad'-wiks) dark blue or purple coloration of vaginal mucous membrane; a presumptive sign of pregnancy.

chal·azion (ka-lā'-zē-on) *n* a cyst on the edge of the eyelid from retained secretion of the Meibomian* glands.

chalk (chawk) *n* native calcium carbonate. Used with other antacids in peptic ulcer, and with astringents in diarrhea.

chal·one (kā'-lōn) *n* a substance which inhibits rather than stimulates, e.g. enterogastrone inhibits gastric secretions and motility.

chancre (shang'-kėr) *n* the primary syphilitic ulcer, associated with swelling of local lymph glands. The picture of chancre plus regional adenitis constitutes 'primary syphilis'. The chancre is painless, indurated, solitary and highly infectious.

chan·croid (shang'-kroyd) *n* (*syn* soft sore) a type of venereal disease prevalent in warmer climates. Causes multiple, painful, ragged ulcers on the penis and vulva, often associated with bubo* formation. Infection is by *Haemophilus ducreyi.*

charac·ter (kā'-rak-tėr) *n* the sum total of the known and predictable mental characteristics of an individual, particularly his conduct. *character change* denotes change in the form of conduct, to one foreign to the patient's natural disposition, e.g. indecent behavior in a hitherto respectable person. Common in the psychoses.

char·coal (chàr'-kōl) *n* the residue after burning organic substances at a high temperature in an enclosed vessel. Used in medicine for its adsorptive and deodorant properties.

Char·cot's joint (shàr'-kōs) complete disorganization of a joint associated with syringomyelia or advanced cases of tabes dorsalis (locomotor ataxia). The condition is painless. *Charcot's triad* manifestation of disseminated sclerosis—nystagmus, intention tremor and staccato speech.

chei·litis (kī-lī'-tis) *n* inflammation of the lip.

chei·loplasty (kī'-lō-plas-tē) *n* any plastic operation on the lip.

chei·losis (kī-lō'-sis) *n* maceration at the angles of the mouth, fissures occur later. May be due to riboflavin* deficiency.

cheiro·pompholyx (kī-rō-pom'-fo-liks) *n* symmetrical eruption of skin of hands (especially fingers) characterized by the formation of tiny vesicles and associated with itching or burning. On the feet the condition is called 'podopompholyx'.

chelat·ing ag·ents (kē'-lā-ting) soluble organic compounds that can fix certain metallic ions into their molecular structure. When given in cases of poisoning the new complex so formed is excreted in the urine.

chemo·nucle·olysis (kē-mō-nū-klē-ol'-is-is) *n* injection of an enzyme, usually into an invertebral disc, for dissolution of same—**chemonucleolytic** *adj.*

chemo·palli·dectomy (kē-mō-pal-id-ek'-to-mē) *n* the destruction of a predetermined section of globus pallidus in the nucleus of the brain by chemicals.

chemo·prophy·laxis (kē-mō-prō-fil-aks'-is) *n* the prevention of disease (or recurrent attack) by administration of chemicals—**chemoprophylactic** *adj.*

chemo·receptor (kē-mō-rē-sep'-tor) *n* **1** a chemical linkage in a living cell having an affinity for, and capable of combining with, certain other chemical substances. **2** a sensory end-organ capable of reacting to a chemical stimulus.

chem·osis (kē-mō'-sis) *n* an edema or swelling of the bulbar conjunctiva*—**chemotic** *adj.*

chemo·taxis (kēm-ō-taks'-is) *n* movements of a cell (e.g. leukocyte) or an organism in response to chemical stimuli; attraction towards a chemical being *positive chemotaxis*, repulsion is *negative chemotaxis*—**chemotactic** *adj.*

chemo·therapy (kēm-ō-thėr'-à-pē) *n* use of a specific chemical agent to arrest the progress of, or eradicate, disease in the body without causing irreversible injury to healthy tissues. Chemotherapeutic agents are administered mainly by oral, intramuscular and intravenous routes, and are distributed usually by the blood stream.

cheno·deoxy·cholic acid (ken-ō-dē-oks-ē-kōl'-ik) *n* a detergent-like molecule normally present in bile. It can be taken orally to dissolve gallstones.

Cheyne·Stokes respir·ation (chān'-stōks) cyclical waxing and waning of breathing, characterized at one extreme by deep fast breaths and at the other by apnea; it generally has an ominous prognosis.

CHF *abbr* congestive* heart failure.

chi·asma (kī-az'-mà) *n* an X-shaped crossing or decusation. *optic chiasma* the meeting of the optic nerves; where the fibers from the medial or nasal half of each retina cross the middle line to join the optic tract of the opposite side (⇒ Figure 1)—**chiasmata** *pl*.

chicken·pox *n* (*syn* varicella) a mild, specific infection with varicella zoster virus. Successive crops of vesicles appear first on the trunk; they scab and heal.

chigger (chig'-gèr) *n* a flea that burrows under the skin to lay its eggs, causing intense irritation. Secondary infection is usual.

chikun·gunya (chik-un-gun'-ya) *n* one of the mosquito*-transmitted hemorrhagic fevers occuring in the tropics.

chil·blain (chil'-blān) *n* (*syn* crythema pernio) congestion and swelling attended with severe itching and burning sensation in reaction to cold.

child abuse ⇒ battered baby syndrome.

chim·ney sweep's can·cer scrotal ephithelioma. ⇒ epithelioma.

Chin·ese rest·aurant syn·drome *n* postprandial disturbance due to eating monosodium* glutamate.

chinio·fon (kin'-i-ō-fen) *n* an amebicide used in prophylaxis and the treatment of acute and chronic amebiasis, often in association with emetine*.

chirop·odist (kī-rop'-o-dist) *n* a person who is qualified in chiropody.

chirop·ody (kī-rop'-o-dē) *n* the theory and practice relating to the promotion and maintenance of normal feet.

chiro·practic (kī-rō-prak'-tik) *n* the manual movement of the vertebrae to relieve the impingement of subluxated transverse processes on the nerve roots.

chiro·practor (kī'-rō-prak-tor) *n* a person who believes that many diseases are due to interference with nerve flow and is skilled in vertebral manipulation.

Chlam·ydia (kla-mid'-ē-à) *n* a genus of virus-like microorganisms which can cause disease in man and birds. Some *Chlamydia* infections of birds can be transmitted to man. *Chlamydia trachomatis* causes trachoma*. There can be sexual transmission of chlamydial infec-

tion and there is an increasing number of babies who acquire neonatal chlamydial ophthalmia ⇒ ornithosis, psittacosis.

chlo·asma (klō-az'-mà) *n* patchy brown discoloration of the skin, especially the face. Can appear during pregnancy.

chloral hy·drate (klōr'-al hī'-drāt) *n* rapid acting sedative and hypnotic of value in nervous insomnia.

chlor·ambucil (klōr-am'-bū-sil) *n* an oral alkylating agent used in lymphoproliferative disorders. (Leukeran.)

chlor·amine (klōr'-am-ēn) *n* an organic compound that slowly liberates chlorine in solution. It has been used as a general surgical antiseptic in a 0.25%–2% solution.

chloram·phenicol (klōr-am-fen'-ik-ol) *n* an orally effective wide range antibiotic. Drug of choice in typhoid and paratyphoid fevers, valuable in many infections resistant to other drugs. Used locally in eye and ear infections. Can cause aplastic anemia*. (Chloromycetin.)

chlorcyc·lizine (klōr-sīk'-li-zēn) *n* a long-acting antihistamine with few side effects. Also used in travel sickness.

chlor·diazepoxide (klōr-dī-az-e-poks'-īd) *n* a drug which relieves anxiety and tension and has a muscle relaxant function. It can be administered by mouth or by injection. (Librium.)

chlor·hexidine (klōr-heks'-i-dēn) *n* a bactericidal solution which is effective against a wide range of bacteria. Used as 1:2000 solution as a general antiseptic, 1:5000 for douches and irrigation. Hand cream (1%) is effective in reducing cross infection. (Hibiclens, Hibistat.)

chlor·ine (klōr'-ēn) *n* a greenish-yellow, irritating gaseous element. Powerful germicide, bleaching and deodorizing agent in the presence of moisture when nascent oxygen is liberated. Used chiefly as hypochlorites, chloramine* or other compounds which slowly liberate active chlorine.

chlor·methia·zole (klōr-meth-ī'-à-zōl) *n* a hypnosedative drug available in capsules and as an injection. Effective in controlling restless excitement; it does not have parkinsonian side effects. (Heminevrin.)

chlor·ocresol (klōr'-ō-krē'-sol) *n* a bactericidal phenolic cresol* particularly useful as a preservative for injections in multiple dose vials.

chloro·form (klōr'-ō-fōrm) *n* a heavy liquid, once used extensively as a general anesthetic. Much used in the form of chloroform water as a flavoring and preservative in aqueous mixtures.

chlor·oma (klōr-ō'-mà) *n* a condition in which multiple greenish-yellow growths grow on the periosteum of facial and cranial bones, and on vertebrae, in association with acute* myeloid leukemia.

Chlor·omycetin (klōr-ō-mī-sē'-tin) proprietary name for chloramphenicol*.

chlorophenothane (klōr-ō-fen'-ō-thān) *n* dichloro-diphenyl-tri-chloroethane, DDT, well known insecticide that is rarely used due to its high toxicity.

chloro·phyll (klōr'-ō-fil) *n* the green coloring matter which assists in photosynthesis in plants. Now prepared medicinally and for external use as a deodorant.

chloro·quine (klōr'-ō-kwin) *n* a potent antimalarial effective in the treatment and suppression of the disease. It is being added to the salt in some endemic areas. Also used in amebic hepatitis and collagen diseases. Can cause ocular complications. Has a mild anti-inflammatory effect and in the long term will lower the titer of the rheumatoid factor in the serum. (Aralen.)

chlorothiazide (klōr-ō-thī'-à-zīd) *n* diuretic with a mild blood pressure lowering action which changes little with posture and rarely gives rise to symptoms of hypotension. (Diuril.)

chloro·trian·isene (klōr-ō-trī-an'-i-sēn) *n* can be used as an alternative to stilbestrol*. Prescribed for some menopausal symptoms, because of its prolonged estrogenic action by slow release, but this is not an advantage if side effects occur, as the effect of the hormone cannot be immediately discontinued. (Tace.)

chlor·oxylenol (klōr-oks'-i-len'-ol) *n* a phenolic cresol* used as a germicide.

chlor·phenir·amine (klōr-fen-ēr'-à-mēn) *n* an antihistamine of high potency and of value in allergic conditions and also in the treatment of transfusion reactions. Can be given orally or by injection.

chlor·promazine (klōr-prō'-mà-zēn) *n* a drug of exceptional pharmacological action, as it is a sedative, antiemetic, antispasmodic and hypotensive. It increases the effectiveness of hypnotics, anesthetics, alcohol and analgesics. Valuable in psychiatric conditions and management of senile patients. May cause skin sensitization, leukopenia, parkinsonism, jaundice and hypothermia. (Thorazine.)

chlor·propamide (klōr-prō'-pa-mīd) *n* an antidiabetic agent; one of the sulfonylureas*. (Diabinese.)

chlor·prothixene (klōr-prō-thicks'-ēn) *n* a tranquilizer which is useful in acute schizophrenic conditions, but is less effective when treatment is prolonged. (Taractan.)

chlor·tetra·cycline (klōr-tet-rà-sī'-klin) *n* a preparation of tetracyline*. (Aureomycin.)

chlor·thalidone (klōr-thal'-i-dōn) *n* an oral diuretic given on alternate days. Its action lasts up to 48 h. (Hygroton.)

cho·anae (kō-ān'-ī) *npl* funnel-shaped openings. ⇒ nares*—**choana** *sing,* **choanal** *adj.*

choc·olate cyst an endometrial cyst* containing altered blood. The ovaries are the most usual site.

choked disc ⇒ papilledema.

chola·gogue (kōl'-a-gog) *n* a drug which causes an increased flow of bile into the intestine.

chol·angi·ography (kōl-an-jē-og'/-raf-ē) *n* the radiographic examination of hepatic, cystic and bile ducts. Can be performed: (a) after oral or intravenous administration of radioopaque substance (b) by direct injection at operation to detect any further stones in the ducts (c) during or after operation by way of a T-tube in the common bile duct (d) by means of an injection via the skin on the anterior abdominal wall and the liver when it is called percutaneous transhepatic cholangiography ⇒ endoscopic retrograde cholangio-pancreatography—**cholangiographic** *adj,* **cholangiograph** *n,* **cholangiographically** *adv.*

chol·angio·hepat·itis (kōl-an'-jē-ō-hep-à-tī'-tis) *n* inflammation of the liver and bile ducts.

cholan·gitis (kōl-an-jī'-tis) *n* inflammation of the bile ducts.

cholecystangiography (kōl-e-sist-anj-ē-og'-raf-ē) *n* radiographic examination of the gallbladder, cystic and common bile ducts.

chole·cyst·ectomy (kōl-ē-sist-ek'-to-mē) *n* surgical removal of the gallbladder. Usually advised for stones, inflammation and occasionally for new growths.

chole·cyst·enter·ostomy (kōl-ē-sist-en-tér-os'-to-mē) *n* literally, the establishment of an artificial opening (anastomosis) between the gallbladder and the small intestine. Specific terminology more frequently used.

chole·cystitis (kŏl-ē-sist-ī'-tis) *n* inflammation of the gallbladder.

chole·cysto·duodenal (kŏl-ē-sist-ō-dū-ō-dēn'-ăl) *adj* pertaining to the gallbladder and duodenum as an anastomosis between them.

chole·cysto·duoden·ostomy (kŏl-ē-sist-ō-dū-ō-dēn-os'-to-mē) *n* the establishment of an anastomosis* between the gallbladder and the duodenum. Usually necessary in cases of stricture of common bile duct, which may be congenital, due to previous inflammation or operation.

chole·cystography (kŏl-ē-sis-tog'-rà-fē) *n* radiographic examination of the gallbladder after administration of opaque medium—**cholecystographic** *adj*, **cholecystogram** *n*, **cholecystograph** *n*, **cholecystographically** *adv*.

chole·cysto·jejun·ostomy (kŏl-ē-sis-tō-je-jūn-os'-tō-mē) *n* an anastomosis between the gallbladder and the jejunum. Performed for obstructive jaundice due to growth in head of pancreas.

chole·cysto·kinin (kŏl-ē-sis-to-kī'-nin) *n* a hormone which contracts the gallbladder. Secreted by the upper intestinal mucosa.

chole·cysto·lith·iasis (kŏl-ē-sis-tō-lith-ī'-à-sis) *n* the presence of stone or stones in the gallbladder.

chole·cystostomy (kŏl-ē-sis-tos'-to-mē) *n* a surgically established fistula between the gallbladder and the abdominal surface; used to provide drainage, in empyema of the gallbladder or after the removal of stones.

chole·cystotomy (kŏl-ē-sis-tot'-o-mē) *n* incision into the gallbladder.

chole·docho·duod·enal (kŏl-ē-dok-ō-dū-ō-dēn'-ăl) *adj* pertaining to the bile ducts and duodenum, e.g. *choledochoduodenal fistula*.

chole·dochog·raphy (kŏl-ē-dok-og'-ra-fē) cholangiography*.

chole·docho·lith·iasis (kŏl-ē-dok-ō-lith-ī'-à-sis) *n* the presence of a stone or stones in the bile ducts.

chole·docho·lith·otomy (kŏl-ē-dok-ō-lith-ot'-o-mē) *n* surgical removal of a stone from the common bile duct.

chole·dochostomy (kŏl-ē-dok-os'-to-mē) *n* drainage of the common bile duct using a T tube, usually after exploration for a stone.

chole·dochotomy (kŏl-ē-dok-ot'-o-mē) *n* incision into the common bile duct.

Chole·dyl (kŏl'-e-dil) *n* proprietary name for choline* theophyllinate.

chole·lithiasis (kŏl-ē-lith-ī'-à-sis) *n* the presence of stones in the gallbladder or bile ducts.

cholemia (kŏl-ēm'-ē-à) *n* the presence of bile* in the blood—**cholemic,** *adj*.

chol·era (kol'-ė-rà) *n* an acute epidemic disease, caused by *Vibrio comma*, occurring in the East. The main symptoms are the evacuation of copious 'rice-water' stools accompanied by agonizing cramp and severe collapse. Spread mainly by contaminated water, overcrowding and insanitary conditions. High mortality.

chol·eric temper·ament (kol'-ėr-ik) *n* one of the four classical types of temperament*, hasty and prone to emotional outbursts.

choles·tasis (kŏl-ē-stā'-sis) *n* diminution or arrest of the flow of bile. *intrahepatic cholestasis* a syndrome comprising jaundice of an obstructive type, itching, pale stools and dark urine, but in which the main bile ducts outside the liver are patent—**cholestatic** *adj*.

choles·teatoma (kŏl-es-tē-à-tō'-mà) *n* a benign encysted tumor containing cholesterol. Mainly occurs in the middle ear—**cholesteatomatous** *adj*.

choles·terol (kol-es'-tėr-ol) *n* a crystalline substance of a fatty nature found in the brain, nerves, liver, blood and bile. It is not easily soluble and may crystallize in the gallbladder and along arterial walls. When irradiated it forms vitamin D.

cholester·osis (kol-es-tėr-os'-is) *n* abnormal deposition of cholesterol*.

choles·tyramine (kol-es-tī'-rà-mēn) *n* a basic ion-exchange resin which combines with bile acids in the intestine to give a product which is not absorbed. It therefore lowers the blood levels of cholesterol*. (Questran.)

chol·ine (kŏl'-ēn) *n* a chemical found in animal tissues as a constituent of lecithin* and acetylcholine*. Thought to be part of the vitamin* B complex, and is known to be a growth factor. Appears to be necessary for fat transportation in the body. Useful in preventing fat deposition in the liver in cirrhosis. Richest sources are dairy products.

chol·ine mag·nesium tri·salicylate (kŏl'-ēn mag-nē'-zē-um trī-sal-is'-il-āt) *n* a derivative of salicylic* acid; the drug has a non-steroidal anti-inflammatory action.

chol·ine the·ophyl·linate (kōl'-ēn thē-of'-il-in-āt) *n* this compound resembles aminophylline* in its general effects, but is less erratic in action. The incidence of gastric irritation is much less, and the response more reliable. (Choledyl.)

cholin·ergic (kōl-in-ėr'-jik) *adj* applied to nerves which liberate acetylcholine* at their termination. Includes nerves which cause voluntary muscle to contract and all parasympathetic nerves. ⇒ adrenergic *opp. cholinergic cris* respiratory failure resulting from over-treatment with anticholinesterase* drugs. It is distinguished from myasthenic* crisis by giving 10 mg edrophonium chloride intravenously. If there is no improvement cholinergic crisis is confirmed and 1 mg atropine sulfate is given intravenously together with immediate mechanical respiration. ⇒ edrophonium test.

cholin·esterase (kōl-in-es'-tér-ās) *n* an enzyme which hydrolyzes acetylcholine into choline and acetic acid at nerve endings.

chol·uria (kō-lū'-rē-à) *n* biluria*—**choluric** *adj.*

chon·dritis (kon-drī'-tis) *n* inflammation of cartilage.

chondro·costal (kon-drō-kos'-tàl) *adj* pertaining to the costal cartilages and ribs.

chondro·dynia (kon-drō-dī'-nē-à) *n* pain in a cartilage.

chondro·lysis (kon-drol'-is-is) *n* dissolution of cartilage—**chondrolytic** *adj.*

chon·droma (kon-drō'-mà) *n* a benign tumor of cartilage. Tends to recur after removal.

chondro·malacia (kon-drō-mà-lā'-sē-a) *n* softening of cartilage.

chondro·sarcoma (kon-drō-sàr-kō-ma) *n* malignant neoplasm of cartilage—**chondrosarcomata** *pl,* **chondrosarcomatous** *adj.*

chondro·sternal (kon-drō-stėr'-nàl) *adj* pertaining to the rib cartilages and sternum.

chor·dee (kōr'-dē) *n* painful erection of the penis lately associated with urethritis.

chor·ditis (kōr-dī'-tis) *n* inflammation of the spermatic or vocal cords.

chor·dotomy (kōr-do'-to-mē) ⇒ cordotomy.

chorea (kōr-ē'-à) *n* a disease manifested by irregular and spasmodic movements, beyond the patient's control. Even voluntary movements are rendered jerky and ungainly. The childhood disease is often called rheumatic chorea or 'St. Vitus Dance'; the adult form is part of a cerebral degenerative process called Huntington's* chorea—**choreal, choreic** *adj.*

chorei·form (kōr-ē'-i-fōrm) *n* resembling chorea*.

chorio·carcinoma (kōr-ē-ō-kàr-sin-o'-mà) chorionepithelioma*.

chor·ion (kōr'-ē-on) *n* the outer membrane forming the embryonic sac—**chorial, chorionic** *adj, chorion biopsy* ⇒ chorionic villus biopsy.

chorion·epithel·ioma (kōr-ē-on-ep-i-thē-lē-ō'-mà) *n* a highly malignant tumor arising from chorionic cells, usually after a hydatidiform* mole although it may follow abortion or even normal pregnancy, quickly metastasizing especially to the lungs. Cytotoxic drugs have improved the prognosis.

chor·ionic villi (kōr-ē-on'-ik vil'-lī) projections from the chorion* from which the fetal part of the placenta is formed. Through the chorionic villi diffusion of gases, nutrient and waste products from the maternal to the fetal blood and vice versa occurs.

chor·ionic villus biopsy (kōr-ē-on'-ik vil'-us bī'-op-sē) biopsy of a chorionic villus for the prenatal diagnosis of many disorders.

chor·io·reti·nitis (kōr-ē-ō-ret-in-īt'-is) *n* (*syn* choroidoretinitis) inflammation of the choroid and retina.

cho·roid (kōr'-oyd) *n* the middle pigmented, vascular coat of the posterior five-sixths of the eyeball, continuous with the iris in front (⇒ Figure 15). It lies between the sclera* externally and the retina* internally, and prevents the passage of light rays—**choroidal** *adj.*

choroid·itis (kōr-oyd-īt'-is) *n* inflammation of the choroid. *Tay's choroiditis* degenerative change affecting the retina around the macula* lutea.

choroido·cyclitis (kōr-oyd-ō-sīk-lī'-tis) *n* inflammation of the choroid and ciliary body.

choroido·retinal (kōr-oyd-ō-ret'-in-àl) *adj* pertaining to the choroid and the retina.

choroidoretinitis (kōr-oyd-ō-ret-in-īt'-is) *n* ⇒ chorioretinitis.

Christ·mas dis·ease ⇒ hemophilias.

chromato·gram (krō-ma'-tō-gram) *n* any recording of the results of chromatography.

chroma·tography (krō-ma-tog′-raf-ē) *n* a method of separating and identifying substances in a complex mixture based on their differential movement through a two-phase system effected by a flow of liquid or gas (mobile phase) which percolates through an absorbent (stationary phase). The stationary phase may be solid (e.g. paper), liquid or a mixture of both. The mobile phase may be liquid or gaseous and fills the spaces of the stationary phase through which it flows. The stationary and mobile phases are so selected that the compounds which are to be separated have different distribution coefficients between the phases due to differences in their physiochemical properties.

chro·mic acid (krō′-mik as′-id) in a 5% solution it is an astringent, used in the preparation of chromicized catgut; stronger solutions are caustic and can be painted on warts.

chromo·some (krōm′-ō-sōm) *n* one of the staining bodies which can be seen within the cell nucleus as a cell prepares to divide and during cell division (for example, by mitosis). Chromosomes split longitudinally in that process. They carry hereditary factors (genes). The chromosomes are made essentially of DNA*, of which the genes are made, and the chromosome number is constant for each species. In man, there are 46 in each cell, except in the mature ovum and sperm in which the number is halved as a result of reduction division (meiosis). A set of 23 chromosomes is inherited from each parent. The human male produces two types of sperm, with the Y chromosome to generate males and with the X chromosome to generate females—**chromosomal** *adj.*

chronic (kron′-ik) *adj* lingering, lasting, opposed to acute*. The word does not imply anything about the severity of the condition, *chronic lymphocytic leukemia* a proliferation of lymphocytes in the blood, which occurs mainly in the elderly. Little active treatment is necessary and patients may live comfortably for many years. *chronic myelocytic leukemia* proliferation of myelocytes in the blood. The condition may run a static course over several years but eventually an acute phase supervenes (blast crisis). *chronic obstructive airways disease* chronic obstructive bronchitis*—**chronicity** *n,* **chronically** *adv.*

chrono·logical age (kron-o-loj′-ik-àl) a person's actual age in years.

Chronulac (kron′-ū-lak) *n* proprietary preparation of lactulose*.

Chvostek's sign (shvos′-teks) excessive twitching of the face on tapping the facial nerve; a sign of tetany*.

chyle (kīl) *n* digested fats which, as an alkaline, milky fluid, pass from the small intestine via the lymphatics to the blood stream—**chylous** *adj.*

chylo·thorax (kīl-ō-thō′-raks) *n* leakage of chyle from the thoracic duct into the pleural cavity.

chy·luria (kīl-ūr′-ē-à) *n* chyle* in the urine, which can occur in some nematode infestations, either when a fistulous communication is established between a lymphatic vessel and the urinary tract or when the distension of the urinary lymphatics causes them to rupture—**chyluric** *adj.*

chyme (kīm) *n* partially digested food which as an acid, creamy-yellow, thick fluid passes from the stomach to the duodenum. Its acidity controls the pylorus so that chyme is ejected at frequent intervals—**chymous** *adj.*

chymo·papain (kī-mō-pap′-ān) *n* a proteolytic enzyme obtained from the latex of the pawpaw tree.

Chymoral (kī′-mōr-àl) *n* a proprietary mixture of the enzymes trypsin* and chymotrypsin*.

chymo·trypsin (kī-mō-trip′-sin) *n* a protein-digesting enzyme secreted by the pancreas; it is activated by trypsin. A pharmaceutical preparation is useful in debridment of necrotic tissue, and for loosening secretions, e.g. in respiratory tract. It also facilitates lens extraction. (Avazyme.)

cic·atrix (sik′-à-triks) *n* ⇒ scar.

Cido·mycin (sīd-ō-mī′-sin) *n* proprietary name for gentamicin* sulfate.

cilia (sil′-ē-à) *n* **1** the eyelashes. **2** microscopic hair-like projections from certain epithelial cells. Membranes containing such cells e.g. those lining the trachea and Fallopian tubes, are known as ciliated membranes—**cilium** *sing,* **ciliary, ciliated, cilial** *adj.*

ciliary (sil′-ē-ār-ē) *adj* hair-like. *ciliary body* a specialized structure in the eye connecting the anterior part of the choroid to the circumference of the iris (⇒ Figure 15); it is composed of the ciliary muscles and processes. *ciliary muscles* fine hair-like muscle fibers arranged in a circular manner to form a greyish-white ring immediately behind the corneoscleral junction. *ciliary processes* about 70 in number, are projections on the undersurface of the choroid which are attached to the ciliary muscles.

cimet·idine (sī-met′-i-dēn) *n* a histamine H_2-receptor antagonist which inhibits both resting and stimulated gastric acid secretion. Useful for active peptic ulcers; should be taken after the evening meal; a single daily dose at night gives better control of nocturnal gastric acid output and lowers the mean 24 h acidity as effectively as divided doses. Antacids interfere with its absorption. (Tagamet.)

Cimex (sī′-meks) *n* a genus of insects of the family Cimicidae. *Cimex lectularius* is the common bedbug, parasitic to man and blood-sucking.

CIN *abbr* ⇒ central intra-epithelial neoplasia.

cin·chona (sin-kō′-nà) *n* the bark from which quinine* is obtained. Occasionally used as a bitter tonic.

cinchon·ism (sin′-kon-ism) quininism*.

cine·angio·cardi·ography (sin-ē-an-jē-ō-kàr-dē-og′-raf-ē) *n* the motion picture technique of recording the passage of contrast medium through the heart and blood vessels.

cine·angi·ography (sin-ē-an-jē-og′-raf-ē) *n* motion picture technique of recording images during angiography*.

cinna·mon (sin′-à-mon) *n* an aromatic bark with carminative and mildly astringent properties. Sometimes used with chalk* and other carminatives in diarrhea.

circad·ian rhythm (sir-kā′-dē-an) rhythm with a periodicity of 24 h.

circ·inata (sir-sin-a′-tà) *n* ⇒ tinea.

circi·nate (sir′-sin-āt) *n* in the form of a circle or segment of a circle, e.g. the skin eruptions of late syphilis, ringworm, etc.

circu·lation (sir-kū-lā′-shun) *n* passage in a circle. Usually means circulation of the blood—**circulatory** *adj*, **circulate** *vi*, *vit*. *circulation of bile* the passage of bile from the liver cells, where it is formed, via the gallbladder and bile ducts to the small intestine, where its constituents are partly reabsorbed into the blood and thus return to the liver. *circulation of blood* the passage of blood from heart to arteries to capillaries to veins and back to heart. *circulation of cerebrospinal fluid* takes place from the ventricles of the brain to the cisterna magna, from whence the fluid bathes the surface of the brain and the spinal cord, including its central canal. It is absorbed into the blood in the cerebral venous sinuses. *circulation of lymph* lymph is collected from the tissue spaces and passed in the lymphatic capillaries, vessels, glands and ducts to be poured back into the blood stream. *greater circulation* circulation of blood from left ventricle to aorta, to tissue and back to right atrium of heart. *lesser circulation* circulation of blood from right ventricle to pulmonary artery, to lungs and back to left atrium of heart.

circum·cision (sir-kum-sizh′-un) *n* excision of the prepuce or foreskin of the penis, usually for religious or ethnic reasons. The operation is sometimes required for phimosis* or paraphimosis*. *female circumcision* excision of the clitoris, labia minora and labia majora.

circum·corneal (sir-kum-kōr′-nē-àl) *adj* around the cornea.

circum·oral (sir-kum-ōr′-àl) *adj* surrounding the mouth. *circumoral pallor* a pale appearance of the skin around the mouth, in contrast to the flushed cheeks. A characteristic of scarlatina*—**circumorally** *adv*.

circum·vallate (sir-kum-val′-āt) *adj* surrounded by a raised ring, as the large circumvallate papillae at the base of the tongue.

cir·rhosis (sir-ō′-sis) *n* hardening of an organ. There are degenerative changes in the tissues with resulting fibrosis. *cirrhosis of liver* Increasing in prosperous countries. Damage to liver cells can be from virus, microorganisms or toxic substances and dietary deficiencies interfering with the nutrition of liver cells—often the result of alcoholism. Associated developments include ascites*, obstruction of the circulation through the portal vein with hematemesis*, jaundice and enlargement of the spleen—**cirrhotic** *adj*.

cir·soid (sir′-soyd) *adj* resembling a tortuous, dilated vein (varix*). *cirsoid aneurysm* a tangled mass of pulsating blood vessels appearing as a subcutaneous tumor, usually on the scalp.

cis·platin (sis′-pla-tin) *n* a platinum compound used in the treatment of malignant conditions.

cis·terna (sis-tèr′-nà) *n* any closed space serving as a reservoir for a body fluid. *cisterna magna* is a subarachnoid space in the cleft between the cerebellum and medulla oblongata—**cisternal** *adj*.

cister·nal puncture ⇒ puncture.

Cita·nest (sīt'-à-nest) *n* proprietary name for prilocaine*.

cit·ric acid (sit'-rik) the acid present in lemons. Widely used as potassium* citrate, a diuretic. *citric acid cycle* ⇒ Kreb's cycle.

citrin (sit'-rin) *n* (*syn* vitamin P) thought to enhance the action of vitamin* C in the prevention of scurvy in human beings. Capillary fragility is associated with lack of this substance. It is found in rose hips, citrus fruits and black currants.

CJD *abbr* Creutzfeldt-Jakob* disease.

clap *n* a slang term for gonorrhea*.

claudi·cation (klaw-di-kā'-shun) *n* limping caused by interference with the blood supply to the legs. The cause may be spasm or disease of the vessels themselves. In *intermittent claudication* the patient experiences severe pain in the calves when he is walking; after a short rest he is able to continue.

claustro·phobia (klaws-trō-fō'-bē-à) *n* a form of mental disturbance in which there is a morbid fear of enclosed spaces—**claustrophobic** *adj.*

clav·icle (klav'-ik-l) *n* the collar-bone (⇒ Figures 2, 3)—**clavicular** *adj.*

clavu·lanic acid (klav-ū-lan'-ik) *n* used in combination with amoxycillin* to inhibit the enzyme penicillinase produced by penicillin-resistant bacteria.

cla·vus (klā'-vus) *n* a corn*.

claw-foot *adj. n* (*syn* pes cavus) a deformity where the longitudinal arch of the foot is increased in height and associated with clawing of the toes. It may be acquired or congenital in origin.

claw-hand *n* the hand is flexed and contracted giving a claw-like appearance; the condition may be due to injury or disease.

cleft pal·ate congenital failure of fusion between the right and left palatal processes. Often associated with hare-lip*.

Cleocin (klē'-ō-sin) *n* proprietary name for clindamycin*.

climac·teric (kli-mak'-te-rik) *n* in the female, the menopause*. A corresponding period occurs in men and is called the *male climacteric.*

clinda·mycin (klin-dà-mī'-sin) *n* a derivative of lincomycin* that is much more active than the parent compound.

clini·cal (klin'-ik-àl) *adj* pertaining to a clinic. Describes the practical observation and treatment of sick persons as opposed to theoretical study.

Clistin (klis'-tin) *n* proprietary name for carbinoxamine* maleate.

clitori·dectomy (klit-ōr-i-dek'-to-mē) *n* the surgical removal of the clitoris.

clitori·ditis (klit-ōr-id-ī'-tis) *n* inflammation of the clitoris.

clit·oris (klit'-ōr-is) *n* a small erectile organ of the female genitalia situated just below the mons veneris at the junction anteriorly of the labia minora.

cloaca (klō-ā'-kà) in osteomyelitis*, the opening through the involucrum* which discharges pus—**cloacal** *adj.*

clo·betasol propi·onate (klō-bet'-a-sol prō'-pē-on-āt) *n* soothing steroid application for such skin conditions as eczema. (Temovate.)

clofaz·imine (klō-faz'-i-mēn) *n* a red dye, given orally. Controls symptoms of erythema nodosum leprosum reaction in lepromatous leprosy better than prednisolone*.

clofib·rate (klō-fī'-brāt) *n* lowers blood cholesterol and is used to prevent fat embolism, particularly in patients with bone injury. (Atromid-S.)

Clo·mid (klō'-mid) *n* proprietary name for clomiphene*.

clomi·phene (klō'-mi-phēn) *n* a synthetic non-steroidal compound which induces ovulation and subsequent menstruation in some otherwise anovulatory women thereby enhancing their fertility. (Clomid.)

clonic (klōn'-ik) *adj* ⇒ clonus.

cloni·dine (klōn'-i-dēn) *n* similar to methyldopa*, but causes less postural hypotension though it gives some patients a very dry mouth. In small doses it is of value in preventing migraine. (Catapres, Dixarit.)

clonus (klō'-nus) *n* a series of intermittent muscular contractions and relaxations. ⇒ tonic *opp.* ankle clonus—**clonic** *adj.* **clonicity** *n.*

closed frac·ture ⇒ fracture.

Clostrid·ium (klos-trid'-ē-um) *n* a bacterial genus. Clostridia are large Gram-positive anaerobic bacilli found as commensals of the gut of animals and man and as saprophytes in the soil. Endospores* are produced which are widely distributed. Many species are pathogenic because of the exotoxins produced e.g. *Clostridium tetani* (tetanus), *C. botulinum* (botulism): *C. perfringens (welchii)* (gas gangrene), *C. difficile* (pseudomembranous colitis).

clot (klot) *v* to coagulate. *n* a thrombus or coagulation.

clotting time the time taken by shed blood to coagulate.

clove oil oil extracted from cloves, which has antiseptic, carminative and anodyne properties. Used to relieve toothache.

cloxa·cillin (kloks-à-sil′-lin) *n* a semisynthetic penicillin* which is active against penicillin-resistant staphylococci. It is acid-stable and can be given orally or parenterally.

club·bed fingers a thickening and broadening of the bulbous fleshy portion of the fingers under the nails. The cause is not known but it occurs in people who have heart and/or lung disease.

club-foot *n* a congenital malformation, either unilateral or bilateral. ⇒ talipes.

clump·ing agglutination*.

Clut·ton's joints (klut′-ons) joints which show symmetrical swelling, usually pain less, the knees often being involved. Associated with congenital syphilis.

clysis (klī′-sis) *n* **1** the cleansing or washing out of a cavity. **2** term used when administering fluids by other than oral route: subcutaneously (hypodermoclysis); intravenously (venoclysis); and rectally (proctoclysis).

CMV *abbr* cytomegalovirus*.

CNS *abbr* central nervous* system.

coagu·lase (kō-ag′-ū-lās) *n* an enzyme produced by some bacteria of the genus *Staphylococcus:* it coagulates plasma and is used to classify staphylococci as coagulase-negative or coagulase-positive.

coagulate (kō-ag′-ū-lāt) *v* to form a clot or solidify–**coagulation,** *n*.

coagu·lum (kō-ag′-ū-lum) *n* any coagulated mass: a scab.

co·alesce (kō-à-les′) *vt* to grow together; to unite into a mass. Often used to describe the development of a skin eruption, when discrete areas of affected skin coalesce to form sheets of a similar appearance—**coalescence** *n*. **coalescent** *adj*.

coal tar the black substance obtained by the distillation of coal. It is used in an ointment for psoriasis and eczema.

coarc·tation (kō-ark-tā′-shun) *n* contraction, stricture, narrowing; applied to a vessel or canal.

coarse tremor *n* violent trembling.

cobal·amin (kō-bal′-à-min) *n* a generic term for the vitamin B_{12} group. ⇒ cyanocobalamin.

cobalt (kō′-balt) *n* a mineral element considered nutritionally essential in minute traces; a constituent of vitamin B_{12} (cobalamin)—the anti-pernicious anemia factor. It is therefore linked with iron and copper in the prevention of anemia. *cobalt-58* a radioactive isotope of cobalt used as a tracer in the study of cobalt metabolism. *cobalt-60* a radioactive isotope of cobalt which is superseding radium* in radiotherapy. *cobalt edetate* used in cyanide poisoning.

COC *abbr* combined* oral contraceptive.

co·caine (kō-kān′) *n* a powerful local anesthetic obtained from the leaves of the coca plant. Toxic, especially to the brain; may cause agitation, disorientation, convulsions and can induce addiction. It has vasoconstrictor properties, hence the blanching which occurs when it is applied to mucous membranes. It is now largely replaced by less toxic compounds such as procaine* and xylocaine*, but is still used as eye drops, often with homatropine*. It can be obtained illegally as purified uncut cocaine, which is ground to a white powder and sniffed in small doses ('cocaine abuse/addiction').

cocain·ism (kō-kān′-izm) *n* mental and physical degeneracy caused by a morbid craving for, and excessive use of, cocaine*.

coc·cus (kok′-us) *n* a spherical or nearly spherical bacterium—**cocci** *pl*. **coccal, coccoid** *adj*.

coccy·dynia (koks-ē-din′-ē-a) *n* pain in the region of the coccyx.

coccy·geal (koks-ē-jē′-ål) **nerve** ⇒ Figure 11.

coccy·gectomy (koks-ē-jek′-to-mē) *n* surgical removal of the coccyx.

coc·cyx (kok′-siks) *n* the last bone of the vertebral column (⇒ Figure 3). It is triangular in shape and curved slightly forward. It is composed of four rudimentary vertebrae, cartilaginous at birth, ossification being completed at about the 30th year—**coccygeal** *adj*.

coch·lea (kōk′-lē-à) *n* a spiral canal resembling the interior of a snail shell, in the anterior part of the bony labyrinth of the ear (⇒ Figure 13)—**cochlear** *adj*.

cocoa (kō′-kō) *n* the seeds of *Theobroma cacao*. The powder is made into a nourishing pleasant beverage. Contains theobromine* and caffeine*. *cocoa butter* is obtained from the roasted seeds; it does not become rancid and melts at body temperature; it is therefore used as a base for suppositories, ointments and as an emollient.

co·deine (kō′-dēn) *n* an alkaloid of

opium*. It has mild analgesic properties, and is often combined with aspirin*. Valuable as a cough sedative in dry and unproductive cough.

cod liver oil contains vitamins A and D and is used on that account as a dietary supplement in mild deficiency. It can be applied as a dressing to promote healing.

co-enzyme (kō-en′-zīm) n an enzyme activator.

cof·fee ground vomit vomit containing blood, which in its partially digested state resembles coffee grounds. Indicative of slow upper gastro-intestinal bleeding ⇒ hematemesis.

Cogen·tin (kō-jen′-tin) proprietary name for benztropine*.

cog·nition (kog-ni′-shun) n awareness: one of the three aspects of mind, the others being affection (feeling or emotion), and conation (willing or desiring). They work as a whole but any one may dominate any mental process.

co·itus (kō′-it-us) n insertion of the erect penis into the vagina: the act of sexual intercourse or copulation. *coitus interruptus* removal from the vagina of the penis before ejaculation of semen as a means of contraception. The method is considered unsatisfactory as it is not only unreliable but can lead to sexual disharmony—**coital** adj.

Colace (kō′-lās) n proprietary name for docusate* sodium.

colchicine (kŏl′-chi-sēn) n drug used to treat gout.

colchi·cum (kŏl′-chi-kum) n the dried seed of the autumn crocus. It contains colchicine, and is of value in the treatment of acute gout.

cold ab·scess ⇒ abscess.

cold sore n oral herpes*.

col·ectomy (kō-lek′-to-mē) n excision of part or the whole of the colon.

colic (kol′-ik) n severe pain resulting from periodic spasm in an abdominal organ. *biliary colic* ⇒ biliary. *intestinal colic* abnormal peristaltic movement of an irritated gut. *painter's (lead) colic* spasm of intestine and constriction of mesenteric vessels, resulting from lead poisoning. *renal colic* spasm of ureter due to a stone. *uterine colic* dysmenorrhea*—**colicky** adj.

coli·form (kol′-i-fôrm) adj a word used to describe any bacterium of fecal origin which is morphologically similar to *Escherichia coli.*

col·istin (kol′-is-tin) n an antibiotic which is active against many Gram-negative organisms. Useful in *Pseudomonas aeruginosa* infections. Less toxic than polymyxin* B. (Coly-Mycin-S.)

col·itis (kol-ī′-tis) n inflammation of the colon. May be acute or chronic, and may be accompanied by ulcerative lesions. *ulcerative colitis* an inflammatory and ulcerative condition of the colon. Etiologically the evidence is accumulating for an immunological basis for the condition rather than a psychosomatic one, as was previously thought. Characteristically it affects young and early middle-aged adults, producing periodic bouts of diarrheal stools containing mucus and blood, and it may vary in severity from a mild form with little constitutional upset to a severe, dangerous and prostrating illness.

col·lagen (kol′-à-jen) n the main protein constituent of white fibrous tissue (skin, tendon, bone, cartilage and all connective tissue). It is composed of bundles of tropocollagen molecules, which contain three intertwined polypeptide chains. The *collagen diseases* are characterized by an inflammatory lesion of unknown etiology affecting collagen and small blood vessels. Said to be due to development of a hypersensitivity state, they include dermatomyositis, lupus erythematosus, polyarteritis (periarteritis) nodosa, purpura, rheumatic fever, rheumatoid arthritis and scleroderma—**collagenic, collagenous** adj. *collagen proline hydroxylase* an enzyme which is necessary for wound healing, and vitamin* C is necessary for this enzyme's maintenance and function. Research indicates that tissues which are rapidly synthesizing collagen (e.g. healing wounds) have high levels of this enzyme.

col·lapse (kol-aps′) 1 the 'falling in' of a hollow organ or vessel, e.g. collapse of lung from change of air pressure inside or outside the organ. 2 physical or nervous prostration.

col·laps·ing pulse the water-hammer pulse of aortic incompetence with high initial upthrust which quickly falls away.

col·lar·bone (kol′-ar-bōn) n the clavicle (⇒ Figures 2, 3).

col·lateral circul·ation (kol-lat′-ėr-er) n an alternative route provided for the blood by secondary blood vessels when a primary vessel is blocked.

Colles' frac·ture (kol′-ēz) a break at the lower end of the radius following a fall on the outstretched hand. The backward displacement of the hand produces the 'dinner fork' deformity.

colliquative (ko-lik'-wå-tiv) *adj.* profuse, excessive.

col·lodion (ko-lō'-dē-on) *n* solution of pyroxylin* with ether and alcohol. It forms a flexible film on the skin, and is used mainly as a protective dressing.

col·loid (kol'-oyd) *n* a glue-like non-crystalline substance; diffusible but not soluble in water; unable to pass through an animal membrane. Some drugs can be prepared in their colloidal form. *colloid degeneration* mucoid degeneration of tumors. *colloid goiter* abnormal enlargement of the thyroid gland, due to the accumulation in it of viscid, iodine-containing colloid.

col·loidal gold test (kol-oyd'-ål) carried out on cerebrospinal fluid to assist the diagnosis of neurosyphilis.

colo·boma (kol-ō-bō'-må) *n* a congenital fissure or gap in the eyeball or one of its parts, particularly the uvea—**colobomata** *pl.*

colocysto·plasty (kol-ō-sis'-to-plas-tē) *n* an operation to increase the capacity of the urinary bladder by using part of the colon—**colocystoplastic** *adj.*

Cologel (kol'-ō-jel) *n* proprietary name for methylcellulose*.

colon (kō'-lon) *n* the large bowel extending from the cecum* to the rectum* (⇒ Figure 18). In its various parts it has appropriate names—ascending, transverse, descending and sigmoid colon. ⇒ flexure. *spasmodic colon* megacolon*—**colonic** *adj.*

colon·ize (kol'-on-īz) *vt* of commensals*, to establish a presence on or in the human body. Soon after birth commensals form a natural flora and do not usually cause infection*. Tissue can therefore be 'colonized' but not infected. Infection results when there is imbalance between the commensals and defense mechanisms.

colon·oscopy (kol-on-os'-ko-pē) *n* use of a fiberoptic colonoscope to view the inner membrane of the colon—**colonoscopic** *adj.* **colonoscopically** *adv.*

col·ony (kol'-on-ē) *n* a mass of bacteria which is the result of multiplication of one or more organisms. A colony may contain many millions of individual organisms and may become macroscopic*; its physical features are often characteristic of the species.

colo·rectal (kol-ō-rek'-tål) *adj* pertaining to the colon and the rectum.

col·ostomy (kol-os'-to-mē) *n* a surgically established fistula between the colon and the surface of the abdomen; this acts as an artificial anus.

col·ostrum (kol-os'-trum) *n* the relatively clear fluid secreted in the breasts during the first 3 days after parturition, before the formation of true milk is established. Also may be secreted during pregnancy.

col·otomy (kol-ot'-o-mē) *n* incision into the colon.

color blind·ness applies to various conditions in which certain colors are confused with one another. Inability to distinguish between reds and greens is called daltonism. ⇒ achromatopsia.

col·pitis (kol-pī'-tis) *n* inflammation of the vagina. Syn., vaginitis.

col·pocele (kol'-pō-sēl) *n* protrusion or prolapse of either the bladder or rectum so that it presses on the vaginal wall.

colpocen·tesis (kol-pō-sen-tē'-sis) *n* withdrawal of fluid from the vagina, as in hematocolpos*.

colpo·hyster·ectomy (kol-pō-his-tėr-ek'-to-mē) *n* removal of the uterus through the vagina.

colpo·perineor·rhaphy (kol-pō-pėr-in-ē-ōr'-af-ē) *n* the surgical repair of an injured vagina and deficient perineum.

colpo·photography (kol-pō-fō-tog'-raf-ē) *n* filming the cervix using a camera and colposcope.

colpor·rhaphy (kol-pōr'-af-ē) *n* surgical repair of the vagina. An anterior colporrhaphy repairs a cystocele* and a posterior colporrhaphy repairs a rectosele*.

colpo·scope (kolp'-ō-skōp) *n* an instrument which, when inserted into the vagina, holds the walls apart thereby permitting inspection of the cervix and upper vagina—**colposcopy** *n.* **colposcopically** *adv.*

colpot·omy (kol-pot'-om-ē) *n* incision of the vaginal wall. A posterior colpotomy drains an abscess in the pouch* of Douglas through the vagina.

Coly-Mycin-S *n* proprietary name for colistin.*

coma (kō'-må) *n* a state of unrousable unconsciousness the severity of which can be assessed by corneal and pupillary reflexes and withdrawal responses to painful stimuli.

coma·tose (kōm'-å-tōs) *adj* in a state of coma*.

com·bined oral contra·ceptive commonly referred to as 'the pill'. Many different brands are available: each contains varying concentrations of the two hormones—estrogen and progestogen. ⇒ contraceptive.

com·edo (kŏm'-ē-dō) *n* a worm-like cast formed of sebum* which occupies the outlet of a hair follicle in the skin, a feature of acne* vulgaris. Comedones have a black color because of pigmentation (blackheads)—**comedones** *pl*.

commen·sals (kom-en'-sàls) *npl* parasitic microorganisms adapted to grow on the skin and mucous surfaces of the host, forming part of the normal flora. Some commensals are potentially pathogenic.

commin·uted frac·ture (kom-in-ū'-ted) ⇒ fracture.

communi·cable (kom-ūn'-ik-à-bl) *adj* transmissible directly or indirectly from one person to another.

compati·bility (kom-pat-ib-il'-it-ē) *n* suitability; congruity. The power of a substance to mix with another without unfavorable results, e.g. two medicines, blood plasma and cells—**compatible** *adj*.

Compazine (kom'-pà-zēn) *n* proprietary name for prochlorperazine*.

compen·sation (kom-pen-sā'-shun) *n* **1** a mental mechanism, employed by a person to cover up a weakness, by exaggerating a more socially acceptable quality. **2** In psychiatry the term *compensation neurosis* denotes symptoms motivated by a wish for monetary compensation for accident or injury. In many cases it is difficult to decide whether an element of malingering is involved or if the mechanism is entirely unconscious. **3** The state of counterbalancing a functional or structural defect, e.g. cardiac compensation.

comple·ment (kom'-ple-ment) *n* a normal constituent of plasma which is of great importance in immunity mechanisms, as it combines with antigen-antibody complex (complement fixation), and this leads to the completion of reactions such as bacteriolysis and the killing of bacteria. *complement fixation test* measures the amount of complement fixed by any given antigen-antibody complex. It can confirm infection with a specific microorganism.

comple·mental air (kom-ple-men'-tàl) the extra air that can be drawn into the lungs by deep inspiration.

comple·mentary feeding a bottle feeding given to an infant to complement breast milk, if this is an insufficient amount.

com·plete abor·tion ⇒ abortion.

com·plex (kom'-pleks) *n* a series of emotionally charged ideas, repressed because they conflict with ideas acceptable to the individual. e.g. *Oedipus* complex*, Electra* complex.

compli·cated frac·ture (kom'-plik-ā-ted) ⇒ fracture.

compli·cation (kom-plik-ā'-shun) *n* in medicine, an accident or second disease arising in the course of a primary disease; it can be fatal.

com·pos men·tis (kom'-pŏs, men'-tis) of sound mind.

com·pound (kom'-pownd) *n* a substance composed of two or more elements, chemically combined in a definitive proportion to form a new substance with new properties.

com·pound (open) frac·ture ⇒ fracture.

comprehen·sion (kom-prē-hen'-shun) *n* mental grasp of meaning and relationships.

com·press (kom'-press) *n* usually refers to a wet dressing of several layers of lint. A cold compress on the forehead relieves headache.

com·pression (kom-presh'-un) *n* the state of being compressed. The act of pressing or squeezing together. *compression bandage* function is as the name implies. Specially used to give support without constriction of vessels after an ankle sprain. It can also be used to shrink a part such as an amputation stump. *compression fracture* ⇒ *fracture*.

compro·mise (kom'-prom-īz) *n* in psychiatry, a mental mechanism whereby a conflict* is evaded by disguising the repressed wish to make it acceptable in consciousness.

compul·sion (kom-pul'-shun) *n* an urge to carry out an act, recognized to be irrational. Resisting the urge leads to increasing tension which is only relieved by carrying out the act.

com·puted axial tomo·graphy (kom-pū'-ted aks'-ē-al tom-og'-ra-fē) computed* tomography (CAT.)

com·puted tomography (CT) (kom-pū'-ted tom-og'-ra-fē) computer-constructed imaging technique of a thin slice through the body, derived from X-ray absorption data collected during a circular scanning motion.

co·nation (kō-nā'-shun) *n* willing or desiring. The conscious tendency to action. One of the three aspects of mind, the others being cognition (awareness, understanding) and affection (feeling or emotion).

con·cept (kon'-sept) *n* an abstract generalization resulting from the mental process of abstracting and recombining certain qualities or characteristics of a number of ideas, to produce e.g. the individual's concept of honor, love, a rose, a house etc.

con·ception (kon-sep'-shun) *n* **1** the creation of a state of pregnancy; impregnation of the ovum by the spermatozoon. **2** an abstract mental idea of anything—**conceptive** *adj*.

concha *n* ⇒ Figure 14.

con·cretion (kon-krē'-shun) *n* a deposit of hard material; a calculus*.

con·cussion (kon-kush'-un) *n* a condition resulting from a violent jar or shock. *cerebral concussion* characterized by loss of consciousness, pallor, coldness and usually an increase in the pulse rate. There may be incontinence of urine and feces.

conden·sation (kon-den-sā'-shun) *n* the process of becoming more compact, e.g. the changing of a gas to a liquid.

con·ditioned re·flex (kon-dish'-und rē'-fleks) a reflex in which the response occurs, not to the sensory stimulus which caused it originally, but to another stimulus which the subject has learned to associate with the original stimulus; it can be acquired by training and repetition. In Pavlov's classic experiments, dogs learned to associate the sound of a bell with the sight and smell of food; even when food was not presented, salivation occurred at the sound of a bell.

con·dition·ing (kon-dish'-un-ing) *n* the encouragement of new (desirable) behavior by modifying the stimulus/response associations. *operant conditioning* the term used when there is a program to reward (or punish) a response each time it occurs, so that given time, it occurs more (or less) frequently. ⇒ deconditioning.

con·dom (kon'-dom) *n* a rubber sheath used as a male contraceptive*. It helps protect both partners against sexually transmitted disease.

con·duction (kon-duk'-shun) *n* the transmission of heat, light, or sound waves through suitable media; also the passage of electrical currents and nerve impulses through body tissues—**conductivity** *n*.

con·ductor (kon-duk'-tor) *n* a substance or medium which transmits heat, light, sound, electric current, etc. The words bad, good or nonconductor designate the degree of conductivity.

condyl·oma (kon-dil-ō'-mà) *n* papilloma*. *Condylomata acuminato* are acuminate (pointed) dry warts found under prepuce (male), on the vulva and vestibule (female) or on the skin of the perianal region (both sexes). *Condylomata lata* are highly infectious, moist, warty excrescences found in moist areas of the body (vulva, anus, axilla etc) as a manifestation of late secondary syphilis*—**condylomata** *pl*. **condylomatous** *adj*.

confabu·lation (kon-fab-ū-lā'-shun) *n* a symptom common in confusional states when there is impairment of memory for recent events. The gaps in the patient's memory are filled in with fabrications of his own invention, which nevertheless he appears to accept as fact. Occurs in senile and toxic confusional states, cerebral trauma and Korsakoff* syndrome.

confec·tion (kon-fek'-shun) *n* a preparation in which drugs are mixed with sugar, syrup and honey.

con·flict (kon'-flikt) *n* in psychiatry, presence of two incompatible and contrasting wishes or emotions. When the conflict becomes intolerable, repression* of the wishes may occur. Mental conflict and repression form the basic causes of many neuroses, especially hysteria.

con·fluence (kon'-flū-ens) *n* becoming merged; flowing together; a uniting, as of neighboring pustules—**confluent** *adj*.

con·fusion (kon-fū-zhun) *n* a mental state which is out of touch with reality and associated with a clouding of consciousness. Can occur in many illnesses but particularly associated with post-epileptic fits, cerebral arteriosclerosis, dementia, infection, trauma and severe toxemia.

con·genital (kon-jen'-it-al) *adj* of abnormal conditions, present at birth, often genetically determined ⇒ genetic. *congenital dislocation of the hip* is due to laxity of the hip capsule. Recognized in the neonate by limitation of hip abduction. *congenital heart disease* developmental abnormalities in the anatomy of the heart, resulting postnatally in imperfect circulation of blood and often manifested by murmurs, cyanosis, breathlessness and sweating. Later there may be clubbing of the fingers ⇒ 'blue baby'. *congenital syphilis* ⇒ syphilis.

conges·tion (kon-jest'-yun) *n* hyperemia*. Passive congestion results from obstruction or slowing down of venous return, as in the lower limbs or the lungs—**congestive** *adj*. **congest** *vi, vt*.

69

con·gestive heart fail·ure a chronic inability of the heart to maintain an adequate output of blood from one or both ventricles resulting in manifest congestion and overdistension of certain veins and organs with blood, and in an inadequate blood supply to the body tissues.

coniz·ation (kŏn-īz-ā'-shun) *n* removal of a cone-shaped part of the cervix by the knife or cautery.

con·jugate (kon'-jū-gāt) *n* a measurement of the bony pelvis. *diagonal conjugate* the clinical measurement taken in pelvic assessment, from the lower border of the symphysis pubis to the sacral promontory = 12.5 cm. It is 1.5–2 cm. greater than *obstetrical conjugate*, the available space for the fetal head, i.e. the distance from the sacral promontory to the posterior surface of the top of the symphysis pubis = 10.6 cm. *true conjugate* the distance from the sacral promontory to the summit of the symphysis pubis = 11 cm.

conjunc·tiva (kon-jungk-tī'-vá) *n* the delicate transparent membrane which lines the inner surface of the eyelids (palpebral conjunctiva) and reflects over the front of the eyeball (bulbar or ocular conjunctiva)—**conjunctival** *adj*.

conjuncti·vitis (kon-jungk-ti-vī'-tis) *n* inflammation of the conjunctiva ⇒ pinkeye. TRIC. *inclusion conjunctivitis* (*syn* inclusion blennorrhea) occurs in countries with low standards of hygiene. The reservoir of infection is the urogenital tract ⇒ TRIC.

Conn syn·drome (kon) hyperplasia or adenoma of the adrenal cortex producing increased aldosterone*. Results in hypertension, hypokalemia and muscular weakness.

Conradi–·Hüner·mann syn·drome (konrad'-ē hun'-èr-man) a skeletal dysplasia which is genetically transmitted as an autosomal dominant trait. Skeletal abnormalities are variable; they are present at birth. After the first few weeks, life expectancy is normal. Mental development is not retarded.

con·sanguin·ity (kon-sang-gwin'-i-tē) *n* blood relationship. This varies in degree from close (as between siblings) to less close (as between cousins etc)—**consanguineous** *adj*.

conserva·tive treat·ment (kon-sèr'-va-tiv) aims at preventing a condition from becoming worse without using radical measures.

consoli·dation (kon-sol-id-ā'-shun) *n* becoming solid, as, for instance, the state of the lung due to exudation and organization in lobar pneumonia.

consti·pation (kon-sti-pā'-shun) *n* an implied chronic condition of infrequent and often difficult evacuation of feces due to insufficient food or fluid intake, or to sluggish or disordered action of the bowel musculature or nerve supply, or to habitual failure to empty the rectum. *Acute constipation* signifies obstruction or paralysis of the gut of sudden onset.

consump·tion (kon-sump'-shun) *n* 1 act of consuming or using up. 2 a once popular term for pulmonary tuberculosis* (which 'consumed' the body)—**consumptive** *adj*.

con·tact (kon'-takt) *n* 1 direct or indirect exposure to infection. 2 a person who has been so exposed. *contact lens* of glass or plastic, worn under the eyelids in direct contact with conjunctiva (in place of eyeglasses) for therapeutic or cosmetic purposes.

con·tagious (kon-tāj'-us) *adj* capable of transmitting infection or of being transmitted.

contain·ment isol·ation (kon-tān'-ment ī-sō-lā'-shun) separation of a patient with any sort of infection to prevent spread of the condition to others. ⇒ exclusion isolation.

continu·ous ambu·latory perito·neal dialy·sis (CAPD) *n* the patient remains ambulant while on peritoneal* dialysis.

continu·ous posi·tive air·ways pres·sure (CPAP) a treatment for babies with a tendency to alveolar collapse from hyaline membrane disease. ⇒ respiratory distress syndrome.

continu·ous sub·cutaneous insul·in in·fusion the use of a pump to deliver a continuous controlled dose of insulin subcutaneously to achieve almost physiological control of diabetes mellitus. Currently it is used mainly in research programs.

contra·ceptive (kon-trá-sep'-tiv) *n. adj* describes an agent used to prevent conception, e.g. condom, spermicidal vaginal pessary or cream, rubber cervical cap, intrauterine device, ⇒ intrauterine device, combined oral contraceptive—**contraception** *n*.

con·tract (kon'-trakt) *vb* 1 draw together; shorten; decrease in size. 2 acquire by contagion or infection.

contrac·tile (kon-trak'-tīl) *adj* possessing the ability to shorten—usually when stimulated, special property of muscle tissue—**contractility** *n*.

contrac·tion (kon-trak'-shun) *n* shortening, especially applied to muscle fibers.

contrac·ture (kon-trak'-tūr) *n* shortening of muscle or scar tissue, producing deformity ⇒ Dupuytren's contracture, Volkmann's ischemic contracture.

contra·indication (kon-trȧ-in-dik-ā'-shun) *n* a sign or symptom suggesting that a certain line of treatment (usually used for that disease) should be discontinued or avoided.

contra·lateral (kon-trȧ-lat'-ėr-ȧl) *adj* on the opposite side—**contralaterally** *adv*.

contre-coup (kon'-tre-kōō) *n* injury or damage at a point opposite the impact, resulting from transmitted force. It can occur in an organ or part containing fluid, as the skull.

con·trolled-dose trans·dermal ab-sorp·tion of drugs application of a drug patch to the skin; gradual absorption gives a constant level in the blood.

con·trolled drugs drugs which are defined in the Drug Abuse Prevention and Control Act of 1971.

con·tusion (kon-tū'-zhun) *n* ⇒ bruise—**contuse** *vt*.

con·vection (kon-vek'-shun) *n* transfer of heat from the hotter to the colder part; the heated substance (air or fluid), being less dense, tends to rise. The colder portion, flowing in to be heated, rises in its turn; thus *convection currents* are set in motion.

con·version (kon-vėr'-zhun) *n* a psychological conflict* manifesting as a physical symptom.

con·volutions (kon-vol-ū'-shuns) *npl* folds, twists or coils as found in the intestine, renal tubules and the surface of the brain—**convoluted** *adj*.

con·vulsions (kon-vul'-shunz) *npl* involuntary contractions of muscles resulting from abnormal cerebral stimulation; there are many causes. They occur with or without loss of consciousness. *clonic convulsions* show alternating contraction and relaxation of muscle groups. *tonic convulsions* reveal sustained rigidity—**convulsive** *adj*.

con·vulsive ther·apy (kon-vul'-siv) electroconvulsive* therapy.

Cooley's anemia (kōō'-lēz ȧ-nē'-mē-ȧ) thalassemia*.

Coombs' test (kōōmz) a highly sensitive test used to detect antibodies to red blood cells; the 'direct' method detects those bound to the red cells; the 'indirect' method detects those circulating unbound in the serum. The 'direct' method is especially useful in the diagnosis of hemolytic syndromes.

co-ordi·nation (kō-ör-din-ā'-shun) *n* moving in harmony, *muscular coordination* is the harmonious action of muscles, permitting free, smooth and efficient movements under perfect control.

COPD *abbr* chronic obstructive pulmonary disease. ⇒ bronchitis.

cop·per (kop'-pėr) *n* essential trace element in all animal tissues, being a component of certain proteins and enzymes. Copper salts have little use in medicine except the sulfate which is used occasionally: (a) as an emetic (orally) in cases of phosphorus poisoning (b) for the treatment of phosphorus burns of the skin (topical application, 1% solution) and (c) as a catalyst with iron in the treatment of iron deficiency anemia. Copper sulfate is used in Benedict's and Fehling's tests to detect glucose in urine.

copro·lalia (kop-rō-lā'-lē-ȧ) *n* filthy or obscene speech. Occurs as a symptom most commonly in cerebral deterioration or trauma affecting frontal lobes of the brain.

copro·lith (kop'-rō'lith) *n* fecalith*.

copro·porphyrin (kop-rō-pȯr-fī'-rin) *n* naturally occurring porphyrin* in the feces, formed in the intestine from bilirubin.

copu·lation (kop-ū-lā'-shun) *n* coitus*.

coraco·brachialis muscle (kȯr-ȧ-kō-brā-kē-al'-is) ⇒ Figure 14.

Cor·amine (kȯr'-ȧ-mēn) *n* proprietary name for nikethamide*.

cord (kȯrd) *n* a thread-like structure. *spermatic cord* that which suspends the testicles in the scrotum. *spinal cord* a cord-like structure which lies in the spinal column, reaching from the foramen magnum to the first or second lumbar vertebra. It is a direct continuation of the medulla oblongata and is about 45 cm long in the adult. *umbilical cord* the navel-string, attaching the fetus to the placenta. *vocal cord* the membranous bands in the larynx, vibrations of which produce the voice.

cor·dectomy (kȯr-dek'-to-mē) *n* surgical excision of a cord, usually reserved for a vocal cord.

cor·dotomy (kȯr-dot'-o-mē) *n* (*syn* chordotomy) division of the anterolateral nerves in the spinal cord to relieve intractable pain in the pelvis or lower limbs.

core (kŏr) *n* central portion, usually applied to the slough in the center of a boil.

corn (kŏrn) *n* a painful, cone-shaped overgrowth and hardening of the epidermis, with the point of the cone in the deeper layers; it is produced by friction or pressure. A *hard corn* usually occurs over a toe joint. a *soft corn* occurs between the toes.

cor·nea (kŏr'-nē-à) *n* the outwardly convex transparent membrane forming part of the anterior outer coat of the eye. It is situated in front of the iris and pupil and merges backwards into the sclera (⇒ Figure 15)—**corneal** *adj*.

cor·neal graft (kŏr'-nē-al graft) (*syn* corneoplasty, keratoplasty) a corneal opacity is excised and replaced by healthy, transparent, human cornea from a donor.

corneo·plasty (kŏr-nē-ō-plas'-tē) *n* corneal* graft.

corneo·scleral (kŏr'-nē-ō-sklē'-ràl) *adj* pertaining to the cornea and sclera, as the circular junction of these structures.

coronal suture (kŏr'-ō-nàl sū'-chur) the transverse line of union between the parietal and frontal bones in the skull.

coron·ary (kŏr'-on-ār-ē) *adj* crown-like; encircling, as of a vessel or nerve. *coronary arteries* those supplying the heart, the first pair to be given off by the aorta as it leaves the left ventricle. Spasm or narrowing of these vessels produces angina pectoris. *coronary sinus* channel receiving most cardiac veins and opening into the right atrium. *coronary thrombosis* occlusion of a coronary vessel by a clot of blood. The area deprived of blood becomes necrotic and is called an infarct*. ⇒ ischemic heart disease, myocardial infarction.

corona·viruses (kŏr-ōn-à-vī'-rus-es) *npl* a group of viruses that can cause the common cold.

cor·oner (kŏr'-on-ėr) *n* a person who investigates the cause of death when violence is a possibility or suspected. When doubt exists a doctor is advised to consult the coroner and act on his advice. He must be notified if a patient is admitted to hospital and dies within 24 h. Likewise all surgery/anesthetic deaths must be reported to the coroner. Any death where the deceased has not consulted a doctor recently means that a coroner's postmortem may be ordered.

cor pulmon·ale (kŏr-pul-mon-al'-ē) heart disease following on disease of lung (em-

physema*, silocosis* etc.) which strains the right ventricle.

cor·pus (kŏr'-pus) *n* any mass of tissue which is easily distinguishable from its surroundings—**corpora** *pl*. *corpus callosum* ⇒ Figure 1. *corpus cavernosa* ⇒ Figure 16. *corpus luteum* ⇒ luteum. *corpus quadrigemina* ⇒ Figure 1. *corpus spongiosum* ⇒ Figure 16.

cor·puscle (kŏr'-pus-l) *n* a microscopic mass of protoplasm. There are many varieties but the word generally refers to the red and white blood cells—**corpuscular** *adj*. ⇒ erythrocytes, leukocytes.

correc·tive (kŏr-ek'-tiv) *adj, n* something which changes, counteracts or modifies something harmful.

Corrigan's pulse (kŏr'-i-gans) the waterhammer pulse of aortic incompetence with high initial upthrust, which quickly falls away.

cor·tex (kŏr'-teks) **1** the outer bark or covering of a plant. **2** the outer layer of an organ beneath its capsule or membrane—**cortices** *pl*. **cortical** *adj*. *cortex of the cerebellum* ⇒ Figure 1. *cortex of the kidney* ⇒ Figure 20.

corticoids (kŏr'-ti-koyds) *npl* a name for the several groups of natural hormones produced by the adrenal cortex and for synthetic compounds with similar actions.

corti·coster·oids (kŏr-tik-ō-ster'-oyds) *npl* hormones produced by the adrenal cortex. The word is also used for synthetic steroids such as prednisolone* and dexamethasone*.

cortico·trophin, corticotropin (kŏr-ti-kō-trōf'-in) *n* the hormone of the anterior pituitary gland which specifically stimulates the adrenal cortex to produce corticosteroids. Synthetic 1–34 corticotrophin is available as tetracosactrin*, given by injection, usually for test purposes.

corti·sol (kŏr'-ti-zol) *n* hydrocortisone, one of the principal adrenal cortical steroids. It is increased in Cushing's disease and syndrome and decreased in Addison's disease. It is essential to life. It is given as physiological replacement treatment in Addison's disease and hypopituarism. Synthetic steroids such as prednisolone* and dexamethasone* are usually used when larger doses are required for antiinflammatory or immunosuppressive purposes, e.g. in asthma, some skin conditions or following transplant surgery.

corti·sone (kŏr'-ti-zōn) *n* one of the hormones of the adrenal gland. It is converted into cortisol* before use by the body. *cortisone suppression test* differentiates primary from secondary hypercalcemia*. Sarcoidosis causes secondary hypercalcemia; primary hyperparathyroidism causes primary hypercalcemia.

Cortisporin (kŏr-ti-spōr'-in) *n* an antibacterial preparation containing Polymixin B, Neomycin, Bacitracin and Hydrocortisone; comes in the form of cream, ointment or eye drops.

Coryne·bacterium (kŏr-nē-bak-tēr'-ē-um) *n* a bacterial genus: Gram-positive, rod-shaped bacteria averaging 3 μm in length, showing irregular staining in segments (metachromatic granules). Many strains are parasitic and some are pathogenic, e.g. *Corynebacterium diphtheriae*, producing a powerful exotoxin.

cor·yza (kŏr-ī'-zà) *n* an acute upper respiratory infection of short duration; highly contagious; causative viruses include rhinoviruses, coronaviruses and adenoviruses.

Corzide (kŏr'-zīd) *n* proprietary name for bendroflumethazide.

cos·metic (kos-met'-ik) *adj, n* that which is done to improve the appearance or prevent disfigurement.

Cosmogen (kos'-mō-jen) *n* proprietary name for dactinomycin.

cos·tal (kos'-tal) *adj* pertaining to the ribs. *costal cartilages* those which attach the ribs to the sternum.

cos·tive (kos'-tiv) *adj* lay term for constipated. ⇒ constipation—**costiveness** *n*.

costo·chondral (kos-tō-kon'-dràl) *adj* pertaining to a rib and its cartilage.

costo·chondritis (kos-tō-kon-drī'-tis) *n* inflammation of the costochondral cartilage. ⇒ Tietze syndrome.

costo·clavicular (kos-tō-klav-ik'-ū-làr) *adj* pertaining to the ribs and the clavicle. *costoclavicular syndrome* is a synonym for cervical rib syndrome ⇒ cervical.

Cota·zym (kot'-à-zim) *n* a proprietary pancreatic enzyme preparation.

co-trimox·azole (kō-trī-moks'-à-zōl) *n* an antibacterial agent comprising sulfamethoxazole*, an early folic acid blocking agent, and trimethoprim*, a late folic acid blocking agent. It is particularly useful for urinary infections. (Bactrim, Septra.)

coty·ledon (kot-il-ē'-don) *n* one of the subdivisions of the uterine surface of the placenta*.

Coumadin (kōō'-mà-din) *n* derivative of dicoumarol*.

counsel·ing (kown'-sel-ing) *n* a professional helping relationship with a client who is experiencing psychological problems. The counselor listens actively and helps the client to identify and clarify the problems and supports him as he makes a positive attempt to overcome them.

counter·irritant (kown-tèr-ir'-it-ant) *n* an agent which, when applied to the skin, produces a mild inflammatory reaction (hyperemia) and relief of pain and congestion associated with a more deep-seated inflammatory process—**counter-irritation** *n*.

counter·traction (kown-ter-trak'-shun) *n* traction upon the proximal extremity of a fractured limb opposing the pull of the traction apparatus on the distal extremity.

cou·vade (kōō-vahd') *n* a custom in some cultures whereby a father exhibits the symptoms of his partner's pregnancy and childbirth.

Cowper's glands (kow'-perz) bulbourethral* glands.

cowpox (kow'-poks) *n* vaccinia; virus disease of cows. Lymph is used in vaccination of humans against smallpox (variola).

coxa (koks'-à) *n* the hip joint—**coxae** *pl*. *coxa valga* an increase in the normal angle between neck and shaft of femur. *coxa vara* a decrease in the normal angle plus torsion of the neck, e.g. slipped femoral epiphysis.

cox·algia (koks-al'-jē-à) *n* pain in the hip joint.

Cox·iella (koks-ē-el'-là) *n* a genus closely related to *Rickettsia* including *Coxiella burneti* which causes Q fever.

cox·itis (koks-īt'-is) *n* inflammation of the hip joint.

cox·sackie virus (koks'-ak-ē vī'-rus) *n* first isolated at Coxsackie, NY. One of the three groups included in the family of enteroviruses. Divided into groups A and B. Many in group A appear to be non-pathogenic. Others cause aseptic meningitis and herpangina. Those in group B also cause aseptic meningitis Bornholm* disease and myocarditis.

CPAP *abbr* continuous* positive airways pressure.

73

CPD *abbr* cephalopelvic* disproportion.

CPK *abbr* creatinephosphokinase ⇒ creatine kinase.

CPR *abbr* cardiopulmonary resuscitation. ⇒ resuscitation.

crab louse pediculus* pubis.

cradle cap (krā'-dl kap) *n* scaling of the scalp of infants, often due to atopic dermatitis* or seborrheic dermatitis.

cramp *n* spasmodic contraction of a muscle or group of muscles; involuntary and painful; may result from fatigue. Occurs in tetany, food poisoning and cholera. *occupational cramp* is such as occurs amongst miners and other workers who use the same muscles continuously.

cranial (krā'-nē-ȧl) *adj* pertaining to the cranium*.

cranio·facial (krā-nē-ō-fā'-shȧl) *adj* pertaining to the cranium and the face. *craniofacial resection* a relatively new procedure which can be used in all age groups for the removal of paranasal sinus tumors, particularly those inaccessible through a usual nasal approach. It avoids the need for a total neurosurgical approach.

crani·ometry (krā-nē-om'-et-rē) *n* the science which deals with the measurement of skulls.

cranio·pharyngioma (krā-nē-ō-fār-in-jē-ōm'-ȧ) *n* a tumor which develops between the brain and the pituitary gland.

cranio·plasty (krā-nē-ō-plas'-tē) *n* operative repair of a skull defect—**cranioplastic** *adj*.

cranio·sacral (krā-nē-ō-sāk'-rȧl) *adj* pertaining to the skull and sacrum. Applied to the parasympathetic nervous system.

cranio·stenosis (krā-nē-ō-sten-ōs'-is) *n* a condition in which the skull sutures fuse too early and the fontanels close. It may cause increased intracranial pressure requiring surgery.

cranio·synostosis (krā-nē-ō-sin-ō-stō'-sis) *n* premature ossification of skull bones with closure of suture lines, giving rise to facial deformities. ⇒ Apert syndrome.

cranio·tabes (krā-nē-ō-tā'-bēz) *n* a thinning or wasting of the cranial bones occurring in infancy and usually due to rickets*—**craniotabetic** *adj*.

crani·otomy (krā-nē-ot'-o-mē) *n* a surgical opening of the skull in order to remove a growth, relieve pressure, evacuate blood clot or arrest hemorrhage.

cran·ium (krā'-nē-um) *n* the part of the skull enclosing the brain. It is composed of eight bones: the occipital, two parietals, frontal, two temporals, sphenoid and ethmoid—**cranial** *adj*.

c-reactive protein test c-reactive protein is a normal constituent of plasma; it is raised in bacterial meningitis.

cream of tartar *n* potassium bitartrate.

creatin·ase (krē-at'-in-ās) *n* ⇒ creatine kinase.

cre·atine (krē'-at-ēn) *n* a nitrogenous compound synthesized in vitro. *Phosphonylated creatine* is an important storage form of high-energy phosphate. *creat·ine kin·ase* (*syn* ATP: creatine phosphotransferase) occurs as three isoenzymes each having two components labelled M and B; the form in brain tissue is BB, in skeletal muscle and serum MM and in myocardial tissue both MM and MB. *creatine kinase test* the MB isoenzyme is raised in serum only in acute myocardial infarction and not in other cardiopathies. *creatine test* estimation of the amount of creatine in the blood. Serum creatine is raised in hyperthyroidism and values above 0.6 mg per 100 ml of blood (40 μmol/l) suggest hyperthyroidism. It is also raised in muscle wasting disorders and in renal failure.

creat·inine (krē-at'-in-ēn) *n* an anhydride of creatine*, a waste product of protein (endogenous) metabolism found in muscle and blood and excreted in normal urine.

creatin·uria (krē-at-in-ūr'-rē-ȧ) *n* an excess of the nitrogenous compound creatine* in the urine. Occurs in conditions in which muscle is rapidly broken down, e.g. acute fevers, starvation.

creator·rhea (krē-at-ōr-ē'-ȧ) *n* the presence of excessive nitrogen in the feces. It occurs particularly in pancreatic dysfunction.

Crede's method (krē-dāz') a method of delivering the placenta by gently rubbing the fundus uteri until it contracts and then, by squeezing the fundus, expressing the placenta into the vagina whence it is expelled.

creosote (krē'-ō-sōt) *n* a phenolic antiseptic obtained from beechwood. Occasionally used as an antiseptic deodorant and expectorant.

crepi·tation (krep-i-tā'-shun) *n* **1** (crepitus) grating of bone ends in fracture. **2** crackling sound in joints, e.g. in osteoarthritis. **3** crackling sound heard via stethoscope. **4** crackling sound elicited by pressure on tissue containing air (surgical emphysema).

cre·sol (krē'-sol) *n* chemically related to phenol* but it is a more powerful germicide. Cresol and/or related phenols are present in a wide range of general disinfectants.

cretin·ism (krē'-tin-izm) *n* due to congenital thyroid deficiency; results in a dull-looking child, underdeveloped mentally and physically, dwarfed, large head, thick legs, pug nose, dry skin, scanty hair, swollen eyelids, short neck, short thick limbs, clumsy uncoordinated gait—**cretin** *n*.

Creutz-feldt-Jakob dis·ease (krutz'-feld-Jā'-kob) a presenile dementia and psychosis; the cause is now thought to be a transmissible agent known as a 'slow virus'.

CRF *abbr* chronic renal failure. ⇒ renal.

crib death (*syn* sudden infant death syndrome) the unexpected sudden death of an infant, usually occurring overnight while sleeping in a crib. The commonest mode of death in infants between the ages of 1 month and 1 year, neither clinical nor post-mortem findings being adequate to account for death. Commoner in late winter among low-birth-weight male infants around the age of 2 months.

cribri·form (krib'-ri-fōrm) *adj* perforated, like a sieve. *cribriform plate* that portion of the ethmoid bone allowing passage of fibers of olfactory nerve.

cri·coid (krī'-koyd) *adj* ring-shaped. Applied to the cartilage forming the inferior posterior part of larynx.

'cri du chat' syn·drome (krē-dū-shah') produced by partial loss of one of the number 5 chromosomes leading to mental subnormality. There are certain physical abnormalities and a curious flat, toneless cat-like cry in infancy.

crimi·nal abor·tion (krim'-in-al ab-ōr'-shun) ⇒ abortion.

crisis (krī'-sis) **1** the turning point of a disease—as the point of defervescence in fever, the arrest of an anemia. ⇒ lysis *opp*. **2** muscular spasm in tabes dorsalis referred to as visceral crisis (gastric, vesical, rectal, etc.)—**crises** *pl*.

Crohn's dis·ease (krōnz) ⇒ regional ileitis.

cromolyn sodium (krōm'-ō-lin sō'-dē-um) an antihypersensitivity agent useful in prevention of asthma in some individuals with allergic responses. (In tal.)

Crosby cap·sule (kroz'-bē) a special tube

which is passed through the mouth to the small intestine; maneuver of the tube selects tissue for biopsy.

cross infec·tion ⇒ infection.

crota·miton (krō-tà-mī'-ton) *n* an agent which is effective for scabies, especially in infants, as it kills the mite and prevents itching. (Eurax.)

croup (kroop) *n* laryngeal obstruction. Croupy breathing in a child is often called 'stridulous', meaning noisy or harsh-sounding. Narrowing of the airway which gives rise to the typical attack with crowing inspiration may be the result of edema or spasm, or both.

CRP *abbr* ⇒ c-reaction protein test.

cru·ciate (kroo'-shē-āt) *adj* shaped like a cross.

crus (kroos) *n* a structure which is leg-like or root-like. Applied to various parts of body, e.g. crus of the diaphragm—**crura** *pl*. **crural** *adj*.

'crush' syn·drome traumatic uremia. Following an extensive trauma to muscle, there is a period of delay before the effects of renal damage manifest themselves. There is an increase of non-protein nitrogen in the blood, with oliguria, proteinuria and urinary excretion of myohemoglobin. Loss of blood plasma to damaged area is marked. Where hypotension has occurred the renal failure will be exacerbated by tubular* necrosis.

crutch palsy paralysis* of extensor muscles of wrist, fingers and thumb from repeated pressure of a crutch upon the radial nerve in the axilla.

cry·esthesia (krī-es-thē'-zē-à) *n* **1** the sensation of coldness. **2** exceptional sensitivity to a low temperature.

cryo·analgesia (krī-ō-an-al-jē'-zē-à) *n* relief of pain achieved by use of a cryosurgical probe to block peripheral nerve function.

cryo·extractor (krī-ō-eks-trak'-tor) *n* a type of cryoprobe* used for removal of a cataractous lens.

cryo·genic (krī-ō-jen'-ik) *adj, n* anything produced by low temperature. Also used to describe any means or apparatus involved in the production of low temperature.

cryo·globulins (krī-ō-glob'-ū-lins) *n* abnormal proteins—immunoglobulins—which may be present in the blood in some diseases. Their characteristic is that they are insoluble at low temperatures which can lead to obstruction of small blood vessels such as those in the fingers and toes.

cry·opexy (krī'-ō-peks-ē) *n* surgical fixation by freezing, as replacement of a detached retina.

cryo·phake (krī'-ō-fāk) *n* cataract extraction using freezing.

cryo·precipi·tate therapy (krī-ō-prē-sip'-i-tāt) use of Factor VIII to prevent or treat bleeding in hemophilia. The term refers to the preparation of Factor VIII for injection. Subarctic temperatures make it separate from plasma. $\Rightarrow$ blood clotting.

cryo·probe (krī'-ō-prōb) *n* freezing probe. Can be used for biopsy. A flexible metal tube attached to liquid nitrogen equipment. The cryoprobe has tips of various sizes which can be cooled to a temperature of $-180°C$. Causes less tissue trauma and 'seeding' of malignant cells.

cryo·surgery (krī-ō-sur'-je-rē) *n* the use of intense, controlled cold to remove or destroy diseased tissue. Instead of a knife a cryoprobe* is used.

cryo·thalamec·tomy (krī-ō-thal-a-mek'-to-mē) *n* freezing applied to destroy groups of neurons within the thalamus in the treatment of Parkinson's disease and other hyperkinetic conditions.

cryo·therapy (krī-ō-ther'-á-pē) *n* the use of cold for the treatment of disease.

crypto·coccosis (krip-tō-kok-ō'-sis) *n* the disease resulting from infection of a human with the yeast *Cryptococcus neoformans*. It has a marked predilection for the central nervous system causing subacute or chronic disease.

Crypto·coccus (krip-tō-kok'-kus) *n* a genus of fungi. *Cryptococcus neoformans* is pathogenic to man.

crypto·genic (krip-tō-jen'-ik) *adj* of unknown or obscure cause.

crypto·menorrhea (krip-tō-men-ōr-ē'-á) *n* retention of the menses due to a congenital obstruction, such as an imperforate hymen or atresia of the vagina. $\Rightarrow$ hematocolpos.

crypt·orchism (krip-tor'-kizm) *n* a developmental defect whereby the testes do not descend into the scrotum; they are retained within the abdomen or inguinal canal—**cryptorchid, cryptorchis** *n*.

crys·tal violet (kris'-tal vī'-ō-let) *n* (*syn* gentian violet) a brilliant, violet-colored, antiseptic aniline dye, used as 0.5% solution for ulcers and skin infections and also as a stain.

crystal·lin (kris'-tá-lin) *n* a globulin*, principal constituent of the lens of the eye.

crystal·line (kris'-tá-lēn) *adj* like a crystal; transparent. Applied to various structures. *crystalline lens* a biconvex body, oval in shape, which is suspended just behind the iris of the eye, and separates the aqueous from the vitreous humor. It is slightly less convex on its anterior surface and it refracts the light rays so that they focus directly on the retina.

crystal·luria (kris-tá-lū'-rē-à) *n* excretion of crystals in the urine—**crystalluric** *adj*.

Crystodigin (kris-tō-dij'-in) *n* proprietary name for digitoxin*.

CSF *abbr* cerebrospinal* fluid.

CSII *abbr* continuous* subcutaneous insulin infusion.

CSSD *abbr* central sterile supplies department.

CSSU *abbr* central sterile supply unit.

CT *abbr* computed* tomography.

CTAB *abbr* cetyltrimethylammonium bromide—i.e. cetrimide*.

CTG *abbr* cardiotocograph*.

cubi·tal tun·nel exter·nal com·pression syn·drome ulnar paralysis* resulting from compression of the ulnar nerve within the cubital tunnel situated on the inner and posterior aspect of the elbow—sometimes referred to as the 'funny bone'.

cubi·tal vein (kū'-bi-tal) $\Rightarrow$ Figure 9.

cubi·tus (kū'-bi-tus) *n* the forearm; elbow—**cubital** *adj*.

cu·boid (kū'-boyd) *adj* shaped like a cube.

cuir·ass (kwir-as') *n* a mechanical apparatus fitted to the chest for artificial respiration.

cul de sac (kul-de-sak') *n* a blind cavity or pouch. *cul de sac of Douglas* an extension of the peritoneal cavity which lies behind the uterus between the posterior uterine wall and the rectum.

culdo·centesis *n* aspiration of the cul de sac of Douglas via the posterior vaginal wall.

culdo·scope (kul'-do-skōp) *n* an endoscope* used via the vaginal route.

culd·oscopy (kul-dos'-kō-pe) *n* a form of peritoneoscopy or laparoscopy. Passage of a culdoscope* through the posterior vaginal fornix, behind the uterus to enter the peritoneal cavity, for viewing same—**culdoscopic** *adj*. **culdoscopically** *adv*.

cul·ture (kul'-tūr) *n* the growth of microorganisms on artificial media under ideal conditions.

cumu·lative action (kŭm'-ū-là-tiv) if the dose of a slowly excreted drug is repeated too frequently, an increasing action is obtained. This can be dangerous as, if the drug accumulates in the system, toxic symptoms may occur, sometimes quite suddenly. Long acting barbiturates, strychnine, mercurial salts and digitalis are examples of drugs with a cumulative action.

cup·ping (kup'-ping) *n* a method of counterirritation. A small bell-shaped glass (in which the air is expanded by heating, or exhausted by compression of an attached rubber bulb) is applied to the skin, resultant suction producing hyperemia—*dry cupping*. When the skin is scarified before application of the cup it is termed *wet cupping*.

cu·rare (kū-ràr'-ē) *n* the crude extract from which tubocurarine* is obtained.

curet·tage (kūr-ett-azh') *n* the scraping of unhealthy or exuberant tissue from a cavity. This may be treatment or may be done to establish a diagnosis after laboratory analysis of the scrapings.

cu·rette (kūr-et') *n* a spoon-shaped instrument or a metal loop which may have sharp, and/or blunt edges for scraping out (curetting) cavities.

curet·tings (kū-ret'-ingz) *npl* the material obtained by scraping or curetting and usually sent for examination in the pathology department.

Curling's ulcer (kur'-lingz ul'-ser) an ulcer* which occurs either in the stomach or duodenum as a complication of extensive burns or scalds.

cushing·oid (koosh'-ing-oyd) *adj* used to describe the moon face and central obesity common in people with elevated levels of plasma corticosteroid from whatever cause.

Cushing's dis·ease (koosh'-ingz) a rare disorder, mainly of females, characterized principally by functional obesity, hyperglycemia, glycosuria, hypertension and hirsutism. Due to excessive cortisol production by hyperplastic adrenal glands as a result of increased corticotrophin secretion by a tumor or hyperplasia of the anterior pituitary gland.

Cushing's reflex (koosh'-ingz) a rise in blood pressure and a fall in pulse rate; occurs in cerebral space-occupying lesions.

Cushing's syn·drome (koosh'-ingz) a disorder clinically similar to Cushing's* disease and also due to elevated levels of plasma corticosteroid, but where the primary pathology is not in the pituitary gland. It can be due to adenoma or carcinoma of the adrenal cortex and to the secretion of ACTH* by non-endocrine tumors such as bronchial carcinoma. It can also be iatrogenic due to excessive administratiion of corticosteroids.

cusp (kusp) *n* a projecting point, such as the edge of a tooth or the segment of a heart valve. The cardiac tricuspid valve has three, the mitral valve two cusps.

cu·taneous (kū-tān'-ē-us) *adj* relating to the skin. *cu·taneous nerve* ⇒ Figure 12. *cu·taneous ureter·ostomy* the ureters are transplanted so that they open on to the skin of the abdominal wall.

cut·icle (kū'-tik-l) *n* the epidermis* or dead epidermis, as that which surrounds a nail—**cuticular** *adj*.

CVA *abbr* cerebrovascular* accident.

CVP *abbr* central* venous pressure.

cyan·ocobalamin (sī-an-ō-kō-bal'-a-mēn) *n* vitamin* B$_{12}$, found in liver, fish, meat and eggs. Needed for maturation of erythrocytes. It can only be absorbed in the presence of the intrinsic* factor secreted in the gastric juice. ⇒ cobalamin.

cyan·osis (sī-an-ō'-sis) *n* a bluish tinge manifested by hypoxic tissue, observed most frequently under the nails, lips and skin. It is always due to lack of oxygen, and the causes of this are legion—**cyanosed, cyanotic** *adj*. *central cyanosis* blueness seen on the warm surfaces such as the oral mucosa and tongue. It increases with exertion. *peripheral cyanosis* blueness of the limb extremities, the nose and the ear lobes.

cycla·mates (sī'-kla-māts) *npl* salts of cyclamic acid which are 30 times as sweet as sugar and are stable to heat. Banned as food additives because they were suspected of causing cancer.

cyclan·delate (sī-klan-del'-āt) *n* a vasodilator used particularly for cerebral vascular disorders. (Cyclospasmol.)

cycle (sī'-kl) *n* a regular series of movements or events; a sequence which recurs ⇒ cardiac. menstrual—**cyclic** *adj*.

cycli·cal syn·drome (si'-klik-al) some people prefer this term to that of premenstrual* syndrome, because it emphasizes that these symptoms are due to normal physiological interaction between several endocrine glands under the cyclical control of the hypothalamus and pituitary.

cycli·cal vomit·ing (si'-klik-al vom'-it-ing) periodic attacks of vomiting in children, usually associated with ketosis and usually with no demonstrable pathological cause. Occurs mainly in highly-strung children.

cy·clitis (sī-klī'-tis) n inflammation of the ciliary body of the eye, shown by deposition of small collections of white cells on the posterior cornea called 'keratitic precipitates' (KP). Often co-existent with inflammation of the iris. ⇒ iridocyclitis.

cy·clizine (sī'-kli-zēn) n an antihistamine. (Marezine.)

cyclobenzaprine (sī-klō-benz'-à-prēn) n a muscle relaxant. (Flexeril.)

cyclo·dialysis (sī-klō-dī-al'-is-is) n establishment of communication between anterior chamber and perichoroidal or suprachoroidal space to relieve intraocular pressure in glaucoma.

cyclo·diathermy (sī-klō-dī-à-thèr'-mē) n destruction of the ciliary body by diathermy*.

Cyclogyl (sī'-klō-jl) n proprietary name for cyclopentolate hydrochloride*.

cyclo·pentolate hydro·chloride (sī-klō-pen'-tō-lāt hī-drō-klōr'-īd) a synthetic, spasmolytic drug. Causes cycloplegia and mydriasis. (Cyclogyl.)

cyclo·phosphamide (sī-klō-fos'-fà-mīd) n a cytotoxic agent, a nitrogen mustard. Alkylating agent that interferes with synthesis of nucleic acid in cell chromosomes, particularly in rapidly dividing cells such as those which occur in bone marrow, skin, gastrointestinal tract and fetal tissues. The main side effects therefore occur in these tissues causing anorexia, nausea, vomiting, diarrhea, depression of bone marrow and alopecia. Main indications are malignancy of lymphoid tissue. (Cytoxan.)

cyclo·plegia (sī-klō-pē'-jē-à) n paralysis of the ciliary muscle of the eye—**cyclo·plegic** adj.

cyclo·plegics (sī-klō-pē'-jiks) npl drugs which cause paralysis of the ciliary muscle, e.g. atropine, homatropine, and scopolamine.

cyclopropane (sī-klō-prō'-pān) n a highly inflammable, gaseous anesthetic, supplied in orange-colored cylinders. Induction is rapid and recovery prompt. Used with closed circuit system apparatus. Largely discontinued.

cyclo·serine (sī-klō-sēr'-ēn) n an antibiotic which is active against many microorganisms. Its main use is for severe pulmonary tuberculosis caused by microorganisms which are resistant to other antitubercular drugs. It must be used together with other antitubercular compounds.

Cyclo·spasmol (sī-klō-spaz'-mol) n proprietary name for cyclandelate*.

cyclo·sporine (sī-klō-spōr'-ēn) n a selective immunosuppressive agent which does not suppress the production of antibodies. It is used prophylactically in graft versus lost reactions. (Sandimmune.)

cyclo·thymia (sī-klō-thī'-mē-à) n a tendency to alternating but relatively mild mood swings between elation and depression—**cyclothymic** adj.

cyclot·omy (sī-klot'-o-mē) n a drainage operation for the relief of glaucoma, consisting of an incision through the ciliary body.

cyclo·tron (sī'-clō-tron) n an apparatus in which radioactive isotopes can be prepared.

cy·esis (sī-ē'-sis) n pregnancy. When there are signs and symptoms of pregnancy in a woman who believes she is pregnant, and this is not so, it is called pseudocyesis. ⇒ phantom pregnancy.

cylin·droma (sil-in-drō'-mà) a tumor of the endothelial element of apocrine tissue such as a sweat gland or a salivary gland. The supporting stroma is hyalinized.

cyllosis (sil-ō'-sis) n club foot.

cyproheptadine (sī-prō-hep'-tà-dēn) n an antihistamine* with antiserotonin* action. (Periactin.)

cyst (sist) n a sac with membranous wall, enclosing fluid or semisolid matter—**cystic** adj.

cyst·adenoma (sist-ad-en-ō'-mà) n an innocent cystic new growth of glandular tissue. Liable to occur in the female breast.

cyst·algia (sist-al'-jē-à) n pain in the urinary bladder.

cyst·athion·inuria (sist-à-thī-on-in-ū'-rē-à) n inherited disorder of cystathionine metabolism marked by excessive excretion of cystathionine in the urine, an intermediate product in conversion of methionine to cysteine. Sometimes associated with mental subnormality.

cys·tectomy (sis-tek'-to-mē) n usually refers to the removal of part or the whole of the urinary bladder. This necessitates urinary diversion. The ureters may then be implanted into an isolated ileal segment (ileal conduit) or into the sigmoid colon.

cys·teine (sis'-tē-in) *n* a sulfur-containing amino acid produced by the breaking down of proteins during the digestive process. Easily oxidized to cystine*.

cysti·cercosis (sis-ti-sėr-kō'-sis) *n* infection of man with cysticercus*.

cysti·cercus (sis-ti-sėr'-kus) *n* the larval form of taenia*. After ingestion, the ova do not develop beyond this form in man, but form 'cysts' in subcutaneous tissues, skeletal muscles and the brain where they provoke epilepsy.

cys·tic fi·brosis (sis'-tik fī-brō'-sis) (*syn* fibrocystic disease of the pancreas, mucoviscidosis) the commonest genetically-determined disease in Caucasian populations; there is abnormality of secretion of the exocrine glands. Thick mucus can block the intestinal glands and cause meconium ileus in a baby; later it can cause steatorrhea, creatorrhea and malabsorption. Thick mucus in the respiratory glands predisposes to repeated infections and bronchiectasis. Abnormality of the sweat glands increases the chloride content of sweat which is a diagnostic tool. ⇒ sweat test.

cys·tine (sis'-tēn) *n* sulfur-containing amino acid, produced by the breakdown of proteins during the digestive process. It is readily reduced to two molecules of cysteine*.

cystin·osis (sis-tin-ō'-sis) *n* a recessively inherited metabolic disorder in which crystalline cystine* is deposited in the body. Cystine and other aminoacids are excreted in the urine.

cystin·uria (sis-tin-ū'-rē-à) *n* metabolic disorder in which cystine* and other amino acids appear in the urine. A cause of renal stones—**cystinuric** *adj*.

cys·titis (sis-tī'-tis) *n* inflammation of the urinary bladder; cause is usually bacterial. The condition may be acute or chronic, primary or secondary to stones, etc. More frequent in females, as the urethra is short.

cys·titome (sis'-ti-tōm) *n* delicate ophthalmic instrument for incision of the lens capsule.

cysto·cele (sis'-tō-sēl) *n* prolapse of the posterior wall of the urinary bladder into the anterior vaginal wall. ⇒ colporrhaphy.

cysto·diathermy (sis'-tō-dī-ath-ėr'-mē) *n* the application of a cauterizing electrical current to the walls of the urinary blad-

der through a cystoscope, or by open operation.

cyst·ography (sis-tog'-ra-fē) *n* radiographic examination of the urinary bladder, after it has been filled with a contrast medium—**cystographic** *adj*, **cystograph** *n*, **cystogram** *n*, **cystographically** *adv*.

cysto·lithiasis (sis-tō-lith-ī'-à-sis) *n* the presence of a stone or stones in the urinary bladder.

cyst·ometer (sis-to'-me-tėr) *n* an apparatus for measuring the pressure under various conditions in the urinary bladder.

cysto·metro·gram (sis-tō-met'-rō-gram) *n* a record of the changes in pressure within the urinary bladder under various conditions; used in the study of voiding disorders.

cyst·ometry (sis-to'-me-trē) *n* the study of pressure changes within the urinary bladder—**cystometric** *adj*.

cysto·pexy (sis'-tō-peks-ē) *n* a 'sling' operation for stress incontinence whereby the bladder neck is supported from the back of the symphysis pubis.

cysto·plasty (sis'-tō-plas-tē) *n* surgical repair of the urinary bladder—**cystoplastic** *adj*.

cysto·scope (sis'-tō-skōp) *n* an endoscope* used in diagnosis and treatment of bladder, ureter and kidney conditions—**cystoscopic** *adj*. **cystoscopically** *adv*.

cyst·oscopy (sis-tos'-kō-pē) *n* use of a cystoscope* to view the internal surface of the urinary bladder. It can also incorporate a biopsy or fulguration of a bladder tumor.

cyst·ostomy (sis-tos'-to-mē) *n* (*syn* vesicostomy) an operation whereby a fistulous opening is made into the urinary bladder via the abdominal wall. Usually the fistula can be allowed to heal when its purpose has been achieved.

cyst·otomy (sis-to'-to-mē) *n* incision into the urinary bladder via the abdominal wall, often done to remove a large stone or tumor or to gain access to the prostate gland in the operation of transvesical prostatectomy*.

cysto·urethritis (sis-tō-ū-rē-thrī'-tis) *n* inflammation of the urinary bladder and urethra.

cysto·urethr·ography (sis-tō-ū-rē-thro'-grà-fē) *n* radiographic examination of the urinary bladder and urethra, after they have been rendered radioopaque—**cys-**

tourethrographic *adj*, **cystourethrogram** *n*, **cystourethrograph** *n*, **cystourethrographically** *adv*.

cysto·urethro·pexy (sis-tō-ū-rē'-thrō-peks-ē) *n* forward fixation of the urinary bladder and upper urethra in an attempt to combat incontinence of urine.

Cytadren (sī'-tå-dren) *n* proprietary name for aminoglutethimide*.

cytar·abine (sī-tār'-a-bēn) *n* an antimetabolite which interferes with DNA synthesis. It is used for treating the acute leukemias. (Cytosar.)

cyto·diagnosis (sī-tō-dī-ag-nō'-sis) *n* diagnosis by the microscopic study of cells—**cytodiagnostic** *adj*.

cyto·genetics (sī-tō-jen-et'-iks) *n* The science concerned with the study of normal and abnormal chromosomes, and of their behavior. In man a person's chromosomes can be studied by culture techniques, using either lymphocytes or a piece of tissue such as skin, or cells such as those of the amniotic fluid (fetal cells). Chromosome abnormalities of either number or make-up (structure) can be associated with physical and mental disorder or with spontaneous abortion or stillbirth—**cytogenesis** *n*.

cy·tology (sī-tol'-o-jē) *n* the microscopic study of cells. The term *exfoliative cytology* is used when the cells studied have been shed, or exfoliated, from the surface of an organ or lesion—**cytological** *adj*.

cy·tolysis (sī-tol'-is-is) *n* the degeneration, destruction, disintegration or dissolution of cells—**cytolytic** *adj*.

cyto·megalovirus (sī-tō-meg'-å-lō-vī'-rus) *n* belongs to the same group of viruses as herpes simplex. Can cause latent and symptomless infection. Virus excreted in urine and saliva. Congenital infection is the most severe form of *cytomegalovirus infection,* can infect the fetus in utero, sometimes causing microcephaly, intracranial calcification and mental defect, or an illness at birth characterized by hepatosplenomegaly and thrombocytopenia. Infection can also be transmitted by blood transfusion, especially in patients with impaired immunity, in whom it causes a glandular fever-like illness and pneumonia.

Cytomel (sī'-tō-mel) *n* a preparation of liothyranine* that has a standardized activity.

cyto·pathic (sī-tō-path'-ik) *adj* pertaining to abnormality of the living cell.

cyto·plasm (sī'-tō-plazm) *n* (*syn* protoplasm) the complex chemical compound constituting the main part of the living substance of the cell, other than the contents of the nucleus—**cytoplasmic** *adj*.

Cyt·osar (sī'-tō-sår) *n* proprietary name for cytarabine*.

cyto·stasis (sī-tō-stā'-sis) *n* arrest or hindrance of cell development—**cytostatic** *adj*.

cyto·toxic (sī-tō-toks'-ik) *adj* any substance which is toxic to cells. Applied to the drugs used for the treatment of carcinomas and the reticuloses. Two main groups: (a) antimetabolites which block action of an enzyme system, e.g. methotrexate, fluorouracil mercaptopurine; (b) alkylating agents which poison cell directly, e.g. cyclophosphamide, mustine. There are known and potential dangers while handling cytotoxic drugs—dermatitis, nasal sores, pigmentation of the skin, blisters and excessive lacrimation have been reported.

cyto·toxins (sī-tō-toks'-ins) *npl* antibodies which are toxic to cells

Cytoxan (sī-toks'-an) *n* proprietary name for cyclophosphamide*.

D

D and C *abbr* dilatation* and curettage.

Da Costa syn·drome (då-kos'-tå) cardiac neurosis. An anxiety* state in which palpitations and left-sided chest pain are the most prominent symptoms.

dacryoadenitis (dak-rē-ō-ad-en-ī'-tis) *n* inflammation of a lacrimal gland. It is a rare condition which may be acute or chronic. May occur in mumps*.

dacryo·cyst (dak'-rē-ō-sist) *n* an old term for the lacrimal sac (tear sac). The word is still used in its compound forms (see below).

dacryo·cystectomy (dak-rē-ō-sis-tek'-to-mē) *n* excision of any part of the lacrimal sac.

dacryo·cystitis (dak-rē-ō-sis-tī'-tis) *n* inflammation of the lacrimal sac, which usually results in abscess formation and obliteration of the tear duct, giving rise to epiphora*.

dacryo·cystography (dak-rē-ō-sis-tog'-raf-ē) *n* radiographic examination of the tear drainage apparatus after it has been rendered radio-opaque—**dacryocystographic** *adj*. **dacryocystogram** *n*. **dacryocystographically** *adv*.

dacryo·cystorhinostomy (dak-rē-ō-sis'-tō-rīn-os'-to-mē) *n* (*syn* Toti's operation) an operation to establish drainage from the lacrimal sac into the nose when there is obstruction of the nasolacrimal duct.

dacryo·lith (dak'-rē-ō-lith) *n* a concretion in the lacrimal passages.

dactinomycin (dak-tin-ō-mī'-sin) *n* an intravenous cytostatic antibiotic useful in Wilm's tumor, Burkitt's lymphona, soft tissue sarcomas and teratomas; a potent radiosensitizer. (Cosmogen.)

dactyl (dak'-tl) *n* a digit, finger or toe— **dactylar, dactylate** *adj*.

dactyl·ion (dak-til'-i-on) *n* syndactyly*.

dactyl·itis (dak-til-ī'-tis) *n* inflammation of finger or toe. The digit becomes swollen due to periostitis. Met with in congenital syphilis, tuberculosis, sarcoid etc.

dactyl·ology (dak-til-ol'-o-gē) *n* the finger sign method of communication with deaf and dumb people.

Dakin's solution (dā'-kinz) an aqueous solution of sodium hypochlorite used to irrigate wounds and as a wet dressing.

Dal·mane (dal'-mān) *n* proprietary name for flurazepam*.

dalton·ism (dal'-ton-izm) *n* red/green color* blindness.

dan·druff (dan'-druf) *n* (*syn* scurf) the common scaly condition of the scalp. May be the forerunner of skin diseases of the seborrheic type, such as flexural dermatitis.

dandy fever (dan'-dē) dengue*.

dan·thron (dan'-thron) *n* a drug which contains fecal-softening agent and laxative for constipation. Available as capsules and in two strengths of highly palatable liquid. (Doxidan.)

Dan·trium (dan'-trē-um) proprietary name for dantrolene*.

dan·trolene (dan'-trō-lēn) *n* an antispasmodic which is useful in severe spasticity, multiple sclerosis, spinal cord injury and stroke. (Dantrium.)

dap·sone (dap'-sōn) *n* a sulfone derivative used mainly in leprosy. Prolonged treatment may produce hemolytic anemia with Heinz body formation, clinical signs of which are cyanosis of the lips, the patient is generally off-color.

Dara·nide (dār'-à-nīd) *n* proprietary name for dichlorphenamide*.

Dara·prim (dār'-à-prim) *n* proprietary name for pyrimethamine*.

Darvon (dàr'-von) *n* proprietary name for dextropropoxyphene.

dauno·rubicin (daw-nō-roo'-bi-sin) *n* similar to doxorubicin*. An antibiotic used in acute leukemia. Believed to act by inhibiting DNA synthesis. Can cause severe bone marrow depression and toxicity of heart muscle.

day hos·pital a center which patients attend daily. Recreational and occupational therapy and physiotherapy often provided. Greatest use is in the geriatric and psychiatric fields.

DBH *abbr* dopamine*-β-hydroxylase.

DDST *abbr* Denver Developmental Screening Test*.

DDT *abbr* chlorophenothane*.

deaf·ness (def'-nes) *n* a partial or complete loss of hearing. *Conductive deafness* is due to an obstruction which prevents the conduction of sound waves from the atmosphere to the inner ear. *Perceptive* or *nerve deafness* is due to a lesion in the inner ear. The auditory nerve or the auditory centers in the brain. *Congenital deafness* can be caused by the mother contracting german measles in early pregnancy.

deamin·ation (dē-am-in-ā'-shun) *n* removal of the amino group from organic compounds such as amino acids.

death (deth) *n* cessation of the body's vital functions usually assessed by the absence of a pulse and breathing. Mechanical ventilation may maintain vital functions despite the fact that the brain stem is fatally and irreversibly damaged. Consequently stringent tests are necessary to diagnose death. ⇒ coroner. *brain death* a new concept used when the brain stem is fatally and irreversibly damaged. In different countries, different criteria are used to diagnose brain death.

de·bility (dē-bil'-it-ē) *n* a condition of weakness with lack of muscle tone.

débride·ment (dē-brēd'-mong) *n* the removal of foreign matter and injured or infected tissue from a wound. *chemical medical debridement* is accomplished by the external application of a substance to the wound. *surgical debridement* is accomplished by using surgical instruments and aseptic technique.

Debri·san (deb'-ri-san) *n* a proprietary brand of hydrophilic porous beads of dextran* polymer which when applied to a suppurating wound provide drainage and removal of bacteria while protecting the tissue from dehydration.

Deca·dron (dek'-à-dron) *n* proprietary name for dexamethasone*.

Deca·Durabolin (dek'-à-dūr-à'-bo-lin) *n* a proprietary synthetic androgen*: anabolic. Given intramuscularly. Neutralizes estrogen uptake by cancer cells.

de·calcifi·cation (dē-kal-si-fi-kā'-shun) *n* the removal of mineral salts, as from teeth in dental caries, bone in disorders of calcium metabolism.

de·cannu·lation (dē-kan-ū-lā'-shun) *n* a word currently in use for the introduction of decreasingly smaller tubes to wean an infant from reliance on the original tracheostomy tube.

de·capsu·lation (dē-kap-sū-lā'-shun) *n* the surgical removal of a capsule.

Deca·spray (dek'-a-sprā) *n* a proprietary brand of aerosol containing dexamethasone* and neomycin* for topical application.

decere·brate (dē-sèr'-e-brāt) *adj* without cerebral function: a state of deep unconsciousness, *decerebrate posture* a condition of the unconscious patient in which all four limbs are spastic and which indicates severe damage to the cerebrum.

Decholin (dek'-ō-lin) *n* proprietary name for dehydrocholic acid*; cholagogue*.

de·cidua (dē-sid'-ū-à) *n* the endometrial lining of the uterus thickened and altered for the reception of the fertilized ovum. It is shed when pregnancy terminates. *decidua basalis* that part which lies under the embedded ovum and forms the maternal part of the placenta, *decidua capsularis* that part that lies over the developing ovum. *decidua vera* the decidua lining the rest of the uterus—**decidual** *adj*.

decidu·ous (dē-sid'-ū-us) *adj* by custom refers to the primary teeth which on shedding are normally replaced by permanent teeth.

Declomycin (dek-lō-mī'-sin) *n* proprietary name for demethylchlortetracycline*.

decompen·sation (dē-kom-pen-sā'-shun) *n* a failure of compensation usually referring to heart disease.

decom·pression (dē-kom-presh'-un) *n* removal of pressure or a compressing force. *decompression of brain* achieved by trephining the skull: *decompression of bladder* in cases of chronic urinary retention, by continuous or intermittent drainage via catheter inserted per urethra. *decompression chamber* used when returning deep-sea divers to the surface ⇒ caisson disease.

deconditioning (de-kon-di'-shun-ing) eliminating an unwanted particular response to a particular stimulus ⇒ aversion therapy, conditioning.

deconges·tants (dē-kon-jes'-tants) *npl* agents which reduce or eliminate congestion, usually referring to nasal congestion. They can be taken by mouth, or they can be applied locally as drops or sprays.

deconges·tion (dē-kon-jest'-yun) *n* relief of congestion—**decongestive** *adj*.

decorti·cation (dē-kòrt-ik-ā'-shun) *n* surgical removal of cortex or outer covering of an organ. *decortication of lung* carried out when thickening of the visceral pleura prevents re-expansion of lung as may occur in chronic emphysema. The visceral pleura is peeled off the lung, which is then re-expanded by positive pressure through an anesthetic apparatus.

decubi·tus (dē-kū'-bit-us) *n* the recumbent position; lying down. *decubitus ulcer* ⇒ pressure sore—**decubiti** *pl*, **decubital** *adj*.

decuss·ation (dē-kus-ā'-shun) *n* intersection; crossing of nerve fibers at a point beyond their origin, as in the optic and pyramidal tracts.

deep muscles ⇒ Figures 4, 5.

def·ecation (de-fe-kā'-shun) *n* voiding of feces per anus—**defecate** *vi*.

defer·ent duct ⇒ Figure 16.

deferoxamine (de-fèr-oks'-à-mēn) *n* an iron chelating agent which can be used in iron poisoning. (Desferal.)

defer·vescence (def-ĕr-ves'ens) *n* the time during which a fever is declining. If the body temperature falls rapidly it is spoken of as 'crisis'; if it falls slowly the term 'lysis' is used.

defibril·lation (dē-fib-ril-lā'-shun) *n* the arrest of fibrillation* of the cardiac muscle (atrial or ventricular), and restoration of normal cycle—**defibrillate** *vt*.

defibril·lator (dē-fib'-ril-ā-tor) *n* any agent, e.g. an electric shock, which arrests ventricular fibrillation* and restores normal rhythm.

defibrin·ated (dē-fī'-brin-ā-ted) *adj* rendered free from fibrin*. A necessary process in the preparation of serum from whole blood ⇒ blood—**defibrinate** *v*.

de·ficiency dis·ease (dē-fish'-ens-ē) disease resulting from dietary deficiency of any substance essential for good health, especially the vitamins.

degener·ation (dē-jen-èr-ā'-shun) *n* deterioration in quality or function. Regression from more specialized to less specialized type of tissue—**degenerative** *adj.* **degenerate** *vi.*

deglu·tition (dē-gloo-tish′-un) *n* the process of swallowing, partly voluntary, partly involuntary.

de·hiscence (dē-his′-ens) *n* the process of splitting or bursting open, as of a wound.

de·hydration (dē-hī-drā′-shun) *n* loss or removal of fluid. In the body this condition arises when the fluid intake fails to replace fluid loss. This is liable to occur when there is bleeding, diarrhea, excessive exudation from a raw area, excessive sweating, polyuria or vomiting, and usually upsets the body's electrolyte balance. If suitable fluid replacement cannot be achieved orally then parenteral administration must be instituted—**dehydrate** *vt, vi.*

dehydrocholic acid (de-hīd-rō-kōl′-ik as′-id) a cholagogue*.

déjà vu phenom·enon (dā′-zhà voo) occurs in epilepsy involving temporal lobes of the brain and in certain epileptic dream states. An intense feeling of familiarity as if everything had happened before.

Delalutin (del-à-loo′-tin) *n* proprietary name for hydroxy progesterone* caproate.

Delhi boil (del′-hī boyl) ⇒ oriental sore.

deli·quescent (del-i-kwes′-ent) *adj* capable of absorption, thus becoming fluid.

de·lirium (dē-lir′-ē-um) *n* abnormal mental condition based on hallucinations or illusion. May occur in high fever, in mental disease, or be toxic in origin. *delirium tremens* results from alcoholic intoxication and is represented by a picture of confusion, terror, restlessness and hallucinations—**delirious** *adj.*

Deltacortef (del-ta-kōr′-tef) *n* proprietary name for prednisolone*.

Deltasone (del′-tà-sōn) *n* proprietary name for prednisone*.

del·toid (del′-toyd) *adj* triangular. *deltoid muscle* (⇒ Figures 4, 5).

del·usion (dē-lū′-zhun) *n* a false belief, inconsistent with the individual's culture, use and level of intelligence, which cannot be altered by argument or reasoning. Found as a psychotic symptom in several types of mental disease, notably schizophrenia, paraphrenia, paranoia, senile psychoses, mania and depressive states including involutional melancholia.

demar·cation (dē-mår-kā′-shun) *n* an outlining of the junction of diseased and healthy tissue, often used when referring to gangrene.

de·mentia (dē-men′-shē-à) *n* (*syn* organic brain syndrome—OBS) an irreversible organic brain disease causing memory and personality disorders, deterioration in personal care, impaired cognitive ability and disorientation. ⇒ Jakob-Creutzfeldt disease. *dementia praecox* early but obsolete description of what is now called schizophrenia*. *presenile dementia* signs and symptoms of dementia* occurring in people between 50 and 60 years of age. It is due to early hyaline degeneration of both the medium and small cerebral blood vessels. ⇒ Alzheimer's disease. Pick's disease.

Demerol (dem′-ėr-ol) *n* proprietary name for meperidine* hydrochloride.

demethyl·chlor·tetra·cycline (dē-meth-l-klōr-tet-ra-sī′-klin) *n* one of the tetracyclines*. (Declomycin.)

de·mography (dem-og′-ra-fē) *n* social science, including vital statistics.

Dem·ser (dem′-sėr) *n* proprietary name for metyrosine*.

de·mulcent (dē-mul′-sent) *n* a slippery, mucilaginous fluid which allays irritation and soothes inflammation, especially of mucous membranes.

demyelin·ization (dē-mī-el-in-īz-ā′-shun) *n* destruction of the myelin* sheaths surrounding nerve fibers; occurs in multiple sclerosis.

den·drite (den′-drīt) *n* (*syn* dendron) one of the branched filaments which are given off from the body of a nerve cell. That part of a neuron which transmits an impulse to the nerve cell—**dendritic** *adj.*

den·dritic ul·cer (den-dri′-tik ul′-sėr) a linear corneal ulcer that sends out treelike branches. Caused by herpes simplex. Treated with idoxuridine.

den·dron (den′-dron) *n* ⇒ dendrite.

dener·vation (dē-nėr-vā′-shun) *n* the means by which a nerve supply is cut off. Usually refers to incision, excision or blocking of a nerve.

dengue (deng′-gä) *n* (*syn* 'break-bone fever') one of the mosquito*-transmitted hemorrhagic fevers, a disease of the tropics. Causative agent is an arbovirus conveyed by a mosquito. Characterized by rheumatic pains, fever and a skin eruption. The hemorrhagic form has a high mortality.

Dennis Browne splints (den′-nis brown) splints used to correct congenital talipes equinovarus (club* foot). The splints are of metal padded with felt, with a joining bar to which the baby's feet are strapped.

den·tal amal·gam (den'-tal à-mal'-gam) ⇒ amalgam.

dental plaque (den'-tal plak) *n* non-calcified deposit on the surface of a tooth composed of a soft mass of bacteria and cellular debris which accumulates rapidly in the absence of oral hygiene.

dentate (den'-tāt) *adj* having teeth present.

den·tine (den'-tēn) *n* the calcified tissue forming the body of the tooth beneath the enamel and cementum enclosing the pulp chamber and root canals.

den·tition (den-ti'-shun) refers to the teeth. In man the primary or deciduous* teeth are called *primary dentition* and are normally 20 in number. The adult, permanent teeth are called the *secondary dentition*, and are normally 32 in number.

den·ture (den'-chūr) *n* a removable dental prosthesis*: it may contain one or several teeth, or it can be a complete upper or lower denture.

Denver Developmental Screening Test (DDST) developmental test for young children.

de·odor·ant (dē-ō'-dōr-ant) *n, adj* any substance which destroys or masks an (unpleasant) odor. Potassium permanganate and hydrogen peroxide are deodorants by their powerful oxidizing action; chlorophyll has some reputation as a deodorant for foul-smelling wounds, but its value in masking other odors is doubtful—**deodorize** *vt*.

deoxy·genation (dē-oks-i-jen-ā'-shun) *n* the removal of oxygen—**deoxygenated** *adj*.

deoxy·ribonucleic acid (dē-oks-i-rī-bō-nū-klē'-ik) **(DNA)** polymers of deoxyribonucleotides which occur in complex molecules called chromosomes* found in cell nuclei and viruses. DNA carries, in coded form, instructions for passing on hereditary characteristics.

depersonal·ization (dē-pèrs-on-al-īz-ā'-shun) *n* a subjective feeling of having lost one's personality, sometimes that one no longer exists. Occurs in schizophrenia and more rarely in depressive states.

depi·late (dep'-il-āt) *vt* to remove hair from—**depilatory** *adj, n*, **depilation** *n*.

depila·tories (dē-pil'-àt-ōr-ēz) *npl* substances usually made in pastes (e.g. barium sulfide) which remove excess hair only temporarily; they do not act on the papillae, consequently the hair grows again. ⇒ epilation—**depilatory** *sing*. Preoperative depilation lessens the risk of wound infection because it is non-abrasive.

Depo·Provera (dep'-ō prŏ-vèr'-à) *n* proprietary name for medroxyprogesterone* acetate.

de·pressed frac·ture (dē-presd' frak'-tūr) ⇒ fracture.

de·pres·sion (dē-presh'-un) *n* **1** a hollow place or indentation. **2** diminution of power or activity. **3** an emotional disorder characterized by feelings of profound sadness. Most clinicians recognize two distinct types, neurotic and psychotic. The neurotic type is called *reactive depression*; it occurs as a reaction to stress. The psychotic type is called *endogenous depression*: it arises spontaneously in the mind. The symptoms vary from mild to fatal and arc: insomnia, headaches, exhaustion, anorexia, irritability, emotionalism or loss of affect, loss of interest, impaired concentration, feelings that life is not worth living and suicidal thoughts. The symptoms of endogenous depression are more severe, but paradoxically respond better to treatment. When the condition occurs in middle life it is sometimes referred to as climacteric depression or involutional melancholia. An alternative theory suggests that endogenous and reactive depression are really both part of the same syndrome, the former being merely more serious than the latter.

depri·vation syn·drome (dep-riv-ā'-shun) usually the result of parental rejection. Includes stunted growth, malnutrition with potbelly, gluttonous appetite, superficial affectionate attachment to any adult, diaper rash or old healed sores on buttocks, chilblain scars on fingers and toes, very thin hair. Affected children usually put on weight rapidly in hospital.

derangement (dē-rānj'-ment) *n* insanity, mental disorder.

Derby·shire neck (der'-bē-shēr) goiter*.

derealiz·ation (dē-rē-àl-īz-ā'-shun) *n* feelings that people, events or surroundings have changed and are unreal. Similar sensations may occur in normal people during dreams. May sometimes be found in schizophrenia and depressive states.

de·reistic (dē-rē-is'-tik) *adj* of thinking, not adapted to reality. Describes autistic thinking.

derma·brasion (dèr-mà-brā'-zhun) *n* ⇒ abrasion.

derma·titis (dèr-mà-tī'-tis) *n* inflammation of the skin (by custom limited to an eczematous reaction). ⇒ eczema. *atopic dermatitis* that variety of infantile eczema which may be associated with asthma of hay fever. *dermatitis herpetiformis* (*syn* hydroa) an intensely itchy skin eruption of unknown cause, most commonly characterized by vesicles, bullae and pustules on urticarial plaques, which remit and relapse. Associated with gluten-sensitive enteropathy. *juvenile dermatitis herpetiformis* recurrent bullous eruption on the genitalia, lower abdomen, buttocks and face, mainly in children under 5, boys being affected more than girls.

dermato·glyphics (dèr-mà-tō-glif'-iks) *n* study of the ridge patterns of the skin of the fingertips, palms and soles to discover developmental anomalies.

dermato·graphia (dèr-mà-tō-graf'-ē-à) *n* ⇒ dermographia.

derma·tologist (dèr-mà-to'-lō-jist) *n* one who studies skin diseases and is skilled in their treatment. A skin specialist.

derma·tology (dèr-mà-to'-lō-jē) *n* the science which deals with the skin, its structure, functions, diseases and their treatment—**dermatological** *adj*. **dermatologically** *adv*.

dermatome (dèr'-mat-ōm) *n* an instrument for cutting slices of skin of varying thickness, usually for grafting.

dermato·mycosis (dèr-mat-ō-mī-kō'-sis) *n* a fungal infection of the skin—**dermatomycotic** *adj*.

dermato·myositis (dèr'-mat-ō-mī-ōs-īt'-is) *n* an acute inflammation of the skin and muscles which presents with edema and muscle weakness. May result in the atrophic changes of scleroderma*. ⇒ collagen.

dermato·phytes (dèr'-ma-tō-fīts) *npl* a group of fungi which invade the superficial skin.

dermato·phytosis (dèr-ma-tō-fī-tō'-sis) *n* infection of the skin with dermatophyte species.

derma·tosis (dèr-ma-tō'-sis) *n* generic term for skin disease—**dermatoses** *pl*.

der·mis (dèr'-mis) *n* the true skin; the cutis vera; the layer below the epidermis (⇒ Figure 12)—**dermal** *adj*.

dermo·graphia (dèr-mō-graf'-ē-à) *n* (*syn* dermatographia, factitial urticaria) a condition in which weals occur on the skin after a blunt instrument or fingernail has been lightly drawn over it. Seen in vasomotor instability and urticaria—**dermographic** *adj*.

der·moid (dèr'-moyd) *adj* pertaining to or resembling skin. *dermoid cyst* a cyst* which is congenital in origin and usually occurs in the ovary. It contains elements of hair, nails, skin, teeth etc.

Dermoplast (dèr'-mō-plast) *n* a proprietary preparation of benzocaine* for use as a topical anesthetic and antipruritic.

DES *abbr*. diethylstilbestrol*.

descend·ing colon (dē-send'-ing) ⇒ Figure 18.

de·sensitiz·ation (dē-sen-sit-īz-ā'-shun) *n* **1** injection of antigens* to diminish or cancel out hypersensitivity to insect venoms, drugs, pollen and other causes of acute hypersensitivity reactions. **2** of phobic patients, using intravenous methohexital sodium to achieve psychological relaxation. In this state the phobic situation is imagined without fear and the patient 'unlearns' his irrational fear—**desensitize** *vt*.

deser·pidine (dē-sèr'-pi-dīn) *n* a drug related to reserpine*; has an antihypertensive function.

Desferol (des'-fer-ol) *n* proprietary name for deferoxamine*.

desic·cation (de-sik-ā'-shun) *n* drying out. There can be desiccation of the nucleus pulposus, thus diminishing the 'water cushion' effect of a healthy intervertebral disc.

des·ipramine (de-sip'-ra-mēn) *n* an antidepressant. (Pertofrane.)

deslano·side (des-lan'-ō-sīd) *n* a natural glycoside; cardiac therapeutic agent. (Cedilanid-D.)

desloughing (dē-sluf'-ing) the process of removing slough* from a wound.

desmo·pressin (des-mō-pres'-in) *n* antidiuretic ⇒ vasopressin.

desoxy·corticosterone (dez-oks'-ē-kōr-ti-kō-stē'-rōn) *n* (**DOCA**) an important hormone of the adrenal cortex, controlling the metabolism of sodium and potassium. (Percorten.)

desqua·mation (des-kwà-mā'-shun) *n* shedding; flaking off, casting off—**desquamate** *vi. vt*.

de·tached ret·ina separation of the neuroretina from the pigment epithelium, usually accompanied by retinal tears or holes (thegmatogenous retinal detachment). Exudative retinal detachment is separation of the combined neuroretina and pigment epithelium from the choroid. Treatment aims to produce scar tissue between all layers of the retina and choroid.

deter·gent (dē-tėr'-jent) *n. adj* describes a cleansing agent. Term often applied to drugs of the cetrimide type, which have both antiseptic and cleaning properties, and so are valuable in removing grease, dirt sec. from skin and wounds, and scabs and crusts from skin lesions.

deterio·ration (dē-tėr-ē-ōr-ā'-shun) *n* progressive impairment of function: worsening of the patient's condition.

detoxi·cation (dē-toks-i-kā'-shun) *n* the process of removing the poisonous property of a substance—**detoxicant** *adj, n,* **detoxicate** *vt.*

de·tritus (dē-trī'-tus) *n* matter produced by detrition; waste matter from disintegration.

de·trusor (dē-trōō'-sėr) *n* the muscle of the urinary bladder.

detu·mescence (de-tū-mes'-ens) *n* subsidence of a swelling.

devi·ance (de'-vē-ans) *n* a variation from normal.

dexa·methasone (deks-à-meth'-à-sōn) *n* 30 times as active as cortisone* in suppressing inflammation. Less likely to precipitate diabetes than the other steroids. Sometimes used to prevent cerebral edema. (Decadron.)

Dexe·drine (deks'-e-drin) *n* proprietary name for dextroamphetamine*.

dex·tran (deks'-tran) *n* a blood plasma substitute, obtained by the action of a specific bacterium on sugar solutions. Used as a 6% or 10% solution in hemorrhage, shock, etc.

dextran·ase (deks'-tran-ās) *n* an enzyme that reduces the formation of dextran* from sucrose and has been used to prevent the formation of dental plaque.

dex·trin (deks'-trin) *n* a soluble polysaccharide formed during the hydrolysis of starch.

dextroamphetamine (deks-trō-am-fet'-à-mēn) *n* central nervous system stimulant similar to amphetamine* and used for similar purposes. Sometimes used as an appetite suppressant in obesity. (Dexedrine.)

dextro·cardia (deks-trō-kàr'-dē-à) *n* transposition of the heart to the right side of the thorax—**dextrocardial** *adj.*

dextro·methorphan (deks-trō-meth-ōr'-fàn) *n* a cough suppressant; available as lozenges, syrup and a linctus.

dextro·propoxyphene (deks-trō-prō-

poks'-i-fēn) *n* milder type of analgesic used as morphine substitute. (Darvon.)

dex·trose (deks'-trōs) *n (syn* glucose) a soluble carbohydrate (monosaccharide) widely used by intravenous infusion in dehydration, shock and postoperatively. Also given orally as a readily absorbed sugar in acidosis and other nutritional disturbances.

dextroxy·lase test (deks-troks'-i-lās) xylose* test.

DFP *abbr* dyflos*.

dhobie itch (dō'-bē) *n* tinea* cruris. Derived from belief that ringworm of the groin originated from infection of the Indian laundryman (dhobie).

DHT *abbr* dihydrotachysterol*.

dia·betes (dī-à-bē'-tēz) *n* a disease characterized by polyuria. Used without qualification it means diabetes mellitus—**diabetic** *adj. diabetes insipidus* polyuria and polydipsia caused by deficiency of ADH. Usually due to trauma or tumor involving posterior pituitary but may be idiopathic. Treated with desmopressin. *nephrogenic diabetes insipidus* polyuria resulting from abnormality or disease rendering renal tubules insensitive to ADH. *diabetes mellitus* a condition characterized by hyperglycemia due to deficiency or diminished effectiveness of insulin. The hyperglycemia leads to glycosuria, which in turn causes polyuria and polydipsia. Severe dehydration, sometimes sufficient to cause unconsciousness (hyperglycemic hyperosmolar nonketoacidotic diabetic coma. HHNK), may occur. Impaired utilization of carbohydrate is associated with increased secretion of antistorage hormones such as glucagon and growth hormone in an attempt to provide alternative metabolic substrate. Glycogenolysis, gluconeogenesis and lipolysis are all increased. The latter results in excessive formation of ketone bodies which in turn leads to acidosis. If untreated this will eventually cause coma (ketoacidotic diabetic coma) and death. Under the new classification diabetic patients are either *insulin dependent* or *non-insulin dependent,* irrespective of the patient's age at the onset of the condition. *Potential diabetics* have a normal glucose tolerance test but are at increased risk of developing diabetes for genetic reasons. *Latent diabetics* have a normal glucose tolerance test but are known to have had an abnormal test under conditions imposing a burden on the pancreatic beta cells, e.g. during infection or pregnancy. In the latter instance the term *gestational diabetes* is commonly used. ⇒ hyperosmolar diabetic coma, insulin dependent diabetes mellitus—**diabetic** *adj, n.*

diabeto·genic (dī-à-bĕt-ō-jen'-ik) *adj* 1 causing diabetes*. 2 applied to an anterior pituitary hormone.

Diab·inese (dī-ab'-in-ēs) *n* proprietary name for chlorpropamide*.

dia·cetic acid (dī-à-sē'-tik) ⇒ acetoacetic acid.

diacetylmorphine (dī-à-sē'-tl-mōr'-fēn) (*syn* heroin) *n* narcotic derived from morphine. Because it is highly addictive, its sale and use are illegal in the U.S.

diag·nosis (dī-àg-nō'-sis) *n* the art or act of distinguishing one disease from another. *differential diagnosis* is the term used when making a correct decision between diseases presenting a similar clinical picture—**diagnoses** *pl.* **diagnose** *vt.*

diag·nostic (dī-àg-nos'-tik) *adj* 1 pertaining to diagnosis. 2 serving as evidence in diagnosis—**diagnostician** *n.*

diaguan·ides (dī'-à-gwan-īds) *npl* ⇒ biguanides.

dia·lysand (dī-al'-i-sand) *n* a word used for the patient in some renal dialysis* units.

dia·lysate (dī-al'-i-sāt) *n* the type of fluid used in dialysis*.

dia·lyser (dī'-à-lī-zėr) *n* (*syn* artificial kidney) contains two compartments, one for blood and the other for dialysate; these are separated by a semipermeable membrane. ⇒ hemodialysis.

dialy·sis (dī-al'-is-īs) *n* separation of substances in solution by taking advantage of their differing diffusability through a porous membrane as in the artificial kidney. ⇒ hemodialysis—**dialyses** *pl.* **dialyse** *vt. peritoneal dialysis* the peritoneum is used as the porous membrane in achieving dialysis for the removal of urea and other waste products into the irrigation fluid which is then withdrawn from the abdominal cavity. Peritoneal dialysis can be used intermittently or continuously.

Dia·mox (dī'-à-moks) *n* proprietary name for acetazolamide*.

dia·pedesis (dī-à-pe-dē'-sis) *n* the passage of cells from within blood vessels through the vessel walls into the tissues—**diapedetic** *adj.*

diaper rash (dī'-à-pėr rash) *n* an erythema of the diaper area. Usual causes are ammoniacal decomposition of urine,

thrush, infantile psoriasis, allergy to detergents, or excoriation from diarrhea.

dia·phoresis (dī-à-fōr-ē'-sis) *n* perspiration.

diaphor·etic (dī-à-fōr-et'-ik) *adj, n* an agent which induces diaphoresis (sweating). ⇒ sudorific.

dia·phragm (dī'-à-fram) *n* 1 the dome-shaped muscular partition between the thorax above and the abdomen below. 2 any partitioning membrane or septum. 3 a rubber cap which encircles the cervix to act as a contraceptive. It should be used with a spermicidal jelly or cream—**diaphragmatic** *adj.*

diaphy·sis (dī-à'-fī-sis) *n* the shaft of a long bone—**diaphyses** *pl.* **diaphysea** *adj.*

dia·placental (dī-à-plà-sen'-tal) *adj* through the placenta*.

diar·rhea (dī-à-rē'-à) *n* deviation from established bowel rhythm characterized by an increase in frequency and fluidity of the stools. Epidemic diarrhea of the newborn is a highly contagious infection of maternity hospitals. The gastroenteritis is probably the result of virus infection. ⇒ arthropathy spurious diarrhea.

diar·throsis (dī-àr-thrō'-sis) *n* a synovial, freely movable joint—**diarthroses** *pl.* **diarthrodial** *adj.*

dias·tase (dī'-às-tās) *n* an amylase* produced by animal, plant and bacterial cells. *pancreatic diatase* is excreted in the urine (and saliva) and therefore estimation of urinary diastase may be used as a test of pancreatic function.

diasta·sis (dī-as'-tas-is) *n* a separation of bones without fracture; dislocation. *diastasis recti* a separation of the rectus abdominus muscle, seen in pregnancy and the postpartum period.

di·astole (dī-as'-to-lē) *n* the relaxation period of the cardiac cycle, as opposed to systole*—**diastolic** *adj.*

dia·thermy (dī'-à-thėr-mē) *n* the passage of a high frequency electric current through the tissues whereby heat is produced. When both electrodes are large, the heat is diffused over a wide area according to the electrical resistance of the tissues. In this form it is widely used in the treatment of inflammation, especially when deeply seated (e.g. sinusitis, pelvic cellulitis). When one electrode is very small the heat is concentrated in this area and becomes great enough to destroy tissue. In this form (surgical diathermy) it is used to stop bleeding at operation by coagulation of blood, or to

87

cut through tissue in operation for malignant disease.

diaz·epam (dī-az′-e-pam) *n* tranquilosedative with muscle relaxant properties. Useful in intravenous infusion for status epilepticus and tetanus and as a premedicant. (Valium.)

diaz·oxide (dī-az-oks′-īd) *n* suppresses activity of insulin-producing beta cells, therefore useful in hypoglycemia from pancreatic tumor. Its main use is as a hypotensive agent by rapid intravenous injection in hypertensive emergencies. (Hyperstat.)

Dibenzy·line (dī-benź-il-ēn) *n* proprietary name for phenoxybenzaminc*.

dibucaine (dī′-bū-kān) *n* powerful local anesthetic used for surface anesthesia, infiltration and spinal anesthesia. Available as cream, ointment and suppositories. (Nupercainal.)

DIC *abbr* disseminated* intravascular coagulation.

dicepha·lous (dī-sef′-à-lus) *adj* two-headed.

dichloral·phenazone (dī-klōr-al-fen′-à-zōn) *n* causes less gastric irritation than chloral* hydrate. Hypnotic of the chloral group. Particularly suitable for children. (Midrin.)

dichlor·phenamide (dī-klōr-fen′-à-mīd) *n* oral diuretic of short duration. Carbonic anhydrase inhibitor. Used for systemic treatment of glaucoma. (Daranide.)

di·chuchwa *n* word for non-venereal syphilis used in Botswana.

Dicloxacillin (dī-cloks-à-sil′-lin) *n* a penicillin active against infections caused by penicillinase-producing staphylococci.

di·crotic (dī-krot′-ik) *adj, n* pertaining to, or having a double beat, as indicated by a second expansion of the artery during diastole. *dicrotic wave* the second rise in the tracing of a dicrotic pulse.

dicu·marol (dī-kōō′-mà-rol) *n* an early orally effective anticoagulant. Now largely replaced by more controllable drugs.

dicyclo·mine (dī-sī′-klō-mēn) *n* an antispasmodic resembling atropine*, but less potent. Used in pylorospasm and gastric hypermotility. (Bentyl.)

Didrex (dī′-dreks) *n* proprietary name for benzphetamine*.

dien·estrol (dī-en-es′-trol) *n* a synthetic estrogen similar to stilbestrol*, but less active.

diet·ary fiber coarse food containing much indigestible vegetable fiber composed mainly of cellulose. It provides bulk in the diet and this helps to stimulate peristalsis and eliminate feces. It is now thought to be useful in preventing diseases in the Western world such as constipation, obesity, diabetes mellitus and bowel cancer. ⇒ bran.

diet·etics (dī-et-et′-iks) *n* the interpretation and application of the scientific principles of nutrition to feeding in health and disease.

diethyl·propion hydro·chloride (dī-ethyl-prō′-pē-on hī-drō-klōf-īd) a central nervous system stimulant used as an appetite suppressant. (Tenuate.)

diethyl·stilbestrol (DES) (dī-eth-yl-stilbes′-trol) *n* a hormone preparation used to treat symptoms of the menopause, menstrual disorders, inflammation of the female reproductive organs and cancer of the breast and prostate. Was previously used to prevent miscarriage in pregnancy but is no longer due to the possibility that its use caused cancer of the reproductive organs in the children born of these pregnancies.

diet·itian (dī-et-ish′-un) *n* one who applies the principles of nutrition* to the feeding of an individual or a group of individuals in a heterogeneous setting of economics or health, e.g. in schools, hospitals, institutions, restaurants, hotels, food factories and in the World Health Organization.

Dietl's crisis (dēt′-lz krī′-sis) a rare complication of 'floating' kidney. Kinking of the ureter is thought to be responsible for the severe colic produced in the lumbar region.

differen·tial blood count (dif-ėr-en′-shal) ⇒ blood count.

differen·tial diag·nosis (dif-ėr-en′-shal) ⇒ diagnosis.

dif·fusion (dif-fū′-zhun) *n* **1** the process whereby gases and liquids of different concentrations intermingle when brought into contact, until their concentration is equal throughout. **2** dialysis.

diflun·isal (dif-lūn′-is-al) *n* a non-steroidal, anti-inflammatory analgesic drug which is derived from salicylic* acid. (Dolobid.)

diges·tion (dī-jest′-chun) *n* the process by which food is rendered absorbable—**digestible, digestive** *adj*. **digestibility** *n*. **digest** *vt*.

digest·ive system (dī-jest′-iv) ⇒ Figure 18.

digit (dij′-it) *n* a finger or toe—**digital** *adj*.

digi·tal compres·sion (dij'-it-al kom-presh'-un) pressure applied by the fingers, usually to an artery to stop bleeding.

digi·talis (dij-it-al'-is) n leaf of the common foxglove. Powerful cardiac tonic, used in congestive heart failure and atrial fibrillation. The active principle of the Australian foxglove, digoxin*, is now preferred as the action is more consistent and reliable.

digital·ization (dij-it-al-īz-ā'-shun) n physiological saturation with digitalis* to obtain optimum therapeutic effect.

digi·toxin (dij-it-oks'-in) n a glycoside of digitals*. (Crystodigin.)

di·goxin (dij-oks'-in) n glycoside of digitalis*. (Lanoxin.)

diguan·ides (dī'-gwan-īds) npl ⇒ biguanides.

dihydro·codeine tar·trate (dī-hī-drō-kō'-dēn tar'-trāt) non-habit forming analgesic, useful for suppression of cough, respiratory infections and painful wounds. Can be given orally or by injection.

dihydro·ergotamine (dī-hī-drō-ėr-got'-à-mēn) n derived from ergotamine*, used in migraine.

dihydro·morphinone (dī-hī-drō-mōr'-fin-ōn) n a morphine*-like analgesic of high potency but short action. It has little hypnotic effect. Occasionally used as a depressant in severe cough. Considered less habit-forming than morphine. (Dilaudid.)

dihydro·tachysterol (dī-hī-drō-tak-is'-tėr-ol) n prepared in oil; used to raise the blood calcium, especially in parathyroid tetany.

diiodo·hydroxy·quin (dī-ī-ō'-dō-hī-droks'-i-kwin) n iodoquinol; used chiefly in amoebic dysentery in association with emetine*. (Diodoquin.)

diiodo·tyrosine (dī-ī-ō-dō-tī'-rō-sēn) n an organic iodine-containing precursor of thyroxine*.

Dilantin (dī-lan'-tin) n proprietary name for phenytoin* sodium.

dilat·ation (dī-là-tā'-shun) n stretching or enlargement. May occur physiologically, pathologically or be induced artificially. dilatation and curettage by custom refers to artificial stretching of the cervical os to procure scrapings of the uterine epithelium.

Di·laudid (dī-law'-did) n proprietary name for dihydromorphinone*.

dill water (aqua anethi) popular preparation of a volatile oil used as a carminative for infants.

dimen·hydrinate (dī-men-hīd'-rin-āt) n powerful antiemetic for travel sickness and vertigo. (Dramamine.)

dimer·caprol (BAL) (dī-mėr-kap'-rol) n an organic compound used as an antidote for poisoning by arsenic and gold. Also useful in mercury poisoning if treatment is prompt, but it is not suitable for lead poisoning. It forms soluble compounds with the metals, which are then rapidly excreted.

Dimetane (dī'-me-tān) n proprietary name for brompheniramine* maleate.

dio·done (dī'-o-dōn) n organic iodine compound used as X-ray contrast agent in intravenous pyelography.

Diogenes syn·drome (dī-oj'-en-ēz) gross self-neglect.

di·opter (dī-op'-tėr) n a unit of measurement in refraction. A lens of one diopter has a focal length of 1 meter.

diox·ide (dī-oks'-īd) n oxide with two atoms of oxygen in each molecule.

diphen·hydramine (dī-fen-hīd'-rà-mēn) n one of the first antihistamines*. Widely used in allergic conditions and travel sickness. Also has a sedative action. (Benadryl.)

diphen·oxylate (dī-fen-oks'-il-āt) n prescribed for acute and chronic diarrhea, and gastrointestinal upsets. It has some morphine*-like actions: (a) it depresses the respiratory center (b) it acts as a cortical depressant (c) it reduces intestinal mobility. Atropine* is included (Lomotil) to provide dryness of the mouth should patient take an overdose.

diph·theria (dif-thē'-rē-à) n an acute, specific, infectious notifiable disease caused by Corynebacterium diptheriae. Characterized by a grey, adherent, false membrane growing on a mucous surface, usually that of the upper respiratory tract. Locally there is pain, swelling and may be suffocation. Systemically the toxins attack the heart muscle and nerves—**diphtheritic** adj.

diph·theroid (dif'-thėr-oyd) adj any bacterium morphologically and culturally resembling Corynebacterium diphtheriae.

di·plegia (dī-plē'-jē-à) n symmetrical paralysis of legs, usually associated with cerebral damage—**diplegic** adj.

diplo·coccus (dip-lō-kok'-us) n a coccal bacterium characteristically occurring in pairs. *Diplococcus* may be used in a binomial to describe a characteristically paired coccus. e.g. *Diplococcus pneumoniae (Streptococcus pneumoniae) =* pneumococcus.

dip·loid (dip'-loyd) *adj* refers to the chromosome complement of organisms, like man, in which each chromosome exists in duplicate form, one member of each pair being derived from the mother, the other from the father. The two sets are united at fertilization. May has a diploid number of 46 chromosomes. 23 pairs.

dip·lopia (dip-lō'-pē-à) *n* the word used alone infers the seeing of two objects when only one exists (double vision). There are several binomials which locate or describe the disability in more detail.

dipso·mania (dip-sō-mān'-ē-à) *n* alcoholism* in which the drinking occurs in bouts, often with long periods of sobriety between—**dipsomaniac** *adj, n.*

dipyrid·amole (dī-pī-rid'-à-mōl) *n* **1** a drug which has antianginal, and antihypertensive properties. It also reduces blood platelet aggregation. **2** a vasodilator which can be taken by mouth or given by injection. (Persantine.)

disac·charide (dī-sak'-à-rīd) *n* a sugar (i.e. carbohydrate) e.g. lactose, maltose, sucrose, which yields two molecules of monosaccharide on hydrolysis.

Di·salcid (dī-sal'-sid) *n* proprietary name for salsalate*.

disarticu·lation (dis-àr-tik-ū-lā'-shun) *n* amputation at a joint.

disc·ectomy (disk-ek'-to-mē) *n* surgical removal of a disc, usually an intervertebral disc.

dis·cission (dis-si'-zhun) *n* (*syn* needling) rupturing of lens capsule to allow absorption of lens substance in the condition of cataract.

dis·closing tab·let (dis-klō'-sing) *n* contains erythrosine* and is used to identify dental* plaque.

disco·genic (dis-kō-jen'-ik) *adj* arising in or produced by a disc, usually an intervertebral disc.

discography (dis-kog'-rà-fē) *n* x-ray of an intervertebral disc after it has been rendered radio-opaque.

dis·crete (dis-krēt') *adj* distinct, separate, not merging.

dis·ease (dis-ēz') *n* any deviation from or interruption of the normal structure and function of any part of the body. It is manifested by a characteristic set of signs and symptoms and in most instances the etiology, pathology and prognosis is known.

dis·impaction (dis-im-pak'-shun) *n* separation of the broken ends of a bone which have been driven into each other during the impact which caused the fracture. Traction may then be applied to maintain the bone ends in good alignment and separate.

dis·infec·tants (dis-in-fek'-tants) *npl* a word usually reserved for germicides which are too corrosive or toxic to be applied to tissues, but which are suitable for application to inanimate objects.

dis·infec·tion (dis-in-fek'-shun) *n* the removal or destruction of harmful microbes but not usually bacterial spores. It is commonly achieved by using heat or chemicals.

dis·infesta·tion (dis-in-fes-tā'-shun) *n* extermination of infesting agents, especially lice (delousing).

Dis·ipal (dis'-i-pal) *n* proprietary name for orphenadrine*.

dis·location (dis-lō-kā'-shun) *n* a displacement of organs or articular surfaces, so that all apposition between them is lost. It may be congenital, spontaneous, traumatic, or recurrent—**dislocated** *adj.* **dislocate** *vt.*

dis·obliter·ation (dis-ob-lit-ér-ā'-shun) *n* rebore. Removal of that which blocks a vessel, most often intimal plaques in an artery, when it is called endarterectomy*.

diso·pyramide (dī-sō-pī'-rà-mīd) *n* a drug with an antiarrhythmic action similar to that of quinidine*.

dis·orienta·tion (dis-ōr-ē-en-tā'-shun) *n* loss of orientation*.

dissec·tion (dīs-sek'-shun) *n* separation of tissues by cutting. When a group of lymph nodes are totally excised it is referred to as a *block dissection of glands*: it is usually part of the treatment for carcinoma.

dis·seminated (dis-em'-in-āt-ed) Widely spread or scattered. *disseminated intravascular coagulation (DIC)* a condition in which there is overstimulation of the body's clotting and anticlotting process in response to disease or injury. *disseminated sclerosis* ⇒ multiple sclerosis.

dis·sociation (dis-sō-shē-ā'-shun) *n* in psychiatry, an abnormal mental process by which the mind achieves non-recognition and isolation of certain unpalatable facts. This involves the actual splitting off from consciousness of all the unpalatable ideas so that the individual is no longer aware of them. Dissociation is a common symptom in hysteria but is seen in its most exaggerated form in delusional psychoses, e.g. a woman who, being deluded, believes she is the Queen cheerfully scrubbing the ward floor. Her royal status and the fact that she is charring are completely separated or dissociated in her mind and she does not recognize the incongruity.

dis·tal (dis'-tàl) *adj* farthest form the head or source—**distally** *adv*.

disti·chiasis (dis-tik-ī'-as-is) *n* an extra row of eyelashes at the inner lid border, which is turned inward against the eye.

distract·ibility (dis-trak-ti-bil'-i-tē) *n* a psychiatric term applied to a disorder of the power of attention when it can only be applied momentarily.

disulf·iram (dī-sulf'-ir-am) *n* a sulfur compound that in the presence of alcohol causes nausea and vomiting. Hence it is used in the treatment of alcoholism. (Antabuse.)

di·uresis (dī-ū-rē'-sis) *n* increased secretion of urine. It is sometimes part of intensive therapy particularly in poisoning when it is termed *forced diuresis*.

di·uretics (dī-ū-ret'-iks) *npl* drugs which increase the flow of urine. Those which enhance the excretion of sodium and other ions thereby increasing urinary output are called *saluretic diuretics* and comprise the thiazide group of drugs. Those which act on the loop of Henle are called *loop diuretics*; they produce a rapid diuresis, onset of action being 5–10 min when given parenterally or 20–30 min if given orally; the duration of action is 4–6 h.

Diuril (dī'-ū-ril) *n* proprietary name for chlorothiazide*.

divari·cation (dī-vār-i-kā'-shun) *n* separation of two points on a straight line.

divari·cator (dī-vār'-i-kā-tor) *n* a hinged wooden splint, permitting various degrees of divarication in congenital dislocation of the hip.

divers' paral·ysis (dī'-verz par-al'-is-is) caisson* disease.

diver·ticulitis (dī-vèr-tik-ū-lī'-tis) *n* inflammation of a diverticulum*.

diver·ticulosis (dī-vér-tik-ū-lō'-sis) *n* a condition in which there are many diverticula, especially in the intestines.

diver·ticulum (dī-vèr-tik'-ū-lum) *n* a pouch or sac protruding from the wall of a tube or hollow organ. May be congenital or acquired—**diverticula** *pl*.

Dix·arit (diks'-à-rit) *n* proprietary name for clonidine*.

dizzi·ness (diz'-i-nes) *n*, a feeling of unsteadiness, usually accompanied by anxiety.

DMPA medroxyprogesterone acetate, long-acting progesterone injections for contraceptive use.

DNA *abbr* deoxyribonucleic* acid. *DNA probe* blood from a finger prick is applied to a radioactively labelled probe; malarial DNA combines with the human DNA causing a dark spot to appear on X-ray film and is diagnostic of malaria.

DOA *abbr* dead on arrival.

dobut·amine (dō-bū'-tà-mēn) *n* a directly acting stimulant of heart muscle which augments myocardial contractility in severe cardiac failure and shock syndrome, e.g. after myocardial infarction. (Dobutrex.)

Dobu·trex (dō'-bū-treks) *n* proprietary name for dobutamine*.

DOCA *abbr* ⇒ deoxycorticosterone acetate.

docusate sodium (do'-kū-sāt sō'-dē-um) stool softener helpful in the prevention of fecal impaction. Formerly dioctyl sodium sulfosuccinate.

Doderlein's bacil·lus (dod'-er-lēnz) *n* a non-pathogenic Gram-positive rod which normally lives in the vagina and by its action provides an acid medium.

Dogger Bank itch (dog'-gèr) sensitization dermatitis due to *Alcyonidum* (seaweed family). Clinical features include a papular and vesicular rash on hands and forearms with facial erythema and edema.

Dolo·bid (dol'-ō-bid) *n* proprietary name for diflunisal*.

Dolophine (dol'-ō-fēn) *n* proprietary name for methadone* hydrochloride.

dolor (dō'-lor) *n* pain; usually used in the context of being one of the four classical signs of inflammation—the others being calor*, rubor*, tumor*.

domi·nant (dom'-in-ant) *adj* describes a character possessed by one parent which, in the offspring, overrides the corresponding alternative character derived from the other parent. The words, and concepts, of dominance and recessivity are now often extended to the genes themselves which control the respective characters, recessive *opp* ⇒ Mendel's law.

domi·nant hemi·sphere (dom'-in-ant hem'-is-fēr) on the opposite side of the brain to that of the preferred hand. The dominant hemisphere for language is the left in 90% of right-handed and 30% of left-handed people.

do·nor (dō'-nor) *n* a person who gives blood for transfusion, or semen for AID*, or donates an organ for transplantation.

Donovan bodies (don'-ō-van bod'-ēz) Leishman-Donovan* bodies.

dopa (dō-på) *n* dihydroxyphenylalanine— an important compound formed in the intermediate stage in the synthesis of catecholamines* from tyrosine*.

dop·amine (dōp'-å-mēn) *n* a catecholamine neurotransmitter, closely related to adrenalin* and noradrenalin*. Increases cardiac output and renal blood flow but does not produce peripheral vasoconstriction. Most valuable in hypotension and shock of cardiac origin. Normally present in high concentration in those regions of the brain which are selectively damaged in Parkinsonism. *dopamine-β-hydroxylase* an enzyme present in blood; it is increased in high blood pressure.

Dop·pler ultra·sound tech·nique (dop'-ler) a machine sends out ultrasounds, which pick up the velocity of blood flow through the vein and are transmitted as sound. If the vein is completely occluded, no sound is transmitted as there is no flow.

Dopram (dō'-pram) proprietary name for doxapram*.

Dop·tone (dop'-tōn) *n* a trade name for an instrument using echo-sound principles to detect the fetal heart at a very early stage.

Doriden (dōr'-i-den) *n* proprietary name for glutethimide*.

Dornier litho·tryptor (dōr'-nē-er lith-ō-trip'-tor) a piece of equipment which can destroy certain types of kidney stones by shock waves thereby rendering invasive surgery unnecessary. The technique is called extra corporeal shockwave lithotrypsy (ESWL).

dor·sal (dōr'-sål) *adj* pertaining to the back, or the posterior part of an organ. *dorsal position* lying on the back with the head supported on a pillow.

dorsi·flexion (dōr-si-flek'-shun) *n* bending backwards. In the case of the great toe— upwards ⇒ Babinski's reflex.

dorso·central (dōr-sō-sen'-trål) *adj* at the back and in the center.

dorso·lumbar (dōr-sō-lum'-bår) *adj* pertaining to the lumbar region of the back.

dosi·meter, dose·meter (dō-sim'-e-tėr) *n* an instrument worn by personnel or placed within equipment to measure incident X-rays or gamma rays. Commonly a small photographic film in a special filter holder.

double vision (du'-bl vi'-zhun) ⇒ diplopia.

douche (doosh) *n* a stream of fluid directed against the body externally or into a body cavity.

Dover's pow·der (dō'-verz pow'-der) a time-honored remedy containing 10% of opium* and ipecacuanha*. Once used extensively as a diaphoretic, but is now prescribed less often.

Down syn·drome (*syn* mongolism) a congenital condition in which there is generally severe mental subnormality and facial characteristics vaguely resembling the Mongoloid races; stigma include oval tilted eyes, squint and a flattened occiput. The chromosome abnormality is of two types: (a) primary trisomy, caused by abnormal division of chromosome 21 (atmeiosis). This results in an extra chromosome instead of the normal pair; the infant has 47 chromosomes and is often born of an elderly mother (b) Structural abnormality involving chromosome 21, with a total number of 46 chromosomes, one of which has an abnormal structure as the result of a special translocation. Such infants are usually born of younger mothers and there is a higher risk of recurrence in subsequent pregnancies.

dox·apram (doks'-å-pram) *n* a stimulant of the vital medullary centers, useful in barbiturate poisoning.

dox·epin (doks'-e-pin) *n* one of the tricyclic antidepressants*. Effective after 3–15 days medication. (Sinequan.)

Doxidan (doks'-i-dan) *n* proprietary name for danthron*.

doxorub·icin (doks-ō-roo'-bi-sin) *n* a cytotoxic antibiotic which is particularly effective in childhood malignancies. It is similar to daunorubicin* but is less cardiotoxic. (Adriamycin.)

doxy·cycline (doks-i-sī'-klin) *n* a rapidly absorbed, slowly excreted tetracycline*. (Vibramycin.)

doxylamine (doks-yl'-å-mēn) *n* an antihistamine useful in the treatment of allergies.

Doylman's procedure (doyl'-mans) application of diathermy* through the esophagus to divide the wall between the esophagus and the lower end of a pharyngeal pouch, thereby draining the food from the pouch into the esophagus.

DP *abbr* Depo-Provera ⇒ medroxyprogesterone acetate.

DPT *abbr* a combination immunization providing immunity against diphtheria, pertussis, and tetanus.

draconti·asis (drak-on-tī'-à-sis) *n* infestation with *Dracunculus* medinensis* common in India and Africa.

Dracun·culus medin·ensis (drak-un'-kū-lus med-in-en'-sis) *n* (*syn* Guinea worm), a nematode parasite which infests man from contaminated drinking water. From the patient's intestine the adult female migrates to the skin surface to deposit her larvae, producing a cordlike thickening which ulcerates.

drain (drān) *n* a word used in surgery ⇒ wound.

Dram·amine (dram'-à-mēn) *n* proprietary name for dimenhydrinate*.

draw·sheet *n* a sheet in which the shortest side is about one-third the length of a bed and the longest side is at least twice the width of a bed. It is placed underneath the buttocks in such a way that a dry cool portion can be drawn through when necessary. It can also help to roll a patient from one side to the other.

dres·sings (dres'-ingz) *npl* ⇒ wound.

drip *n* ⇒ intravenous.

Dro·moran (drŏ'-mōr-an) *n* proprietary name for levorphanol*.

drop attacks periodic falling because of sudden loss of postural control of the lower limbs, without vertigo or loss of consciousness. Usually followed by sudden return of normal muscle tone, allowing the person to rise, if uninjured ⇒ vertebrobasilar insufficiency.

droper·idol (drŏ-pèr'-i-dol) *n* a neuroleptic agent. Can be used as a pre-operative premedication. Induces a state of mental detachment without loss of consciousness or effect upon respiratory system. (Inapsine.)

dropsy (drop'-sē) *n* ⇒ edema—**dropsical** *adj*.

drug *n* the generic name for any substance used for the prevention, diagnosis and treatment of diagnosed disease and also for the relief of symptoms. The term 'prescribed drug' describes such usage. The word medicine is usually preferred for therapeutic drugs to distinguish them from the addictive drugs which are used illegally. For alleviating unpleasant symptoms of self-limiting illnesses, any remedy which does not require a medical prescription is termed an 'over-the-counter' medicine. ⇒ non-compliance, non-comprehension. *drug dependence* a state arising from repeated administration of a drug on a periodic or continuous basis (WHO, 1964). Now a preferable term to drug addiction and drug habituation. *drug-fast* a term used to describe resistance of microbial cells to the action of antimicrobial drugs. *drug interaction* occurs when the pharmacological action of one drug is affected by another drug taken previously or simultanteously.

dry eye syn·drome ⇒ Sjögren's syndrome.

Dubowitz score (dū'-bō-wits) assesses gestational age.

Duchenne muscu·lar dys·trophy (dū-shen') an x-linked recessive disorder affecting only boys. The disorder usually begins to show between 3 and 5 years and is characterized by progressive muscle weakness and loss of locomotor skills. Death usually occurs during the teens or early twenties from respiratory or cardiac failure.

duck bill spec·ulum ⇒ Sim's speculum.

Ducrey's bacillus (dū-krāz') *Haemophilus* ducreyi*.

duct (dukt) *n* a tube or duct for carrying away the secretions from a gland.

duct·less glands endocrine* glands.

ductus arter·iosus (duk'-tus àr-tēr-ē-ō'sus) a blood vessel connecting the left pulmonary artery to the aorta, to bypass the lungs in the fetal circulation. At birth the duct closes, but if it remains open it is called *persistent ductus arteriosus*, a congenital heart defect.

Duhamel's oper·ation (dū-ham'-els) a surgical operation for Hirschsprung's* disease.

Duke's test (dōoks) the skin is pricked and the blood is continuously removed with absorbent paper until it ceases to flow. The normal bleeding time is 3–5 min.

Dulco·lax (dūl'-kō-laks) *n* proprietary name for bisacodyl*.

dumb·ness (dum'-nes) *n* ⇒ mutism.

'dump·ing syn·drome' (dump'-ing) the name given to the symptoms which sometimes follow a partial gastrectomy, epigastric fullness and a feeling of faintness and sweating after meals.

duo·denal intuba·tion (dū-ō-dē'-nàl, dū-od'-en-àl) ⇒ intubation.

duodenal ulcer an ulcer* which occurs in the duodenal lining caused by the action of acid and pepsin. Pain occurs several hours after meals, so they are described as hunger pains. Food relieves the pain so the patient does not usually lose weight. The ulcer can bleed, leading to occult blood in the stools, or it can perforate, constituting an abdominal emergency. Severe scarring following chronic ulceration may produce pyloric stenosis. Cimetidine* is the drug of choice for uncomplicated duodenal ulcers.

duoden·itis (dū-o-den-ī'-tis) *n* inflammation of the duodenum.

duodeno·jejunal (dū-ō-dēn-ō-je-jōō'-nàl) *adj* pertaining to the duodenum and jejunum.

duodeno·pancreat·ectomy (dū-ō-dē'-nō-pan-krē-at-ek'-to-mē) *n* surgical excision of the duodenum and part of the pancreas, carried out in cases of cancer arising in the region of the head of the pancreas.

duodeno·scope (dū-ō-dē'-nō-skōp) *n* a side-viewing flexible fiberoptic endoscope*—**duodenoscopic** *adj.* **duodenoscopy** *n*.

duoden·ostomy (dū-ō-dē-nos'-to-mē) *n* a surgically made fistula between the duodenum and another cavity, e.g. cholecystoduodenostomy, a fistula between the gallbladder and duodenum made to relieve jaundice in inoperable cancer of the head of the pancreas.

duo·denum (dū-ō-dē'-num, dū-o'-de-num) *n* the fixed, curved, first portion of the small intestine, connecting the stomach* above to the jejunum* below (⇒ Figure 18)—**duodenal** *adj.*

Dupuytren's contrac·ture (dū'-pwi-trens) painless, chronic flexion of the digits of the hand, especially the third and fourth, towards the palm. The etiology is uncertain but some cases are associated with hepatic cirrhosis.

Dura·bolin (dūr'-à-bol-in) *n* proprietary name for nandrolone* phenylpropionate.

dura mater (dū'-rà-mà'-ter) the outer fibrous membrane of the meninges which surround the brain and spinal cord.

DVT *abbr* deep vein thrombosis ⇒ phlebothrombosis.

dwarf *n* person of stunted growth. May be due to growth hormone deficiency. Also occurs in untreated congenital hypothyroidism (cretinism*) and juvenile hypothyroidism, achondroplasia and other conditions.

dwarf·ism (dwarf'-izm) *n* arrested growth and development as occurs in cretinism*, and in some chronic diseases such as intestinal malabsorption, renal failure and rickets.

dyazide (dī'-a-zīd) *n* proprietary name for triamterene* and hydrochlorothiazide*.

dyflos (DFP) (dī'-flōs) *n* a fluorine derivative with an action similar to that of eserine and neostigmine*. Used mostly as a 0.1% solution in oil for glaucoma, when a very long action is required. As an organophosphorous compound, it is used as an insecticide in agriculture. It has a powerful and irreversible anticholinesterase action which makes it potentially dangerous to man.

Dymelor (dī'-me-lōr) *n* proprietary name for acetohexamide*.

dy·namic psych·ology (dī-nam'-ik sī-kol'-o-jē) a psychological approach which stresses the importance of (typically unconscious) energy or motives, as in Freudian or psychoanalytic theory.

dyna·mometer (dī-nà-mo'-me-tèr) *n* apparatus to test the strength of grip.

Dyrenium (dī-ren'-ē-um) *n* proprietary name for triamterine*.

dys·arthria (dis-àrth'-rē-à) *n* a neuromuscular disorder affecting the actual formation and articulation of words, and therefore the listener's understanding of such speech to varying degrees; the patient's linguistic ability remains unimpaired. Generally, such speech is slow and monotonous with indistinct consonants and long intervals between words—**dysarthric** *adj.*

dys·calculia (dis-kal-kū'-lē-à) *n* impairment of numeral ability.

dys·chezia (dis-kē'-zē-à) *n* difficult or painful defecation.

dys·chondro·plasia (dis-kon-drō-plāz'-ē-à) *n* a disorder of bone growth resulting in normal trunk, short arms and legs.

dys·coria (dis-kōr'-ē-à) *n* abnormality of the pupil of the eye.

dys·crasia (dis-krā'-zē-à) *n* a morbid general state resulting from presence of toxic materials in the blood.

dys·entery (dis'-en-tèr-ē) *n* inflammation of the bowel with evacuation of blood and mucus, accompanied by tenesmus and colic—**dysenteric** *adj* amoebic dysentery is caused by the protozoon en-

tamoeba histolytica ⇒ amoebiasis. *bacillary dysentery* is caused by *Shigella shigae*. *S. Flexneri* or *S. sonnei*. Disease results from poor sanitation and the house-fly carries the infection from feces to food.

dysesthesia (dis-es-thēz'-ē-à) *n* impairment of touch sensation.

dys·function (dis-fungk'-shun) *n* abnormal functioning of any organ or part.

dysfunctional uterine bleeding any unusual uterine bleeding without organic uterine cause.

dys·gamma·globulin·emia (dis-gam'-mà-glob'-ū-lin-ē'-mē-à) *n* (*syn* antibody deficiency syndrome) disturbance of gammaglobulin production. Can be transient, congenital or acquired. Normally there is transfer of IgG from mother to baby, the amount so transferred gradually falls. This can lead to transient hypogammaglobulinemia with repeated respiratory infections. Injections of gammaglobulin are given until normal blood levels occur. Congenital agammaglobulinemia is a sex-linked recessive genetic variety and is the commonest type of total deficiency. The lymph nodes and spleen are abnormal. Males are solely affected, females being carriers of the abnormal gene. As yet there is no means of detecting carriers. The disease usually presents in the second or third year as severe, recurrent bacterial infections with high fever. Virus infections are handled well, because the defense mechanism is different. Acquired agammaglobulinemia occurs at any age and in either sex. Cause unknown. Secondary agammaglobulinemia may occur in lymphoma. Leukemia and myeloma, especially after chemotherapy or radiation. It may also be found in bullous skin disorders such as pemphigus and eczema and after burns when it is due to excessive loss of protein in the exuded fluid.

dys·genesis (dis-jen'-e-sis) *n* malformation during embryonic development—**dysgenetic** *adj.* **dysgenetically** *adv.*

dysgerminoma (dis-jèr-min-ō'-mà) *n* a tumor of the ovary of low grade malignancy. It is not hormone secreting, as it is developed from cells which date back to the undifferentiated state of gonadal development, i.e. before the cells have either male or female attributes.

dys·hidrosis (dis-hīd-rō'-sis) *n* a vesicular skin eruption, formerly thought to be caused by blockage of the sweat ducts at their orifice, histologically an eczematous process.

dys·karyosis (dis-kār-ē-ōs'-is) *n* a word used for the first stage of abnormality in a cervical smear. Follow-up tests may revert to normal, but some may become positive and demand biopsy.

dys·kinesia (dis-kin-ēz'-ē-à) *n* impairment of voluntary movement—**dyskinetic** *adj.* *tardive dyskinesia* uncontrollable movements often of the face and mouth which are a side-effect of antipsychotic medication.

dys·lalia (dis-lal'-ē-à) difficulty in talking due to defect of speech organs. Immature articulation—**dyslalic** *adj.*

dys·lexia (dis-leks'-ē-à) *n* a condition affecting the ability to read, write and spell in persons of the intelligence normally associated with such abilities. Can be acquired by brain injury or be the consequence of early sensory/neural disorders which prevent consistency of sensory input at the 'abinitio' stage of learning. This learning is later needed for identification procedures and maturity of function. Weaknesses placing a child at risk of remaining dyslexic can be genetically transmitted—**dyslexic** *adj.*

dysmaturity (dis-ma-tū'-ri-tē) *n* signs and symptoms of growth retardation at birth. ⇒ low birth-weight.

dys·melia (dis-mēl'-ē-à) *n* limb deficiency.

dys·menorrhea (dis-men-ōr-ē'-à) *n* painful menstruation, which in some women responds to an oral antiprostaglandin and in others to an oral contraceptive. *spasmodic dysmenorrhea* comes during the first day of a period, often within an hour or two of the start of bleeding. It comes in spasms of acute colicky pain in the lower part of the abdomen, and sometimes in the back and inner part of the thighs. The spasms can be bad enough to cause fainting and vomiting. *congestive dysmenorrhea* sufferers know several days in advance that their period is coming, because they have a dull aching pain in the lower abdomen, increasing heaviness, perhaps constipation, nausea and lack of appetite. There may also be breast tenderness, headache and backache. Fluid retention at this time leads to typical edema and weight gain; this can be helped by the use of diuretics.

dys·morpho·genic (dis-mōrf-ō-jen'-ik) *adj* now preferred to teratogenic when applied to drugs taken during pregnancy. ⇒ teratogen.

dysopia (dis-ō'-pē-à) *n* painful or defective vision.

95

dys·orexia (dis-ōr-eks'-ē-à) *n* an abnormal or unnatural appetite.

dys·pareunia (dis-pàr-ū'-nē-à) *n* painful or difficult coitus, experienced by the woman.

dys·pepsia (dis-pep'-sē-à) *n* indigestion—**dyspeptic** *adj.*

dys·phagia (dis-fā'-jē-à) *n* difficulty in swallowing—**dysphagic** *adj.*

dys·phasia (dis-fā'-zē-à) *n* in this disorder it is not the physical production of speech which is affected but the mental processes which permit formulation and understanding of language. *expressive dysphasia* results in disturbance of the memory of motor speech pattern, and the patient is therefore unable to communicate his thoughts even though comprehension is intact. Such speech is characterized by hesitancy, slowness and lack of grammar. Articulation and pronunciation are sometimes poor and thus may lead to an associated dysarthria*.

dys·plasia (dis-plā'-zē-à) *n* formation of abnormal tissue—**dysplastic** *adj.*

dysp·nea (disp'-nē-à) *n* difficulty in, or labored, breathing, can be mainly of an inspiratory or expiratory nature—**dyspponeic** *adj.*

dys·praxia (dis-praks'-ē-à) *n* lack of voluntary control over muscles, particularly the orofacial ones—**dyspraxic** *adj.*

dys·rhythmia (dis-rith'-mē-à) *n* disordered rhythm, usually of heart, e.g. atrial fibrillation*—**dysrhythmic** *adj.*

dys·taxia (dis-taks'-ē-à) *n* difficulty in controlling voluntary movements—**dystaxic** *adj.*

dys·tocia (dis-tōs'-ē-à) *n* difficult or slow labor.

dys·trophy (dis'-tro-fē) *n* defective nutrition of an organ or tissue, usually muscle. The word is applied to several unrelated conditions ⇒ muscular dystrophy. Duchenne muscular dystrophy.

dys·uria (dis-ūr'-ē-à) *n* painful micturition*—**dysuric** *adj.*

E

ear ⇒ Figure 13.

eardrum ⇒ Figure 13.

Eaton agent (ē'-ton) *Mycoplasmia* *pneumoniae.*

EBM *abbr* expressed breast milk.

EBV Epstein* Barr virus.

ebola (ē-bōl'-a) *n* one of the viral* hemorrhagic fevers, usually transmitted by ticks.

ec·bolic (ek-bol'-ik) *adj* describes any agent which stimulates contraction of the gravid uterus and hastens expulsion of its contents.

ECC external cardiac compressions.

ecchon·droma (ek-kon-drō'-mà) *n* a benign tumor composed of cartilage which protrudes from the surface of the bone in which it arises—**ecchondromata** *pl.*

ecchy·mosis (ek-i-mō'-sis) *n* an extravasation of blood under the skin. ⇒ bruise—**ecchymoses** *pl.*

ECG *abbr* electrocardiogram ⇒ electrocardiograph. Also electrocorticography*.

Echino·coccus (ek-in'-ō-kok'-us) *n* a genus of tapeworms, the adults infecting a primary host, e.g. a dog. In man (secondary host) the encysted larvae cause 'hydatid* disease'.

echo·cardiography (ek-ō-kàr-dē-og'-raf-ē) *n* the use of ultrasound as a diagnostic tool for studying the structure and motion of the heart.

echo·encephalography (ek-ō-en-sef-àl-og'-raf-ē) *n* passage of ultrasound waves across the head. Can detect abscess, blood clot, injury or tumor within brain.

echo·lalia (ek-ō-lāl'-ē-à) *n* repetition, almost automatically of words or phrases heard. Occurs most commonly in schizophrenia and dementia; sometimes in toxic delirious states. A characteristic of all infants' speech—**echolalic** *adj.*

echophony (ek'-ō-fō'-nē) *n* the echo of a vocal sound heard during auscultation of the chest.

echo·praxia (ek-ō-praks'-ē-à) *n* involuntary mimicking of another's movements.

echo·viruses (ek'-ō-vī'-rus-es) *npl* the name derives from Enteric Cytopathic Human Orphan. It was given because these viruses were originally found in the stools of diseaseless children. Echoviruses have caused meningitis and mild respiratory infection in children. At least 30 types have been identified.

eclamp·sia (ē-klamp'-sē-à) *n* **1** a severe manifestation of toxemia of pregnancy, associated with fits and coma. **2** a sudden convulsive attack—**eclamptic** *adj.*

ecm·nesia (ek-nē'-zē-à) *n* impaired memory for recent events with normal memory of remote ones. Common in old age and in early cerebral deterioration.

ecraseur (ă-krä-zēr') *n* an instrument with a wire loop that can be tightened round the pedicle of a new growth to sever it.

ECT *abbr* ⇒ electroconvulsive therapy.

ecthyma (ek-thī'-mà) *n* a crusted eruption of impetigo* contagiosa on the legs, producing necrosis of the skin, which heals with scarring. A similar condition occurs in syphilis.

ecto·derm (ek'-tō-dèrm) *n* the external primitive germ layer of the embryo. From it are developed the skin structures, the nervous system, organs of special sense, pineal gland and part of the pituitary and adrenal glands—**ectodermal** *adj*.

ecto·dermosis (ek-tō-dèrm-ō'-sis) *n* disease of any organ or tissue derived from the ectoderm.

ecto·genesis (ek-tō-jen'-e-sis) *n* the growth of the embryo outside the uterus (in* vitro fertilization).

ecto·parasite (ek-tō-pār'-a-sīt) *n* a parasite that lives on the exterior surface of its host—**ectoparasitic** *adj*.

ec·topia (ek-tō'-pē-à) *n* malposition of an organ or structure, usually congenital. *ectopia vesicae* an abnormally placed urinary bladder which protrudes through or opens on to the abdominal wall—**ectopic** *adj*.

ec·topic beat (ek-top'-ik) ⇒ extrasystole.

ec·topic preg·nancy (ek-top'-ik) (*syn* tubal pregnancy) extrauterine gestation, the fallopian tube being the most common site. At about the 6th week the tube ruptures, constituting a 'surgical emergency'.

ecto·zoa (ek-tō-zō'-à) *n* external parasites.

ectro·dactyly, ectrodactylia (ek-trō-dak'-til-ē) *n* congenital absence of one or more fingers or toes or parts of them.

ec·tropion (ek-trō'-pē-on) *n* an eversion or turnover outward, especially of the lower eyelid or of the pupil margin—*ectropion uveae*.

ECV *abbr* external cephalic version*.

ec·zema (ek'-ze-mà) *n* the eczema skin reaction begins with erythema, then vesicles appear. These rupture, forming crusts or leaving pits which ooze serum. This is the exudative or weeping stage. In the process of healing, the area becomes scaly. Some authorities limit the word 'eczema' to the cases with internal (endogenous) causes while those caused by external (exogenous) contact factors are called dermatitis or eczematous dermatitis. The skin of inpatients may be colonized or infected with hospital strains of *Staphylococcus aureus*. Due to the exfoliative nature of eczema, modification of patient management is required to protect others from infection. ⇒ dermatitis—**eczematous** *adj*.

eczema·asthma syndrome (ek'-ze-mà-az'-mà) affected infants begin with infantile eczema and in childhood develop asthma as the eczema remits; frequently the asthma remits at puberty.

EDC *abbr* ⇒ expected date of confinement.

Ede·crin (e'-de-krin) *n* proprietary name for ethacrinic* acid.

edema (e-dē'-mà) *n* abnormal infiltration of tissues with fluid. There are many causes–it can be in the blood, or disease of the cardiopulmonary system, the urinary system and the liver. → anasarca, angioneurotic edema, ascites–**edematous**, *adj*.

edent·ulous (ē-dent'-ū-lus) *adj* without natural teeth.

edro·phonium test (ed-rō-fō'-nē-um) in patients with myasthenia* gravis, a small intramuscular dose of edrophonium chloride will immediately relieve symptoms, albeit temporarily, while quinine sulfate will increase the muscular weakness.

EDTA *abbr* ethylenediaminetetraacetic acid, a chelating agent, the calcium and sodium salts of which have been used to remove harmful metal ions from the body, e.g. lead, excess calcium and radioactive heavy metals. The newly formed stable chelate compounds are excreted in the urine.

Edward syn·drome (ed'-ward) an autosomal trisomy* associated with mental subnormality. The cells have 47 chromosomes. Sometimes called trisomy E.

EEG *abbr* electroencephalogram* ⇒ electroencephalograph.

EENT *abbr* eye, ear, nose and throat.

EFAs *abbr* ⇒ essential fatty acids.

effec·tor (ĕf-fek'-tor) *n* a motor or secretory nerve ending in a muscle, gland or organ.

effer·ent (ef'-fèr-ent) *adj* carrying, conveying, conducting away from a center ⇒ afferent *opp*.

effleu·rage (ef-floo-razh') *n* a massage technique of using long, whole-hand strokes in one direction only, with the aim of assisting the venous return of blood which then increases arterial blood supply; edematous swelling can be reduced by this method. Alternatively, circular, finger-only movements can be applied, as in the Lamaze method of natural childbirth.

effort syn·drome (ef'-ort) a form of anxiety neurosis, manifesting itself in a variety of cardiac symptoms including precordial pain, for which no pathological explanation can be discovered.

effus·ion (ē-fū'-zhun) n extravasation of fluid into body tissues or cavities.

ego (ē'-gō) n refers to the conscious self, the 'I', which according to Freud, deals with reality, is influenced by social forces and controls unconscious instinctual urges (the id*).

Ehrlich's theory of immunity (ār'-liks) postulated that tissue cells received molecules of antigen by means of receptors. Under certain conditions these receptors were overproduced and released into the body fluids. The free receptor groups became the antibodies and were capable of combining specifically with antigen molecules.

EIA *abbr* exercise induced asthma. ⇒ asthma.

ejacu·lation (ē-jak-ū-lā'-shun) n the sudden emission of semen from the erect penis at the moment of male orgasm.

ejacu·latory duct (ē-jak'-ū-la-tōr-ē) ⇒ Figure 16.

Elase oint·ment (ē'-lās) a proprietary cleansing agent used in the debridement of necrotic debris and purulent exudates from wounds.

Elasto·plast (ē-last'-ō-plast) n a proprietary brand of elastic cotton cloth without rubber threads, with porous adhesive and non-fray edges. *Elastoplast bandages* are applied firmly in the ambulatory treatment of varicose ulcers and after injection treatment of veins; the compression reduces edema and pain and promotes healing. Removal of the bandages should be carefully carried out by cutting with special flat-bladed scissors. *Elastoplast dressings* are elastic, porous, adhesive dressings for surgical purposes. *Elastoplast extension plaster* 2.75 m length of elastic cotton cloth spread with porous adhesive in which the stretch is *across* the width; rigid lengthwise for skin traction in orthopedic conditions.

Elavil (el'-à-vil) n proprietary name for amitriptyline*.

elderly abuse non-accidental injury to the elderly, usually carried out in the domestic setting by those relatives responsible for their care → battering.

Electra com·plex (ē-lek'-trà) excessive emotional attachment of daughter to father. The name is derived from Greek mythology.

electro·cardio·gram (ECG) (ē-lek-trō-kàr'-de-ō-gram) n a recording of the electrical activity of the heart on a moving paper strip, made by an electrocardiograph*.

electro·cardio·graph (ē-lek-tro-kàr'-dē-ō-graf) n an instrument which records the electrical activity of the heart from electrodes on the limbs and chest—**electrocardiographic** adj, **electrocardiography** n, **electrocardiographically** adv.

electro·coagu·lation (ē-lek-trō-kō-ag-ū-lā'-shun) n technique of surgical diathermy*. Coagulation, especially of bleeding points, by means of electrodes.

electro·cochle·ography (ECoG) (ē-lek-trō-kō-klē-og'-raf-ē) n direct recording of the action potential generated following stimulation of the cochlear nerve.

electro·convulsive ther·apy (ECT) (ē-lek-trō-kon-vul'-siv) a form of physical treatment still used by psychiatrists mainly in the treatment of depression. An apparatus is used which delivers a definite voltage for a precise fraction of a second to electrodes placed on the head, producing a convulsion. *modified ECT* the convulsion is modified with an intravenous anesthetic and a muscle relaxant, thus reducing the risk of unpleasant sequelae. ECT is currently invariably modified. *unilateral ECT* avoids the sequela of amnesia for recent events. The mechanism for memory of recent events is probably in the dominant cerebral hemisphere which is the left in practically all people. ECT is therefore applied to the right hemisphere to minimize memory disturbance.

electro·cortic·ography (ē-lek-trō-kor-tik-og'-raf-ē) n direct recording from the cerebral cortex during operation—**electrocorticographic** adj, **electrocorticogram** n, **electrocorticograph** n, **electrocorticographically** adv.

elec·trode (ē-lek'-trōd) n in medicine, a conductor in the form of a pad or plate, whereby electricity enters or leaves the body in electrotherapy.

electro·desic·cation (ē-lek-trō-des-i-kā'-shun) n a technique of surgical diathermy*. There is drying and subsequent removal of tissue, e.g. papillomata.

electro·diag·nosis (ē-lek'-trō-dī-ag-nō'-sis) n the use of graphic recording of electrical irritability of tissues in diagnosis—**electrodiagnostic** adj.

electro·encephalo·gram (ē-lek'-trō-en-sef'-al-ō-gram) *n* (EEG) a recording of the electrical activity of the brain on a moving paper strip, made by an electroencephalograph*.

electro·encephalo·graph (ē-lek'-trō-en-sef'-al-ō-graf) *n* an instrument by which electrical impulses derived from the brain can be amplified and recorded on paper, in a fashion similar to that of the electrocardiograph—**electroencephalographic** *adj*, **electroencephalograph** *n*, **electroencephalographically** *adv*.

electroly·sis (ē-lek-trol'-is-is) *n* **1** chemical decomposition by electricity, with migration of ions shown by changes at the electrodes. **2** term used for the destruction of individual hairs (epilation), eradication of moles, spider naevi, etc, using electricity.

electro·lyte (ē-lek'-trō-līt) *n* a liquid or solution of a substance which is capable of conducting electricity because it dissociates into ions. In medical usage it refers to the ion itself, for example sodium, potassium, chloride and potassium ions in the serum. Various diseases can cause serum electrolyte imbalance; deficient ones can be replaced orally or by intravenous drip; those in excess can be removed by dialysis or by resins which can be taken by mouth or given by enema—**electrolytic** *adj*.

electro·myography (ē-lek-trō-mī-og'-raf-ē) *n* the use of an instrument which records electric currents generated in active muscle—**electromyographical** *adj*, **electromyogram** *n*, **electromyograph** *n*, **electromyographically** *adv*.

electro·oculo·graphy (ē-lek-trō-ok-ū-lo'-graf-ē) *n* the use of an instrument which records eye position and movement, and potential difference between front and back of the eyeball using electrodes placed on skin near socket. Can be used as an electrodiagnostic test—**electrooculographical** *adj*, **electro-oculogram** *n*, **electro-oculograph** *n*, **electro-oculographically** *adv*.

electro·pyrexia (ē-lek-tro-pī-reks'-ē-à) *n* a high body temperature produced by an electrical apparatus.

electro·retinogram (ERG) (ē-lek-trō-ret'-in-ō-gram) *n* graphic record of electrical currents generated in active retina.

electrosection (ē-lek'-trō-sek'-shun) *n* technique of surgical diathermy for cutting the skin or parting soft tissues.

electroshock therapy (ē-lek-trō-shok') electroconvulsive therapy*.

element (el'-e-ment) *n* one of the constituents of a compound. The elements are the primary substances which in pure form, or combined into compounds, constitute all matter.

elephan·tiasis (el-ef-an-tī'-a-sis) *n* the swelling of a limb, usually a leg, as a result of lymphatic obstruction (lymphedema), followed by thickening of the skin (pachydermia) and subcutaneous tissues. A complication of filariasis in tropical countries, or may be a result of syphilis or recurring streptococcal infection (elephantiasis nostras).

elimin·ation (ē-lim-in-ā'-shun) *n* the passage of waste from the body, usually reserved for urine and feces—**eliminate** *vt*.

ELISA *abbr* ⇒ enzyme-linked immunosorbent assay.

elixir (ē-liks'-ėr) *n* a sweetened, aromatic solution of a drug, often containing an appreciable amount of alcohol. Elixirs differ from syrups in containing very little sugar and in requiring dilution before use.

ellipto·cytosis (ē-lip-tō-sī-tō'-sis) *n* anemia in which the red blood cells are oval.

emaci·ation (ē-mā-shē-ā'-shun) *n* excessive leanness, or wasting of body tissue—**emaciate** *vt*.

emascu·lation (ē-mas-kū-lā'-shun) *n* castration*.

embol·ectomy (em-bol-ek'-to-mē) *n* surgical removal of an embolus*. Usually a fine balloon catheter is used to extract the embolus.

em·bolic (em-bol'-ik) *adj* pertaining to an embolism or an embolus.

embol·ism (em'-bol-izm) *n* the condition in which there is obstruction of a blood vessel by the impaction of a solid body (e.g. thrombi, fat globules, tumor cells) or an air bubble. ⇒ therapeutic embolization.

embolo·genic (em-bol-ō-jen'-ik) *adj* capable of producing an embolus*.

em·bolus (em'-bol-us) *n* solid body or air bubble transported in the circulation. ⇒ embolism—**emboli** *pl*.

embro·cation (em-brō-kā'-shun) *n* a liquid which is applied topically by rubbing.

em·bryo (em'-brē-ō) *n* the word applied to the developing ovum during the early months of gestation—**embryonic** *adj*.

embry·ology (em-brē-ol'-o-jē) *n* study of the development of an organism from fertilization to extrauterine life—**embryological** *adj*. **embryologically** *adv*.

embry·oma (em-brē-ōm′-à) *n* teratoma*.

embry·opathy (em-brē-op′-à-thē) *n* disease or abnormality in the embryo. More serious if it occurs in the first 3 months. Includes the 'rubella* syndrome'—**embryopathic** *adj*, **embryopathically** *adv*.

embry·otomy (em-brē-ot′-o-mē) *n* mutilation of the fetus to facilitate removal from the womb, when natural birth is impossible.

em·esis (em′-is-is) *n* vomiting.

em·etic (ē-met′-ik) *n* any agent used to produce vomiting.

em·etine (em′-i-tēn) *n* the principal alkaloid of ipecacuanha*. Used in amoebic dysentery, often in association with other amoebicides.

emiss·ion (ē-mish′-un) *n* an ejaculation or sending forth, especially an involuntary ejaculation of semen.

emme·tropia (em-met-rō′-pē-à) *n* normal or perfect vision—**emmetropic** *adj*.

emol·lient (ē-mol′-ē-ent) *adj, n* an agent which softens and soothes skin or mucous membrane.

emotion (ē-mō′-shun) *n* the tone of feeling recognized in ourselves by certain bodily changes, and in others by tendencies to certain characteristic behavior. Aroused usually by ideas or concepts.

emotion·al (ē-mō′-shun-al) *adj* characteristic of or caused by emotion. *emotional bias* tendency of emotional attitude to affect logical judgement. *emotional lability* ⇒ lability. *emotional state* effect of emotions on normal mood. e.g. agitation.

empa·thy (em′-path-ē) *n* identifying oneself with another person or the actions of another person. 'Putting oneself in another person's shoes'—**empathic** *adj*.

emphy·sema (em-fis-ēm′-à) *n* gaseous distension of the tissues. ⇒ crepitation, pulmonary, surgical emphysema—**emphysematous** *adj*.

empiri·cal (em-pir′-ik-àl) *adj* based on observation and experience and not on scientific reasoning.

em·pyema (em-pī-ēm′-à) *n* a collection of pus in a cavity, hollow organ or space.

EMT *abbr* emergency medical technician.

emul·sion (ē-mul′-shun) *n* a uniform suspension of fat or oil particles in an aqueous continuous phase (*O/W emulsion*) or aqueous droplets in an oily continuous phase (*W/O emulsion*).

en·amel (ē-nam′-el) *n* the hard, acellular external covering of the crown of a tooth.

encapsul·ation (en-kap-sū-lā′-shun) *n* enclosure within a capsule.

encepha·lins, enkephalins (en-sef′-à-lins, en-kef′-à-lins) *n* two pentapeptides which are neuroleptic and relieve pain. They are *methionine-encephalin* and *isoleucine encephalin*. Researchers have isolated them in the brain, gastrointestinal tract and the pituitary gland ⇒ endorphins.

encephal·itis (en-sef-àl-ī′-tis) *n* inflammation of the brain.

encephalo·cele (en-sef-al′-ō-sēl) *n* protrusion of brain substance through the skull. Often associated with hydrocephalus when the protrusion occurs at a suture line.

encepha·lography (en-sef-àl-og′-ra-fē) *n* a technique to examine the brain, to produce a printed or visible record of the investigation ⇒ echoencephalography, electroencephalography, pneumoencephalography—**encephalogram** *n*.

encephaloma (en-sef-àl-ō′-mà) *n* a tumor of the brain—**encephalomata**, *pl*.

encephalo·malacia (en-sef-àl-ō-mà-lās′-ē-à) *n* softening of the brain.

encephalo·myelitis (en-sef-à-lō-mī-el-ī′-tis) *n* inflammation of the brain and spinal cord.

encephalo·myelopathy *n* disease affecting both brain and spinal cord—**encephalomyelopathic** *adj*.

encepha·lon (en-sef′-à-lon) *n* the brain.

encepha·lopathy (en-sef-à-lop′-à-thē) *n* any disease of the brain—**encephalopathic** *adj*.

enchon·droma (en-kon-drō′-mà) *n* a cartilaginous tumor—**enchondromata** *pl*.

enco·presis (en-kō-prē′-sis) *n* involuntary passage of feces; the word is usually reserved for fecal incontinence associated with mental illness—**encopretic** *adj, n*.

encoun·ter group (en-kown′-ter) a form of psychotherapy. Members of a small group focus on becoming aware of their feelings and developing the ability to express them openly, honestly and clearly. The objectives are to increase self-awareness, promote personal growth and improve interpersonal communication.

Enda·moeba (end-à-mē′-bà) ⇒ Entamoeba.

endarter·ectomy (end-àr-tėr-ek′-to-mē) *n* the surgical removal of an atheromatous core from an artery, sometimes called disobliteration or 'rebore'. Carbon dioxide gas can be used to separate the occlusive core.

endarter·itis (end-år-tėr-īt'-is) *n* inflammation of the intima or inner lining coat of an artery. *endarteritis obliterans* the new intimal connective tissue obliterates the lumen.

endaural (end-ōr'-ål) *adj* pertaining to the inner portion of the external auditory canal.

en·demic (en-dem'-ik) *adj* recurring in an area ⇒ epidemic *opp*.

endemi·ology (en-dē-mē-ol'-o-jē) *n* the special study of endemic diseases.

Endep (en'-dep) *n* proprietary name for amitriptyline.

endo·cardial map·ping (en-dō-kår'-dē-al) the recording of electrical potentials from various sites on the endocardium to determine the site of origin of cardiac arrhythmia.

endo·cardial resect·ion (en-dō-kår'-dē-al rē-sek'-shun) surgical removal of that part of the endocardium causing cardiac arrhythmia.

endo·carditis (en-dō-kår-dī'-tis) *n* inflammation of the inner lining of the heart (endocardium*) due to infection by microorganisms (bacteria, fungi or *Rickettsia*), or to rheumatic fever. There may be temporary or permanent damage to the heart valves.

endo·cardium (en-dō-kår'-dē-um) *n* the lining membrane of the heart, which covers the valves.

endo·cervical (en-dō-sėr'-vi-kål) *adj* pertaining to the inside of the cervix uteri.

endo·cervi·citis (en-dō-sėr-vi-sī'-tis) *n* inflammation of the mucous membrane lining the cervix uteri.

endo·crine (en'-dō-krin) *adj* secreting internally ⇒ exocrine *opp*—**endocrinal** *adj, endocrine glands* the ductless glands of the body; those which make an internal secretion or hormone which passes into the blood stream and has an important influence on general metabolic processes: e.g. the pineal, pituitary, thyroid, parathyroids, adrenals, ovaries, testes and pancreas. The last-mentioned has both an internal and external secretion.

endocrin·ology (en'-dō-krin-ol'-o-jē) *n* the study of the ductless glands and their internal secretions.

endocrin·opathy (en-dō-krin-op'-a-thē) *n* abnormality of one or more of the endocrine glands or their secretions.

endoderm (en'-dō-dėrm) *n* the inner layer of cells which form during the early development of the embryo—**endodermal,** *adj*.

endogen·ous (en-do'-jen-us) *adj* originating within the organism. ⇒ ectogenous, exogenous *opp*.

endo·lymph (en'-dō-limf) *n* the fluid contained in the membranous labyrinth of the internal ear.

endo·lymphatic shunt (en-dō-limf-at'-ik) drainage of excess endolymph* from the vestibular labyrinth to the subarachnoid space where it flows to join the cerebrospinal fluid. Performed for patients with Ménière's disease.

endo·lysin (en-dō-lī'-sin) *n* an intracellular, leukocytic substance which destroys engulfed bacteria.

endo·metrioma (en-dō-mēt-rē-ō'-må) *n* a tumor of misplaced endometrium ⇒ chocolate cyst—**endometriomata** *pl*.

endo·metriosis (en-dō-mēt-rē-ōs'-is) *n* the presence of endometrium in abnormal sites ⇒ chocolate cyst.

endo·metritis (en-dō-mēt-rī'-tis) *n* inflammation of the endometrium*.

endo·metrium (en-dō-mēt'-rē-um) *n* the lining mucosa of the uterus—**endometrial** *adj*.

endo·myocardium (en-dō-mī-ō-kår'-dē-um) *n* relating to the endocardium and myocardium—**endomyocardial** *adj*.

endo·neurium (en-dō-nū'-rē-um) *n* the delicate, inner connective tissue surrounding the nerve fibers.

endo·parasite (en-dō-pår'-å-sīt) *n* any parasite living within its host—**endoparasitic** *adj*.

endophlebitis (en-dō-flē-bī'-tis) *n* inflammation of internal lining of vein. Can occur after prolonged intravenous infusion.

endoph·thalmitis (en-dōf-thal-mī'-tis) *n* internal infection of the eye, usually bacterial.

endor·phins (en'-dōr-fins, en-dōr'-fins) *n* a group of neuropeptides elaborated by the pituitary gland; they are said to be involved in both central and peripheral nervous functions. They originate from a multifunctional prohormone which is the common precursor of adrenocorticotrophic hormone and melanocyte-stimulating hormones. ⇒ encephalins.

endo·scope (en'-dō-skōp) *n* an instrument for visualization of body cavities or organs. The older ones are rigid, tubular and made of metal. If of the fiberoptic variety, light is transmitted by means of very fine glass fibers along a flexible tube. It can permit examination, photography and biopsy of the cavities or organs of a relaxed conscious person—**endoscopic** *adj*, **endoscopy** *n*.

endoscopic retrograde cholangio·pancreatography (ERCP) (en-dō-skop'-ik ret'-rō-grăd kŏl-anj'-ē-ō-pan'-krē-a-tog'-raf-ē) *n* introduction of an opaque medium into the pancreatic and bile ducts via a catheter from an endoscope located in the duodenum.

endo·spore (en'-dō-spŏr) *n* a bacterial spore which has a purely vegetative function. It is formed by the loss of water and probably rearrangement of the protein of the cell, so that metabolism is minimal and resistance to environmental conditions, especially high temperature, desiccation and antibacterial drugs, is high. The only genera which include pathogenic species that form spores are Bacillus and Clostridium.

endo·thelioid (en-dō-thē'-lē-oyd) *adj* resembling endothelium*.

endo·thelioma (en-dō-thē-lē-ō'-mà) *n* a malignant tumor derived from endothelial cells.

endo·thelium (en-dō-thē'-lē-um) *n* the lining membrane of serous cavities, heart, blood and lymph vessels—**endothelial** *adj*.

endo·toxin (en-dō-tok'-sin) *n* a toxic product of bacteria which is associated with the structure of the cell, and can only be obtained by destruction of the cell. ⇒ exotoxin *opp*.—**endotoxic** *adj*.

endo·tracheal (en-dō-trăk'-ē-ăl) *adj* within the trachea. *endotracheal anesthesia* the administration of an anesthetic through a special tube passed into the trachea.

End·uron (en'-dū-ron) *n* a proprietary preparation of methyclothiazidc* ⇒ chlorothiazide.

Enduronyl (en-dū'-re-nil) *n* proprietary name for a preparation of methyclothiazide* and deserpidine*.

en·ema (en'-em-à) *n* the introduction of a liquid into the bowel via the rectum, to be returned or retained. The word is usually preceded by the name of the liquid used. It can be further designated according to the function of the fluid. The evacuant enemas are usually prepared commercially in small bulk as a disposable enema; the chemicals attract water into the bowel promoting cleansing and peristatic contractions of the lower bowel. The enemas to be retained are usually drugs, the most common being

cortisone. ⇒ barium enema—**enemas, enemata** *pl*.

enflu·rane (en'-flū-ăn) *n* halogenated ether, a volatilie liquid anesthetic agent. (Ethrane.)

enkepha·lins (en-kef'-à-lins) *n* ⇒ encephalins.

enoph·thalmos (en-of-thal'-mus) *n* abnormal retraction of an eyeball within its orbit.

enostosis (en-os-tō'-sis) *n* a bony growth within the medullary canal of a bone.

ensi·form (en'-si-fōrm) *adj* sword shaped; xiphoid.

ENT *abbr* ear, nose and throat.

Ent·amoeba (ent-à-mē'-ba) *n* (*syn* Endamoeba) a genus of protozoon parasites, three species infesting man: *Entamoeba coli*, nonpathogenic, infesting intestinal tract; *E. gingivalis*, non-pathogenic, infesting mouth; *E. hystolytica*, pathogenic causing amoebic* dysentery.

en·teral (en'-tèr-ăl) *adj* within the gastrointestinal tract. *enteral diets* those which are taken by mouth or through a naso-gastric* tube; low residue enteral diets can be whole protein/polymeric, or amino acid/peptide. *enteral feeding* includes the introduction of nutrients into the gastrointestinal tract by modes other than eating ⇒ gastrostomy, nasogastric.

en·teric (en-tèr'-ik) *adj* pertaining to the small intestine. *enteric fever* includes typhoid* and paratyphoid* fever.

enter·itis (en-tèr-ī'-tis) *n* inflammation of the intestines. The term 'regional enteritis' is currently preferred for Crohn's* disease.

enteroanastomosis (en'-tèr-ō-an-as-to-mō'-sis) *n* intestinal anastomosis.

Enterobacter (en'-tèr-ō-bak'-tèr) *n* a genus of aerobic, nonspore-bearing. Gram-negative bacilli of the family Enterobacteriaceae. Includes two species. *Enterobacter aerogenes* and *Enterobacter cloacae*.

entero·biasis (en'-tèr-ō-bī'-à-sis) *n* infestation with *Enterobius vermicularis* (threadworms).

Entero·bius vermicularis (threadworm) (en'-tèr-ō-bī'-us vèr-mik'-ū-lār'-is) a nematode which infests the small and large intestine. Because of the autoinfective life-cycle, treatment aims at complete elimination. Each member of household given three single dose treatments at weekly intervals of piperazine citrate. 75 mg/kg. Hygiene measures necessary to prevent re-infestation during treatment.

entero·cele (en'-tėr-ō-sēl) *n* prolapse* of intestine. Can be into the upper third of vagina.

entero·clysis (en-tėr-ō-klī'-sis) *n* (*syn* proctoclysis) the introduction of fluid into the rectum.

Entero·coccus (en-tėr-ō-kok'-us) *n* a Gram-positive coccus which occurs in short chains and is relatively resistant to heat. Enterococci belong to Lancefield's group D, and occur as commensals in human and warm-blooded animal intestines, and sometimes as pathogens in infections of the urinary tract, ear, wounds and more rarely, in endocarditis.

entero·colitis (en-tėr-ō-kō-lī'-tis) *n* inflammation of the small intestine and colon ⇒ necrotizing enterocolitis.

entero·kinase (en-tėr-ō-kī'-nās) *n* (*syn* enteropeptidase) an enzyme in intestinal juice. A proteolytic enzyme of the pancreatic juice which converts inactive trypsinogen into active trypsin.

entero·lith (en'-tėr-ō-lith) *n* an intestinal concretion.

entero·lithiasis (en'-tėr-ō-lith-ī'-à-sis) *n* the presence of intestinal concretions.

en·teron (en'-tėr-on) *n* the gut.

entero·peptidase (en'-tėr-ō-pep'-tī-dās) *n* ⇒ enterokinase.

enter·ostomy (en-tėr-os'-to-mē) *n* a surgically established fistula between the small intestine and some other surface ⇒ gastroenterostomy, ileostomy, jejunostomy—**enterostomal** *adj*.

enter·otomy (en-tėr-ot'-om-ē) *n* an incision into the small intestine.

enter·otoxin (en-tėr-ō-toks'-in) *n* a toxin which has its effect on the gastrointestinal tract, causing vomiting, diarrhea and abdominal pain.

entero·tribe (en'-tėr-ō-trīb) *n* a metal clamp which causes necrosis of the spur of a double-barrelled colostomy, as a preliminary to its closure.

entero·viruses (en'-tėr-ō-vī'-rus-es) *npl* viruses which enter the body by the alimentary tract. Comprise the poliomyelitis virus, coxsackie viruses and echo viruses, which tend to invade the central nervous system. Enteroviruses, together with rhinoviruses*, are now called picornaviruses.

enter·ozoa (en-tėr-ō-zō'-à) *n* any animal parasites infesting the intestines—**enterozoon** *sing*.

en·tropion (en-trō'-pē-on) *n* inversion of an eyelid so that the lashes are in contact with the globe of the eye.

enu·cleation (ē-nū-klē-ā'-shun) *n* the removal of an organ or tumor in its entirety, as of an eyeball from its socket.

enur·esis (ē-nū-rē'-sis) *n* incontinence of urine, especially bed-wetting. *nocturnal enuresis* bed wetting during sleep.

environ·ment (en-vī'-ron-ment) *n* external surroundings. Environmental factors are conditions influencing an individual from without—**environmental** *adj*.

en·zyme (en'-zīm) *n* a soluble protein produced by living cells; it acts as a catalyst* without being destroyed or altered, and the substrate is often specific—**enzymatic** *adj*. *enzyme tests* since abnormal levels of particular enzymes can indicate specific underlying disease, tests for various enzymes can be a diagnostic tool.

enzyme-linked immunosorbent assay (en'-zīm-linkd-im-ū'-nō-sōr'-bent as'-ā) a method of testing for AIDS antibodies. The presence of antibodies means that the virus has been in the body; it does not necessarily mean that the virus is still present. Nor does it mean that the person will necessarily develop AIDS* or ARC*.

enzym·ology (en'-zīm-ol'-o-jē) *n* the science dealing with the structure and function of enzymes*—**enzymological** *adj*, **enzymologically** *adv*.

eosin (ē'-ō-sin) *n* a red staining agent used in histology and laboratory diagnostic procedures.

eosino·phil (ē-ō-sin'-ō-fil) *n* **1** cells having an affinity for eosin. **2** a type of polymorphonuclear leukocyte containing eosin-staining granules—**eosinophilic** *adj*.

eosino·philia (ē-ō-sin-ō-fil'-ē-à) *n* increased eosinophils in the blood.

ependy·moma (ep-end-im-ō'-mà) *n* neoplasm arising in the lining of the cerebral ventricles or central canal of spinal cord. Occurs in all age groups.

eph·edrine (ef-ed'-rin) *n* a drug widely used in asthma and bronchial spasm for its relaxant action on bronchioles; raises blood pressure by peripheral vasoconstriction. Useful in hay fever.

ephel·ides (e-fe'-līds) *npl* freckles, an increase in pigment granules with a normal number of pigment cells. ⇒ lentigo—**ephelis** *sing*.

epi·canthus (ep-i-kan'-thus) *n* the congenital occurrence of a fold of skin obscuring the inner canthus of the eye—**epicanthal** *adj*.

epi·cardium (ep-i-kår'-dē-um) *n* the visceral layer of the pericardium—**epicardial** *adj*.

epi·critic (ep-i-krit'-ik) *adj* describes cutaneous nerve fibers which are sensitive to fine variations of touch or temperature. ⇒ protopathic *opp*.

epi·demic (ep-i-dem'-ik) *n* simultaneously affecting many people in an area ⇒ endemic *opp*.

epidemi·ology (ep-i-dēm-ē-ol'-o-jē) *n* the scientific study of the distribution of disease—**epidemiological** *adj*, **epidemiologically** *adv*.

epi·dermis (ep-i-dėr'-mis) *n* the external non-vascular layer of the skin (⇒ Figure 12); the cuticle—**epidermal** *adj*.

Epidermo·phyton (ep-i-dėr-mōf'-i-ton) *n* a genus of fungi which affects the skin and nails.

epidermo·phytosis (ep-i-dėr-mō-fī-tō'-sis) *n* infection with fungi of the genus *Epidermophyton*.

epididy·mectomy (ep-id-id-i-mek'-to-mē) *n* surgical removal of the epididymis*.

epididy·mis (ep-id-id'-i-mis) *n* a small oblong body attached to the posterior surface of the testes (⇒ Figure 16). It consists of the tubules which convey the spermatozoa from the testes to the vas deferens.

epididy·mitis (ep-id-id-i-mī'-tis) *n* inflammation of the epididymis*.

epididymo·orchitis (ep-id-id-i-mō-ōr-kī'-tis) *n* inflammation of the epididymis* and the testis*.

epi·dural (ep-i-dū'-rål) *adj* upon or external to the dura. *epidural block* single injection or intermittent injection through a catheter of local anesthetic for maternal analgesia during delivery or for surgical operations. *epidural space* the region through which spinal nerves leave the spinal cord. It can be approached at any level of the spine, but the administering of anesthetic is commonly done at the lumbar level or through the sacral cornua for caudal epidural block.

epi·gastrium (ep-i-gas'-trē-um) *n* the abdominal region laying directly over the stomach—**epigastric** *adj*.

epi·glottis (ep-i-glot'-tis) *n* the thin leaf-shaped flap of cartilage behind the tongue which, during the act of swallowing, covers the opening leading into the larynx (⇒ Figure 6).

epiglot·titis (ep-i-glot-ī'-tis) *n* inflammation of the epiglottis*.

epi·lation (ep-i-lā'-shun) *n* extraction or destruction of hair roots, e.g. by coagulation necrosis, electrolysis or forceps. ⇒ depilation—**epilate** *vi*.

epi·latory (ep-il'-à-tōr-ē) *adj, n* describes an agent which produces epilation*.

epi·lepsy (ep'-il-ep-sē) *n* correctly called the epilepsies, a group of conditions resulting from disordered electrical activity of brain. The seizure is caused by an abnormal electrical discharge that disturbs cerebration and usually results in loss of consciousness. *major epilepsy* (*syn* grand mal), loss of consciousness with generalized convulsions. When patient does not regain consciousness between attacks the term status* epilepticus is used. *flicker epilepsy* one or more convulsions occurring as a result of exposure to flickering light, particularly liable to occur with multicolored light. *focal epilepsy* (*syn* Jacksonian epilepsy) motor seizure begins in one part of body, can spread to other muscle groups so that the fit is similar to clonic stage of major epilepsy. Fits can be sensory, i.e. abnormal *feeling* in one part, which spread to other parts. In *psychomotor epilepsy, temporal lobe epilepsy* 'psychic' warning of seizure consists of feelings of unreality, déjà vu; auditory, visual, gustatory or olfactory hallucinations. Jerking not as severe as in major epilepsy. *minor epilepsy* (*syn* petit mal) characterized by transitory interruption of consciousness without convulsions. Characteristic spike and wave pattern on EEG. Any seizure not conforming to this definition is not petit mal. The term is widely misused. All except petit mal can be symptomatic or idiopathic, but focal and temporal lobe epilepsy carry a higher incidence of symptomatic causes. Petit mal is always idiopathic. ⇒ akinetic.

epilep·tic (ep-il-ep'-tik) **1** *adj* pertaining to epilepsy. **2** *n* a person with epilepsy. *epileptic aura* premonitory subjective phenomena (tingling in the hand or visual or auditory sensations) which precede an attack of major epilepsy. ⇒ aura. *epileptic cry* the croak or shout heard from the epileptic person as he falls unconscious.

epilepti·form (ep-il-ep'-ti-fŏrm) *adj* resembling epilepsy.

epilepto·genic (ep-il-ep-tō-jeń-ik) *adj* capable of causing epilepsy.

epiloia (ep-il-oy'-à) *n* ⇒ tuberous sclerosis.

epimenor·rhea (ep-i-men-or-rē'-à) *n* reduction of the length of the menstrual cycle.

epi·nephrine (ep-in-ef'-rin) *n* a hormone produced by the adrenal medulla in mammals. It can be prepared synthetically. Solutions may darken in color and lose activity if stored for long periods. Applied locally in epistaxis; given by subcutaneous injection, it is invaluable in relieving serum sickness, asthmatic attacks, urticaria and other allergic states. It is added to local anesthetic solutions to reduce diffusion and so prolong the anesthetic effect. Also used in circulatory collapse, but only in very dilute solution (1:100,000) by slow intravenous infusion. (*syn* Adrenalin).

epi·phora (ē-pif'-ōr-à) *n* pathological overflow of tears on to the cheek.

epi·physis (ē-pif'-i-sis) *n* the end of a growing bone. Separated from the shaft by a plate of cartilage (epiphyseal plate) which disappears due to ossification when growth ceases—**epiphyses** *pl*, **epiphyseal** *adj*.

epiphysitis (e-pif-is-īt'-is) *n* inflammation of an epiphysis*.

epi·ploon (ep-i-plō'-on) *n* the greater omentum*—**epiploic** *adj*.

epi·sclera (ep-i-sklèr'-à) *n* loose connective tissue between the sclera and conjunctiva—**episcleral** *adj*.

epi·scleritis (ep-i-sklèr-ī'-tis) *n* inflammation of the episclera*.

episior·rhaphy (ep-ēs-ē-ōr'-a-fē) *n* surgical repair of a lacerated perineum.

episi·otomy (ep-ēs-ē-ot'-om-ē) *n* a perineal incision made during the birth of a child when the vaginal orifice does not stretch sufficiently.

epi·spadias (ep-i-spā'-dē-às) *n* a congenital opening of the urethra on the anterior (upper side) of the penis, often associated with ectopia* vesicae. ⇒ hypospadias.

epi·spastic (ep-i-spas'-tik) *n* a blistering agent.

epi·staxis (ep-is-taks'-is) *n* bleeding from the nose—**epistaxes** *pl*.

epithelial·ization (ep-i-thēl'-ē-àl-īz-ā'-shun) *n* the growth of epithelium over a raw area; the final stage of healing.

epi·thelioma (ep-i-thēl-ē-ō'-mà) *n* a malignant growth arising from squamous or transitional epithelium, usually the skin, esophagus or external genital organs.

epi·thelium (ep-i-thēl'-ē-um) *n* the surface layer of cells covering cutaneous, mucous and serous surfaces. It is classified according to the arrangement and shape of the cells it contains—**epithelial** *adj*.

Eppy (ep'-ē) *n* proprietary brand of neutral epinephrine* eye drops for use in open angle glaucoma.

Epsom salts (ep'-som) *n* ⇒ magnesium sulfate.

Epstein Barr virus (EBV) (ep'-stēn-bar' vī'-rus) causative agent of infectious* mononucleosis. A versatile herpes virus which infects many people throughout the world; does not always produce symptoms. Cancer research workers have discovered EBV genome in the malignant cells of Burkitt's lymphoma and nasopharyngeal carcinoma.

Epstein's pearls small white patches on the palate of the newborn.

epulis (e-pū'-lis) *n* a tumor growing on or from the gums.

Equal (ē'-kwàl) *n* proprietary name for aspartame*.

Equanil (e'-kwan-il) *n* proprietary name for meprobamate*.

Erb's palsy (erbs) paralysis* involving the shoulder and arm muscles from a lesion of the fifth and sixth cervical nerve roots. The arm hangs loosely at the side with the forearm pronated ('waiter's tip position'). Most commonly a birth injury.

ERCP *abbr* endoscopic* retrograde cholangiopancreatography.

erec·tile (ē-rek'-tīl) *adj* upright; capable of being elevated; *erectile tissue* highly vascular tissue, which, under stimulus, becomes rigid and erect from hyperemia.

erec·tion (ē-rek'-shun) *n* the state achieved when erectile tissue is hyperemic.

erec·tor (ē-rek'-tōr) *n* a muscle which achieves erection of a part. *erector spinae* ⇒ Figure 5.

erepsin (ē-rep'-sin) *n* a proteolytic enzyme in succus entericus (intestinal fluid).

ERG *abbr* ⇒ electroretinogram.

Ergomar (èr'-gō-mar) *n* proprietary name for ergotamine*.

erg·ometry (er-go'-me-trē) *n* measurement of work done by muscles—**ergometric** *adj*.

ergo·nomics (èr-gō-nom'-iks) *n* the application of various biological disciplines in relation to man and his working environment.

ergonovine (ėr-gō-nō'-vēn) n main alkaloid of ergot*. Widely used in obstetrics to reduce hemorrhage and improve contraction of the uterus. (Ergotrate.)

ergost·erol (ėr-gos'-tėr-ol) n a provitamin present in the subcutaneous fat of man and animals. On irradiation it is converted into vitamin D_2, which has antirachitic properties.

er·got (ėr'-got) n a fungus found on rye. Widely used as ergonovine* for postpartum hemorrhage.

ergot·amine (ėr-got'-à-mēn) n an alkaloid of ergot* used in the treatment of migraine. Early ergotamine treatment of an attack is more effective, especially when combined with antiemetics. (Ergomar.)

ergo·tism (ėr'-got-izm) n poisoning by ergot*, which may cause gangrene, particularly of the fingers and toes.

Ergo·trate (ėr'-gō-trāt) n proprietary name for ergonovine*.

erosion (ē-rō'-zhun) n a wearing away or a kind of ulceration. *cervical erosion* a destruction of the tissue of the external layer of the cervix.

eruc·tation (ē-ruk-tā'-shun) n ⇒ belching.

erup·tion (ē-rup'-shun) n the process by which a tooth emerges through the alveolar bone and gingiva.

erysip·elas (e-ri-sip'-e-las) n an acute, specific infectious disease, in which there is a spreading, streptococcal inflammation of the skin and subcutaneous tissues, accompanied by fever and constitutional disturbances.

erysipel·oid (e-ri-sip'-ė-loyd) n a skin condition resembling erysipelas*. It occurs in butchers, persons who handle fish or cooks. The infecting organism is the *Erysipelothrix* of swine erysipelas.

ery·thema (e-ri-thē'-mà) n reddening of the skin—**erythematous** adj. *erythema induratum* Bazin's* disease. *erythema multiforme* a form of toxic or allergic skin eruption which breaks out suddenly and lasts for days; the lesions are in the form of violet-pink papules or plaques and suggest urticarial weals. Severe form called Stevens-Johnson syndrome. *erythema nodosum* an eruption of painful red nodules on the front of the legs. It occurs in young women, and is generally accompanied by rheumatoid pains. It may be a symptom of many diseases including tuberculosis, acute rheumatism, gonococcal septicemia, etc. *erythema pernio* ⇒ chilblain.

erythr·emia (e-ri-thē'-mē-à) n ⇒ polycythemia.

erythro·blast (er-ith'-rō-blast) n a nucleated red blood cell found in the red bone marrow from which the erythrocytes* are derived—**erythroblastic** adj.

erythro·blastosis fet·alis (er-ith-rō-blast-ōs'-is) ⇒ hemolytic disease of the newborn. Immunization of women at risk, using immunoglobulin containing a high titer of anti-D, prevents the condition.

Ery·throcin (er-ith'-rō-sin) n proprietary name for erythromycin*.

erythro·cyanosis frigida (er-ith-rō-sī-an-ōs'-is) n vasospastic disease with hypertrophy of arteriolar muscular coat—**erythrocyanotic** adj.

erythro·cytes (e-rith'-rō-sītz) npl the normal non-nucleated red cells of the circulating blood; the red blood corpuscles—**erythrocytic** adj. *erythrocyte sedimentation rate (ESR)* citrated blood is placed in a narrow tube. The red cells fall, leaving a column of clear supernatant serum, which is measured at the end of an hour and reported in millimeters. Tissue destruction and inflammatory conditions cause an increase in the ESR.

erythro·cythemia (e-rith-rō-sī-thē'-mē-à) n overproduction of red cells. This may be: (a) a physiological response to a low atmospheric oxygen tension (high altitudes), or to the need for greater oxygenation of the tissues (congenital heart disease), in which case it is referred to as erythrocytosis; or (b) an idiopathic condition—polycythemia* vera—**erythrocythemic** adj.

erythro·cytopenia (e-rith-rō-sī-tō-pēn'-ē-à) n deficiency in the number of red blood cells—**erythrocytopenic** adj.

erythro·cytosis (e-rith-rō-sī-tōs'-is) ⇒ erythrocythemia.

erythro·derma (e-rith'-rō-dėr-mà) n excessive redness of the skin.

erythr·oedema poly·neuritis (e-rith'-rō-e-dē'-mà-pol-ē-nū-rī'-tis) n (syn pink disease) a former disease of infancy characterized by red, swollen extremities, photophobia and irritability, caused by mercury poisoning.

erythro·genic (e-rith-rō-jen'-ik) adj 1 producing or causing a rash. 2 producing red blood cells.

erythro·mycin (e-rith-rō-mī'-sin) n an orally active antibiotic, similar to penicillin* in its range of action. Best reserved for use against organisms resistant to other antibiotics. Risk of jaundice, particularly with erythromycin estolate. (Erythrocin.)

erythro·penia (e-rith-rō-pē'-nē-à) *n* a reduction in the number of red blood cells; it usually, but not necessarily, occurs in anemia.

erythro·poiesis (e-rith-rō-pī-ē'-sis) *n* the production of red blood cells ⇒ hemopoiesis.

erythro·poietin (e-rith-rō-pī-ē'-tin) *n* a hormone secreted by certain cells in the kidney in response to a lowered oxygen content in the blood. It acts on the bone marrow, stimulating erythropoiesis*.

erythro·sine (e-rith'-rō-sēn) *n* a red dye used in dental disclosing tablets.

Esbach's albumin·ometer (es'-baks al-bū'-min-ō'-me-tèr) a graduated glass tube in which albumin in urine is precipitated by the addition of Esbach's reagent (picric acid) and the result read after 24 h.

es·char (es'-kàr) *n* a slough, as results from a burn, application of caustics, diathermy etc.

eschar·otic (es-kàr-ot'-ik) *adj* describes any agent capable of producing a slough.

Escher·ichia (esh-èr-ēk'-ē-à) *n* a genus of bacteria. Motile, Gram-negative rods which are widely distributed in nature, especially in the intestinal tract of vertebrates. Some strains are pathogenic to man, causing enteritis, peritonitis, pyelitis, cystitis and wound infections. The type species is *Escherichia coli*.

Esi·drix (e'-si-driks) *n* proprietary name for hydrochlorothiazide*.

Eskalith (es'-kà-lith) *n* proprietary name for lithium carbonate.

Esmarch's ban·dage (es'marks) a rubber roller bandage used to procure a bloodless operative field in the limbs.

eso·phageal (ē-sof-a-je'-al) *adj* pertaining to the esophagus*. *esophageal ulcer* ulceration of the esophagus due to gastroesophageal reflux caused by hiatus hernia*. *esophageal varices* varicosity of the veins in the lower esophagus due to portal hypertension, they often extend below the cardia into the stomach. These varices can bleed and cause a massive hematemesis, but this occurs only in a minority of patients. Others present with iron deficiency anemia or melena.

esopha·gectasis (ē-sof-a-jek'-ta-sis) *n* a dilated esophagus*.

esopha·gectomy (ē-sof-a-jek'-to-mē) *n* excision of part of the whole of the esophagus*.

esopha·gitis (ē-sof-a-gī'-tis) *n* inflammation of the esophagus*.

esophago·scope (ē-sof'-a-gō-skōp) *n* an endoscope* for passage into the esophagus*—**esophagoscopy** *n*, **esophagoscopic** *adj*.

esophag·ostomy (ē-sof-a-gos'-to-mē) *n* a surgically established fistula between the esophagus and the skin in the root of the neck. Used temporarily for feeding after excision of the pharynx for malignant disease.

esophag·otomy (ē-sof-a-got'-o-mē) *n* an incision into the esophagus.

esoph·agus (ē-sof'-a-gus) *n* the musculomembranous canal. 23 cm in length, extending from the pharynx* to the stomach* (⇒ Figure 18)—**esophageal** *adj*.

espun·dia (es-pun'-dē-a) *n* South American mucocutaneous leishmaniasis*.

ESR *abbr* erythrocyte* sedimentation rate.

ESRD *abbr* end stage renal disease ⇒ renal.

es·sence (es'-ens) *n* a solution of a volatile oil in rectified spirit.

essen·tial amino acids ⇒ amino acids.

essen·tial fatty acids (EFAs) (arachidonic, tinoleic and linolenic acids). Polyunsaturated acids which cannot be synthesized in the body. They have diverse functions, the most important being that they are precursors of prostaglandins, fulfill an important role in fat metabolism and transfer and are thought to prevent and break up cholesterol deposits on arterial walls. They are present in natural vegetable oils and fish oils. Research suggests that deficiency contributes to premenstrual syndrome.

estra·diol (es-trà-dī'-ol) *n* synthetic estrogen. Given in amenorrhea kraurosis, menopause and other conditions of estrogen deficiency, orally and by injection.

estriol (es'-trē-ol) *n* estrogen metabolite present in the urine of pregnant women. The fetus and placenta are concerned in its production. Estriol excretion is an indicator of fetal well being.

estro·gen (es'-trō-jen) *n* a generic term referring to ovarian hormones. Three 'classical' ones: estriol, estrone, and estradiol. Urinary excretion of these substances increases throughout normal pregnancy—**estrogenic** *adj*.

estrone (es'-trōn) *n* an ovarian hormone.

Estro·vis (es'-trō-vis) proprietary name for quinestrol*.

ESWL *abbr* extracorporeal shock-wave lithotrypsy. ⇒ Dornier lithotryptor.

etha·crynic acid (eth-à-krin'-ik) a loop diuretic with a wider range of effectiveness than the thiazide group of saluretics. (Edecrin.) ⇒ diuretics.

etham·butol (eth-am′-bū-tol) *n* a synthetic antituberculosis drug which can be taken by mouth. It is highly effective when used with isoniazid* for tuberculosis. Almost non-toxic, but occasionally its toxic effect results in retrobulbar neuritis. (Myambutol.)

etha·nol (eth′-a-nol) *n* alcohol*.

ether (ē′-thėr) *n* an inflammable liquid, one of the oldest volatile anesthetics and less toxic than chloroform. Rarely used today in the Western world as a general anesthetic.

eth·ics (eth′-iks) *n* a code of moral principles derived from a system of values and beliefs.

ethinyl·estradiol (eth′-in-yl-es-trà-dī′-ol *n* a powerful orally effective estrogen, usually well tolerated.

ethion·amide (eth-ī-on′-à-mīd) *n* expensive synthetic antitubercular compound. Hepatotoxicity guarded against by twice weekly SGOT tests. Like isoniazid*, ethionamide can be neurotoxic. It can produce gastrointestinal side effects. (Trecator.)

eth·moid (eth′-moyd) *n* a spongy bone forming the lateral walls of the nose and the upper portion of the bony nasal septum (⇒ Figure 14).

ethmoid·ectomy (eth-moyd-ek′-to-mē) *n* surgical removal of a part of the ethmoid bone, usually that forming the lateral nasal walls.

eth·nic (eth′-nik) *adj* pertaining to racial or cultural groups.

eth·nology (eth-nol′-o-jē) *n* a branch of anthropology which has implications for health care; it studies mainly the cultural differences between groups, particularly the attitudes, values and beliefs relating to such life events as birth, contraception, abortion, marriage, diet, health care and death—**ethnological** *adj*, **ethnologically** *adv*.

etho·heptazine (eth-ō-hep′-tà-zēn) *n* an analgesic which relieves muscle spasm. Related to pethidine*.

etho·propazine (eth-ō-prō′-pà-zēn) *n* an antispasmodic used chiefly in rigidity of parkinsonism. May have more side effects than other drugs.

etho·suximide (eth-ō-suks′-i-mīd) *n* an anti-convulsant useful in minor epilepsy. (Zarontin.)

etho·toin (eth-ō-tō′-in) *n* an antiepileptic

drug which is useful for major, focal and psychomotor epilepsy. (Peganone.)

Eth·rane (eth′-rān) *n* proprietary name for enflurane*.

ethyl chlor·ide (eth′-yl klōr′īd) *n* a volatile general anesthetic for short operations, and a local anesthetic by reason of the intense cold produced when applied to the skin; useful in sprains.

ethyl·estrenol (eth-yl-es′-tren-ol) *n* an anabolic steroid; useful for treating severe weight loss, debility and osteoporosis.

ethylnorepinephrine (eth′-yl-nōr-e-pin-ef′-rin) *n* bronchodilator useful for asthma. (Bronkephrine.)

ethy·nodiol diacetate (eth′-i-nō-dī′-ol dī-as′-e-tāt) controls uterine bleeding.

eti·ology (ē-tē-ol′-o-jē) *n* a science dealing with the causation of disease. **etiological** *adj*, **etiologically** *adv*.

etreti·nate (e-tre′-tin-āt) *n* a vitamin A derivative used in severe psoriasis and some other serious skin disorders. Many adverse effects including fetal damage.

eucalyp·tus oil (ū-kà-lip′-tus) has mild antiseptic properties and is sometimes used in nasal drops for catarrh.

eu-flavine (ū-flā′-vēn) ⇒ acriflavine.

eu·genics (ū-jen′-iks) *n* the study of agencies and measures aimed at improving the hereditary qualities of human generations—**eugenic** *adj*.

eu·nuch (ū′-nuk) *n* a human male from whom the testes have been removed; a castrated male.

eu·pepsia (ū-pep′-sē-à) *n* normal digestion.

eu·phoria (ū-fōr′-ē-à) *n* in psychiatry, an exaggerated sense of well-being—**euphoric** *adj*.

Eurax (ū′-raks) *n* proprietary name for crotamiton*.

eurhyth·mics (ū-rith′-miks) *n* harmonious bodily movements performed to music.

eustachian tube (ūs-tāsh′-ē-àn (*syn* pharyngotympanic tube) a canal, partly bony, partly cartilaginous, measuring 40–50 mm in length, connecting the pharynx with the tympanic cavity (⇒ Figure 13). It allows air to pass into the middle ear, so that the air pressure is kept even on both sides of the eardrum. *eustachian catheter* an instrument used for insufflating the eustachian tube when it becomes blocked.

eutha·nasia (ū-than-ās′-ē-à) *n* **1** a good, inferring a painless, death. **2** frequently interpreted as the painless killing of a person suffering from an incurable disease.

euthyr·oid state (ū-thī′-royd) denoting normal thyroid function.

eu·tocia (ū-tō′-shē-à) *n* a natural and normal labor and childbirth without any complications.

Eutonyl (ū′-to-nyl) *n* proprietary name for monoamine* oxidase inhibitor.

EVA *abbr* evacuation (of the uterus) under anesthetic.

evacu·ant (ē-vak′-ū-ant) *n* an agent which causes an evacuation; particularly of the bowel ⇒ enema.

evacu·ation (ē-vak′-ū-ā′-shun) *n* the act of emptying a cavity; generally refers to the discharge of fecal matter from the rectum. *manual evacuation* digital removal of feces from the rectum.

evacu·ator (ē-vak′-ū-ā-tor) *n* an instrument for procuring evacuation, e.g. the removal from the bladder of a stone, crushed by a lithotrite.

evap·orate (ē-vap′-ōr-āt) *vt, vi* to convert from the liquid to the gaseous state by means of heat.

evapor·ating lotion (ē-vap′-ōr-ā-ting lō′-shun) one which, applied as a compress, absorbs heat in order to evaporate and so cools the skin.

evers·ion (ē-vėr′-zhun) *n* a turning outwards as of the upper eyelid to expose the conjunctival sac.

eviscer·ation (ē-vis-ėr-ā′-shun) *n* removal of internal organs.

evul·sion (ē-vul′-shun) *n* forcible tearing away of a structure.

Ewing's tumor (ū′-ings tū′-mor) (*syn* reticulocytoma sarcoma) involving the marrow of a long bone in a child or young person. May be difficult to distinguish it from a secondary bone deposit from a malignant neuroblastoma.

exacer·bation (ex-as-ėr-bā′-shun) *n* increased severity, as of symptoms.

exan·thema (ex-an-thēm′-mà) *n* a skin eruption—**exanthemata** *pl,* **exanthematous** *adj.*

ex·cision (ek-sizh′-un) *n* removal of a part by cutting—**excise** *vt.*

excit·ability (ek-sīt-à-bil′-i-tē) *n* rapid response to stimuli; a state of being easily irritated—**excitable** *adj.*

excit·ation (ek-sīt-ā′-shun) *n* the act of stimulating an organ or tissue.

ex·clusion isol·ation (eks-klū′-zhun) separation of a patient so that he can be

protected from infection. This may be necessary when the patient is immunodeficient (immunocompromised*, immunosuppressed) most commonly from taking such things as steroids and cytotoxic drugs for whatever reason. ⇒ containment isolation.

excori·ation (eks-kŏr-ē-ā′-shun) *n* ⇒ abrasion.

excre·ment (eks′-krē-ment) *n* feces*.

ex·crescence (eks-kres′-ens) *n* an abnormal protuberance or growth of the tissues.

ex·creta (eks-krē′-tà) *n* the waste matter which is normally discharged from the body, particularly urine and feces.

ex·cretion (eks-krē′-shun) *n* the elimination of waste material from the body, and also the matter so discharged—**excretory** *adj,* **excrete** *vt.*

exenter·ation (eks-en-tėr-ā′-shun) *n* removal of the viscera from its containing cavity, e.g. the eye from its socket, the pelvic organs from the pelvis.

exfoli·ative cyto·ology (eks-fō′-lē-à-tiv-si-tol′-o-jē) ⇒ cytology.

exfoli·ation (eks-fō-lē-a′-shun) *n* **1** the scaling off of tissues in layers. **2** the shedding of the primary teeth—**exfoliative** *adj.*

exhibition·ism (eks-i-bi′-shun-izm) *n* **1** any kind of showing off, extravagant behavior to attract attention. **2** a psychosexual disorder confined to males and consisting of repeated exposure of the genitals to a stranger. No further contact is sought with the victim, who is usually a female adult or a child—**exhibition·ist** *n.*

Exna (eks′-nà) *n* proprietary name for benzthiazide*.

exo·crine (eks′-ō-krin) *adj* describes glands from which the secretion passes via a duct; secreting externally. ⇒ endocrine *opp*—**exocrinal** *adj.*

exo·genous (eks-o′-jen-us) *adj* of external origin. ⇒ endogenous *opp.*

exom·phalos (eks-om′-fàl-us) *n* a condition present at birth and due to failure of the gut to return to the abdominal cavity during fetal development. The intestines protrude through a gap in the abdominal wall, still enclosed in peritoneum.

exoph·thalmos (eks-of-thal′-mus) *n* protrusion of the eyeball—**exophthalmic** *adj.*

exo·stosis (eks-os-tō′-sis) *n* an overgrowth of bone tissue forming a benign tumor.

exo·toxin (eks'-ō-toks'-in) *n* a toxic product of bacteria which is passed into the environment of the cell during growth. ⇒ endotoxin *opp*—**exotoxic** *adj*.

expect·ed date of confinement (EDC) usually dated from the first day of the last normal menstrual period, even though for the next 14 days there is really no pregnancy.

expec·torant (eks-pek'-tōr-ant) *n* a drug which promotes or increases expectoration*.

expector·ation (eks-pek-tōr-ā'-shun) *n* 1 the elimination of secretion from the respiratory tract by coughing. 2 sputum*—**expectorate** *vt*.

expir·ation (eks-pėr-ā'-shun) *n* the act of breathing out air from the lungs—**expiratory** *adj*, **expire** *vt, vi*.

explor·ation (eks-plōr-ā'-shun) *n* the act of exploring for diagnostic purposes, particularly in the surgical field—**exploratory** *adj*.

ex·pression (eks-presh'-un) *n* 1 expulsion by force as of the placenta from the uterus; milk from the breast, etc. 2 facial disclosure of feelings, mood, etc.

expres·ive motor apha·sia (eks-pres'-iv mō'-tor ă-fā'-zē-ă) a type of aphasia* in which the patient is aware of what is said and knows what he wants to reply, but is unable to assemble the symbols of language (speech) in any coherent order, thus giving the impression that he does not understand.

exsangui·nation (eks-sang-gwin-ā'-shun) *n* the process of rendering bloodless—**exsanguinate** *vt*.

exten·sion (eks-ten'-shun) *n* 1 traction upon a fractured or dislocated limb. 2 the straightening of a flexed limb or part.

exten·sor (eks-ten'-sor) *n* a muscle which on contraction extends or straightens a part ⇒ Figures 4, 5, flexor *opp*.

exter·nal cepha·lic ver·sion (ECV) (eks-tėr'-nal sef-al'-ik vėr'-zhun) ⇒ version.

external respi·ration (eks-tėr'-nal res-per-ā'-shun) ⇒ respiration.

extir·pation (eks-tėr-pā'-shun) *n* complete removal or destruction of a part.

extra·anatomic by·pass (EAB) (eks'-trà-an-à-tom'-ik bī-pas) a prosthetic vascular graft is threaded subcutaneously to carry a limb-preserving blood supply from an efficient proximal part of an artery to a distal one, thus bypassing the inefficient part of the artery.

extra·articular (eks'-trà-àr-tik'-ū-làr) *adj* outside a joint.

extra·capsular (eks'-trà-kap'-sū-làr) *adj* outside a capsule. ⇒ intracapsular *opp*.

extra·cardiac (eks'-trà-kar'-dē-ak) *adj* outside the heart.

extra·cellular (eks'-trà-sel'-ū-lar) *adj* out side the cell membrane. ⇒ intracellular *opp*.

extra·corporeal (eks-trà-kōr-pōr'-ē-àl) *adj* outside the body. *extracorporeal circulation* blood is taken from the body, directed through a machine ('heart-lung' or 'artificial kidney') and returned to the general circulation.

extracorpo·real shock wave litho·trypsy ⇒ Dornier lithoptryptor.

extra·corpuscular (eks-trà-kōr-pus'-kū-làr) *adj* outside corpuscles.

ex·tract (eks'-trakt) *n* a preparation obtained by evaporating a solution of a drug.

extrac·tion (eks-trak'-shun) *n* the removal of a tooth. *extraction of lens* surgical removal of the lens. *extracapsular extraction* the capsule is ruptured prior to delivery of the lens and preserved in part. *intracapsular extraction* the lens is removed within its capsule.

extra·dural (eks-trà-dū'-ràl) *adj* external to the dura mater.

extra·genital (eks-trà-jen'-i-tàl *adj* on areas of the body apart from genital organs. *extragenital chancre* is the primary ulcer of syphilis when it occurs on the finger, the lip, the breast etc.

extra·hepatic (eks-trà-hep-at'-ik) *adj* outside the liver.

extra·mural (eks'-trà-mūr'-al) *adj* outside the wall of a vessel or organ—**extramurally** *adv*.

extra·peritoneal (eks'-trà-per'-it-on-ē'-al) *adj* outside the peritoneum—**extraperitoneally** *adv*.

extra·pleural (eks-trà-plū'-ràl) *adj* outside the pleura, i.e. between the parietal pleura and the chest wall. ⇒ plombage—**extrapleurally** *adv*.

extra·pyramidal side effects (eks'-trà-pėr-am'-id-al) unwanted effects from drugs which interfere with the function of the extrapyramidal* tracts.

extra·pyramidal tracts those comprised of motor neurons from the brain to the spinal cord except for the fibers in the pyramidal* tracts. They are functional rather than anatomical units; they control and coordinate the postural, static mechanisms which cause contractions of muscle groups in sequence or simultaneously.

extra·renal (eks-trà-rē′-nàl) *n* outside the kidney—**extrarenally** *adv*.

extra·systole (eks-trà-sis′-to-lē) *n* premature beats (ectopic beats) in the pulse rhythm: the cardiac impulse is initiated in some focus apart from the sinoatrial node.

extra·thoracic (eks-trà-thōr-as′-ik) *adj* outside the thoracic cavity.

extra·uterine (eks-trà-ū′-tèr-in) *n* outside the uterus. *extrauterine pregnancy* ⇒ ectopic pregnancy.

extra·vasation (eks-trà-va-sā′-shun) *n* an escape of fluid from its normal enclosure into the surrounding tissues.

extra·venous (eks-trà-vē′-nus) *adj* outside a vein.

extra·vert, extrovert (eks′-trà-vèrt, eks′-trō-vèrt) *adj* Jungian description of an individual whose characteristic interests and modes of behavior are directed outwards to other people and the physical environment. ⇒ introvert *opp*.

extrin·sic (eks-trin′-sik) *adj* developing or having its origin from without; not internal. *extrinsic factor* now known to be vitamin B_{12}. It is absorbed in the presence of the internal factor secreted by the stomach.

extro·version (eks′-trō-vèr-shun) *n* turning inside out. *extroversion of the bladder* ectopia* vesicae*. In psychology, the direction of thoughts to the external world.

exu·date (eks′-ū-dāt) *n* the product of exudation*.

exu·dation (eks-ū-dā′-shun) *n* the oozing out of fluid through the capillary walls, or of sweat through the pores of the skin—**exudate** *n*, **exude** *vt,vi*.

eye (ī) ⇒ Figure 15.

eye·teeth (ī-tēth′) the canine teeth* in the upper jaw.

F

facet (fa′-set) *n* a small, smooth, flat surface of a bone or a calculus. *facet syndrome* dislocation of some of the gliding joints between vertebrae causing pain and muscle spasm.

facial (fāsh′-al) *adj* pertaining to the face. *facial nerve* seventh pair of the 12 pairs of cranial nerves which arise directly from the brain. *facial paralysis* paralysis of muscles supplied by the facial nerve.

facies (fā′-sēz) *n* the appearance of the face, used especially of the subject of congenital syphilis with saddle nose, prominent brow and chin. *adenoid facies* open mouthed, vacant expression due to deafness from enlarged adenoids. *facies hippocratica* the drawn, pale, pinched appearance indicative of approaching death. *Parkinson facies* a mask-like appearance; saliva may trickle from the corners of the mouth.

fac·tor P (fak′-tor) one component of the complement system.

facult·ative (fak′-ul-tā-tiv) *adj* conditional; having the power of living under different conditions.

Fahren·heit (far′-en-hīt) *n* a thermometric scale; the freezing point of water is 32° and its boilding point 212°.

fail·ure to thrive a blanket term replacing marasmus*. Afflicted children do not progress because of malnutrition or difficulty in absorbing the basic nutritional requirements.

faint (fānt) *n* syncope—**faint** *vi*.

falci·form (fal′-si-fôrm) *adj* sickle-shaped.

fall·opian tubes (fal-lō′-pē-àn) (*syn* oviducts, uterine tubes) two tubes opening out of the upper part of the uterus. Each measures 10 cm and the distal end is fimbriated (⇒ Fig. 17) and lies near the ovary. Their function is to convey the ova into the uterus.

Fallot's tetral·ogy (fal-lōz′-tet-rol′-o-jē) congenital heart defect comprising interventricular septal defect, pulmonary stenosis, right ventricular hypertrophy and malposition of the aorta.

falx (falks) *n* a sickle-shaped structure. *falx cerebri* that portion of the dura mater separating the two cerebral hemispheres.

fam·ilial (fam-il′-ē-àl) *adj* pertaining to the family, as of a disease affecting several members of the same family.

fam·ily plann·ing the use of contraceptives to space or limit the number of children born to a couple.

Fan·coni syn·drome (fan-kōn′-ē) an inherited or acquired dysfunction of the proximal kidney tubules. Large amounts of amino acids, glucose and phosphates are excreted in the urine, yet the blood levels of these substances are normal. Symptoms may include thirst, polyuria, bone abnormalities and muscular weakness ⇒ aminoaciduria, cystinosis.

fang (fāng) *n* the root of a tooth.

fan·tasy (fan'-tas-ē) *n* a 'day dream' in which the thinker's conscious or unconscious desires and impulses are fulfilled. May be accompanied by a feeling of unreality. Occurs pathologically in schizophrenia.

fari·naceous (far-i-nā'-shus) *adj* pertaining to cereal substances, i.e. made of flour or grain. Starchy.

farmer's lung a form of alveolitis due to allergy to certain spores (e.g. *Micropolyspora faeni*) that occur in the dust of moldy hay or other moldy vegetable produce. Recognized as an industrial disease.

far-sightedness (far-sī'-ted-nes) *n* hyperopia*.

FAS *abbr* fetal* alcohol syndrome.

fascia (fash'-ē-à) *n* a connective tissue sheath consisting of fibrous tissue and fat which unites the skin to the underlying tissues. It also surrounds and separates many of the muscles, and, in some cases, holds them together—**fascial** *adj*.

fascicu·lation (fas-ik-ū-lā'-shun) *n* visible flickering of muscle; can occur in the upper and lower eyelids.

fas·ciculus (fas-ik'-ū-lus) *n* a little bundle, as of muscle or nerve—**fascicular** *adj*, **fasciculi** *pl*.

fasci·otomy (fash-ē-ot'-o-mē) *n* incision of a fascia.

fas·tigium (fas-tij'-ē-um) *n* the highest point of a fever; the period of full development of a disease.

fat *n* **1** an ester of glycerol with fatty acids which may be of animal or vegetable origin, and may be either solid or liquid. Vitamins A, D, E and K are fat-soluble. **2** adipose tissue, which acts as a reserve supply of energy and smooths out body contours—**fatty** *adj*.

fatigue (fà-tēg') *n* weariness. Term used in physiological experiments on muscle to denote diminishing reaction to stimulus applied—**fatigability** *n*.

fatty degener·ation (fat'-ē dē-jen-ėr-ā'-shun) degeneration* of tissues which results in appearance of fatty droplets in the cytoplasm; found especially in disease of liver, kidney and heart.

fauces (faw'-sēz) *n* the opening from the mouth into the pharynx, bounded above by the soft palate, below by the tongue. Pillars of the fauces anterior and posterior, lie laterally and enclose the tonsil—**faucial** *adj*.

favism (fā'-vizm) *n* reduced amount of enzyme G6PD (glucose-6-phosphate dehydrogenase) in red blood cells. Afflicted people develop a severe hemolytic anemia when they eat fava beans.

favus (fā'-vus) *n* a type of ringworm caused by *Trichophyton schoenleini*. Yellow cup-shaped crusts (scutula) develop especially on the scalp.

FDA *abbr* Food and Drug Administration.

fear (fēr) *n* an intense emotional state involving a feeling of unpleasant tension, and a strong impulse to escape, which is natural in response to a threat of danger but is unnatural as a continuous state ⇒ anxiety.

fe·brile (fēb'-rīl) *adj* feverish; accompanied by fever. *febrile convulsions* occur in children who have an increased body temperature; they do not usually result in permanent brain damage. Most common between the ages of 6 months and 5 years. ⇒ convulsions.

fe·calith (fē'-kà-lith) *n* a concretion formed in the bowel from fecal matter; it can cause obstruction and/or inflammation.

fecal-oral route (fē'-kàl-ōr'-àl) a term that describes the ingestion of microorganisms from feces which can be transmitted directly or indirectly.

fe·ces (fē'-sēz) *n* the waste matter excreted from the bowel, consisting mainly of indigestible cellulose, unabsorbed food, intestinal secretions, water and bacteria—**fecal** *adj*.

fecund·ation (fe-kund-ā'-shun) *n* impregnation. Fertilization.

fec·undity (fe-kund'-it-ē) *n* the power of reproduction; fertility.

feed-back treat·ment (fēd'-bak) physiological activities such as excessive muscle tension and raised blood pressure are measured graphically so that patients can benefit from the information and learn to relax muscles and lower blood pressure.

Fehling's solution (fā'-lingz) an alkaline copper solution used for the detection and estimation of amount of sugars.

Feldene (fel'-dēn) *n* proprietary name for piroxicam*.

Felty syn·drome (fel'-tē) enlargment of the liver, spleen and lymph nodes as a complication of rheumatoid* arthritis.

fem·oral artery (fem'-ōr-àl) ⇒ Figure 9.

fem·oral vein ⇒ Figure 10.

femoro·popliteal (fem'-ér-ō-pop-li-tē'-ál) *adj* usually, referring to the femoral and popliteal vessels.

femur (fē'-mur) *n* the thigh bone (⇒ Figures 2, 3); the longest and strongest bone in the body—**femora** *pl*, **femoral** *adj*.

fen·estra (fen-es'-trá) *n* a window-like opening. *fenestra ovalis* an oval opening between the middle and internal ear. Below it lies the *fenestra rotunda* a round opening.

fen·estration (fen-es-trā'-shun) *n* 1 the surgical creation of an opening (of fenestra) in the inner ear for the relief of deafness in otosclerosis. 2 (*syn* festination) a type of walking seen in such nervous diseases as paralysis agitans, when the patient trots along in little bursts, getting faster and faster until he has to stop and then start off again, otherwise he would fall over.

fen·fluramine hydro·chloride (fen-flōōr'-a-mēn) an appetite suppressant. It does not possess the central stimulant effects of the amphetamines. (Ponderal.)

fen·tanyl (fen'-tan-yl) *n* a morphine*-like short-acting narcotic analgesic but of considerably higher potency. Can be used in conjunction with other drugs to promote anesthesia in children and the aged. (Sublimaze.)

fer·ment (fér'-ment) ⇒ catalyst.

ferment·ation (fér-men-tā'-shun) *n* the glycolysis of carbohydrates to produce ATP in which simple organic compounds (not molecular oxygen) act as the terminal electron acceptors (e.g. alcohol). Excellent examples are the making of bread, cheese and wine.

ferric (fér'-ik) *adj* pertaining to trivalent iron, as of its salts and compounds.

ferrous (fér'-us) *adj* pertaining to divalent iron, as of its salts and compounds. *Ferrous carbonate, ferrous fumarate, ferrous gluconate, ferrous succinate and ferrous sulfate* are oral preparations for iron-deficiency anemias.

fertiliz·ation (fér-til-ī-zā'-shun) *n* the impregnation of an ovum by a spermatozoon.

fester (fes'-tér) *vi* to become inflamed; to suppurate.

festin·ation (fes-tin-ā'-shun) *n* ⇒ fenestration.

fetal alco·hol syn·drome (FAS) (fē'-tal al'-ko-hol) stillbirth and fetal abnormality due to prenatal growth retardation caused by the mother's consumption of alcohol during pregnancy.

fetal circul·ation (fē'-tal sir-kū-lā'-shun) circulation* of blood through the fetus, umbilical cord and placenta.

fetal monitor measures the fetal heart rate either by an external microphone or by the application of an electrode to the fetal scalp, recording the fetal ECG and from it the fetal heart rate. Also measures maternal contractions.

fetish·ism (fet'-ish-izm) *n* a condition in which a particular material object is regarded with irrational awe or a strong emotional attachment. Can have a psychosexual dimension in which such an object is repeatedly or exclusively used in achieving sexual excitement.

fetor (fē'-tor) *n* offensive odor, stench. *fetor oris* bad breath.

fet·oscopy (fē-tos'-ko-pē) *n* direct visual examination of the fetus by using a suitable fiberglass endoscope.

fetus (fē'-tus) an unborn child—**fetal** *adj*. *fetus papyraceous* a dead fetus, one of a twin which has become fattened and mummified.

FEV *abbr* forced expiratory volume. ⇒ respiratory function tests.

fever (fē'-vér) *n* (*syn* pyrexia) an elevation of body temperature above normal. Designates some infectious conditions, e.g. *paratyphoid fever, scarlet fever, typhoid fever.* etc.

FHR *abbr* fetal heart rate.

fiber (fī'-bér) *n* a thread-like structure—**fibrous** *adj*.

fiber·optics (fī-bér-op'-tiks) *n* light is transmitted through flexible glass fibers which enable the user to 'see round corners'. Incorporation of fiberoptics into endoscopes* has contributed to (a) increased knowledge through their use in research and (b) reliable diagnosis of pathological conditions.

fib·ril (fī'-bril) *n* a component filament of a fiber; a small fiber.

fibril·lation (fi-bril-lā'-shun) *n* uncoordinated quivering contraction of muscle; referring usually to atrial fibrillation in the myocardium wherein the atria beat very rapidly and are not synchronized with the ventricular beat. The result is a total irregularity of the pulse.

fi·brin (fī'-brin) *n* the matrix on which a blood clot is formed. The substance is formed from soluble fibrinogen* of the blood by the catalytic (enzymatic) action of thrombin*—**fibrinous** *adj*. *fibrin foam* a white, dry, spongy material made from fibrinogen. It is used in conjunction with

113

thrombin as a hemostatic in brain and lung surgery.

fibrin·ogen (fī-brin'-ō-jen) *n* a soluble protein of the blood from which is produced the insoluble protein called fibrin* which is essential to blood coagulation.

fibrinogen·openia (fī-brin-ō-jen-ō-pē'-nē-à) *n* (*syn* fibrinopenia) lack of blood plasma fibrinogen*. Can be congenital or due to liver disease.

fibrin·olysin (fī-brin-ō-lī'-sin) *n* blood stream enzyme thought to dissolve fibrin* occurring after minor injuries. It has been administered intravenously in thrombosis.

fibrin·olysis (fī-brin-ol'-is-is) *n* the dissolution of fibrin* which can precede hemorrhage. There is normally a balance between blood coagulation and fibrinolysis in the body—**fibrinolytic** *adj*.

fibrino·penia (fī-brin-ō-pē-nē-à) *n* ⇒ fibrinogenopenia.

fibro·adenoma (fī-brō-ad-en-ōm'-à) *n* a benign tumor containing fibrous and glandular tissue.

fibro·blast (fī'-brō-blast) *n* (*syn* fibrocyte) a cell which produces collagen, a major constituent of the connective tissues—**fibroblastic** *adj*.

fibro·cartilage (fī-brō-kàr'-ti-laj) *n* cartilage containing fibrous tissue—**fibrocartilaginous** *adj*.

fibro·caseous (fī-brō-kā'-sē-us) *adj* a soft, cheesy mass infiltrated by fibrous tissue, formed by fibroblasts.

fibro·chondritis (fī-brō-kon-drī'-tis) *n* inflammation of fibrocartilage.

fibro·cyst (fī'-brō-sist) *n* a fibroma which has undergone cystic degeneration.

fibro·cystic (fī-brō-sis'-tik) *adj* pertaining to a fibrocyst* *fibrocystic disease of bone* cysts may be solitary or generalized. If generalized and accompanied by decalcification of bone, it is symptomatic of hyperparathyroidism. *fibrocystic disease of breast* the breast feels lumpy due to the presence of cysts, usually caused by hormone imbalance. *fibrocystic disease of pancreas* cystic* fibrosis.

fibro·cyte (fī'-brō-sīt) *n* ⇒ fibroblast—**fibrocytic** *adj*.

fi·broid (fī'-broyd) *n* a fibromuscular benign tumor usually found in the uterus. An *interstitial uterine fibroid* is embedded in the wall of the uterus (intramural)—if extended to the outer surface it becomes a *subperitoneal fibroid* (subserous), if to the inner or endometrial surface it becomes submucous or even a *fibroid polypus*.

fi·broma (fī-brō'-mà) *n* a benign tumor composed of fibrous tissue—**fibromata** *pl*, **fibromatous** *adj*.

fibro·muscular (fī-brō-mus'-kū-làr) *adj* pertaining to fibrous and muscle tissue.

fibro·myoma (fī-brō-mī-ōm'-à) *n* a benign tumor consisting of fibrous and muscle tissue—**fibromyomata** *pl*, **fibromyomatous** *adj*.

fibro·plasia (fī-brō-plāz'-ē-à) *n* the production of fibrous tissue which is a normal part of healing ⇒ retrolental fibroplasia. *retrolental fibroplasia* the presence of fibrous tissue in the vitreous and retina extending in an area from the ciliary body to the optic disc, causing blindness. Noticed shortly after birth, more commonly in premature babies who have had continuous oxygen therapy.

fibro·sarcoma (fī-brō-sàr-kō'-mà) *n* a form of sarcoma. A malignant tumor derived from fibroblastic cells—**fibrosarcomata** *pl*, **fibrosarcomatous** *adj*.

fi·brosis (fī-brō'-sis) *n* the formation of excessive fibrous tissues in a structure—**fibrotic** *adj*.

fibro·sitis (fī-brō-sī'-tis) *n* (*syn* muscular rheumatism) pain of uncertain origin which affects the soft tissues of the limbs and trunk. It is generally associated with muscular stiffness and local tender points—fibrositic nodules. Cause unknown; some disturbance in immunity may be a factor, as may be gout. Nonspecific factors include chill, postural trauma, muscular strain and psychological stress especially in tense, anxious people.

fibro·vascular (fī-brō-vas'-kū-làr) *adj* pertaining to fibrous tissue which is well supplied with blood vessels.

fib·ula (fi'-bū-là) *n* one of the longest and thinnest bones of the body, situated on the outer side of the leg and articulating at the upper end with the lateral condyle of the tibia and at the lower end with the lateral surface of the talus (astragalus) and tibia (⇒ Figures 2, 3)—**fibular** *adj*.

field of vison the area in which objects can be seen by the fixed eye.

Filaria (fi-làr'-ē-à) *n* a genus of parasitic, thread-like worms, found mainly in the tropics and subtropics. The adults of *Filaria bancrofti* and *Brugia malayi* live in the lymphatics, connective tissues or mesentery, where they may cause obstruction, but the embryos migrate to the blood stream. Completion of the life-cycle is dependent upon passage through a mosquito. ⇒ loiasis—**filarial** *adj.*

filari·asis (fil-·ar-ī´-à-sis) *n* infestation with *Filaria* ⇒ elephantiasis.

filari·cide (fil-ār´-i-sīd) *n* an agent which destroys *Filaria.*

fili·form (fil´-i-fōrm) *adj* threadlike. *filiform papillae* small projections ending in several minute processes; found on the tongue.

fili·puncture (fil-i-pungk´-tūr) *n* insertion of wire thread etc. into an aneurysm to produce coagulation of contained blood.

filix mas (fil´-iks mas) *n* male fern extract, used to expel taenia*.

fil·trate (fil´-trāt) *n* that part of a substance which passes through the filter.

fil·tration (fil-trā´-shun) *n* the process of straining through a filter under gravity, pressure or vacuum. The act of passing fluid through a porous medium. *filtration under pressure* occurs in the kidneys, due to the pressure of blood in the glomeruli.

filum (fī´-lum) *n* any filamentous or thread-like structure. *filum terminale* a strong, fine cord blending with the spinal cord above, and the periosteum of the sacral canal below.

fim·bria (fim´-brē-à) *n* a fringe or frond; resembling the fronds of a fern; e.g. the fimbriae of the fallopian tubes (⇒ Figure 17)—**fimbriae** *pl.* **fimbrial, fimbriated** *adj.*

fine tremor *n* slight trembling as seen in the outstretched hands or tongue of a patient suffering from thyrotoxicosis.

finger (fing´-gėr) *n* a digit. *clubbed finger* swelling of terminal phalanx which occurs in many lung and heart diseases.

fis·sion (fish´-un) *n* a method of reproduction common among the bacteria and protozoa.

fis·sure (fish´-ur) *n* a split or cleft. *palpebral fissure* the opening between the eyelids.

fis·tula (fis´-tū-là) *n* an abnormal communication between two body surfaces or cavities, e.g. gastrocolic fistula between the stomach and the colon; colostomy, between the colon and the abdominal surface—**fistulae** *pl,* **fistular, fistulous** *adj.*

fits ⇒ convulsions.

fix·ation (fiks-ā´-shun) *n* 1 in optics, the direct focusing of one or both eyes on an object so that the image falls on the retinal disc. 2 as a psychoanalytical term, an emotional attachment, generally sexual, to a parent, causing difficulty in forming new attachments later in life.

flac·cid (flas´-id) *adj* soft, flabby, not firm—**flaccidity** *n flaccid paralysis* results mainly from lower motor neuron lesions. There are diminished or absent tendon reflexes.

flagel·lation (flaj-el-lā´-shun) *n* 1 the act of whipping oneself or others to gain sexual pleasure. Can be a component of masochism and sadism. 2 a form of massage in which the skin is rhythmically tapped by either the outstretched hand or the little-finger side of the hand.

flagel·lum (fla-jel´-um) *n* a fine, hair-like appendage capable of lashing movement. Characteristic of spermatozoa, certain bacteria and protozoa—**flagella** *pl.*

Flagyl (fla´-jl) *n* proprietary name for metronidazole*.

flail chest (flāl chest) unstable thoracic cage due to fracture ⇒ respiration.

Flama·zine (flam´-a-zēn) *n* proprietary name for silver* sulfadiazine.

flap *n* partially-removed tissue, retaining blood and nerve supply, used to repair defects in other parts of the body. Common in plastic surgery to treat burns and other injuries; skin flaps used to cover amputation stumps.

flat-foot *n* (*syn* pes planus) a congenital or acquired deformity marked by depression of the longitudinal arches of the foot.

flat pelvis a pelvis in which the antero-posterior diameter of the brim is reduced.

flatu·lence (flat´-ū-lens) *n* gastric and intestinal distension with gas—**flatulent** *adj.*

flatus (flāt´-us) *n* gas in the stomach or intestines.

flav·oxate (fla-voks´-āt) *n* an oral urinary antiseptic which is useful for controlling urinary spasm. (Urispas.)

Flax·edil (flaks´-e-dil) *n* proprietary name for gallamine*.

flea (flē)*n* a blood-sucking wingless insect of the order Siphonaptera; it acts as a host and can transmit disease. Its bite leaves a portal of entry for infection. *human flea Pulex irritans. rat flea Xenopsylla cheopis.* transmitter of plague*.

flec·ainide (flek-´ān-īd) *n* a cardiac antiarrhythmic drug.

Fleet enema a laxative and bowel evacuant contained in a disposable plastic squeeze bottle. Contains sodium biphosphate and sodium phosphate.

flex (fleks) *vi, vt* bend.

Flexeril (fleks'-er-il) *n* proprietary name for cyclobenzaprine*.

flexibilitas cerea (fleks-i-bil'-i-tas-sē'-rē-à) literally waxy flexibility. A condition of generallized hypertonia of muscles found in catatonic schizophrenia*. When fully developed, the patient's limbs retain positions in which they are placed, remaining immobile for hours at a time. Occasionally occurs in hysteria as hysterical rigidity.

flex·ion (flek'-shun) *n* the act of bending by which the shafts of long bones forming a joint are brought towards each other.

Flex·ner's bacil·lus (fleks'-ners) *Shigella* flexneri.

flexor (fleks'-or) *n* a muscle which on contraction flexes or bends a part ⇒ Figures 4, 5, extensor *opp*.

flex·ure (fleks'-ūr) *n* a bend, as in a tube-like structure, or a fold, as on the skin—it can be obliterated by extension or increased by flexion in the locomotor system—**flexural** *adj. left colic (splenic) flexure* is situated at the junction of the transverse and descending parts of the colon. It lies at a higher level than the *right colic* or *hepatic flexure* the bend between the ascending and transverse colon, beneath the liver. *sigmoid flexure* the S-shaped bend at the lower end of the descending colon. It is continuous with the rectum below.

flight of ideas succession of thoughts with no rational connection. A feature of manic disorders.

float·ers (flōt'-ers) *npl* floating bodies in the vitreous humor (of the eye) which are visible to the person.

float·ing kid·ney (flōt'-ing kid'-nē) abnormally mobile kidney. ⇒ nephropexy.

floccu·lation (flok-ūl-ā'-shun) *n* the coalescence of colloidal particles in suspension resulting in their aggregation into larger discrete masses which are often visible to the naked eye as cloudiness. *flocculation test* serum is set up against various salts such as gold, thymol, cephalin or cholesterol. When the presence of abnormal serum proteins results in cloudiness. Abnormal forms of albumin and globulin are produced by diseased liver cells.

flood·ing (flud'-ing) *n* a popular term to describe excessive bleeding from the uterus.

floppy baby syn·drome (flop'-ē bā'-bē) ⇒ amyotonia congenita.

flora (flōr'-à) *n* in medicine the word is used to describe the colonization of various parts of the body by microorganisms which in most instances are non-pathogenic but which in particular circumstances can become pathogenic.

florid (flōr'-id) *adj* flushed, high colored.

flow·meter (flō'-mē-tèr) *n* a measuring instrument for flowing gas or liquid.

fluctu·ation (fluk-tū-ā'-shun) *n* a wave-like motion felt on digital examination of a fluid-containing tumor, e.g. abscess—**fluctuant** *adj.*

flucytosine (flū-sī'-tō-sēn) *n* an antifungal agent effective against Candida and Cryptococcus. (Ancobon.)

fludrocortisone (floo-drō-kōr'-ti-sōn) *n* sodium-retaining tablets. Useful in some cases of Addison's disease.

fluke (flook) *n* a trematode worm of the order Digenea. The *European* or *sheep fluke (Fasciola hepatica)* usually ingested from watercress. There is fever, malaise, a large tender liver and eosinophilia. The *Chinese fluke (Clonorchis sinensis)* is usually ingested with raw fish. The adult fluke lives in the bile ducts and, while it may produce cholangitis, hepatitis and jaundice, it may be asymptomatic or be blamed for vague digestive symptoms. *lung fluke (Paragonimus)* usually ingested with raw crab in China and Far East. The symptoms are those of chronic bronchitis, including blood in the sputum.

fluocin·olone (floo-ō-sin'-ō-lōn) *n* a cortisone derivative for topical application. (Synalar.)

fluor·escein (floo-ōr'-es-ēn) *n* red substance which forms a green fluorescent solution. Used as eye drops to detect corneal lesions, which stain green. It can be used in retinal angiography by injection into a vein, followed by viewing and photographing its passage through the retinal blood vessels. *fluorescein string test* used to detect the site of obscure upper gastrointestinal bleeding. The patient swallows a radioopaque knotted string. Fluorescein is injected intravenously and after a few minutes the string is withdrawn. If staining has occurred the site of bleeding can be determined.

fluorescent treponemal antibody test (FTA) carried out for syphilis: virulent

Treponema pallidum is used as the antigen.

fluori·dation (floo-ôr-i-dā'-shun) *n* ⇒ fluoride.

fluor·ide (floo'-ôr-īd) *n* an iron sometimes present in drinking water. It can be incorporated into the structure of bone and then provides protection against dental caries but in gross excess it causes mottling of the teeth. As a preventive measure it can be added to a water supply in a strength of 1 part fluoride in a million parts of water (fluoridation).

5-fluoro·cystosine (fīv-floo-ôr'-ō-sist'-ō-sēn) *n* an antifungal agent.

fluor·oscopy (floo-ôr-os'-ko-pē) *n* X-ray examination of movement in the body, observed by means of fluorescent screen and TV system.

fluor·ouracil, 5-FU (floo-ôr-ûr'-à-sil) *n* an antimetabolic cytotoxic agent.

Fluo·thane (flū'-ō-thān) *n* proprietary name for halothane*.

flu·phenazine (floo-fen'-à-zēn) *n* a phenothiazine* tranquilizer with anti-emetic properties. Can be given as a depot injection. A newer preparation is *fluphenazine deconoate* which is longer acting. (Permitil, Prolixin.)

flur·azepam (floor-az'-e-pam) *n* a drug which is chemically related to mitrazepam* and has basically similar properties. (Dalmane.)

flux (fluks) *n* any excessive flow of any of the body excretions.

folic acid (fō'-lik as'-id) (*syn* pteroylglutamic acid) a member of the vitamin* B complex which is abundant in green vegetables, yeast and liver. It is absorbed from the small intestine and is an essential factor for normal hemopoiesis and cell division generally. Used in the treatment of megaloblastic anemias other than those due to vitamin B_{12} deficiency.

folie à deux (fō-lē'-à-duh') a rare psychiatric syndrome, in which one member of a close pair suffers a psychotic illness and eventually imposes his delusions on the other.

fol·licle (fol'-li-kl) *n* 1 a small secreting sac. 2 a simple tubular gland—**follicular** *adj. follicle stimulating hormone (FSH)* secreted by the anterior pituitary gland; it is trophic to the ovaries in the female, where it develops the ovum-containing (graafian) follicles; and to the testes in the male, where it is responsible for sperm production.

folliculi·tis (fol-li-kū-lī'-tis) *n* inflammation of follicles, such as the hair follicles. ⇒ alopecia.

folliculosis (fol-ik-ūl-ō'-sis) *n* hypertrophy of follicles.

Folvite (fōl'-vīt) *n* proprietary brand of folic acid* and antianemia compounds especially for anemia in pregnancy.

fomen·tation (fō-men-tā'-shun) *n* a hot, wet application to produce hyperemia. When the skin is intact, strict cleanliness is observed (medical fomentation); when the skin is broken, aseptic technique is used (surgical fomentation).

fo·mite (fō'-mīt) *n* any article which has been in contact with infection and is capable of transmitting same.

fonta·nel (fon-tà-nel') *n* a membranous space between the cranial bones. The diamond-shaped anterior fontanel (bregma) is at the junction of the frontal and two parietal bones. It usually closes in the second year of life. The triangular posterior fontanel (lambda) is at the junction of the occipital and two parietal bones. It closes within a few weeks of birth.

food allergy a term which has come to be used to cover all adverse reactions to food, whether or not the underlying mechanism has been identified ⇒ allergy.

food poison·ing vomiting, with or without diarrhea, resulting from eating food contaminated with chemical poison, preformed bacterial toxin or live bacteria or poisonous natural vegetation, e.g. berries, toadstools (fungi).

foot *n* that portion of the lower limb below the ankle. *foot drop* inability to dorsiflex foot, as in severe sciatica and nervous disease affecting lower lumbar regions of the cord. Can be a complication of being bedfast.

for·amen (fōr-ā'-men) *n* a hole or opening. Generally used with reference to bones—**foramina** *pl. foramen magnum* the opening in the occipital bone through which the spinal cord passes. *foramen ovale* a fetal cardiac interatrial communication which normally closes at birth.

forced expira·tory volume *n* ⇒ forced vital capacity.

forced gut lav·age the fluid is introduced via a nasogastric tube to give continuous perfusion of the large bowel lining.

forced vital capacity (FVC), forced expiratory volume the maximum gas volume that can be expelled from the lungs in a forced expiration.

for·ceps (fōr'-seps) *n* surgical instruments with two opposing blades which are used to grasp or compress tissues, swabs, needles and many other surgical appliances. The two blades are controlled by direct pressure on them (tong-like), or by handles (scissor-like). *obstetrical forceps* forceps used to extract the fetal head during delivery.

forebrain (fōr'-brān) ⇒ Figure 1.

foren·sic med·icine (for-en'-sik) (*syn* medical jurisprudence) also called 'legal medicine'. The application of medical knowledge to questions of law.

fore·skin (fōr'-skin) *n* the prepuce or skin covering the glans* penis.

formal·dehyde (fōr-mal'-de-hīd) *n* powerful germicide. Formalin* is a 40% solution; used mainly for room disinfection and the preservation of pathological specimens.

formi·cation (fōr-mi-kā'-shun) *n* a sensation as of ants running over the skin. Occurs in nerve lesions, particularly in the regenerative phase.

for·mula (fōr'-mū-là) *n* a prescription. A series of symbols denoting the chemical composition of a substance—**formulae, formulas** *pl.*

for·mulary (fōr'-mū-lā-rē) *n* a collection of formulas. The *National Formulary* is published by the U.S. Pharmacopeial Convention and contains standards for drugs enforced by the U.S. government.

for·nix (fōr'-niks) *n* an arch; particularly referred to the vagina, i.e. the space between the vaginal wall and the cervix of the uterus—**fornices** *pl.*

fossa (fos'-sà) *n* a depression or furrow—**fossae** *pl.*

foster·ing (fos'-tėr-ing) *n* placing an 'at risk' child with a compatible family as a short or long term measure. The aims are (a) to provide a child in need of care with the security of a home environment (b) to reunite child and natural family as soon as practical. Long term fosterings can be 'with a view to adoption'.

Father·gill's oper·ation (foth'-ėr-gilz) (*syn* Manchester operation) anterior colporrhaphy* amputation of part of the cervix and posterior colpoperineorrhaphy, performed for genital prolapse.

fourch·ette (foor'-shet) *n* a membranous fold connecting the posterior ends of the labia minora.

fovea (fō'-vē-à) *n* a small depression or fossa; particularly the fovea centralis retinae, the site of most distinct vision.

frac·ture (frak'-tūr) *n* breach in continuity of a bone as a result of injury. *Bennett's* fracture, closed fracture there is no communication with external air. *Colles' fracture* ⇒ Colles'. *comminuted fracture* a breach in the continuity of a bone which is broken into more than two pieces. *complicated fracture* a breach in the continuity of a bone when there is injury to surrounding organs and structures. *compression fracture* usually of lumbar or dorsal region due to hyperflexion of spine; the anterior vertebral bodies are crushed together. *depressed fracture* the broken bone presses on an underlying structure, such as brain or lung. *impacted fracture* one end of the broken bone is driven into the other. *incomplete fracture* the bone is only cracked or fissured—called 'green-stick fracture' when it occurs in children. *open (compound) fracture* there is a wound permitting communication of broken bone end with air. *pathological fracture* occurring in abnormal bone as a result of force which would not break a normal bone. *spontaneous fracture* one occurring without appreciable violence; may be synonymous with pathological fracture.

fragil·itas (fra-jil'-i-tàs) *n* brittleness. *fragilitas ossium* congenital disease characterized by abnormal fragility of bone, multiple fractures and a china-blue coloring of the sclera.

fram·besia (fram-bē'-zē-à) *n* yaws*.

Fre·amine (frē-à-mēn) *n* a proprietary, mainly synthetic preparation of those amino acids normally ingested as protein in egg, meat and fish.

free associaton a psychoanalytic procedure of having the patient say whatever comes to mind.

Frei·berg's infarc·tion (frī'-bergz in-fark'-shun) an aseptic necrosis of bone tissue which most commonly occurs in the head of the second metatarsal bone.

Frei test (frī) an intradermal test using antigen from those infected with lymphogranuloma venereum and a control. A positive skin reaction to the killed antigen confirms diagnosis.

French chalk talc*.

Frenkel's exer·cises (fren'-kls) special exercises for tabes* dorsalis to teach muscle and joint sense.

fren·otomy (fren-ot'-o-mē) *n* surgical severance of a frenum, particularly for tongue-tie.

frenum (fren'-um) *n* a fold of membrane

which checks or limits the movement of an organ. *frenum linguae* from the undersurface of the tongue to the floor of the mouth.

Freud, Sigmund (1856–1939) (froyd sig'-mund) the originator of psychoanalysis* and the psychoanalytical theory of the causation of neuroses. He first described the existence of the unconscious mind, censor, repression and the theory of infantile sexuality, and worked out in detail many mental mechanisms of the unconscious which modify normal, and account for abnormal human behavior.

Freyer's oper·ation (frī'-erz) suprapubic transvesical type of prostatectomy*.

fri·able (frī'-à-bl) *adj* easily crumbled; readily pulverized.

Friar's bal·sam (frī'-àrz bal'-sam) ancient remedy for bronchitis. Contains benzoin, aloes and balsam of Tolu, dissolved in alcohol. It is added to hot water and the vapor is inhaled. Of dubious value.

fric·tion (frik'-shun) *n* rubbing. Can cause abrasion of skin, loading to superficial pressure sore; the adhesive property of friction, increased in the presence of moisture, can contribute to shearing force which can cause a deep pressure sore. *friction massage* a form of massage in which strong circular manipulation of deep tissue is followed by centripetal stroking. The friction applied in drying after bating can be therapeutic. *friction murmur* heard through the stethoscope when two rough or dry surfaces rub together, as in pleurisy and pericarditis.

Friedlander's bacillus (frēd'-lan-dèrz) a large Gram-negative rod bacterium occasionally found in the upper respiratory tract, of which it can cause inflammation.

Friedman's curve (frēd'-manz) a graphic analysis of labor which correlates the length of labor with the degree of cervical dilatation. Aids in evaluating the normalcy of the progression of an individual labor by referring to this curve.

Friedreich's ataxia (frēd'-riks) a progressive familial disease of childhood, in which there develops a sclerosis of the sensory and motor columns in the spinal cord, with consequent muscular weakness and staggering (ataxia). The heart may also be affected.

frig·idity (frij-id'-it-ē) *n* lack of normal sexual desire. Used mainly in relation to the female.

frog plaster conservative treatment of a congenital dislocation of the hip,

whereby the dislocation is reduced by gentle manipulation and both hips are immobilized in plaster of Paris, both hips abducted to 80 degrees and externally rotated.

Frohlich's syndrome (fro'-liks) (*syn.* adiposogenital dystrophy) uncommon syndrome resulting from anterior pituitary insufficiency secondary to hypothalamine neoplasm. Characterized by obesity, stunted growth, arrested sexual development and knock-knees.

frontal (fron'-tàl) *adj* **1** pertaining to the front of a structure. **2** the forehead bone (⇒ Figure 14). *frontal sinus* a cavity at the inner aspect of each orbital ridge on the frontal bone (⇒ Figure 14).

frostbite (frost'-bīt) *n* freezing of the skin and superficial tissues resulting from exposure to extreme cold. The lesion is similar to a burn and may become gangrenous. ⇒ trench foot.

frozen shoulder (frō'-zen shōl'-dèr) initial pain followed by stiffness, lasting several months. As pain subsides, exercises are intensified until full recovery is gained. Cause unknown.

fruc·tose (fruk'-tōs) *n* ⇒ evulose.

FSH follicle* stimulating hormone.

FTA *abbr* fluorescent* treponemal antibody.

fugue (fūg) *n* A period of loss of memory in which a journey takes place. The behavior of the person involved may appear normal or unspectacular to the casual observer. May occur in hysteria or in some forms of epilepsy.

fulgur·ation (ful-gūr-ā'-shun) *n* destruction of tissue by diathermy.

full-term *adj* mature—when pregnancy has lasted 40 weeks.

fulmi·nant (ful'-min-ant) *adj* developing quickly and with an equally rapid termination.

fumi·gation (fū-mi-gā'-shun) *n* disinfection by exposure to the fumes of a vaporized disinfectant.

func·tion (fungk'-shun) *n* the special work performed by an organ or structure in its normal state.

func·tional (fungk'-shun-al) *adj* **1** in a general sense, pertaining to function. **2** of a disorder, of the function but not the structure of an organ. **3** as a psychiatric term, of neurotic origin, i.e. psychogenic, without primary organic disease.

fundo·plication (fun-dô-plik-ā'-shun) *n* surgical folding of the gastric fundus to prevent reflux of gastric contents into the esophagus.

fun·dus (fun'-dus) *n* the basal portion of a hollow structure; the part which is distal to the opening *fundus uteri* the top of the uterus between the openings to the fallopian tubes.—**fundi** *pl.* **fundal** *adj.*

fungi·cide (fun'-ji-sīd) *n* an agent which is lethal to fungi—**fungicidal** *adj.*

fungi·form (fun'-ji-förm) *adj* resembling a mushroom, like the fungiform papillae found chiefly in the dorsocentral area of the tongue.

fungi·static (fun-ji-stat'-ik) *adj* describes an agent which inhibits the growth of fungi.

Fungi·zone (fun'-ji-zōn) *n* proprietary name for amphotericin B.

fun·gus (fung'-gus) *n* a low form of vegetable life including many microscopic organisms capable of producing superficial and systemic disease in man. The *ray fungus* was the original term for the genus *Actinomyces*, descriptive of the radial arrangement of the filaments which make up the sulfur granules or colonies of the organism in pus—**fungi** *pl.* **fungal** *adj.*

funicu·litis (fū-nik-ū-lī'-tis) *n* inflammation of the spermatic cord.

funicu·lus (fun-ik'-ū-lus) *n* a cord-like structure.

funnel chest (fun'-nl chest) (*syn* pectus excavatum) a congenital deformity in which the breast-bone is depressed towards the spine.

Fur·acin (fūr'-á-sin) *n* proprietary name for nitrofurazonc*.

Fura·dantin (fūr-á-dan'-tin) *n* proprietary name for nitrofurantoin*.

furazol·idone (fūr-á-zol'-i-dōn) *n* used for non-specific diarrheas, bacillary dysentery and bacterial food poisoning. (Furoxone.)

fu·ror (fūr'-or) *n* a sudden outburst of uncontrolled fury or rage during which an irrational act of violence may be committed.

Fur·oxone (fūr-oks'-ōn) proprietary name for furazolidone*.

fu·runcle (fur'-ung-kl) *n* ⇒ boil.

furun·culosis (fur-un-kū-lō'-sis) *n* an affliction due to boils.

furun·culus orient·alis (fur-un'-kū-lus ōr'-ē-ent-al'-is) oriental* sore.

fusi·form (fū'-si-förm) *adj* resembling a spindle.

FVC *abbr* forced* vital capacity ⇒ respiratory function tests.

G

gag *n* an instrument placed between the teeth to keep the mouth open.

gait (gāt) *n* a manner or style of walking. *ataxic gait* an incoordinate or abnormal gait. *cerebellar gait* reeling, staggering, lurching. *scissors gait* one in which the legs cross each other in progressing. *spastic gait* stiff, shuffling, the legs being held together. *tabetic gait* the foot is raised high then brought down suddenly, the whole foot striking the ground.

galacta·gogue (ga-lak'-ta-gog) *n* an agent inducing or increasing the flow of milk.

galacto·cele (ga-lak'-tō-sēl) *n* a cyst containing milk, or fluid resembling milk.

galactor·rhea (gal-ak-tor-ē'-á) *n* excessive flow of milk. Usually reserved for abnormal or inappropriate secretion of milk.

galac·tose (ga-lak'-tōs) *n* a monosaccharide found with glucose in lactose or milk sugar. *galactose test* after fasting, the patient drinks 40 g of galactose dissolved in 500 ml of water. 5 hours later urine is collected; if it contains 2 g or more galactose it indicates liver damage.

galactos·emia (gal-ak-tos-ēm'-ē-á) *n* excess of galactose in the blood and other tissues. Normally lactase in the small intestine converts lactose into glucose and galactose. In the liver another enzyme system converts galactose into glucose. Galactosemia is the result of a congenital enzyme deficiency in this system (two types) and is one cause of mental subnormality—**galactosemic** *adj.*

gall (gol) *n* bile*.

gall·amine (gol'-á-mēn) *n* a non-polarizing muscle relaxant resembling curare, but with a shorter action. Now superceded by alcuronium* and other synthetic drugs. (Flaxedil.)

gallblad·der (gol'-blad'-ėr) a pear-shaped bag on the undersurface of the liver (⇒ Figure 18). It concentrates and stores bile.

Gallie's oper·ation (gal'-ēz) the use of fascial strips from the thigh for radical cure after reduction of a hernia.

galli·pot (gal'-lē-pot) *n* a small vessel for lotions.

gallows trac·tion (gal'-ōwz) ⇒ Bryant's traction.

galls *n* the excrescences which form on certain oak trees, and from which tannic* acid is obtained. Ung. Gallae c Opio is an astringent ointment used mainly for hemorrhoids.

gall·stones (gol'-stōnz) *n* concretions formed within the gallbladder or bile ducts; they are often multiple and faceted.

galvano·cauterization (gal-van-ō-kaw-tėr-ī-zā'-shun) *n* the use of a wire heated by galvanic current to destroy tissue.

galva·nometer (gal-van-o'-me-tėr) *n* an instrument for measuring an electrical current.

Gam·blers Anony·mous an organization which exists to help compulsive gamblers to resist the compulsion.

ga·mete (gam'-ēt) *n* a male or female reproductive cell ⇒ ova, spermatazoon.

gam·gee (gam'-jē) *n* a brand of absorbent, white cotton wool enclosed in a fine gauze mesh.

gamma·ben·zenehexa·chloride (gam-à-ben'-zēn-heks-à-klōr'-īd) used as shampoo for treatment of head lice. Less irritant than benzyl* benzoate for scabies; requires only one application. (Kwell.)

gamma·en·cephal·ography (gam'-ma-en-sef-àl-og'-ra-fē) *n* a small dose of isotope is given. It is concentrated in many cerebral tumors. The pattern of radioactivity is then measured.

gamma·globulin (gam-mà-glo'-bū-lin) *n* a group of plasma proteins (IgA, IgD, IgE, IgG and IgM) which have antibody activity, referred to as immunoglobulins*. They are responsible for the humeral aspects of immunity.

gamma rays (gam'-mà rāz) short wavelength, penetrating rays of the electromagnetic spectrum produced by disintegration of the atomic nuclei of radioactive elements.

ganglion (gang'-lē-on) *n* **1** a mass of nerve tissue forming a subsidiary nerve center which receives and sends out nerve fibers, e.g. the ganglionic masses forming the sympathetic nervous system. **2** localized cyst-like swelling near a tendon, sheath or joint. Contains a clear, transparent, gelatinous or colloid substance; sometimes occurs on the back of the wrist due to strain such as excessive practice on the piano. **3** an enlargement on the course of a nerve such as is found on the receptor nerves before they enter the spinal cord—**ganglia** *pl*, **ganglionic** *adj*. *Gasserian ganglion* deeply situated within the skull, on the sensory root of the fifth cranial nerve. It is involved in trigeminal neuralgia.

ganglion·ectomy (gang-lē-on-ek'-to-mē) *n* surgical excision of a ganglion.

gangliosid·osis (gang-lē-ō-sīd-ō'-sis) *n* ⇒ Tay-Sachs' disease.

gangrene (gang'-rēn) *n* death of part of the tissues of the body. Usually the result of inadequate blood supply, but occasionally due to direct injury (traumatic gangrene) or infection (e.g. gas* gangrene). Deficient blood supply may result from pressure on blood vessels (e.g. tourniquets, tight bandages and swelling of a limb); from obstruction within healthy vessels (e.g. arterial embolism, frostbite where the capillaries become blocked); from spasm of the vessel wall (e.g. ergot poisoning); or from thrombosis due to disease of the vessel wall (e.g. arteriosclerosis in arteries, phlebitis in veins)—**gangrenous** *adj*. *dry gangrene* occurs when the drainage of blood from the affected part is adequate; the tissues become shrunken and black. *moist gangrene* occurs when venous drainage is inadequate so that the tissues are swollen with fluid.

gangre·nous stoma·titis (gang'-ren-us stō-mà-tī'-tis) ⇒ cancrum oris.

Ganser syn·drome (gan'-sėr) (nonsense syndrome) a hysterical condition in which approximate answers to questions are given which show that the correct answers are known; e.g. a horse may be said to have six legs.

Gan·trisin (gan'-tris-in) *n* proprietary name for sulfisoxazole*.

Garamycin (gār-à-mī'-sin) *n* proprietary name for gentamicin*.

Gar·denal (gàr'-den-al) *n* proprietary name for phenobarbital.

gargle (gàr'-gl) *n*, *vi* to wash the throat, a solution used for washing the throat.

gar·goylism (gàr'-goul-izm) *n* (*syn* Hunter-Hurler syndrome) congenital disorder of mucopolysaccharide metabolism with recessive or sex-linked inheritance. The polysaccharides chondroitin sulfate 'B' and heparitin sulfate are excreted in the urine. Characterized by skeletal abnormalities, coarse features, enlarged liver and spleen, mental subnormality. ACTH is useful.

Gärtner's bacillus (gàrt'-nerz) *Salmonella* enteritidis.

gas *n* one of the three states of matter, the others being solid and liquid. A gas retains neither shape nor volume when released—**gaseous** *adj*. *gas gangrene* a wound infection caused by anaerobic organisms of the genus *Clostridium*, especially *Clostridium perfringens (welchii),* a soil microbe often harbored in the intestine of man and animals; consequently there are many sources from which infection can arise. ⇒ gangrene.

gasser·ectomy (gas-sėr-ek'-to-mē) *n* surgical excision of the Gasserian ganglion*.

gas·tralgia (gas-tral'-jē-à) *n* pain in the stomach.

gas·trectomy (gas-trek'-to-mē) *n* removal of a part or the whole of the stomach. *Billroth I gastrectomy* is a partial gastrectomy least commonly performed and usually reserved for ulcer on the lesser curvature. *Billroth II gastrectomy* is the most commonly performed gastrectomy. Used for duodenal ulcer and as a palliative procedure for gastric cancer. Transverse colon and its mesentery intervene between stomach and jejunum. A hole can be made in the mesentery so that the anastomosis lies behind the transverse colon (retrocolic gastrectomy); or the loop of jejunum can be lifted up anterior to the transverse colon (antecolic gastrectomy). *total gastrectomy* is carried out only for cancer of the stomach. ⇒ roux-en-y operation.

gas·tric (gas'-trik) *adj* pertaining to the stomach. *gastric crisis* ⇒ crisis. *gastric influenza* a term used when gastrointestinal symptoms predominate. *gastric juice* is acid in reaction and contains two proteolytic enzymes. *gastric suction* may be intermittent or continuous to keep the stomach empty after some abdominal operations. *gastric ulcer* an ulcer in the gastric mucous membrane. Characteristically there is pain shortly after eating food which may be so severe that the person fails to eat adequately and loses weight. H_2 antagonists are the drugs of choice. Can be complicated by hematemesis or perforation constituting an abdominal emergency.

gas·trin (gas'-trin) *n* a hormone secreted by the gastric mucosa on entry of food, which causes a further flow of gastric juice.

gas·tritis (gas-trī'-tis) *n* inflammation of the stomach, especially the mucous membrane lining.

gastro·cnemius (gas-trŏk-nē'-mē-us) *n* the large two-headed muscle of the calf (⇒ Figures 4,5).

gastro·colic (gas-trŏ-kol'-ik) *adj* pertaining to the stomach and the colon.

gastro·duodenal (gas-trŏ-dū-o-dēn'-àl) *adj* pertaining to the stomach and the duodenum.

gastro·duodenostomy (gas-trŏ-dū-ŏ-dēn-os'-to-mē) *n* a surgical anastomosis between the stomach and the duodenum.

gastro·dynia (gas-trŏ-dī'-nē-à) *n* pain in the stomach.

gastro·enteritis (gas-trŏ-en-tėr-ī'-tis) *n* inflammation of mucous membranes of the stomach and the small intestine; although sometimes the result of dietetic error, the cause is usually a microbiological one. Infant gastroenteritis is usually caused by viruses, particularly the rotavirus although enteropathic *Escherichia coli* is still a common cause. Infection is spread by the fecal-oral route, either directly or indirectly.

gastro·enterology (gas-trŏ-en-tėr-ol'-o-jē) *n* study of the digestive tract, including the liver, biliary tract and pancreas and the accompanying diseases—**gastroenterological** *adj*, **gastroenterologically** *adv*.

gastro·enteropathy (gas-trŏ-en-tėr-op'-ath-ē) *n* disease of the stomach and intestine—**gastroenteropathic** *adj*.

gastro·enteroscope (gas-trŏ-en'-tėr-o-skōp) *n* an endoscope* for visualization of stomach and intestine—**gastroenteroscope** *adj*, **gastroenteroscopically** *adv*.

gastroenterostomy (gas-trŏ-en-tėr-os'-to-mē) *n* a surgical anastomosis between the stomach and small intestine.

gastro·esophageal (gas'-trŏ-ē-sof-à-jē'-àl) *adj* pertaining to the stomach and esophagus, as gastric reflux in heartburn.

gastro·esophagostomy (gas'-trŏ-ē-sof-à-gos'-to-mē) *n* a surgical operation in which the esophagus is joined to the stomach to bypass the natural juncture.

Gastrografin (gas-trŏ-gra'-fin) *n* a proprietary contrast medium composed of sodium and meglumine diatrizoates. Can be used early in patients with hematemesis. Its detergent and purgative effects are used in meconium ileus, when it is given as an enema.

gastrointestinal (gas-trŏ-in-tes'-tin-àl) *adj* pertaining to the stomach and intestine.

gastrojejunostomy (gas-trŏ-je-jŭn-os'-to-mē) *n* a surgical anastomosis between the stomach and the jejunum.

gastrop·athy (gas-tro'-path-ē) *n* any disease of the stomach.

gastro·pexy (gas'-trō-peks-ē) *n* surgical fixation of a displaced stomach.

gastro·phrenic (gas-trō-fren'-ik) *adj* pertaining to the stomach and diaphragm.

gastro·plasty (gas'-trō-plas-tē) *n* any plastic operation on the stomach. Currently used for reconstruction of the cardiac orifice of the stomach, where fibrosis prevents replacement of the stomach below the diaphragm in cases of hiatus hernia.

gastroplication (gas-trō-plik-ā'-shun) *n* an operation for the cure of dilated stomach by pleating the wall.

gastrop·tosis (gas-trop-tō'-sis) *n* downward displacement of the stomach.

gastropylorectomy (gas-trō-pī-lōr-ek'-to-mē) *n* excision of the pyloric end of the stomach.

gastro·schisis (gas-trō-skiz'-is) *n* a congenital incomplete closure of the abdominal wall with consequent protrusion of the viscera uncovered by peritoneum.

gastro·scope (gas'-trō-skōp) *n* ⇒ endoscope—**gastroscopic** *adj*, **gastroscopy** *n*.

gas·trostomy (gas-tros'-to-mē) *n* a surgically established fistula between the stomach and the exterior abdominal wall; usually for artificial feeding.

gas·trotomy (gas-trot'-o-mē) *n* incision into the stomach during an abdominal operation for such purposes as removing a foreign body, securing a bleeding blood vessel, approaching the esophagus from below to pull down a tube through a constricting growth.

gas·trula (gas'-trū-là) *n* the next stage after blastula in embryonic development.

Gaucher's dis·ease (go'-shāz) a rare familial disorder, mainly in Jewish children, characterized by a disordered lipid metabolism (lipid reticulosis) and usually accompanied by very marked enlargement of the spleen. Diagnosis follows sternal marrow puncture and the finding of typical Gaucher cells (distended with lipoid).

gauze (gawz) *n* a thin open-meshed absorbent material used in operations to dry the operative field and facilitate the procedure.

gavage feeding (ga-vazh') by custom refers to introducing fluid and nutrients into the stomach either by an esophageal tube passed orally or by a fine-bore nasogastric tube. Currently includes the use of mercury-weighted tubes to ensure nasojejunal feeding.

Gaviscon (gav'-is-kon) *n* a proprietary antacid containing aluminum* hydroxide and magnesium* carbonate.

Geiger counter (gī'-gèr kown'-tèr) a device for detecting and registering radioactivity.

gela·tin(e) (jel'-à-tin) *n* the protein-containing, glue-like substance obtained by boiling bones, skins and other animal tissues. Used as a base for pessaries, as the adhesive constituent of Unna's paste and in jellies and pastilles—**gelatinous** *adj*.

gemellus muscles (jem-el'-us) ⇒ Figure 5.

gene (jēn) a specific unit, located at a specific place (locus) of a specific chromosome. Genes are responsible for determining specific characteristics or traits. According to how they influence these characteristics, different forms of genes (alleles) may act as dominant (i.e. they manifest their presence in single doses of such alleles as are required). It is now known that each gene is a special and discrete coiled segment of the chemical DNA*, which is the principal and essential component of chromosomes.

gener·ative (jen-èr'-à-tiv) *adj* pertaining to reproduction.

generic (jen-èr'-ik) *adj* pertaining to a genus. *generic name* in reference to a drug, the distinctive, identifying name, not proprietary and not protected by a trademark.

gen·etic (jen-et'-ik) *adj* that which pertains to heredity. For example, disorders the basis of which resides in abnormalities of the genetic material, genes and chromosomes. ⇒ congenital.

gen·etic code (jen-et'-ik kōd) the name given to arrangement of genetic material stored in the DNA molecule of the chromosome. It is in this coded form that the information contained in the genes is transmitted to the cells to determine their activity.

gen·etics (jen-et'-iks) *n* the science of heredity and variation, namely the study of the genetic material, its transmission (from cell to cell and generation to generation) and its changes (mutations).

geni·tal (jen'-i-tàl) *adj* pertaining to the organs of generation. *genital herpes* ⇒ herpes.

geni·talia (jen-i-tā'-lē-à) *n* the external organs of generation.

genito·crural (jen-i-tō-krōō'-ràl) *adj* pertaining to the genital area and the leg.

genito·urinary (jen-i-tŏ-ûr'-i-nàr-ē) *adj* pertaining to the reproductive and urinary organs.

genome (jen'-ōm) *n* the basic set of chromosomes*, with the genes contained therein, equivalent to the sum total of gene types possessed by different organisms of a species.

geno·type (jēn'-ō-tīp) *n* the total genetic information encoded in the chromosomes* of an individual (as opposed to the phenotype*). Also, the genetic constitution of an individual at a particular locus, namely the alleles* present at that locus.

genta·micin (jen-tà-mī'-sin) *n* an antibiotic produced by *Micromonospora purpurea*. Antibacterial, especially against *Pseudomonas* and staphylococci resistant to other antibiotics. Given intramuscularly and as eye and ear drops. Ototoxic and dangerous in renal failure. (Garamycin.)

gen·tian violet (jen'-shun) ⇒ crystal violet.

genu (jen'-ū) *n* the knee.

genu·pectoral pos·ition (jen-ū-pek'-tŏr-àl) the knee-chest position, i.e. the weight is taken by the knees, and by the upper chest, while the shoulder girdle and head are supported on a pillow in front.

ge·nus (jē'-nus) *n* a classification ranking between the family (higher) and the species (lower).

genu valgum (jen'-ū-val'-gum) (knock knee) abnormal incurving of the legs so that there is a gap between the feet when the knees are in contact.

genu varum (jen'-ū-vār'-um) (bow legs) abnormal outward curving of the legs resulting in separation of the knees.

geo·phagia (jē-ō-fā'-jē-à) *n* the habit of eating clay or earth.

geria·trician (jer-ē-à-trish'-un) *n* one who specializes in geriatrics.

geri·atrics (jer-ē-a'-triks) *n* the branch of medical science dealing with old age and its diseases together with the medical care and nursing required by 'geriatric' patients.

germ (jerm) *n* a unicellular micro-organism, especially used for a pathogen.

German measles (jerm'-an mē'-zls) ⇒ rubella.

germi·cide (jer'-mi-sīd) *n* an agent which kills germs—**germicidal** *adj*.

geron·tology (jer-on-tol'-o-jē) *n* the scientific study of aging—**gerontological** *adj*.

gestalt (ge-shtålt') *n* a unified whole with characteristics not derived from the individual parts. *gestalt psychology* a here and now school of psychology which holds that psychological phenomena are gestalts, wholes which are not the sums of their parts, but rather the parts in relationship to each other.

ges·tation (jes-tā'-shun) *n* ⇒ pregnancy—**gestational** *adj*.

GFR *abbr* glomerular* filtration rate.

GH *abbr* growth hormone.

Ghon focus (gon fō'-kus) ⇒ primary complex.

giant cell arteritis ⇒ arteritis.

giar·diasis (jē-àr-dī'-à-sis) *n* (*syn* lambliasis) infection with the flagellate *Giardia intestinalis*. Often symptomless, especially in adults. Can cause diarrhea with steatorrhea. Treatment is quinacrine or metronidazole orally.

gigan·tism (jī-gan'-tizm) *n* an abnormal overgrowth, especially in height. May be associated with anterior pituitary tumor if the tumor develops before fusion of the epiphyses. Due to excess of growth hormone.

Gilliam's oper·ation (gil'-ē-amz) a method of correcting retroversion by shortening the round ligaments of the uterus.

gin·ger (jin'-jėr) *n* an aromatic root with carminative properties. Used as syrup or tincture for flavoring purposes.

gin·giva (jin'-ji-và) *n* the gum; the vascular tissue surrounding the necks of the erupted teeth—**gingival** *adj*.

gingival sulcus (jin'-ji-vàl sul'-kus) the investigation* made by the gingiva as it joins with the tooth surface.

gingi·vectomy (jin-ji-vek'-to-mē) *n* excision of a portion of the gum, usually for pyorrhea.

gingi·vitis (jin-ji-vī'-tis) *n* inflammation of the gum or gingiva usually caused by irritation from dental plaque and calculus. Can occur with the systemic use of some drugs, e.g. dilantin sodium, or mercury and may be associated with pregnancy, due to hormone changes.

girdle (gėr'dl) *n* usually a bony structure of oval shape such as the shoulder and pelvic girdles.

gland (gland) *n* an organ or structure capable of making an internal or external secretion. *lymphatic gland* (node) does not secrete, but is concerned with filtration of the lymph. ⇒ endocrine, exocrine—**glandular** *adj*.

glan·ders (glan'-dèrz) *n* a contagious, febrile, ulcerative disease communicable from horses, mules and asses to man.

glandu·lar fever (gland'-ū-lar fē'-vèr) *n* ⇒ infectious mononucleosis.

glans (glanz) *n* the bulbous termination of the clitoris and penis (⇒ Figure 16).

glau·coma (glaw-kō'-mà) *n* a condition where the intraocular pressure is raised. In the acute stage the pain is severe—**glaucomatous** *adj*.

gleno·humeral (glē-nō-hū'-mèr-àl) *adj* pertaining to the glenoid cavity of scapula and the humerus.

gle·noid (glē'-noyd) *n* a cavity on the scapula* into which the head of the humerus* fits to form the shoulder joint.

glia (glē'-à) *n* ⇒ neuroglia—**glial** *adj*.

glio·blastoma multi·forme (glē-o-blas-tō'-mà-mul'-ti-fōrm) a highly malignant brain tumor.

gli·oma (glē-ō'-mà) *n* a malignant growth which does not give rise to secondary deposits. It arises from neuroglia. One form, occurring in the retina, is hereditary—**gliomata** *pl*.

glio·myoma (glē-ō-mī-ō'-mà) *n* a tumor of nerve and muscle tissue—**gliomyomata** *pl*.

glipi·zide (glip'-i-zīd) *n* an orally active antidiabetic drug. One of the sulfonylureas. ⇒ tolbutamide. (Glucotrol.)

glo·bin (glō'-bin) *n* a protein which combines with hematin to form hemoglobin.

globu·lin (glob'-ū-lin) *n* the fraction of serum or plasma which contains the immunoglobulins* A, D, E, G and M.

globulin·uria (glob-ū-lin-ūr'-ē-à) *n* the presence of globulin in the urine.

globus hystericus (glōb'-us his-tèr'-i-kus) a subjective feeling of neurotic origin of a lump in the throat. Can also include difficulty in swallowing and is due to tension of muscles of deglutition. Occurs in hysteria, anxiety states and depression. Sometimes follows slight trauma to throat, e.g. scratch by foreign body.

globus pallidus (glōb'us pal'-i-dus) literally pale globe; situated deep within the cerebral hemispheres, lateral to the thalamus.

glomer·ular fil·tration rate (GFR) (glom-ėr'-ū-lar fil-trā'-shun) the rate of filtration from blood in the glomerulus of renal capillaries to the fluid in Bowman's capsule. It is usually 120 ml per min and is a fine index of renal function.

glomer·ulitis (glom-ėr-ū-lī'-tis) *n* inflammation of the glomeruli, usually of the kidney. The use of electron microscopes and fluorescent staining of biopsy specimens has improved diagnosis and knowledge of the condition.

glomer·ulonephritis (glom-ėr-ū-lō-nef-rī'-tis) *n* a term which covers several diseases which have as their common denominator damage to the glomeruli of the renal cortex mediated through the immune mechanisms of the body and the immunoglobulins of the blood. Proteinuria and microscopic hematuria are features but no bacteria appear in the urine.

glomerulo·sclerosis (glom-ėr'-ū-lō-sklėr-ō'-sis) *n* fibrosis of the glomeruli of the kidney, usually the result of inflammation. *intercapillary glomerulosclerosis* a common pathological finding in diabetics—**glomerulosclerotic** *adj*.

glomeru·lus (glom-ėr'-ū-lus) *n* a coil of minute arterial capillaries held together by scanty connective tissue. It invaginates the entrance of the uriniferous tubules in the kidney cortex—**glomerular** *adj*, **glomeruli** pl.

glossa (glos'-sà) *n* the tongue—**glossal** *adj*.

gloss·ectomy (glos-sek'-to-mē) *n* excision of the tongue.

gloss·itis (glos-ī'-tis) *n* inflammation of the tongue.

glosso·dynia (glos-ō-dī'-nē-à) *n* a name used for a painful tongue when there is no visible change.

glosso'pharyngeal (glos-ō-fār-in-jē'-àl) *adj* pertaining to the tongue and pharynx. The ninth pair of the 12 pairs of cranial nerves arising directly from the brain.

glosso·plegia (glos-ō-plēj'-ē-à) *n* paralysis of the tongue.

glot·tis (glot'-tis) *n* that part of the larynx associated with voice production—**glottic** *adj*.

gluc·agon (gloo'-kà-gon) *n* hormone produced in alpha cells of pancreatic islets of Langerhans. Causes breakdown of glycogen into glucose thus preventing blood sugar from falling too low during fasting. Can now be obtained commercially from the pancreas of animals. Given to accelerate breakdown of glycogen in the liver and raise blood sugar rapidly. As it is a polypeptide hormone, it must be given by injection.

gluco·corticoid (glōō-kō-kōr'-ti-koyd) *n* any steroid hormone which promotes gluconeogenesis (i.e. the formation of glucose and glycogen from protein) and which antagonizes the action of insulin. Occurring naturally in the adrenal cortex as cortisone and hydrocortisone, and produced synthetically as, for example, prednisone and prednisolone.

gluco·genesis (glōō-kō-jen'-e-sis) *n* production of glucose.

gluconeo·genesis (glōō-kō-nē'-ō-jen'-e-sis) *n* (*syn* glyconeogenesis) the formation of sugar from protein or fat when there is lack of available carbohydrate.

glu·cose (glōō'-kōs) *n* dextrose or grape sugar. A monosaccharide. The form in which carbohydrates are absorbed through the intestinal tract and circulated in the blood. It is stored as glycogen* in the liver. *glucose tolerance test* after a period of fasting, a measured quantity of glucose is taken orally; thereafter blood and urine samples are tested for glucose at intervals. Higher than normal levels are indicative of diabetes mellitus.

Glucotrol (glōō'-ko-trol) *n* proprietary name for glipizide*.

glucu·ronic acid (glōō-kū-ron'-ik) an acid which acts on bilirubin* to form conjugated bilirubin.

glue ear an accumulation of a glue-like substance in the middle ear which bulges the ear drum and impairs hearing.

glue sniff·ing an increasingly popular practice of inhaling the vapors of toluene, a constituent of most glues, from a plastic bag. The sniffers are commonly adolescents. Redness and blistering around the mouth and nose may be evidence. Intoxication results.

glutamic oxalo·acetic trans·aminase (glōō-tam'-ik-oks-al'-ō-à-sēt'-ik-tranz-am'-in-ās) an enzyme present in serum and body tissues, especially the heart and liver. It is released into the serum following tissue damage such as myocardial infarction or acute damage to liver cells. (*abbr,* SGOT.)

glutamic pyr·uvic trans·aminase (glōō-tam'-ik-pī-rōō'-vik) an enzyme present in serum and body tissues, especially the liver. Acute damage to hepatic cells causes an increase in serum concentration. (*abbr,* SGPT.)

glu·taminase (glōō-tam'-in-ās) *n* an amino acid-degrading enzyme, being used in the treatment of cancer.

glu·teal (glōō'-tē-àl) *adj* pertaining to the buttocks* ⇒ Figure 5.

glu·ten (glōō'-ten) *n* a protein constituent of wheat flour insoluble in water but an essential component of the elastic 'dough'. It is not tolerated in celiac disease*.

gluten-induced enteropathy (glōō'-ten in-dūsd') ⇒ celiac.

glutethimide (glōō-teth'-i-mīd) *n* hypnotic of medium action. Useful when an alternative to the barbiturates is required. (Doriden.)

gluteus muscles (glōō'-tē-us) ⇒ Figures 4,5.

glycer·in(e) (gli'-sèr-in) *n* a clear, syrupy liquid prepared synthetically or obtained as a byproduct in soap manufacture. It has a hygroscopic action. *glycerine and borax* useful for softening sordes. *glycerine and honey* useful as a softening agent for oral toilet. *glycerine and ichthyol* applied as a compress to relieve inflammation. *glycerine and magnesium sulfate* useful for boils, etc.

glycero·phosphates (glis'-èr-ō-fos'-fāts) *npl* appetite stimulant.

gly·ceryl trinitrate (glis'-èr-yl trī-nī'-trāt) (*syn,* nitroglycerin) a vasodilator used mainly in angina pectoris. Given mainly as tablets which should be chewed, or dissolved under the tongue; or transdermally by application as a gel to the skin.

gly·cine (glī'-sēn) *n* a non-essential amino* acid.

glycin·uria (glī-sin-ūr'-ē-à) *n* excretion of glycine* in the urine. Associated with mental subnormality.

glyco·gen (glī'-kō-jen) *n* the main carbohydrate storage compound in animals, in which glucose molecules are linked in branched chains. *glycogen storage disease* a metabolic recessive inherited condition caused by various enzyme deficiencies—types 1–13 are now recognized. The liver becomes large and fatty due to the excessive glycogen deposits. Hypoglycemia is a major problem. The body tends to metabolize fat rather than glucose and ketosis and acidosis are prevalent. 3 hourly daytime feeds and overnight intragastric feeding have improved the prognosis.

glyco·genase (glī-ko'-jen-ās) *n* an enzyme necessary for the conversion of glycogen into glucose.

glyco·genesis (glī-kō-jen′-es-is) *n* glycogen formation from blood glucose.

glyco·geno·lysis (glī-kō-jen-ol′-is-is) *n* the breakdown of glycogen to glucose.

glyco·genosis (glī-kō-jen-os′-is) *n* a metabolic disorder leading to increased storage of glycogen*. Leads to glycogen myopathy.

gly·colysis (glī-kol′-is-is) *n* the hydrolysis of sugar in the body—**glycolytic** *adj.*

glyconeo·genesis (glī-kō-nē-ō-jen′-es-is) ⇒ gluconeogenesis*.

glyco·pyrrolate (glī-kō-pī′-rol-āt) *n* a synthetic, atropine-like drug which does not cause such extensive tachycardia as atropine*. (Robinul.)

glyco·sides (glī′-kō-sīdz) *npl* natural substances composed of a sugar with another compound. The non-sugar fragment is termed an 'aglycone,' and is sometimes of therapeutic value. Digoxin is a familiar example of a glycoside.

glyco·suria (glī-kō-sū′-rē-à) *n* the presence of large amounts of sugar in the urine.

glycyr·rhiza (glis-i-rī′-zà) *n* licorice root, demulcent, slightly laxative, expectorant and used as a flavoring agent. Results in an increase in extracellular fluid, retention of sodium and increased excretion of potassium.

gnath·algia (nath-al′-jē-à) *n* pain in the jaw.

gnatho·plasty (nath′-ō-plas-tē) *n* plastic surgery of the jaw.

gob·let cells (gob′-let) special secreting cells, shaped like a goblet, found in the mucous membranes.

Goeckerman régime (gā′-kėr-man) a method of treatment for psoriasis; exposure to ultraviolet light alternating with the application of a tar paste.

goiter (goy′-tèr) *n* an enlargement of the thyroid gland. In *simple goiter* the patient does not show any signs of excessive thyroid activity. In *toxic goiter* the enlarged gland secretes an excess of thyroid hormone. The patient is nervous, loses weight and often has palpitations and exophthalmos. ⇒ colloid.

goi·trogens (goy′-trō-jens) *npl* agents causing goiter. Some occur in plants, e.g. turnip, cabbage, brussels sprouts and peanuts.

golden eye oint·ment ⇒ mercuric oxide.

gold injection ⇒ aurothiomalate.

Goldthwait belt (gōld′-thwāt) wide belt with steel support for back injuries.

gonad (gō′-nad) *n* a male or female sex gland ⇒ ovary, testis—**gonadal** *adj.*

gonado-trophic (gō-nad-ō-trō′-fik) *adj* having an affinity for, or influence on the gonads.

gonado-trophin (gō-nad-ō-trō′-fin) *n* any gonad-stimulating hormone. ⇒ follicle stimulating hormone, human chorionic gonadotrophin test, luteotrophin.

goni·oscopy (gō-nē-os′-ko-pē) *n* measuring angle of anterior chamber of eye with a gonioscope.

goni·otomy (gō-nē-ot′-o-mē) *n* operation for glaucoma incision through the anterior chamber angle to the canal of Schlemm.

gono·coccal comp·lement fix·ation test (go-nō-kok′-al) a specific serological test for the diagnosis of gonorrhea.*

Gono·coccus (gon-ō-kok′-us) *n* a Gram-negative diplococcus (*Neisseria gonorrhea*), the causative organism of gonorrhea. It is a strict parasite. Occurs characteristically inside polymorphonuclear leukocytes in the tissues—**gonococci** *pl*, **gonococcal** *adj.*

gonor·rhea (gon-ōr-rē′-à) *n* a sexually-transmitted disease in adults. In children infection is accidental, e.g. gonococcal ophthalmia of the newborn, gonococcal vulvovaginitis of girls before puberty. Chief manifestations of the disease in the male are a purulent urethritis with dysuria, in the female, urethritis, endocervicitis and salpingitis which may be symptomless. Incubation period is usually 2-5 days—**gonorrheal** *adj.*

gonor·rheal (gon-ōr-rē′-àl) *adj* resulting from gonorrhea. *gonorrheal arthritis* is a metastatic manifestation of gonorrhea *gonorrheal ophthalmia* is one form of ophthalmia neonatorum.

Good·pasture syn·drome association of hemorrhagic lung disorder with glomerulonephritis.

goose flesh contraction of the tiny muscles attached to the sheath of the hair follicles causes the hair to stand on end; it is a reaction to either cold or fear.

Gordh needle (gōrd) an intravenous needle with a rubber diaphragm. Through it repeated injections can be given.

GOT test glutamic* oxalacetic transaminase test.

gouge (gowj) *n* a chisel with a grooved blade for removing bone.

gout (gowt) *n* a form of metabolic disorder in which sodium biurate is deposited in the cartilages of the joints, the ears, and elsewhere. The big toe is characteristically involved and becomes acutely painful and swollen. There are now drugs which increase the excretion of urates; these have largely controlled the disease.

GPI *abbr* ⇒ general paralysis of the insane.

GPT test glutamic-pyruvic* transaminase test.

graafian fol·icle (graf'-ē-àn fol'-li-kl) minute vesicles contained in the stroma of an ovary*, each containing a single ovum. When an ovum is extruded from a Graafian follicle each month the corpus luteum is formed under the influence of luteotrophin from the anterior pituitary gland. If fertilization occurs, the corpus luteum persists for 12 weeks; if not, it only persists for 12–14 days.

gracilis muscle (gra-sil'-lis) ⇒ Figures 4,5.

Graefe's knife (grā'fēs) finely pointed knife with narrow blades used for making incisions across anterior chamber of eye prior to removal of cataract.

graft *n* a tissue or organ which is transplanted to another part of the same animal (autograft), to another animal of the same species (homograft), or to another animal of a different species (heterograft).

gramici·din (gram-is'-i-din) *n* a mixture of antibiotic substances obtained from tyrothricin*. Too toxic for systemic use, but valuable for topical application when local antibiotic therapy is required.

Gram's stain a bacteriological stain for differentiation of microorganisms. Those retaining the blue dye are Grampositive (+), those unaffected by it are Gram-negative (−).

grand mal (grahn' mahl) major epilepsy. ⇒ epilepsy.

granu·lation (gran-ū-lā'-shun) *n* the outgrowth of new capillaries and connective tissue cells from the surface of an open wound. *granulation tissue* the young, soft tissue so formed—**granulate** *vi*.

granulo·cyte (gran'-ū-lō-sīt) *n* a cell containing granules in its cytoplasm. Used for polymorphonuclear leukocytes which have neutrophil, eosinophil or basophil granules.

granulo·cytopenia (gran'-ū-lō-sī-tō-pē'-nē-à) *n* decrease of granulocytes* (polymorphs) not sufficient to warrant the term agranulocytosis*.

granu·loma (gran-ū-lō'-mà) *n* a tumor

formed of granulation tissue. *granuloma venereum* lymphogranuloma* inguinale.

gravel (grav'-el) *n* a sandy deposit which, if present in the bladder, may be passed with the urine.

Graves' disease (grāvs) ⇒ thyrotoxicosis.

gra·vid (gra'-vid) *adj* pregnant; carrying fertilized eggs or a fetus.

Gravindex test (grav'-in-deks) an immunological test for pregnancy.

gravi·tational (grav-it-ā'-shun-àl) *adj* being attracted by force of gravity. *gravitational ulcer* ⇒ varicose ulcer.

grav·ity (grav'-it-ē) *n* weight. The weight of a substance compared with that of an equal volume of water is termed *specific gravity*.

Grawitz tumor (gra'-vits) ⇒ hypernephroma.

green monkey disease ⇒ Marburg disease.

green stick·frac·ture ⇒ fracture.

gregari·ous (greg-ār'-ē-us) *adj* showing a preference for living in a group, liking to mix. The gregarious or herd instinct is an inborn tendency on the part of various species, including man.

Griffith's types (grif'-iths) antigenic subdivisions of Lancefield* group A streptococci by virtue of their characteristic M protein antigens.

grinder's asthma (grīn'-derz az'-mà) one of the many popular names for silicosis* arising from inhalation of metallic dust.

grip (grip) *n* abdominal colic.

griseofulvin (gris-ē-ō-ful'-vin) *n* an oral fungicide, useful in ringworm*.

grocer's itch (grō'-serz ich) contact dermatitis, especially from flour or sugar.

groin (groyn) *n* the junction of the thigh with the abdomen.

grom·met (grom'-et) *n* a type of ventilation tube inserted into the tympanic membrane. Frequently used in the treatment of glue* ear in children ⇒ myringotomy.

group psycho·therapy ⇒ psychotherapy.

grow·ing pains pain in the limbs during youth; the differential diagnosis is rheumatic fever.

growth hormone (GH), growth hormone test (GHT) there is a reciprocal relationship between growth hormone (secreted by the pituitary* gland) and blood glucose. Blood is therefore estimated for

GH during a standard 50 g oral glucose tolerance test. In acromegaly, not only is the resting level of GH higher, but it does not show normal suppression with glucose.

guan·ethidine (gwan-eth'-id-ēn) *n* a hypotensive, sympathetic blocking agent. Gives sustained reduction of intraocular pressure in glaucoma. Applied locally to block the sympathetic fibers to the eye in exophthalmos. (Ismelin.)

guar (gwar) *n* fiber derived from natural sources which disperses readily in fluid to produce a palatable drink.

Guillain-Barré syndrome (gē-yan' bar-ra') (*syn* acute polyneuritis) polyneuritis accompanied by progressive muscular weakness.

guillo·tine (gil'-ō-tēn) *n* a surgical instrument for excision of the tonsils.

Guinea worm (gin'-ē) ⇒ *Dracunculus* *medinensis*.

gul·let (gul'-let) *n* the esophagus*.

gumboil (gum'-boyl) lay term for an abscess of gum tissue and periosteum (dento-alveolar abscess) which is usually very painful.

gumma (gum'-mà) *n* a localized area of vascular granulation tissue which develops in the later stages (tertiary) of syphilis. Obstruction to the blood supply results in necrosis, and gummata near a surface of the body tend to break down, forming chronic ulcers, which are probably not infectious—**gummata** *pl*.

gut *n* the intestines, large and small. *gut decontamination* the use of non-absorbable antibiotics to suppress growth of microorganisms to prevent endogenous infection for patients undergoing bowel surgery or those who are neutropenic or immunocompromised.

Guthrie test (guth'-rē) assay of phenylalanine* from a drop of blood dried on special filter paper. It is necessary to confirm the diagnosis in those infants with a positive test.

gyne·cography (gī-ne-cog'-rà-fē) *n* radiological visualization of internal female genitalia after pneumoperitoneum—**gynecographical** *adj*, **gynecographically** *adv*.

gynecoid (gī'-ne-koyd *adj* resembling a woman. *gynecoid pelvis* the normal shaped female pelvis.

gyne·cologist (gī-ne-kol'-o-jist) *n* a surgeon who specializes in gynecology*.

gyne·cology (gī-ne-kol'-o-jē) *n* the science dealing with the diseases of the fe-

male reproductive system—**gynecological** *adj*.

gyne-comastia (gī-ne-kō-mas'-tē-à) *n* enlargement of the male mammary gland.

gyp·sum (jip'-sym)*n* plaster of Paris (calcium sulfate)*.

gyr·ectomy (jī-rek'-to-mē) *n* surgical removal of a gyrus*.

gyrus (jī'-rus) *n* a convoluted portion of cerebral cortex.

H

habilitation (hab-il-it-ā'-shun) *n* the means by which a child gradually progresses towards the maximum degree of physical and psychological independence of which he is capable. ⇒ rehabilitation.

habit (hab'-it) *n* any learned behavior that has a relatively high probability of occurrence in response to a particular situation or stimulus. Acquisition of habits may depend on both reinforcement and associative learning. *habit training* used in mental hospitals for deteriorated patients who relearn personal hygiene by constant repetition with encouragement.

habit·ual abor·tion (hab-it'-ū-al ab-ōr'-shun) ⇒ abortion.

habitu·ation (hab-it-ū-ā'-shun) *n* the means of acquiring or developing a pattern of behavior as a habit. The word is often used in a negative sense such as a person becoming dependent on sleeping pills. ⇒ drug dependence.

Haemophilus (hē-mo'-fil-us) *n* a genus of bacteria. Small Gram-negative rods which show much variation in shape (pleomorphism). Characteristically intracellular in polymorphonuclear leukocytes in exudate. They are strict parasites, and accessory substances present in blood, are usually necessary for growth. *Haemophilus aegyptius* causes a form of acute infectious conjunctivitis. *Haemophilus ducreyi* causes chancroid. *Haemophilus influenzae* causes respiratory infections; it was thought to cause influenza but is now considered to be a primary and secondary invader and as such causes influenza meningitis, conjunctivitis and septicemia. *Haemophilus pertussis* (now *Bordetella pertussis*) causes whooping cough.

HAI *abbr* hospital acquired infection. ⇒ infection.

hair (hār) *n* thread-like appendage present on all parts of human skin except palms, soles, lips, glans penis and that surrounding the terminal phalanges. The broken-off stump found at the periphery of spreading bald patches in alopecia areata is called an exclamation mark hair, from the characteristic shape caused by atrophic thinning of the hair shaft. *hair bulb* ⇒ Figure 12. *hair follicle* the sheath in which a hair grows. *hair root* ⇒ Figure 12. *hair shaft* ⇒ Figure 12.

Haldol (hal'-dol) *n* proprietary name for haloperidol*.

half-life *n* in reference to a radioactive isotope, the time taken for it to disintegrate by one half or to lose 50 per cent of its energy.

hali·but liver oil (hal'-i-but) a very rich source of vitamins* A and D. The smaller dose required makes it more acceptable than cod liver oil.

hali·tosis (hal-i-tō'-sis) *n* foul smelling breath.

halluci·nation (hal-lū-sin-ā'-shun) *n* a false perception occurring without any true sensory stimulus. A common symptom in severe psychoses including schizophrenia, paraphrenia and confusional states. Also common in delirium, during toxic states and following head injuries.

hallucino·gens (hal-lū-sin'-ō-jens) *npl* ⇒ psychotomimetics.

halluci·nosis (hal-lū-sin-ō'-sis) *n* a psychosis in which the patient is grossly hallucinated. Usually a subacute delirious state; the predominant symptoms are auditory illusions and hallucinations.

hal·lux (hal'-luks) *n* the great toe. *hallus valgus* ⇒ bunion. *hallux varus* the big toe is displaced towards the other foot. *hallux rigidus* ankylosis of the metatarsophalangeal articulation caused by osteoarthritis.

halo (hā'-lō) *n* a splint which encircles the head. ⇒ halopelvic traction.

hal·ogen (hal'-ō-jen) *n* any one of the nonmetallic elements—bromine, chlorine, fluorine, iodine.

halopel·vic trac·tion (hal-ō-pel'-vik) a form of external fixation whereby traction can be applied to the spine between two fixed points. The device consists of three main parts (a) a halo (b) a pelvic loop and (c) four extension bars.

halo·peridol (hal-ō-pèr'-i-dol) *n* a psychotrophic agent used in the treatment of schizophrenia and other psychotic disorders for its tranquilizing properties. It can be taken orally, but if necessary, as in mania, it can be given by injection. (Haldol.)

halo·thane (hal'-ō-thān) *n* a clear colorless liquid used as an inhalation anesthetic. Advantages: non-explosive and non-inflammable in all circumstances. Odor is not unpleasant. It is non-irritant (Fluothane.)

hama·melis (ham-à-mel'-lis) (*syn* witch hazel) a tree whose bark contains an astringent. *aqua hamamelis* extract of witch hazel, made from the bark. Astringent lotion. *hamamelis leaf* incorporated in suppositories for non-inflammatory piles.

ham·mer toe a permanent hyperextension of the first phalanx and flexion of second and third phalanges.

hand *n* that part of the upper limb below the wrist. *hand bandage* made from a smooth-textured flesh-colored yarn. It is available with open fingers to enable observation of the digits. The two-way stretch provides constant pressure over the entire hand.

handi·capped (hand'-i-kapd) *adj* the term applied to a person with a defect that interferes with normal activity and achievement.

Hand-Schüller-Christian dis·ease (hand shil'-èr kris'-chan) a rare condition usually manifesting in early childhood with histiocytic granulomatous lesions affecting many tissues. Regarded as a form of histiocytosis X. Cause unknown and course relatively benign.

hang·nail *n* a narrow strip of skin partly detached from the nail fold.

Hansen's bacillus (han'-senz bà-sil'-us) ⇒ leprosy.

H_2 antagonist an agent which has a selective action against the H_2 histamine receptors and thereby decreases, for example, the secretion of gastric juice.

hap·loid (hap'-loyd) *adj* refers to the chromosome complement of the mature gametes (eggs and sperm) following meiosis (reduction division). This set represents the basic complement of 23 chromosomes in man. Its normal multiple is diploid, but abnormally three or more chromosome sets can be found (triploid, tetraploid, etc).

hare·lip (hār'-lip) *n* a congenital defect in the lip; a fissure extending from the margin of the lip to the nostril; may be single or double, and is often associated with cleft* palate.

Harrington rod (hār'-ing-ton) used in operations for scoliosis*, it provides internal fixation whereby the curve is held by the rod and is usually accompanied by a spinal fusion.

Harrison Narcotic Act (hăr'-i-son) regulates the importing, manufacture, sale, dispensing and prescribing of opium cocaine and their derivatives. Also now includes synthetic drugs that are addicting. Original act was established in 1914 but has since been amended several times.

Harris' oper·ation (hăr'-is-iz) a transvesical, suprapubic type of prostatectomy*.

Hartmann's sol·ution (hărt'-manz) an electrolyte replacement solution. Contains sodium lactate and chloride, potassium chloride and calcium chloride.

Hartnup dis·ease (hart'-nup) an inborn error of protein metabolism, associated with diffuse psychiatric symptoms or mild mental subnormality. It can be treated with nicotinamide and neomycin.

Hashimoto's dis·ease (hash-ē-mō'-tōz) affliction of an enlarged thyroid gland occurring in middle-aged females, and producing mild hypothyroidism. Result of sensitization of patient to her own thyroid protein, thyroglobulin.

hash·ish (hash'-ish) $n \Rightarrow$ cannabis indica.

haus·tration (haws-trā'-shun) n sacculation*, as of the colon—**haustrum** *sing.* **haustra** *pl.*

hay fever a form of allergic rhinitis in which attacks of catarrh of the conjunctiva, nose and throat are precipitated by exposure to pollen.

Haygarth's nodes (hā'-gărths) swelling of joints sometimes seen in the finger joints of patients suffering from arthritis.

HBIG *abbr* hepatitis B immunoglobulin.

HCG *abbr* human* chorionic gonadotrophin.

heal·ing (hēl'-ing) the natural process of cure or repair of the tissues—**heal** *vt. vi. healing by first intention* when the edges of a clean wound are accurately held together, healing occurs with the minimum of scarring and deformity. *healing by second intention* when the edges of a wound are not held together, the gap is filled by granulation tissue before epithelium can grow over the wound.

health (helth) n the World Health Organization states, 'Health is a state of complete physical, mental and social wellbeing and not merely the absence of disease or infirmity.'

Health Maintenance Organization (*abbr

HMO) a group medical practice that offers prepaid health care with an emphasis on complete care, including prevention.

hear·ing tests $\Rightarrow$ auditory acuity*.

heart (hàrt) n the hollow muscular organ which pumps the blood round the body; situated behind the sternum, lying obliquely between the two lungs ($\Rightarrow$ Figure 6). It weighs 2.24–3.36 hg in the female and 2.80–3.36 hg in the male. *heart transplant* surgical transplantation of a heart from a suitable donor who has recently died. *heart block* partial or complete inhibition of the speed of conduction of the electrical impulse from the atrium to the ventricle of the heart. The cause may be an organic lesion or a functional disturbance. In its mildest form, it can only be detected electrocardiographically, whilst in its complete form the ventricles beat at their own slow intrinsic rate uninfluenced by the atria.

heart·burn (hàrt'-burn) $n \Rightarrow$ pyrosis, hotfat heartburn syndrome.

heart-lung machine n a machine by means of which the blood can be removed from a vein for oxygenation, after which it is returned to the vein.

heat exhaus·tion (hēt eks-awst'-yun) (*syn* heat syncope) collapse, with or without loss of consciousness, suffered in conditions of heat and high humidity: largely resulting from loss of fluid and salt by sweating. If the surrounding air becomes saturated, heatstroke will ensue.

heat·stroke n (*syn* sunstroke) final stage in heat exhaustion. When the body is unable to lose heat, hyperpyrexia occurs and death may ensue.

hebe·phrenia (hē-be-frē'-nē-à) n a common type of schizophrenia* characterized by a general disintegration of the personality. The onset is sudden and usually occurs in the teenage years. At present time prognosis tends to be unfavorable—**hebephrenic** *adj.*

Heberden's dis·ease (he'-bėr-denz) Angina* pectoris. *Heberden's nodes* small osseous swellings at terminal phalangeal joints occurring in many types of arthritis.

hedon·ism (hēd'-on-izm) n excessive devotion to pleasure, so that a person's conduct is determined by an unconscious drive to seek pleasure and avoid unpleasant things.

Hegar's sign (hā'-gàrz) marked softening of the cervix in early pregnancy.

Heimlich's maneuver (hīm'-liks) a first

131

aid measure to dislodge a foreign body (e.g. food) obstructing the glottis, performed by holding the patient from behind and jerking the operator's clenched fists into the victim's epigastrium.

Heinz body (Hīnz) refractile, irregularly shaped body present in red blood cells in some hemoglobinopathies.

he·lium (hēl'-ē-um) *n* an inert gas of low density. Sometimes mixed with oxygen for treatment of asthma, as it aids inspiration.

helix (hē'-liks) *n* the outer edge of the external ear. ⇒ Figure 13. *double helix* the double stranded structure of the DNA molecule, consisting of two strands composed of alternating sugar–phosphate units, joined at intervals by four nitrogen bases: adenine, guanine, thymine and cytosine.

Heller's opera·tion (hel'-ėrz) division of the muscle coat at the junction between the esophagus and the stomach; used to relieve the difficulty in swallowing in cases of achalasia*.

helmin·thagogue (hel-minth'-à-gog) *n* an anthelmintic*.

helmin·thiasis (hel-min-thī'-à-sis) *n* the condition resulting from infestation with worms.

helmin·thology (hel-min-thol'-o-jē) *n* the study of parasitic worms.

hemag·glutin·ation tests for pregnancy (hēm-à-glōō-tin-ā'-shun) are all based on the same principle and can be done rapidly. If urine from a pregnant woman contains certain antisera it will prevent hemagglutination occurring between red cells pretreated with human chorionic gonadotrophin and this will confirm pregnancy.

heman·gioma (hē-man-jē-ō'-mà) *n* a malformation of blood vessels which may occur in any part of the body. When in the skin it is one form of birthmark, appearing as a red spot or a 'port wine stain'—**hemangiomata** *pl*.

hemar·throsis (hē-màr-thrō'-sis) *n* the presence of blood in a joint cavity—**hemarthroses** *pl*.

hema·temesis (hē-mà-te-mē'-sis) *n* the vomiting of blood which may be bright red if recently swallowed. Otherwise it is of 'coffee ground' appearance due to the action of gastric juice.

hema·tin (hē'-mà-tin) *n* an iron-containing constituent of hemoglobin. It may crystallize in the kidney tubules when there is excessive hemolysis.

hema·tinic (hē-mà-tin'-ik) *adj* any substance which is required for the production of the red blood cell and its constituents.

hema·tite (hē'-mà-tīt) *n* (*syn* miner's lung) a form of silicosis* occurring in the hematite (iron ore) industry.

hemato·cele (hēm-at'-ō-sēl) *n* a swelling filled with blood.

hemato·colpos (hēm-à-tō-kol'-pos) *n* retained blood in the vagina. ⇒ cryptomenorrhea.

hematogen·ous (hē-mà-toj'-en-us) *adj* **1** concerned with the formation of blood. **2** carried by the blood stream.

hema·tology (hē-mà-tol'-o-je) *n* the science dealing with the formation, composition, functions and diseases of the blood—**hematological** *adj*, **hematologically** *adv*.

hema·toma (hē'-mà-tō'-mà) *n* a swelling filled with blood—**hematomata** *pl*.

hema·tometra (hē-mà-to-mē'-trà) *n* an accumulation of blood (or menstrual fluid) in the uterus.

hemato·poiesis (hē-mà-to-poy-ē'-sis) *n* ⇒ hemopoiesis.

hemato·porphyrin test (hē-mà-tō-pōr'-fir-in) 1–3 h after injection, hematoporphyrin localizes in rapidly multiplying cells and fluoresces under ultraviolet light. In many instances investigators can detect the exact extent of malignant or precancerous tissue.

hemato·salpinx (hē-mà-tō-sal'-pinks) *n* (*syn* hemosalpinx) blood in the fallopian tube.

hemato·zoa (hē-mà-tō-zō'-à) *n* parasites living in the blood—**hematozoon** *sing*.

hema·turia (hē-mà-tū'-rē-à) *n* blood in the urine; it may be from the kidneys, one or both ureters, the bladder or the urethra—**hematuric** *adj*.

hemera·lopia (he-mėr-à-lō'-pē-à) *n* defective vision in a bright light. Term has been incorrectly used for night* blindness.

hemia·nopia (hē-mē-à-nōp'-ē-à) *n* blindness in one half of the visual field of one or both eyes.

hemia·trophy (hē-mē-at'-rof-ē) *n* atrophy of one half or one side. *hemiatrophy facialis* a congenital condition, or a manifestation of scleroderma* in which the structures on one side of the face are shrunken.

hemi·chorea (hem-i-kōr-ē'-à) *n* choreiform movements limited to one side of the body. ⇒ chorea.

hemi·colectomy (hem-i-kō-lek′-to-mē) *n* removal of approximately half the colon.

hemi·crania (hem-i-krăn′-ē-à) *n* unilateral headache, as in migraine.

hemi·diaphor·esis (hem-i-dī-à-fŏr-ē′-sis) *n* unilateral sweating of the body.

hemi·glossectomy (hem-i-glos-sek′-to-mē) *n* removal of approximately half the tongue.

Hemin·evrin (hem-i-nef′-rin) *n* proprietary name for chlormethiazole.

hemi·paresis (hem-i-par-ē′-sis) *n* a slight paralysis or weakness of one half of face or body.

hemi·plegia (hem-i-plē′-jē-à) *n* paralysis of one side of the body, usually resulting from a cerebrovascular accident on the opposite side—**hemiplegic** *adj*.

hemi·spherectomy (hem-i-sfěr-ek′-to-mē) *n* surgical removal of a cerebral hemisphere in the treatment of epilepsy. It may be either subtotal or total.

hemochroma·tosis (hēmō-krō-mà-tō′-sis) *n* (*syn* bronzed diabetes) a congenital error in iron metabolism with increased iron deposition in tissues, resulting in brown pigmentation of the skin and cirrhosis of the liver—**hemochromatotic** *adj*.

hemo·concentration (hē-mō-kon-sen-trā′-shun) *n* relative increase of volume of red blood cells to volume of plasma, usually due to loss of the latter.

hemo·cytometer (hē-mō-sī-to′-me-tèr) *n* an instrument for measuring the number of blood corpuscles.

hemo·dialysis (hē-mō-dī-al′-i-sis) *n* removal of toxic solutes and excess fluid from the blood by dialysis* which is achieved by putting a semipermeable membrane between the blood and a rinsing solution called dialysate*. It is necessary when the patient is either in the end stage of renal failure (irreversible) or in acute renal failure (reversible).

hemodynamics (hē-mō-dī-nam′-iks) *npl* the forces involved in circulating blood round the body.

hemo·filtration (hē-mō-fil-trā′-shun) *n* requires the same access to the blood circulation as hemodialysis*. The patient's cardiac output drives the blood through a small, highly permeable filter; this permits separation of fluid and solutes; this hemofiltrate is measured and discarded and is replaced with an isotonic solution. When large amounts of hemofiltrate are removed, hemodialysis is unnecessary. Particularly useful for patients in acute renal failure, in congestive heart failure with diuretic-resistant overhydration and in hypernatremia resistant to drugs.

hemo·globin (hē′-mō-glō′-bin) *n* the respiratory pigment in the red blood corpuscles. It is composed of an iron-containing substance called 'hem', combined with globin. It has the reversible function of combining with and releasing oxygen. At birth 45–90% of hemoglobin is of the fetal type which is replaced by adult hemoglobin at the end of the first year of life. ⇒ oxyhemoglobin.

hemo·globinemia (hē′-mō-glō-bin-ē′-mē-à) *n* hemoglobin in the blood plasma—**hemoglobinemic** *adj*.

hemoglobin·ometer (hē′-mō-glō-bin-om′-e-tèr) *n* an instrument for estimating the percentage of hemoglobin in the blood.

hemo·globinopathy (hē′-mō-glō-bin-op′-ath-ē) *n* abnormality of the hemoglobin—**hemoglobinopathic** *adj*.

hemo·globinuria (hē′-mō-glō-bin-ū′-rē-à) *n* hemoglobin in the urine—**hemoglobinuric** *adj*.

hemoly·sin (hē-mō-lī′-sin) *n* an agent which causes disintegration of erythrocytes. ⇒ immunoglobulins.

hemoly·sis (hē-mol′-is-is) *n* disintegration of red blood cells, with liberation of contained hemoglobin. Laking—**hemolytic** *adj*.

hemo·lytic dis·ease of the new·born (hē-mō-lit′-ik) (*syn* erythroblastosis fetalis) a pathological condition in the newborn child due to Rhesus incompatibility between the child's blood and that of the mother. Red blood cell destruction occurs with anemia, often jaundice and an excess of erythroblasts or primitive red blood cells in the circulating blood. Immunization of women at risk, using gammaglobulin containing a high titer of anti-D* can prevent hemolytic disease of the newborn. Exchange transfusion of the infant may be essential.

hemo·lytic uremic syn·drome (HUS) (hē-mō-lit′-ik ūr-ē′-mik) a febrile illness resembling gastroenteritis and followed by intravascular hemolysis which may also lead to hypertension and acute renal failure, manifested by oliguria. The longer this persists, the poorer the prognosis—which can be death or chronic renal failure. A third do not develop oliguria and make a good recovery. It may be an autoimmune disease or an abnormal reaction to an uncommon virus.

hemo·pericardium (hē'-mō-pèr-i-kàr'-dē-um) *n* blood in the pericardial sac.

hemo·peritoneum (hē'-mō-pèr-it-on-ē'-um) *n* blood in the peritoneal cavity.

hemo·philias (hē-mō-fil'-ē-as) *npl* a group of conditions with congenital blood coagulation defects. In clinical practice the most commonly encountered defects are *hemophilia A*, factor VIII procoagulant deficiency *hemophilia B* or Christmas disease factor IX procoagulant deficiency. Both these conditions are X-linked recessive disorders exclusively affecting males and resulting in abnormalities in the clotting mechanism only. The bleeding usually occurs into deeply lying structures, muscles and joints. ⇒ hemophilic arthropathy, von Willebrand's disease.

hemo·philic arthrop·athy (hē-mō-fil'-ik àrth-rop'-à-thē) the extent of joint damage has been staged from radiological findings: (a) synovial thickening (b) epiphyseal overgrowth (c) minor joint changes and cyst formation (d) definite joint changes with loss of joint space (e) end-stage joint destruction and secondary changes leading to deformity.

hemoph·thalmia (hē-mof-thal'-mē-à) *n* bleeding into the eyeball.

hemo·pneumothorax (hē-mō-nū-mō-thōr'-aks) *n* the presence of blood and air in the pleural cavity.

hemo·poiesis (hē-mō-poy-ē'-sis) *n* (*syn* hematopoiesis) the formation of blood. ⇒ erythropoiesis—**hemopoietic** *adj*.

hemopty·sis (hē-mop'-tis-is) *n* the coughing up of blood—**hemoptyses** *pl*.

hemor·rhage (hem'-ōr-raj) *n* the escape of blood from a vessel. Arterial, capillary, venous designate the type of vessel from which it escapes—**hemorrhagic** *adj primary hemorrhage* that which occurs at the time of injury or operation. *reactionary hemorrhage* that which occurs within 24 hours of injury or operation. *secondary hemorrhage* that which occurs within 7–10 days of injury or operation. *antepartum hemorrhage* ⇒ placental abruption. *intrapartum hemorrhage* that occurring during labor. *postpartum hemorrhage* excessive bleeding after delivery of child. In the US it must be at least 500 ml to qualify as hemorrhage. *secondary postpartum hemorrhage* excessive uterine bleeding more than 24 h after delivery.

hemor·rhagic disease of the new·born (hem-ōr-raj'-ik) characterized by gastrointestinal, pulmonary or intracranial hemorrhage occurring from the 2nd to the 5th day of life. Caused by a physiological variation in clotting power due to change in prothrombin content, which falls on 2nd day and returns to normal at end of first week when colonization of gut with bacteria results in synthesis of vitamin K, thus permitting formation of prothrombin* by the liver. Responds to administration of vitamin K.

hemor·rhagic fever ⇒ mosquito-transmitted hemorrhagic fevers, viral hemorrhagic fevers.

hemor·rhoidal (hem-ōr-oyd'-al) *adj* 1 pertaining to hemorrhoids*. 2 applied to blood vessels and nerves in the anal region.

hemor·rhoidectomy (hem-ōr-oyd-ek'-to-mē) *n* surgical removal of hemorrhoids.

hemor·rhoids (hem'-ōr-oyds) *npl* (*syn* piles) varicosity of the veins around the anus. *external hemorrhoids* those outside the anal sphincter, covered with skin. *internal hemorrhoids* those inside the anal sphincter, covered with mucous membrane.

hemo·salpinx (hē-mō-sal'-pinks) ⇒ hematosalpinx.

hemo·siderosis (hē-mō-sid-èr-ōs'-is) *n* iron deposits in the tissues.

hemo·spermia (hē-mō-spèr'-mē-à) *n* the discharge of bloodstained semen.

hemo·stasis (hē-mō-stā'-sis) *n* 1 arrest of bleeding. 2 stagnation of blood within its vessel.

hemo·static (hē-mō-stat'-ik) *adj* any agent which arrests bleeding. *hemostatic forceps* artery forceps.

hemo·thorax (hē-mō-thōr'-aks) *n* blood in the pleural cavity.

Henoch-Schonlein purpura (hen'-ok shàn'-līn) *n* a disorder mainly affecting children. It is characterized by purpuric bleeding into the skin, particularly shins and buttocks, and from the wall of the gut, resulting in abdominal colic and melena; and bruising around joints. Recurrence is not uncommon.

hepar (hep'-àr) *n* the liver—**hepatic** *adj*.

hep·arin (hep'-àr-in) *n* an acid present in liver and lung tissue. When injected intravenously it inhibits coagulation of the blood, and it is widely used in the treatment of thrombosis, often in association with orally active anticoagulants such as warfarin*.

heparinize (hep'-à-rin-īz) *v* to administer heparin therapeutically.

hepa·tectomy (hep-à-tek'-to-mē) *n* excision of the liver, or more usually part of the liver.

hep·atic (hep-at'-ik) *adj* pertaining to the liver.

hepatico·choledoch·ostomy (hep-at'-i-kō-kōl'-ē-dō-kos'-to-mē) *n* end-to-end union of the severed hepatic and common bile ducts.

hepatico·enteric (hep-at'-ik-ō-en-tėr'-ik) *adj* pertaining to the liver and intestine.

hepatico·jejunostomy (hep-at'-ik-ō-je-jūn-os'-to-mē) *n* anastomosis of the common hepatic duct to a loop of proximal jejunum*.

hepa·titis (hep-à-tī'-tis) *n* inflammation of the liver in response to toxins or infective agents. It is usually accompanied by fever, gastrointestinal symptoms and an itchy skin. *amoebic hepatitis* can occur as a complication of amoebic dysentery. *infective hepatitis* is caused by hepatitis-A virus spread by the fecal-oral route. The incubation period is 2–6 weeks, the jaundice appearing after a brief influenza-like illness. *serum hepatitis* is caused by hepatitis-B virus and is spread only by contact or inoculation with human blood and its products. The incubation period is 3–5 months; it is followed by three general patterns of clinical response. About 30%–40% of adults develop clinically apparent hepatitis; the majority, 50%–60%, remain asymptomatic but show serological evidence of infection. But 5%–10% develop a chronic infection, the so-called chronic carrier state. Certain minority groups show a higher prevalence of carriers; these include drug addicts, male homosexuals and mentally subnormal patients in institutions. *viral hepatitis* includes infective and serum hepatitis but other viruses including cytomegalovirus, Epstein-Barr virus, herpes simplex virus and rubella virus have also been implicated as causal agents. *hepatitis B immunoglobulin* a blood product for immunization against hepatitis B infection, recommended for at risk populations for hepatitis B infection, e.g. health care workers, emergency medical and fire personnel.

hepatization (hep-à-tī-zā'-shun) *n* pathological changes in the tissues, which cause them to resemble liver. Occurs in the lungs in pneumonia.

hepato·cellular (hep-à-tō-sel'-ū-lar) *adj* pertaining to or affecting liver cells.

hepato·cirrhosis (hep-at'-ō-ser-ō'-sis) *n* cirrhosis of the liver.

hepa·toma (hep-à-tō'-mà) *n* primary carcinoma of the liver—**hepatomata** *pl*.

hepato·megaly (hep-a-tō-meg'-à-lē) *n* enlargement of the liver. It is palpable below the costal margin.

hepato·splenic (hep-at'-ō-splen'-ik) *adj* pertaining to the liver and spleen.

hepato·splenomegaly (hep-at'-ō-splen-ō-meg'-à-lē) *n* enlargement of the liver and the spleen, so that each is palpable below the costal margin.

hepato·toxic (hep-at'-ō-toks'-ik) *adj* having an injurious effect on liver cells—**hepatotoxicity** *n*.

Heptavax-B (hep'-ta-vaks-bē) *n* proprietary name for hepatitis* B immunoglobulin.

heredi·tary (her-ed'-it-âr-ē) *adj* inherited; capable of being inherited.

her·edity (hėr-ed'-it-ē) *n* transmission from parents to offspring of physical and mental attributes by means of the genetic material; the process by which this occurs, and the study of the biological laws that govern this transmission.

hermaphro·dite (hėr-ma'-frō-dīt) *n* individual possessing both ovarian and testicular tissue. Although they may approximate either to male or female type, they are usually sterile from imperfect development of their gonads.

her·nia (hėr'-nē-à) *n* the abnormal protrusion of an organ, or part of an organ, through an aperture in the surrounding structures; commonly the protrusion of an abdominal organ through a gap in the abdominal wall. *diaphragmatic hernia* (*syn* hiatus hernia) protrusion through the diaphragm, the commonest one involving the stomach at the esophageal opening. *femoral hernia* protrusion through the femoral canal, alongside the femoral blood vessels as they pass into the thigh. *inguinal hernia* protrusion through the inguinal canal in the male. *irreducible hernia* when the contents of the sac cannot be returned to the appropriate cavity without surgical intervention. *strangulated hernia* hernia in which the blood supply to the organ involved is impaired, usually due to constriction by surrounding structures. *umbilical hernia* (*syn* omphalocele) protrusion of a portion of intestine through the area of the umbilical scar.

hernio·plasty (hėr'-nē-ō-plas'-tē) *n* an operation for hernia in which an attempt is made to prevent recurrence by refashioning the structures to give greater strength—**hernioplastic** *adj*.

hernior·rhaphy (hėr-nē-ōr'-raf-ē) *n* an operation for hernia in which the weak area is reinforced by some of the patient's own tissues or by some other material.

herni·otome (hėr'-nē-o-tōm) *n* a special knife with a blunt tip, used for hernia operations.

herni·otomy (hėr-nē-ot'-o-mē) *n* operation to cure hernia by the return of its contents to their normal position and removal of the hernial sac.

her·oin (hėr'-ō-in) *n* ⇒ diacetylmorphine.

herpan·gina (hėr-pan-jī'-nà) *n* minute vesicles and ulcers at the back of the palate. Short, febrile illness in children caused by coxsackievirus Group A.

her·pes (hėr'-pēz) *n* a vesicular eruption due to infection with the herpes* simplex virus. *genital herpes* infection with the herpes* simplex virus (HSV) Type I or II; it is a sexually transmitted disease. In the female, ulcers and vesicles can occur on the cervix, vagina, vulva and labia. In the male, these occur on the glans, prepuce and penal shaft and less commonly on the scrotum. In both sexes lesions may be seen on the pharynx, thighs, buttocks and perianal regions. *herpes gestationis* a rare skin disease peculiar to pregnancy. It clears in about 30 days after delivery. *herpes zoster* the virus attacks sensory nerves, with consequent severe pain, and the appearance of vesicles along the distribution of the nerves involved (usually unilateral).

her·pes sim·plex virus (HSV) (hėr'-pēz sim'-pleks) consists of two biologically and immunologically distinct types designated Type I, which generally causes oral disease and lesions above the waist, and Type II, most commonly associated with genital disease and lesions below the waist. Recurrent episodes are common as the virus remains latent in nerve ganglia after the initial infection. ⇒ herpes.

her·petiform (hėr-pet'-i-form) *adj* resembling herpes*.

Herplex (hėr'-pleks) *n* proprietary name for idoxuridine*.

hesperi·din (hes-pėr'-i-den) *n* a crystalline substance found in most citrus fruits. Has similar actions to citrin*.

Hess test (hes) a sphygmomanometer cuff is applied to the arm and is inflated. Petechial eruption in the surrounding area after 5 min denotes weakness of the capillary walls, characteristic of purpura.

hetero·genous (het-ėr-oj'-en-us) *adj* of unlike origin; not originating within the body; derived from a different species. ⇒ homogenous *opp*.

heter·ologous (het-ėr-ol'-o-gus) *adj* of different origin; from a different species. ⇒ homologous *opp*.

hetero·phile (het'-ėr-ō-fil) *n* a product of one species which acts against that of another, for example human antigen against sheep's red blood cells.

heteroplasty (het-ėr-ō-plas'-tē) *n* plastic operation using a graft from another individual—**heteroplastic** *adj*.

hetero·sexual (het-ėr-ō-seks'-ū-àl) *adj, n* literally, of different sexes; often used to describe a person who is sexually attracted towards the opposite sex. ⇒ homosexual *opp*.

hetero·zygous (het-ėr-ō-zī'-gus) *adj* having different genes or alleles at the same locus on both chromosomes of a pair (one of maternal and the other of paternal origin) ⇒ homozygous *opp*.

hexa·chlorophene (heks-à-klōr'-ō-fēn) *n* an antiseptic used in skin sterilization, and in some bactericidal soaps. Under suspicion as being a possible cause of brain damage in babies. Any medicinal product containing hexachlorophene (irrespective of the amount) must bear a warning on the container 'not to be used for babies' or 'not to be administered to a child under 2'. (Phisohex.)

hexamethonium (heks-à-meth-ō'-nē-um) *n* one of the earlier ganglionic blocking agents, used to treat hypertension, given by subcutaneous or intramuscular injection. Now being replaced by oral drugs.

hex·estrol (heks-es'-trol) *n* a synthetic compound related to stilbestrol* and used for similar purposes.

hexo·barbital (heks-ō-bar-bi-tol) *n* a short-acting barbiturate, useful when a prompt but relatively brief action is required. (Sombulex.)

hex·ose (heks'-ōs) *n* a class of simple sugars, monosaccharides containing six carbon atoms ($C_6H_{12}O_6$). Examples are glucose, mannose, galactose.

hexyl·resorcinol (heks-yl-rē-sōrs'-in-ol) *n* an anthelmintic with a wide range of activity, being effective against threadworm, roundworm, hookworm and intestinal fluke. It is followed by a saline purge. Treatment may have to be repeated at 3 day intervals. Also used in cystitis and other infections of the urinary tract.

HGH *abbr* human growth* hormone.

HHNK *abbr* hyperglycemic hyperosmolar non-ketoacidotic coma. ⇒ diabetes.

hi·atus (hī-ā'-tus) *n* a space or opening. *hiatus hernia* ⇒ hernia—**hiatal** *adj*.

Hibb's oper·ation (hibs) operation for spinal fusion, following spinal tuberculosis. No bone graft is used, but the split vertebral spines are pressed outwards and laid in contact with the laminae. Bony union occurs and the spine is rigid.

Hibiclens (hib'-i-klenz) *n* a proprietary preparation of chlorhexidine* gluconate 4% in a detergent base; especially useful for preoperative baths.

Hibistat (hib'-i-stat) *n* proprietary name for chlorhexidine*.

hic·cough (hi'-kuf) *n* (*syn* hiccup). An involuntary inspiratory spasm of the respiratory organs, ending in a sudden closure of the glottis with the production of a characteristic sound.

hic·cup (hi'-kup) ⇒ hiccough.

hi·drosis (hī-drō'-sis) *n* sweat secretion.

Higginson's syr·inge (hig'-in-sonz) compression of the rubber bulb forces fluid forward through the nozzle for irrigation of a body cavity.

high den·sity lipo·protein a plasma protein relatively high in protein, low in cholestrol. It is involved in transporting cholesterol and other lipids from plasma to the tissues.

hi·lum (hī'-lum) *n* a depression on the surface of an organ where vessels, ducts, etc enter and leave—**hili** *pl*. **hilar** *adj*. *hilar adenitis* ⇒ adenitis.

hindbrain (hīnd'-brān) ⇒ Figure 1.

hip bone (innominate bone) formed by the fusion of three separate bones—the ilium, ischium and pubis ⇒ Figures 2, 3.

Hippocrates (hip-po'-kra-tēz) *n* famous Greek physician and philosopher (460–367 BC) who established a school of medicine at Cos, his birthplace. He is often termed the 'Father of Medicine'.

Hirschsprung's dis·ease (hirsh'-sproongz) congenital intestinal aganglionosis, leading to intractable constipation or even intestinal obstruction. There is marked hypertrophy and dilation of the colon (megacolon) above the aganglionic segment. Commoner in boys and children with Down syndrome.

hir·sute (hėr'-sūt) *adj* hairy or shaggy.

hir·suties, hir·sutism (hėr'-sūt-ēz, hėr'-sūt-izm) *n* excessive growth of hair in sites in which body hair is normally found. ⇒ hypertrichosis.

hiru·din (hi-roo'-din) *n* a substance secreted by the medicinal leech*, which prevents the clotting of blood by acting as an antithrombin.

hirudo (hi-roo'-dō) *n* ⇒ leech.

hist·amine (hist'-à-mēn) *n* a naturally occurring chemical substance in body tissues which, in small doses, has profound and diverse actions on muscle, blood capillaries, and gastric secretion. Sudden excessive release from the tissues, into the blood, is believed to be the cause of the main symptoms and signs in anaphylaxis*—**histaminic** *adj*. *histamine receptor cells* there are two types in the body. H_1 in the bronchial muscle and H_2 in the secreting cells in the stomach. *histamine test* designed to determine the maximal gastric secretion of hydrochloric acid. A Levin* tube is positioned in the stomach of the most dependent part of the stomach of a fasting patient who has been weighed. Following the collection of a control specimen and the injection of an antihistamine and a histamine gastric secretions are collected for a further hour. By titrating the collections against a standard alkaline solution, the acidity of the gastric secretions can be determined.

hist·dinemia (his-ti-din-ē'-mē-à) *n* genetically determined increase in histidine* in blood. Gives rise to speech defects without mental retardation.

histi·dine (his'-ti-den) *n* an essential amino acid which is widely distributed and is present in hemoglobin. It is a precursor of histamine*.

histio·cytes (his'-tē-ō-sīts) *n* macrophages derived from reticuloendothelial cells; act as scavengers.

histio·cytoma (his-tē-ō-sī-tō'-mà) *n* benign tumor of histiocytes.

histo·compatibility antigens (his'-tō-kom-pat-i-bil'-i-tē) *n* the antigens on nucleated cells which induce an allograft* response; important in organ transplantation.

his·tology (his-tol'-o-jē) *n* microscopic study of tissues—**histological** *adj*, **histologically** *adv*.

histoly·sis (his-tol'-is-is) *n* disintegration of organic tissue—**histolytic** *adj*.

his·tones (his'-tōns) *n* a special set of proteins closely associated with the chromosomal DNA of higher organisms, which coils and supercoils around histone molecules. These are therefore part and parcel of the way the DNA is organized to form the chromosomes.

histo·plasmosis (his-tō-plaz-mō'-sis) *n* an infection caused by inhaling spores of the fungus *Histoplasma capsulation*.

The primary lung lesion may go unnoticed or be accompanied by fever, malaise, cough and adenopathy. Progressive histoplasmosis can be fatal.

hives (hīvs) *n* nettlerash; urticaria*.

hob·nail liver (hob'-nāl liv'-ér) firm nodular liver which may be found in cirrhosis.

Hodgkin's dis·ease (hoj'-kinz) a malignant lymphoma* causing progressive enlargement of lymph nodes and involvement of reticuloendothelial tissues including bone marrow. Some cases show Pel-Ebstein* fever.

Hofmann re·action (hof'-man) chemical inactivation, without the activity of enzymes, of compounds which occur spontaneously in the blood.

holistic medicine (hōl-is'-tik) (wholistic) medical care which considers the patient as a whole, including his phyical, mental, emotional, social and economic needs.

Homans' sign (Hō'-mans sīn) passive dorsiflexion of foot causes pain in calf muscles. Indicative of incipient or established venous thrombosis of leg.

hom·atropine (hōm-à-trō'-pēn) *n* a mydriatic similar to atropine*, but with a more rapid and less prolonged effect. Often used as a 2% solution with a similar amount of cocaine*, which addition increases the mydriatic action and deadens pain.

home·opathy (hō-mē-op'-à-thē) *n* a method of treating disease by prescribing minute doses of drugs which, in maximum dose, would produce symptoms of the disease. First adopted by Hahnemann—**homeopathic** *adj*.

home·ostasis (hōm-ē-ō-stā'-sis) *n* a physiological regulatory process whereby functions such as blood pressure, body temperature and electrolytes are maintained within a narrow range of normal.

homi·cide (hom'-i-sīd) *n* killing of another person.

homo·cystin·uria (hō-mō-sis-tin-ū'-rē-à) *n* excretion of homocystine (a sulfur containing amino acid, homologue of cystine) in the urine. Caused by an inborn recessively-inherited metabolic error. Gives rise to slow development or mental retardation of varying degree; lens may dislocate and there is overgrowth of long bones with thrombotic episodes which are often fatal in childhood—**homocystinuric** *adj*.

homogen·eous (hōm-ō-jē'-nē-us) *adj* of the same kind; of the same quality or consistency throughout.

homogen·ize —(hom-oj'-en-īz) *vt* to make into the same consistency throughout.

homogen·ous (hom-oj'-en-us) *adj* having a like nature, e.g. a bone graft from another human being. ⇒ heterogenous *opp*.

homo·graft (hō'-mō-graft) *n* a tissue or organ which is transplanted from one individual to another of the same species. ⇒ allograft.

homo·lateral (hō-mō-lat'-ér-àl) *adj* on the same side—**homolaterally** *adv*.

homolo·gous (hom-ol'-o-gus) *adj* corresponding in origin and structure. ⇒ heterologous *opp*. *homologous chromosomes* those that pair during reduction cell division (meiosis) whereby mature gametes are formed. Their DNA has an identical arrangement and sequence of different genes. Of the two homologues, one is derived from the father, the other from the mother.

homony·mous (hom-on'-i-mus) *adj* consisting of corresponding halves.

homo·sexual (hō-mō-seks'-ū-àl) *adj, n* literally, of the same sex; often used to describe a person who indulges in homosexuality*. Homosexuals are at particular risk of contracting infection with hepatitis-B virus, cytomegalovirus and Epstien-Barr virus. ⇒ acquired immune deficiency syndrome. (⇒ heterosexual *opp*.)

homo·sexuality (hō-mō-seks-ū-al'-i-tē) *n* attraction for, and desire to establish an emotional and sexual relationship with a member of the same sex.

homo·transplant (hō-mō-tranz'-plant) *n* (*syn* allotransplant) tissues or organ transplanted from non-identical members of the same species.

homo·zygous (hō-mō-zī'-gus) *adj* having identical genes or alleles in the same locus on both chromosomes of a pair (one of maternal and the other of paternal origin). ⇒ heterozygous *opp*.

Honvol (hon'-vol) *n* stilbestrol diphosphate, broken down by prostatic tissue to release stilbestrol in situ, thus reducing systemic side effects.

hook·worm *n* ⇒ Ancylostoma.

hord·eolum (hōr-dē'-ō-lum) *n* ⇒ sty.

hor·mone (hōr'-mōn) *n* specific chemical substance secreted by an endocrine gland and conveyed in the blood to regulate the functions of tissues and organs elsewhere in the body.

hormono·therapy (hōr-mōn-ō-thér'-à-pē) *n* treatment by hormones.

Horner syn·drome (hôr'-nẽr) clinical picture following paralysis of cervical sympathetic nerves on the one side. There is myosis, slight ptosis with enophthalmos, and anhidrosis.

Horton syn·drome (hôr'-ton) severe headache due to the release of histamine in the body. To be differentiated from migraine*.

hospice (hos'-pis) *n* 1) a homelike facility that provides physical, emotional, spiritual and social care to the dying and their families. 2) a program that provides this care to the dying in their own homes.

hos·pital ac·quired infec·tion ⇒ infection.

hos·pital steriliz·ation and disinfec·tion unit (HSDU) a title being used by some previous central sterile supply units (CSSUs) which have extended their work to include disinfection of equipment.

host (hōst) *n* the organic structure upon which parasites or bacteria thrive. *intermediate host* one in which the parasite passes its larval or cystic stage.

hot·dog head·ache post-prandial; induced by the sodium nitrite content of frankfurters.

hot-fat heart·burn syn·drome due to reflux from stomach to esophagus producing hypersensitivity in the esophageal mucosa; tends to be worse after eating fatty or fried food or drinking coffee. May be associated with hiatus hernia*.

hour-glass contrac·tion a circular constriction in the middle of a hollow organ (usually the stomach or uterus), dividing it into two portions following scar formation.

house·maid's knee ⇒ bursitis.

HSDU *abbr* ⇒ hospital sterilization and disinfection unit.

HSSU *abbr* hospital sterile supply unit. ⇒ hospital sterilization and disinfection units.

HSV *abbr* herpes* simplex virus.

human chori·onic gonado·trophin (HCG) (hū'-man kōr-ē-on'-ik gō-nad'-ō-trō'-fin) a hormone arising from the placenta. Used for cryptorchism, and sometimes for female infertility. The presence of HCG in urine is detectable in an early morning specimen of urine from the 6th week of pregnancy. The result can be given in 2 min and confirmed in 2 h. (Pregnyl.)

Humatin (hūm'-à-tin) *n* proprietary name for paromomycin*.

humer·us (hū'-mẽr-us) *n* the bone of the upper arm, between the elbows and shoulder joint (⇒ Figures 2, 3)—**humeri** *pl*, **humeral** *adj*.

humidi·fier (hū-mid'-i-fī-ẽr) *n* a heated water device for warming and moistening inspired air when a patient has a tracheal tube or tracheostomy in place.

humid·ity (hū-mid'-it-ē) *n* the amount of moisture in the atmosphere, as measured by a hygrometer. *relative humidity* the ratio of the amount of moisture present in the air to the amount which would saturate it (at the same temperature).

humor (hū'-mor) *n* any fluid of the body. ⇒ aqueous, vitreous.

humoral immun·ity (hū'-mor-al im-mū'-ni-tē) ⇒ immunity.

Humulin (hū'-mū-lin) *n* a proprietary preparation of human insulin which is completely free from animal insulin and pancreatic impurities.

hunger (hung'-gẽr) *n* a longing, usually for food. *hunger pain* epigastric pain which is relieved by taking food; associated with duodenal ulcer.

Hunter-Hurler syn·drome (hun'-tẽr hẽr'-lẽr) ⇒ gargoylism.

Hunter syn·drome (hun'-tẽr) one of the mucopolysaccharidoses*, designated Type II. A sex-linked recessive condition.

Hunterian chancre (hun-tẽr'-ē-an shang'-ker) the hard sore of primary syphilis.

Huntington's chorea (hunt'-ing-tunz kōr-ē'-à) genetically determined heredofamilial disease with slow progressive degeneration of the nerve cells of the basal ganglia and cerebral cortex. Affects both sexes, and is due to a dominant gene of large effect. Develops in middle age, or later, and is associated with progressive dementia. ⇒ chorea.

Hurler syn·drome (hẽr'-lẽr) one of the mucopolysaccharidoses*; designated Type II. Inherited as an autosomal recessive trait.

HUS *abbr* hemolytic* uremic syndrome.

Hutchin·son's teeth (huch'-in-sunz) defect of the upper central incisors (second dentition) which is part of the facies of the congenital syphilitic person. The teeth are broader at the gum than at the cutting edge, with the latter showing an elliptical notch.

hya·line (hī'-à-lin) *adj* like glass; transparent. *hyaline degeneration* degeneration of connective tissue especially that of blood vessels in which tissue takes on

139

a homogenous or formless appearance. *hyaline membrane disease* ⇒ respiratory distress syndrome.

hyal·itis (hī-ál-ī′-tis) *n* inflammation of the optical vitreous* humor or its enclosing membrane. When the condition is degenerative rather than inflammatory, there are small opacities in the vitreous and it is called *asteroid hyalitis.*

hya·loid (hī′-á-loyd) *adj* resembling hyaline* tissue. *hyaloid membrane* ⇒ membrane.

hyaluroni·dase (hī-al-ūr-on′-id-āz) *n* an enzyme obtained from testes, which when injected subcutaneously, promotes the absorption of fluid. Given with or immediately before a subcutaneous infusion; 1000 units will facilitate the absorption of 500–1000 ml of fluid. (Wydase.)

Hycal (hī′-kal) *n* proprietary flavored liquid; protein-free; low-electrolytic; carbohydrate preparation based on demineralized liquid glucose, providing 240 kcal per 100 ml.

hy·datid cyst (hī′-dat-id) *n* the cyst formed by larvae of a tapeworm. *Echinococcus*, which is found in dogs. The encysted stage normally occurs in sheep but can occur in man after he eats with soiled hands from petting a dog. The cysts are commonest in the liver and lungs; they grow slowly and only do damage by the space they occupy. If they leak, or become infected, urticaria and fever supervene and 'daughter' cysts can result. The treatment is surgical removal. ⇒ Casoni test.

hydatidi·form (hī-dat-id′-i-förm) *adj* pertaining to or resembling a hydatid* cyst. *hydatidiform mole* a condition in which the chorionic villi of the placenta undergo cystic degeneration and the fetus is absorbed. The villi penetrate and destroy only the decidual layer of the uterus, but a hydatidiform mole may progress to become an invasive mole in which the villi penetrate the myometrium and can destroy the uterine wall and metastasize to the vagina or even the lungs and brain; these regress after evacuation of the mole. Invasive mole is benign but it may convert to choriocarcinoma.

hydral·azine (hī-dral′-á-zēn) *n* a synthetic compound which lowers blood pressure, mainly by its peripheral vasodilator action. Response to treatment may be slow and the use of diuretics* may improve this. (Apresoline.)

hy·dramnios (hī-dram′-nē-os) *n* an excess of amniotic fluid.

hydrargyrum (hīd-rár′-ji-rum) *n* mercury or quicksilver.

hydrar·throsis (hī-drár-thrō′-sis) *n* a collection of synovial fluid in a joint cavity. *intermittent hydrarthrosis* afflicts young women; probably due to allergy. Synovitis develops spontaneously, lasts a few days and disappears as mysteriously.

hy·drate (hī′-drāt) *vi* combine with water—**hydration** *n.*

hydremia (hī-drē′-mē-á) *n* a relative excess of plasma volume compared with cell volume of the blood; it is normally present in late pregnancy–**hydremic,** *adj.*

hy·droa (hī-drō′-á) *n* ⇒ dermatitis herpetiformis. *hydroa aestivale* **1** a vesicular or bullous disease occurring in atopic* children. It affects exposed parts and probably results from photosensitivity. **2** sun-induced dermatitis in some forms of porphyria. *hydroa vacciniforme* is a more severe form of this in which scarring ensues.

hydro·cele (hī′-drō-sēl) *n* a swelling due to accumulation of serous fluid in the tunica vaginalis of the testis or in the spermatic cord.

hydro·cephalus (hī-drō-sef′-á-lus) *n* (*syn* 'water on the brain') an excess of cerebrospinal fluid inside the skull due to an obstruction to normal CSF circulation—**hydrocephalic** *adj. external hydrocephalus* the excess of fluid is mainly in the subarachnoid space. *internal hydrocephalus* the excess of fluid is mainly in the ventricles of the brain. A Spitz*-Holter valve is used in drainage operations for this condition.

hydro·chloric acid (hī-drō-klōr′-ik) secreted by the gastric oxyntic cells and present in gastric juice (0.2%). The strong acid is caustic, but a 10% dilution is used orally in the treatment of achlorhydria.

hydro·chloro·thiazide (hī′-drō-klōr-ō-thī′-á-zīd) *n* a thiazide diuretic. (Esidrex, HydroDiuril.) ⇒ diuretics.

hydro·cortisone (hī-drō-kōr′-ti-sōn) *n* ⇒ cortisol.

hydro·cyanic acid (hī-drō-sī-an′-ik) (*syn* prussic acid) the dilute acid (2%) has a sedative action on the stomach, and has been given with bismuth carbonate and other antacids in the treatment of vomiting. In large doses, both the solution and its vapor are poisonous, and death may occur very rapidly from respiratory paralysis. Prompt treatment with intravenous injections of sodium nitrite, sodium thiosulfate and ketocyanor may be life-saving.

Hydro Diuril (hī-drō-dī′-ūr-il) *n* proprietary name for hydrochlorothiazide*.

hydro·flumethiazide (hī-drō-floo-meth-ī′-à-zīd) *n* a thiazide diuretic.

hydro·gen (hī′-drō-jen) *n* a colorless, odorless, combustible gas. *hydrogen ion concentration* a measure of the acidity or alkalinity of a solution, ranging from pH 1 to pH 14. 7 being approximately neutral; the lower numbers denoting acidity; the higher ones denoting alkalinity. *hydrogen peroxide* H_2O_2, a powerful oxidizing and deodorizing agent, used for cleaning wounds; diluted with 4–8 parts of water as a mouthwash and with 50% alcohol as ear drops.

hydroly·sis (hī-drol′-is-is) *n* the splitting into more simple substances by the addition of water—**hydrolytic** *adj*, **hydrolyze** *vt*.

hydro·meter (hī-drō′-me-tèr) *n* an instrument for determining the specific gravity of fluids—**hydrometry** *n*:

hydrometria (hī-drō-mēt′-rē-à) *n* a collection of watery fluid within the uterus.

Hydromox (hī′-drō-moks) *n* proprietary name for quinethazone*.

hydro·nephrosis (hī-drō-nef-rō′-sis) *n* distension of the kidney pelvis with urine, from obstructed outflow. If unrelieved, pressure eventually causes atrophy of kidney tissue. Surgical operations include nephroplasty and pyelonplasty.

hydro·pericarditis (hī-drō-pèr-ē-kàr-dī′-tis) *n* pericarditis with effusion.

hydro·pericardium (hī-drō-pèr-ē-kàr′-dē-um) *n* fluid in the pericardial sac in the absence of inflammation. Can occur in heart and kidney failure.

hydro·peritoneum (hī-drō-pèr-it-on-ē′-um) *n* ⇒ ascites.

hydro·phobia (hī-drō-fō′-bē-à) *n* ⇒ rabies.

hydro·phylic (hī-drō-fil′-ik) *adj* having an affinity for water.

hydro·pneumo·pericardium (hī-drō-noo-mō-pèr-i-kàr′-dē-um) *n* the presence of air and fluid in the membranous pericardial sac surrounding the heart. It may accompany pericardiocentesis*.

hydro·pneumo·peritoneum (hī-drō-noo′-mō-pèr-i-ton-ē′-um) *n* the presence of fluid and gas in the peritoneal cavity;

it may accompany paracentesis of that cavity; it may accompany perforation of the gut; or it may be due to gas-forming microorganisms in the peritoneal fluid.

hydro·pneumo·thorax (hī-drō-noo-mō-thōr′-aks) *n* pneumothorax further complicated by effusion of fluid into the pleural cavity.

hy·drops (hī′-drops) *n* edema*—**hydropic** *adj*, *hydrops fetalis* a severe form of erythroblastosis fetalis*.

hydro·salpinx (hī-drō-sal′-pinks) *n* distension of a fallopian tube with watery fluid.

hydro·therapy (hī-drō-thèr′-à-pē) *n* the science of therapeutic bathing for diagnosed conditions.

hydro·thorax (hī-drō-thōr′-aks) *n* the presence of fluid in the pleural cavity.

hydro·ureter (hī-drō-ūr′-e-tèr) *n* abnormal distension of the ureter with urine.

hydroxo·cobalamin (hī-droks′-ō-kō-bal′-à-min) *n* a longer-acting form of vitamin* B_{12} given by injection. ⇒ cyanocobalamin.

hydroxy·butyric dehydrog·enase (hī-droks′-ē-bū-tèr′-ik dē-hī-droj′-en-ās) a serum enzyme: high concentrations are indicative of myocardial infarction.

hydroxy·chloroquine (hī-droks′-ē-klōr′-ō-kwin) *n* an antimalarial. ⇒ chloroquine.

hy·droxyl (hī-droks′-il) *n* a monovalent ion (OH), consisting of a hydrogen atom linked to an oxygen atom.

hydroxy·progesterone capro·ate (hī-droks′-ē-prō-jest′-èr-ōn kap′-rō-āt) given intramuscularly for recurrent and threatened abortion. (Delalutin.)

hydroxy·stilbamidine (hī-droks′-ē-stil-bam′-i-dīn) *n* an antiprotozoal drug useful in aspergillosis.

5-hydroxy·tryptamine (5-HT) (fīv-hī-droks′-i-trip′-ta-mēn) *n* ⇒ serotonin.

hydroxy·urea (hī-droks′-i-ū-rē′-à) *n* simple compound given orally. Mode of action uncertain, may be of value in patients with chronic myeloid leukemia who no longer show a response to busulphan*.

hydroxy·zine (hī-droks′-i-zēn) *n* an antihistamine which is also a sedative; useful in treating nausea and vomiting. (Atarax, Vistaril.)

hy·giene (hī′-jēn) *n* the science dealing with the maintenance of health—**hygienic** *adj. communal hygiene* embraces all measures taken to supply the community with pure food and water, good sanitation, housing, etc. *industrial hygiene* (*syn* occupational health) includes all measures taken to preserve the individual's health while he is at work. *mental hygiene* deals with the establishment of healthy mental attitudes and emotional reactions. *personal hygiene* includes all those measures taken by the individual to preserve his own health.

hy·groma (hī-grō'-mȧ) *n* a cystic swelling containing watery fluid, usually situated in the neck and present at birth, sometimes interfering with birth—**hygromata** *pl.* **hygromatous** *adj.*

hy·grometer (hī-gro'-me-tėr) *n* an instrument for measuring the amount of moisture in the air. ⇒ humidity.

hygro·scopic (hī-grō-skop'-ik) *adj* readily absorbing water, e.g. glycerine.

Hy·groton (hī'-grō-ton) *n* proprietary name for chlorthalidone*.

hy·men (hī'-men) *n* a membranous perforated structure stretching across the vaginal entrance. *imperforate hymen* a congenital condition leading to hematocolpos. ⇒ cryptomenorrhea.

hymen·ectomy (hī-men-ek'-to-mē) *n* surgical excision of the hymen.

hymen·otomy (hī-men-ot'-o-mē) *n* surgical incision of the hymen.

hy·oid (hī'-oyd) *n* a U-shaped bone at the root of the tongue ⇒ (Figure 6).

hy·oscine (hī'-ō-sēn) *n* (*syn* scopolamine) a hypnotic alkaloid obtained from belladonna and hyoscyamus.

hy·oscyamus (hī-ō-sī'-ȧ-mus) *n* henbane leaves and flowers. Resembles belladonna in its properties. Sometimes given with potassium citrate for urinary tract spasm.

hyper·acidity (hī-pėr-as-id'-it-ē) *n* excessive acidity. ⇒ hyperchlorhydria.

hyper·activity (hī-pėr-ak-tiv'-i-tē) *n* excessive activity and distractability: modes of treatment incorporate techniques such as behavior modification, diets and drugs.

hyper·aldosteronism (hī-pėr-al-dos'-tėr-ōn-izm) *n* production of excessive aldosterone *primary hyperaldosteronism* Conn* syndrome. *secondary hyperaldosteronism* the adrenal responds to an increased stimulus of extra-adrenal origin.

hyper·algesia (hī-pėr-al-jē'-zē-ȧ) *n* excessive sensibility to pain—**hyperalgesic** *adj.*

hyper·alimentation (hī-pėr-al-i-men-tā'-shun) *n* total* parenteral nutrition.

hyper·baric oxy·gen treat·ment (hī-pėr-bär'-ik oks'-i-jen) carried out by inserting patient into a sealed cylinder, into which O_2 under pressure is introduced. It is used for patients with carbon monoxide poisoning, gas gangrene, prior to radiotherapy and is currently being investigated for multiple sclerosis.

hyper·bilirubin·emia (hī-pėr-bi'-lē-rōō-bin-ēm'-ē-ȧ) *n* excessive bilirubin in the blood. When it rises above 1–1.5 mg per 100 ml, visible jaundice* occurs. Present in physiological jaundice of the newborn. ⇒ phototherapy—**hyperbilirubinemic** *adj.*

hyper·calcemia (hī-pėr-kal-sē'-mē-ȧ) *n* excessive calcium in the blood usually resulting from bone resorption as occurs in hyperparathyroidism, metastatic tumors of bone. Paget's disease and osteoporosis. It results in anorexia, abdominal pain, muscle pain and weakness. It is accompanied by hypercalciuria and can lead to nephrolithiasis—**hypercalcemic** *adj.*

hyper·calciuria (hī-pėr-kal-sē-ūr'-ē-ȧ) *n* greatly increased excretion of calcium in the urine. Occurs in diseases which result in bone resorption. *idiopathic hypercalciuria* is the term used when there is no known metabolic cause. Hypercalciuria is of importance in the pathogenesis of nephrolithiasis—**hypercalciuric** *adj.*

hyper·capnia (hī-pėr-kap'-nē-ȧ) (*syn* hypercarbia) raised CO_2 tension* in arterial blood—**hypercapnic** *adj.*

hyper·carbia (hī-pėr-kȧr'-bē-ȧ) *n* ⇒ hypercapnia.

hyper·catabolism (hī-pėr-kat-ab'-ol-izm) *n* abnormal, excessive breakdown of complex substances into simpler ones within the body. Can occur in fevers and in acute renal failure—**hypercatabolic** *adj.*

hyper·chloremia (hī-pėr-klōr-ēm'-ē-ȧ) *n* excessive chloride in the blood. One form of acidosis*—**hyperchloremic** *adj.*

hyper·chlorhydria (hī-pėr-klōr-hī'-drē-ȧ) *n* excessive hydrochloric acid in the gastric juice—**hyperchlorhydric** *adj.*

hyper·cholesterol·emia (hī'-pėr-kol-es'-tėr-ol-ēm'-ē-ȧ) *n* excessive cholesterol in the blood. Predisposes to atheroma and gall-stones. Also found in myxedema—**hypercholesterolemic** *adj.*

hyperchromic (hī-pėr-krō'-mik) *adj* excessively colored or pigmented. Excessive hemoglobin in a red blood cell.

hyper·electrolyt·emia (hī-pėr-ē-lek'-trō-līt-ēm'-ē-à) *n* dehydration (not manifested clinically), associated with high serum sodium and chloride levels.

hyper·emesis (hī-pėr-em'-es-is) *n* excessive vomiting. *hyperemesis gravidarum* a complication of pregnancy which may become serious.

hyper·emia (hī-pėr-ēm'-ē-à) *n* excess of blood in an area. *active hyperemia* caused by an increased flow of blood to a part. *passive hyperemia* occurs when there is restricted flow of blood from a part—**hyperemic** *adj.*

hyperesthesia (hī-pėr-es-thē'-zē-à) *n* excessive sensitivity of a part–**hyperesthetic**, *adj.*

hyper·extension (hī-pėr-eks-ten'-shun) *n* overextension.

hyper·flexion (hī-pėr-flek'-shun) *n* excessive flexion

hyper·glycemia (hī-pėr-glī-sē'-mē-à) *n* excessive glucose in the blood, usually indicative of diabetes mellitus. The discovery of isolated high blood glucose readings in an otherwise symptomless diabetic is of little value, but during illness raised blood glucose readings may be a valuable guide to the need for extra insulin—**hyperglycemic** *adj.*

hyper·glycinemia (hī-pėr-glī-sin-ēm'-ē-à) *n* excess glycine in the serum. Can cause acidosis and mental retardation—**hyperglycinemic** *adj.*

hyper·hidrosis (hī-pėr-hī-drō'-sis) *n* excessive sweating—**hyperhidrotic** *adj.*

hyper·insulinism (hī-pėr-in'-sul-in-izm) *n* intermittent or continuous loss of consciousness, with or without convulsions (a) due to excessive insulin from the pancreatic islets lowering the blood sugar (b) due to administration of excessive insulin.

hyper·involution (hī'-pėr-in-vol-ū'-shun) *n* reduction to below normal size, as of the uterus after parturition.

hyper·kalemia (hī-pėr-kal-ēm'-ē-à) *n* (*syn* hyperpotassemia) excessive potassium in the blood as occurs in renal failure; early signs are nausea, diarrhea and muscular weakness. ⇒ Resonium—**hyperkalemic** *adj.*

hyper·keratosis (hī-pėr-ke-rà-tō'-sis) *n* hypertrophy of the stratum corneum or the horny layer of the skin—**hyperkeratotic** *adj.*

hyper·kinesis (hī-pėr-kin-ē'-sis) *n* excessive movement—**hyperkinetic** *adj.*

hyper·kinetic syn·drome (hī-pėr-kin-et'-ik) first described as a syndrome in 1962; usually appears between the ages of 2 and 4 years. The child is slow to develop intellectually and displays a marked degree of distractability and a tireless unrelenting perambulation of the environment, together with aggressiveness (especially towards siblings) even if unprovoked. He may appear to be fearless and undeterred by threats of punishment. The parents complain of his cold unaffectionate character and destructive behavior.

hyper·lipemia (hī-pėr-lī-pē'-mē-à) *n* excessive total fat in the blood—**hyperlipemic** *adj.*

hyper·magnesemia (hī-pėr-mag-nēs-ē'-mē-à) *n* excessive magnesium in the blood, found in kidney failure and people who take excessive magnesium-containing antacids—**hypermagnesemic** *adj.*

hyper·metabolism (hī-pėr-met-ab'-ol-izm) *n* production of excessive body heat. Characteristic of thyrotoxicosis—**hypermetabolic** *adj.*

hyper·metropia (hī-pėr-met-rō'-pē-a) *n* (*syn,* hyperopia) longsightedness caused by faulty accommodation of the eye, with the result that the light rays are focused beyond, instead of on, the retina—**hypermetropic** *adj.*

hyper·mobility (hī-pėr-mō-bil'-it-ē) *n* excessive mobility.

hyper·motility (hī-pėr-mō-til'-it-ē *n* increased movement, as peristalsis.

hyper·natremia (hī-pėr-na-trē'-mē-à) *n* excessive sodium in the blood caused by excessive loss of water and electrolytes owing to polyuria, diarrhea, excessive sweating or inadequate fluid intake—**hypernatremic** *adj.*

hyper·nephroma (hī-pėr-nef-rō'-mà) *n* (*syn* Grawitz tumor) a malignant neoplasm of the kidney whose structure resembles that of adrenocortical tissue—**hypernephromata** *pl.* **hypernephromatous** *adj.*

hyper·onychia (hī-pėr-on-ik'-ē-à) *n* excessive growth of the nails.

hyperopia (hī-pėr-ōp'-ē-à) *n* hypermetropia.

hyper·osmolar dia·betic coma (hī-pėr-oz-mol'-ar) coma characterized by a very high blood sugar without accompanying ketosis.

hyper·osmolarity (hī-pėr-oz-mō-lār'-it-ē) *n* (*syn* hypertonicity) a solution exerting a higher osmotic pressure than another, is said to have a hyperosmolarity, with reference to it. In medicine, the comparison is usually made with normal plasma.

hyper·ostosis (hī-pėr-os-tō'-sis) *n* exostosis*.

hyper·oxaluria (hī-pėr-oks-al-ūr'-ē-à) *n* excessive calcium oxalate in the urine—**hyperoxaluric** *adj.*

hyper·parathyroid·ism (hī-pėr-pā-rà-thī'-royd-izm) *n* overaction of the parathyroid* glands with increase in serum calcium levels; may result in osteitis fibrosa cystica with decalcification and spontaneous fracture of bones. ⇒ hypercalcemia, hypercalciuria.

hyper·peristal·sis (hī-pėr-pe-ri-stal'-sis) *n* excessive peristalsis—**hyperperistaltic** *adj.*

hyper·phenyl·alanin·emia (hī-pėr-fen-il-al'-à-nēn-ēm'-ē-à) *n* excess of phenylalanine in the blood which results in phenylketonuria*.

hyper·phagia (hī-pėr-fā'-jē-à) *n* overeating. ⇒ obesity.

hyper·phosphatemia (hī-pėr-fos'-fà-tē'-mē-à) *n* excessive phosphates in the blood—**hyperphosphatemic** *adj.*

hyperpiesis (hī-pėr-pī-ēs'-is) *n* hypertension*.

hyper·pigmentation (hī-pėr-pig-men-tā'-shun) *n* increased or excessive pigmentation.

hyper·pituitarism (hī-pėr-pit-ōō'-it-ar-izm) *n* overactivity of the anterior lobe of the pituitary* producing gigantism or acromegaly*.

hyper·plasia (hī-pėr-plā'-zē-à) *n* excessive formation of cells—**hyperplastic** *adj.*

hyper·pnea (hī-pėrp-nē'-à) *n* rapid, deep breathing; panting; gasping—**hyperpneic** *adj.*

hyper·potassemia (hī-pėr-pō'-tas-ē'-mē-à) *n* ⇒ hyperkalemia—**hyperpotassemic** *adj.*

hyper·pyrexia (hī-pėr-pī-reks'-ē-à) *n* body temperature above 40–41° C (105° F)—**hyperpyrexial** *adj. malignant hyperpyrexia* an inherited condition which presents during general anesthesia; there is progressive rise in body temperature at a rate of 6° C per hour.

hyper·secretion (hī-pėr-sē-krē'-shun) *n* excessive secretion.

hyper·sensitivity (hī-pėr-sen-sit-iv'-it-ē) *n* a state of being unduly sensitive to a stimulus or an allergen*—**hypersensitive** *adj.*

hyper·splenism (hī-pėr-splen'-izm) *n* term used to describe depression of erythrocyte, granulocyte and platelet counts by enlarged spleen in presence of active bone marrow.

Hyperstat (hī'-pėr-stat) *n* proprietary name for diazoxide*.

hyper·telorism (hī-pėr-tel'-or-izm) *n* genetically determined cranial anomaly (low forehead and pronounced vertex) associated with mental subnormality.

hyper·tension (hī-pėr-ten'-shun) *n* abnormally high tension, by custom abnormally high blood pressure involving systolic and/or diastolic levels. There is no universal agreement of their upper limits of normal, especially in increasing age. Many cardiologists consider a resting systolic pressure of 160 mmHg, and/or a resting diastolic pressure of 100 mmHg, to be pathological. The cause may be renal, endocrine, mechanical or toxic (as in toxemia of pregnancy) but in many cases it is unknown and this is then called 'essential hypertension', portal* hypertension, pulmonary* hypertension—**hypertensive** *adj.*

hyper·thermia (hī-pėr-thėr'-mē-à) *n* very high body temperature—**hyperthermic** *adj. local hyperthermia* can be induced by a thermotherapy machine to heat a cancerous tumor for one hour after which the machine is switched off and the tumor cooling curve is recorded. *whole body hyperthermia* is being used in conjunction with chemotherapy for cancer.

hyper·thyroidism (hī-pėr-thī'-royd-izm) *n* thyrotoxicosis*.

hyper·tonia (hī-pėr-tō'-nē-à) *n* increased tone in a muscular structure—**hypertonic** *adj,* **hypertonicity** *n.*

hyper·tonic (hī-pėr-ton'-ik) *adj* 1 pertaining to hypertonia. 2 pertaining to saline. *hypertonic saline* has a greater osmotic pressure than normal physiological (body) fluid.

hyper·tonicity (hī-pėr-ton-is'-it-ē)*n* ⇒ hyperosmolarity.

hypertoxic (hī-pėr-toks'-ik) *adj* very poisonous.

hyper·trichosis (hī-pėr-trik-ōs'-is) *n* excessive hairiness in sites not usually bearing prominent hair, e.g. the forehead.

hyper·trophy (hī-pėr'-tro-fē) *n* increase in the size of tissues or structures, independent of natural growth. It may be congenital, compensatory, complementary or functional. ⇒ stenosis—**hypertrophic** adj.

hyper·uricemia (hī'-pėr-ūr-i-sē'-mē-à) n excessive uric acid in the blood characteristic of gout. Occurs in untreated reticulosis, but is increased by radiotherapy, cytotoxins and corticosteroids. ⇒ Lesch-Nyhan disease—**hyperuricemic** adj.

hyper·ventilation (hī'-pėr-ven-til-ā'-shun) n increased breathing; may be active, as in salicylate poisoning or head injury, or passive as when it is imposed as part of a technique of general anesthesia in intensive care.

hyper·vitaminosis (hī'-pėr-vī-tà-min-ōs'-is) n any condition arising from an excess of vitamins, especially vitamin D.

hyper·volemia (hī'-per-vol-ēm'-ē-à) n an increase in the volume of circulating blood.

hy·phema (hī-fē'-mà) n blood in the anterior chamber of the eye.

hyp·nosis (hip-nō'-sis) n a state resembling sleep, brought about by the hypnotist utilizing the mental mechanism of suggestion. Can be used to produce painless labor and for dental extractions, and is occasionally utilized in minor surgery and in psychiatric practice—**hypnotic** adj.

hypno·therapy (hip-nō-thėr'-à-pē) n treatment by prolonged sleep or hypnosis.

hyp·notic (hip-not'-ik) adj 1 pertaining to hypnotism. 2 a drug which produces a sleep resembling natural sleep.

hypo·calcemia (hī'-pō-kal-sēm'-ē-à) n decreased calcium in the blood—**hypocalcemic** adj.

hypo·capnia (hī-pō-kap'-nē-à) n reduced CO_2 tension* in arterial blood; can be produced by hyperventilation—**hypocapnial** adj.

hypo·chloremia (hī-pō-klōr-ēm'-ē-à) n reduced chlorides in the circulating blood. A form of alkalosis*—**hypochloremic** adj.

hypo·chlorhydria (hī-pō-klōr-hī'-drē-à) n decreased hydrochloric acid in the gastric juice—**hypochlorhydric** adj.

hypo·chlorite (hī-pō-klōr'-īt) n salts of hypochlorous acid. They are easily decomposed to yield active chlorine, and have been widely used on that account in the treatment of wounds—Dakin's solution and eusol being examples.

hypo·chondria (hī-pō-kon'-drē-à) n excessive anxiety about one's health. Common in depressive and anxiety states—**hypochondriac, hypochondriacal** adj, **hypochondriasis** n.

hypo·chondrium (hī-pō-kon'-drē-um) n the upper lateral region (left and right) of the abdomen, below the lower ribs—**hypochondriac** adj.

hypo·chromic (hī-pō-krō'-mik) adj deficient in coloring or pigmentation. Of a red blood cell, having decreased hemoglobin.

hypo·dermic (hī-po-dėr'-mik) adj below the skin; subcutaneous—**hypodermically** adv.

hypoesthesia (hī-pō-es-thē'-zē-à) n diminished sensitivity of a part–**hypoesthetic,** adj.

hypo·fibrinogenemia (hī-pō-fiī-brin'-ō-jen-ēm'-ē-à) n ⇒ acute defibrination syndrome—**hypofibrinogenemic** adj.

hypo·function (hī-pō-fung'-shun) n diminished performance.

hypo·gamma·globulin·emia (hī-pō-gam-mà-glob'-ū-lin-ēm'-ē-à) n decreased gammaglobulin in the blood, occurring either congenitally or, more commonly, as a sporadic disease in adults. Lessens resistance to infection. ⇒ dysgammaglobulinemia—**hypogamma-globulinemic** adj.

hypo·gastrium (hī-pō-gas'-trē-um) n that area of the anterior abdomen which lies immediately below the umbilical region. It is flanked on either side by the iliac fossae—**hypogastric** adj.

hypo·glossal (hī-pō-glos'-àl) adj under the tongue. hypoglossal nerve the 12th pair of the 12 pairs of cranial nerves which arise directly from the brain.

hypo·glycemia (hī-pō-glī-sē'-mē-à) n decreased blood glucose, attended by anxiety, excitement, perspiration, delirium or coma. Hypoglycemia occurs most commonly in diabetes* mellitus when it is due either to insulin overdosage or inadequate intake of carbohydrate—**hypoglycemic** adj.

hypo·kalemia (hī-pō-kal-ēm'-ē-à) n (syn hypopotassemia) abnormally low potassium level of the blood. ⇒ potassium deficiency—**hypokalemic** adj.

hypo·magnesemia (hī-pō-mag-nēs-ēm'-ē-à) n decreased magnesium in the blood—**hypomagnesemic** adj.

hypo·mania (hī-pō-mā'-nē-à) n a less intense form of mania in which there is a mild elevation of mood with restlessness, distractability, increased energy and pressure of speech. The flight of ideas and grandiose delusions of frank mania* are usually absent—**hypomanic** *adj.*

hypo·metabolism (hī-pō-met-ab'-ol-izm) *n* decreased production of body heat. Characteristic of myxedema*.

hypo·motility (hī-po-mō-til'-it-ē) *n* decreased movement, as of the stomach or intestines.

hypo·natremia (hī-pō-nà-trē'-mē-à) *n* decreased sodium in the blood—**hyponatremic** *adj.*

hypo·osmolarity (hī-pō-os-mo-lār'-it-ē) *n* (*syn* hypotonicity) a solution exerting a lower osmotic pressure than another is said to have a hypo-osmolarity with reference to it. In medicine the comparison is usually made with normal plasma.

hypo·parathyroid·ism (hī-pō-pā-rà-thī'-royd-izm) *n* underaction of the parathyroid* glands with decrease in serum calcium levels, producing tetany*.

hypo·pharynx (hī-pō-fār'-inks) *n* that portion of the pharynx* lying below and behind the larynx, correctly called the laryngopharynx.

hypo·phoria (hī-pō-fōr'-ē-à) *n* a state in which the visual axis in one eye is lower than the other.

hypo·phosphatemia (hī-pō-fos-fà-tēm'-ē-à) *n* decreased phosphates in the blood—**hypophosphatemic** *adj.*

hypo·physectomy (hī-pof-i-sek'-to-mē) *n* surgical removal of the pituitary gland.

hypo·physis cerebri (hī-pof'-is-is) *n* ⇒ pituitary gland—**hypophyseal** *adj.*

hypopiesis (hī-pō-pī-ēs'-is) *n* hypotension*.

hypo·pigmentation (hī-pō-pig-men-tā'-shun) *n* decreased or poor pigmentation.

hypo·pituitarism (hī'-pō-pit-ū'-it-ar-izm) *n* pituitary* gland insufficiency, especially of the anterior lobe. Absence of gonadotrophins leads to failure of ovulation, uterine atrophy and amenorrhea in women and loss of libido, pubic and axillary hair in both sexes. Lack of growth hormone in children results in short stature. Lack of corticotrophin (ACTH) and thyrotrophin (TSH) may result in lack of energy, pallor, fine dry skin, cold intolerance and sometimes hypoglycemia. Usually due to tumor of or involving pituitary gland or hypothalamus but in other cases cause is unknown. Occasionally due to postpartum infarction of the pituitary gland.

hypo·plasia (hī-pō-plā'-zē-à) *n* defective development of any tissue—**hypoplastic** *adj.*

hypo·potassemia (hī'-pō-pot-as-ēm'-ē-à) *n* ⇒ hypokalemia.

hypo·protein·emia (hī'-pō-prō-tēn-ēm'-ē-à) *n* deficient protein in blood plasma, from dietary deficiency or excessive excretion (albuminuria*)—**hypoproteinemic** *adj.*

hypo·prothrombin·emia (hī-pō-prō-throm'-bin-ēm'-ē-à) *n* deficiency of prothrombin in the blood which retards its clotting ability—**hypoprothrombinemic** *adj.*

hypo·pyon (hī-pō-pī'-on) *n* a collection of pus in the anterior chamber of the eye.

hypo·secretion (hī-pō-sē-krē'-shun) *n* deficient secretion.

hypo·sensitivity (hī-pō-sen-sit-iv'-it-ē) *n* lacking sensitivity to a stimulus.

hypo·smia (hī-pos'-mē-à) *n* decrease in the normal sensitivity to smell. Has been observed in patients following laryngectomy.

hypo·spadias (hī-pō-spā'-dē-às) *n* a congenital malformation of the male-urethra. Subdivided into two types: (a) penile, when the terminal urethral orifice opens at any point along the posterior shaft of the penis (b) perineal, when the orifice opens on the perineum and may give rise to problems of sexual differentiation—**epispadias** *opp.*

hypo·stasis (hī-pō-stā'-sis) *n* **1** a sediment **2** congestion of blood in a part due to impaired circulation—**hypostatic** *adj.*

hypo·tension (hī-pō-ten'-shun) *n* low blood pressure (systolic below 110 mmHg, diastolic below 70 mmHg); may be primary, secondary (e.g. caused by bleeding, shock, Addison's disease) or postural. It can be produced by the administration of drugs to reduce bleeding in surgery—**hypotensive** *adj.*

hypo·thalamus (hī-pō-thal'-à-mus) *n* literally, below the thalamus. Forms the ventral part of the diencephalon above the midbrain (⇒ Figure 1). It is the highest center of the autonomic nervous system and contains centers controlling various physiological functions such as emotion, hunger, thirst and circadian rhythms. Also has an important endocrine function producing releasing and some inhibiting hormones that act on the anterior pituitary and regulate the release of its hormones. Also produces oxytocin* and vasopressin* that are released by the posterior pituitary.

hypo·thenar emi·nence (hī-po'-then-ar em'-in-ens) the eminence on the ulnar side of the palm below the little finger.

hypothermia (hī-pō-thèr'-mē-à) *n* below normal body temperature, ascertained by a low-reading thermometer. Occurs particularly in the very young and in old people. An artificially induced hypothermia (30° C or 86° F) can be used in the treatment of head injuries and in cardiac surgery. It reduces the oxygen consumption of the tissues and thereby allows greater and more prolonged interference of normal blood circulation. *hypothermia of the newborn* failure of the newborn child to adjust to external cold; may be associated with infection. *local hypothermia* has been tried in the treatment of peptic ulcer.

hypo·thyroidism (hī-pō-thī'-royd-izm) *n* defines those clinical conditions which result from suboptimal circulating levels of one or both thyroid hormones currently classified as: (a) overt, which if present at birth produces a cretin; if it occurs later, it is myxedema* (b) mild (c) preclinical (d) autoimmune thyroid disease (Hashimoto's* disease).

hypo·tonic (hī-pō-ton'-ik) *adj* 1 ⇒ hypoosmolarity. 2 lacking in tone, tension, strength—**hypotonia, hypotonicity** *n*.

hypo·ventilation (hī-pō-ven-til-ā'-shun) *n* diminished breathing or underventilation.

hypo·vitamin·emia (hī-pō-vīt'-à-min-ē'-mē-à) *n* deficiency of vitamins* in the blood—**hypovitaminemic** *adj*.

hypo·vitaminosis (hī-pō-vīt'-à-min-ōs'-is) *n* any condition due to lack of vitamins*.

hypo·volemia (hī-pō-vol-ēm'-ē-à) ⇒ oligemia—**hypovolemic** *adj*.

hypox·emia (hī-poks-ēm'-ē-à) *n* diminished amount of oxygen in the arterial blood, shown by decreased arterial oxygen tension* and reduced saturation—**hypoxemic** *adj*.

hy·poxia (hī-poks'-ē-à) *n* diminished amount of oxygen in the tissues—**hypoxic** *adj*. *anemic hypoxia* resulting from a deficiency of hemoglobin. *histotoxic hypoxia* interference with the cells in their utilization of O_2, e.g. in cyanide poisoning. *hypoxic hypoxia* interference with pulmonary oxygenation. *stagnant hypoxia* a reduction in blood flow, as seen in the finger nails in surgical shock or in cold weather.

hyster·ectomy (his-tèr-ek'-to-mē) *n* surgical removal of the uterus. *abdominal hysterectomy* effected via a lower abdominal incision. *subtotal hysterectomy* removal of the uterine body, leaving the cervix in the vaginal vault. Rarely performed because of the risk of a carcinoma developing in the cervical stump. *total hysterectomy* complete removal of the uterine body and cervix. *vaginal hysterectomy* carried out through the vagina. *Wertheim's hysterectomy* total removal of the uterus, the adjacent lymphatic vessels and glands, with a cuff of the vagina.

hys·teria (his-tèr'-ē-à) *n* a neurosis usually arising from mental conflict and repression and characterized by the production of a diversity of physical symptoms, e.g. tics, paralysis, anesthesia etc. The disorder is characterized by dissociation—**hysterical** *adj*.

hysterography (his-tèr-og'-rä-fē) *n* x-ray examination of the uterus—**hysterograph, hysterogram**, *n*; **hysterographical**, *adj*.; **hysterographically**, *adv*.

hystero·salpingectomy (his'-tèr-ō-salpin-jek'-to-mē) *n* excision of the uterus and usually both fallopian tubes.

hystero·salpingography (his'-tèr-ō-salping-ōg'-raf-ē) ⇒ uterosalpingography.

hystero·salpingostomy (his'-ter-ō-salping-os'-to-mē) *n* anastomosis between a fallopian tube and the uterus.

hyster·otomy (his-tèr-ot'-o-mē) *n* incision of the uterus to remove a pregnancy. The word is usually reserved for a method of abortion*.

hystero·trachelor·raphy (his-tèr-ō-träkel-ōr'-à-fē) *n* repair of a lacerated cervix* uteri.

Hytakerol (hī-tak'-èr-ol) a proprietary name for dihydrotachysterol*.

HZV *abbr* herpes zoster virus.

I

iatro·genic (ī-at-rō-jen'-ik) *adj* describes a secondary condition arising from treatment of a primary condition.

ibu·profen (ī-bū-prō'-fen) *n* non-narcotic analgesic. Can be irritant to the gastrointestinal tract. (Motrin.)

ichtham·mol (ik'-tham-mol) *n* thick black liquid derived from the destructive distillation of shale. Used as a mild antiseptic ointment for skin disorders and as a solution in glycerin to reduce inflammation. (Ichthyol.)

Ich·thyol (ik'-thē-ol) *n* proprietary name for ichthammol*.

ichthy·oses (ik-thē-ōs'-is) *n* a group of congenital conditions in which the skin is dry and scaly. Fish skin. Xeroderma. *ichthyosis hystrix* is a form of congenital nevus with patches of warty excrescences.

ICP *abbr* intracranial* pressure.

ICSH *abbr* interstitial*-cell stimulating hormone.

ic·terus (ik'-tėr-us) *n* ⇒ jaundice. *icterus gravis* acute diffuse necrosis of the liver. *icterus gravis neonatorum* of the clinical forms of hemolytic* disease of the newborn. *icterus neonatorum* excess of the normal, or physiological, jaundice occurring in the first week of life as a result of excessive destruction of hemoglobin ⇒ phototherapy. *icterus index* measurement of concentration of bilirubin in the plasma. Used in diagnosis of jaundice.

id *n* that part of the unconscious mind which consists of a system of primitive urges (instincts) and, according to Freud, persists unrecognized into adult life.

IDDM *abbr* insulin dependent diabetes mellitus.

idea (ī-dē'-å) *n* a concept or plan of something to be aimed at, created or discovered. *ideas of reference* incorrect interpretation of casual incidents and external events as having direct reference to oneself. If of a sufficient intensity may lead to the formation of delusions.

ideation (ī-dē-ā'-shun) *n* the process concerned with the highest function of awareness, the formation of ideas. It includes thought, intellect and memory.

ident·ical twins (ī-dent'-i-kal twinz) two offspring of the same sex, derived from a single fertilized ovum.

identifi·cation (ī-dent'-if-i-kā'-shun) *n* recognition. In psychology, the way in which we form our personality by modeling it on a chosen person, e.g. identification with the parent of same sex—helping to form one's sex role; identification with a person of own sex in the hero-worship of adolescence.

ideo·motor (id-ē-ō-mō'-tor) *n* mental energy, in the form of ideas, producing automatic movement of muscles, e.g. mental agitation producing agitated movement of limbs.

idio·pathic (id-ē-ō-path'-ik) *adj* of a condition, of unknown or spontaneous origin, e.g. some forms of epilepsy. *idiopathic respiratory distress syndrome* ⇒ respiratory.

idio·syncrasy (id-ē-ō-sing'-krà-sē) *n* **1** a peculiar variation of constitution or temperament. **2** Unusual individual response to certain drugs, proteins, etc, whether by injection, ingestion, inhalation or contact.

idioventricular (id-ē-ō-ven-trik'-ū-lår) *adj* pertaining to the cardiac ventricles* and not affecting the atria.

idox·uridine (ī-doks-ūr'-i-dēn) *n* 5-iodo-2-deoxyuridine. An antiviral chemotherapeutic agent for corneal herpetic ulcers. It interferes with synthesis of DNA in herpes simplex virus and prevents it from multiplying. (Herplex.)

Ig *abbr* ⇒ immunoglobulins.

IgE one class of immunoglobulin* which binds to the surface of mast cells and basophils, involved in hay fever, asthma and anaphylaxis.

IHD *abbr* ⇒ ischemic heart disease.

il·eal blad·der (il'-ē-al blad'-dėr) ⇒ ileoureterostomy.

il·eal con·duit (il'-ē-al kon'-dōō-it) ⇒ ileoureterostomy.

il·eitis (il-ē-ī'-tis) *n* inflammation of the ileum*.

ileo·cecal (il-ē-ō-sē'-kàl) *adj* pertaining to the ileum and the cecum.

ileo·colic (il-ē-ō-kol'-ik) *adj* pertaining to the ileum and the colon.

ileo·colitis (il-ē-ō-kol-ī'-tis) *n* inflammation of the ileum and the colon.

ileo·colostomy (il-ē-ō-kol-os'-to-mē) *n* a surgically made fistula between the ileum and the colon, usually the transverse colon. Most often used to bypass an obstruction or inflammation in the cecum or ascending colon.

ileo·cysto·plasty (il-ē-ō-sis'-tō-plas-tē) *n* operation to increase the size of the urinary bladder—**ileocystoplastic** *adj*.

ileo·proctostomy (il-ē-ō-prok-tos'-to-mē) *n* an anastomosis between the ileum and rectum; used when disease extends to the sigmoid colon.

ileo·rectal (il-ē-ō-rek'-tàl) *adj* pertaining to the ileum and the rectum.

ileo·sigmoidostomy (il-ē-ō-sig-moyd-os'-to-mē) *n* an anastomosis between the ileum and sigmoid colon; used where most of the colon has to be removed.

ileos·tomy (il-ē-os'-to-mē) *n* a surgically made fistula between the ileum and the anterior abdominal wall; usually a permanent form of artificial anus when the whole of the large bowel has to be removed, e.g. in severe ulcerative colitis. *ileostomy bags* rubber or plastic bags used to collect the liquid discharge from an ileostomy.

ileoureter·ostomy (il-ē-o-ū′-rē-tèr-os′-to-mē) *n* (*syn* ureteroileostomy) transplantation of the lower ends of the ureters from the bladder to an isolated loop of small bowel (ileal bladder) which, in turn, is made to open on the abdominal wall (ileal conduit).

il·eum (il′-ē-um) *n* the lower three-fifths of the small intestine, lying between the jejunum* and the cecum*—**ileal** *adj*.

il·eus (il′-ē-us) *n* intestinal obstruction. Usually restricted to paralytic as opposed to mechanical obstruction and characterized by abdominal distension, vomiting and the absence of pain ⇒ meconium.

iliac artery (il′-ē-ak àr′-tèr-ē) ⇒ Figure 9.

iliococcygeal (il-ē-ō-koks-i-jē′-àl) *adj* pertaining to the ilium and coccyx.

iliofemoral (il-ē-ō-fem′-or-àl) *adj* pertaining to the ilium and the femur.

iliopectineal (il-ē-ō-pek-tin′-ē-al) *adj* pertaining to the ilium and the pubis.

iliopsoas (il-ē-ō-sō′-as) *adj* pertaining to the ilium and the loin.

ilio·tibial tract muscle (il′-ē-ō-tib′-ē-al) ⇒ Figure 5.

il·ium (il′-ē-um) *n* the upper part of the innominate (hip) bone; it is a separate bone in the fetus—**iliac** *adj*.

il·lusion (il-lū′-zhun) *n* a misidentification of a sensation, e.g. of sight, a white sheet being mistaken for a ghost, the sheet being misrepresented in consciousness as a figure.

Ilo·tycin (il-ō-tī′-sin) *n* proprietary name for erythromycin*.

im·age (im′-aj) *n* a revived experience of a percept recalled from memory (smell and taste).

ima·gery (im′-aj-èr-ē) *n* imagination. The recall of mental images of various types depending upon the special sense organs involved when the images were formed, e.g. *auditory imagery* sound. *motor imagery* movement. *visual imagery* sight. *tactile imagery* touch. *olfactory imagery* smell.

im·balance (im-bal′-ans) *n* want of balance. Term refers commonly to the upset of acid-base relationship and the electrolytes in body fluids.

Imferon (im′-fèr-on) *n* a proprietary iron-dextran complex or parenteral iron therapy. Used as a total dose infusion to obtain a rapid response in marked iron deficiency anemia.

im·ipramine (im-ip′-ra-mēn) *n* tricyclic antidepressant with anticholinergic properties. Cardiotoxic in overdose. (Janimine, Totranil.)

im·mersion foot (im-mèr′-zhun) ⇒ trench foot.

im·mune (im-mūn′) *adj* possessing the capacity to resist infection. *immune body* immunoglobulin*.

im·mune react·ion, re·sponse that which causes a body to reject a transplanted organ, to respond to bacterial disease which develops slowly, and to act against malignant cells; cell mediated immunity*.

immun·ity (im-mūn′-it-ē) *n* an intrinsic or acquired state of resistance to an infectious agent. *active immunity* is acquired, naturally during an infection or artificially by immunization*. *cell mediated immunity* T lymphocyte-dependent responses which cause graft rejection, immunity to some infectious agents and tumor rejection. *humoral immunity* from immunoglobulin produced by B-lymphocytes. Immunity can be innate (from inherited qualities), or it can be acquired, actively or passively, naturally or artificially. *passive immunity* is acquired, naturally when maternal antibody passes to the child via the placenta or in the milk, or artificially by administering sera containing antibodies from animals or human beings.

immun·ization (im-mū-nī-zā′-shun) *n* the administration of antigens to induce immunity*.

immuno·compromised patients (im-mū-nō-kom′-prom-ized) (*syn* immunosuppressed patients) patients with defective immune responses, often produced by treatment with drugs or irradiation. Also occurs in some patients with cancer and other diseases affecting the lymphoid system. Patients are liable to develop infections with opportunistic organisms such as *Candida, Pneumocystis carinii* and *Cryptococcus neoformans*.

immuno·deficiency (im-mū-nō-dē-fish′-ens-ē) *n* the state of having defective immune responses, leading to increased susceptibility to infectious diseases.

immuno·deficiency dis·eases inherited or acquired disorders of the immune system.

immuno·genesis (im-mū-nō-gen′-es-is) *n*

149

the process of production of immunity—**immunogenetic** *adj.*

immuno·genicity (im-mū-nō-jen-is'-it'-ē) *n* the ability to produce immunity*.

immuno·globulins (Igs) (im-mū-nō-glob'-ū-lins) *n* (*syn* antibodies) high molecular weight proteins produced by B lymphocytes which can combine with antigens such as bacteria and produce immunity or interfere with membrane signals to produce autoimmune disease, e.g. thyrotoxicosis.

immunolog·ical re·sponse (im-mūn'-nol-oj'-i-kal) ⇒ immunity.

immu·nology (im-mū-nol'-o-jē) *n* the study of the immune system of lymphocytes, inflammatory cells and associated cells and proteins, which affect an individual's response to antigens—**immunological** *adj,* **immunologically** *adv.*

immuno·pathology (im-mū-nō-path-ol'-o-jē) *n* the study of tissue injury involving the immune system.

immuno-suppressed patients (im-mū-nō-sup-presd') ⇒ immunocompromised patients.

immuno·suppression (im-mū-nō-sup-presh'-un) *n* treatment which reduces immunological responsiveness.

immuno·suppressive (im-mū-nō-sup-pres'-iv) *n* that which reduces immunological responsiveness.

immunotherapy (im-mūn-ō-thėr'-ȧ-pē) *n* any treatment used to produce immunity.

immunotransfusion (im-mūn-ō-trans-fū'-zhun) *n* transfusion of blood from a donor previously rendered immune by repeated inoculations with a given agent from the recipient.

Imodium (im-ō'-dē-um) *n* proprietary name for loperamide*.

impac·ted (im-pak'-ted) *adj* firmly wedged, abnormal immobility, as of feces in the rectum; fracture; a fetus in the pelvis; a tooth in its socket or a calculus in a duct. ⇒ fracture.

impal·pable (im-pal'-pȧ-bl) *adj* not palpable, incapable of being felt by touch (palpation).

imper·forate (im-pėr'-fōr-āt) *adj* lacking a normal opening. *imperforate anus* a congenital absence of an opening into the rectum. *imperforate hymen* a fold of mucous membrane at the vaginal entrance which has no natural outlet for the menstrual fluid. ⇒ hematocolpos.

im·petigo (im-pet-ī'-gō) *n* an inflamma-

tory, pustular skin disease usually caused by *Staphylococcus*, occasionally by *Streptococcus impetigo contagiosa* a highly contagious form of impetigo, commonest on the face and scalp, characterized by vesicles which become pustules and then honey-colored crusts. ⇒ ecthyma—**impetiginous** *adj.*

implan·tation (im-plant-ā'-shun) *n* the insertion of living cells or solid materials into the tissues, e.g. accidental implantation of tumor cells in a wound; implantation of radium or solid drugs; implantation of the fertilized ovum into the endometrium.

im·plants (im'-plants) *npl* tissues or drugs inserted surgically into the human body, e.g. implantation of pellets of testosterone under the skin in treatment of carcinoma of the breast, implants of deoxycortone acetate in Addison's disease, silastic implants in plastic surgery.

impo·tence (im'-po-tens) *n* inability to participate in sexual intercourse, by custom referring to the male. It can be due to lack of erection or premature ejaculation.

impreg·nate (im-preg'-nāt) *v* fill; saturate; render pregnant.

im·pulse (im'-puls) *n* **1** a sudden inclination, sometimes irresistible urge to act without deliberation. **2** the electrochemical process involved in neurotransmission of information and stimuli throughout the body.

impul·sive action (im-pul'-siv) ⇒ action.

Imuran (im'-ūr-an) *n* proprietary name for azathioprine*.

inaccessi·bility (in-ak-ses-i-bil'-i-tē) *n* in psychiatry, absence of patient response.

Inapsine (in-ap'-sēn) *n* proprietary name for droperidol*.

inassim·ilable (in-as-sim'-il-ȧ-bl) *adj* not capable of absorption.

incar·cerated (in-kår'-sėr-āt-ed) *adj* describes the abnormal imprisonment of a part, as in a hernia which is irreducible or a pregnant uterus held beneath the sacral promontory.

in·cest (in'-sest) *n* sexual intercourse between close blood relatives. The most common type of sexual abuse occurs between father and daughter; other types—between mother and son and between siblings—are known to occur.

incipi·ent (in-sip'-ē-ent) *adj* initial, beginning, in its early stages.

in·cised wound (in-sīzd') one which results from cutting with a sharp knife or scalpel; if uninfected it heals by first intention.

in·cision (in-si'-zhun) *n* the result of cutting into body tissue, using a sharp instrument—**incisional** *adj*, **incise** *vt*.

in·cisors (in-sī'-sorz) *npl* the teeth first and second from the midline, four in each jaw used for cutting food.

in·clusion bodies (in-kloo'-zhun) minute particles found in some cells of pathological and normal tissues.

incom·patibility (in-kom-pat-i-bil'-i-tē) *n* usually refers to the bloods of donor and recipient in transfusion, when antigenic differences in the red cells result in reactions such as hemolysis or agglutination. When two or more medicaments are given concurrently or consecutively they can attenuate or counteract the desired effect of each.

incom·petence (in-kom'-pe-tens) *n* inadequacy to perform a natural function, e.g. mitral incompetence—**incompetent** *adj*.

incom·plete abor·tion (in-kom-plēt' ab-ōr'-shun) ⇒ abortion.

incom·plete frac·ture (in-kom-plēt' frak'-tūr) ⇒ fracture.

inconti·nence (in-kon'-tin-ens) *n* inability to control the evacuation of urine or feces. *overflow incontinence* dribbling of urine from an overfull bladder. *stress incontinence* occurs when the intra-abdominal pressure is raised as in coughing, giggling and sneezing; there is usually some weakness of the urethral sphincter muscle coupled with anatomical stretching and displacement of the bladder neck.

inco·ordination (in-kō-ōr-din-ā'-shun) *n* inability to produce smooth, harmonious muscular movements.

incu·bation (in-kū-bā'-shun) *n* **1** the period from entry of infection to the appearance of the first symptom. **2** the process of development, of an egg, or of a bacterial culture. **3** the process to which a baby in an incubator is exposed.

incu·bator (in'-kū-bā-tor) *n* **1** an enclosed cradle kept at appropriate temperatures in which premature or delicate babies can be reared. **2** a low-temperature oven in which bacteria are cultured.

incus (in'-kus) *n* the central bone of the middle ear. ⇒ Figure 13.

indapa·mide (in-dap'-à-mīd) *n* an antihypotensive diuretic.

Inder·al (in'-dèr-al) *n* proprietary name for propranolol*.

Indian hemp (in'-dē-an hemp) cannabis* indica.

indi·can (in'-di-kan) *n* potassium salt excreted in the urine as a detoxification product of indoxyl ⇒ indicanuria.

indican·uria (in-di-kan-ū'-rē-à) *n* excessive potassium salt (indican*) in the urine. There are traces in normal urine; high levels are suggestive of intestinal obstruction ⇒ indole.

indi·cator (in'-di-kā-tor) *n* a substance which, when added in small quantities, is used to make visible the completion of a chemical reaction or the attainment of a certain pH.

indigen·ous (in-dij'-en-us) *adj* of a disease etc., native to a certain locality or country, e.g. Derbyshire neck (simple colloidal goiter).

indiges·tion (in-dij-es'-chun) *n* (*syn* dyspepsia) a feeling of gastric discomfort, including fullness and gaseous distension, which is not necessarily a manifestation of disease.

indigo-carmine (in'-di-gō-kàr'-mīn) *n* a dye used as an 0.4% solution for testing renal function. Given by intravenous or intramuscular injection. The urine is colored blue in about 10 min if kidney function is normal.

Indo·cin *n* proprietary name for indomethacin*.

in·dole (in'-dōl) *n* a product of the decomposition of tryptophan* in the intestines; it is oxidized to indoxyl in the liver and excreted in urine as indican ⇒ indican, indicanuria.

indol·ent (in'-dol-ent) *adj* a term applied to a sluggish ulcer which is generally painless and slow to heal.

indometh·acin (in-dō-meth'-à-sin) *n* a prostaglandin inhibitor with analgesic and anti-inflammatory properties. Useful in the rheumatic disorders. Can be given orally but, to prevent nausea, capsules should be taken with a meal or a glass of milk. Also available as suppositories. (Indocid.)

induced abor·tion (in-dūsd' ab-or'-shun) ⇒ abortion.

induc·tion (in-duk'-shun) *n* the act of bringing on or causing to occur, as applied to anesthesia and labor.

indu·ration (in-dur-ā'-shun) *n* the hardening of tissue, as in hyperemia, infiltration by neoplasm etc—**indurated** *adj*.

indus·trial derma·titis (in-dus'-trē-al dèrm-à-tī'-tis) ⇒ dermatitis.

indus·trial dis·ease (in-dus'-trē-al diz-ēz') (*syn* occupational disease) a disease contracted by reason of occupational exposure to an industrial agent known to be hazardous, e.g. dust, fumes, chemicals, irradiation etc, the notification of, safety precautions against and compensation for which are controlled by law.

iner·tia (in-ėr'-shē-à) *n* inactivity, *uterine inertia* lack of contraction of parturient uterus. It may be primary due to constitutional weakness; secondary due to exhaustion from frequent and forcible contractions.

inevi·table abor·tion (in-ev'-it-à-bl à-bōr'-shun) ⇒ abortion.

in extremis (in eks-trē'-mis) at the point of death.

in·fant (in'-fant) *n* a baby or a child of less than 1 year old

infan·tile paral·ysis (in'-fant-īl pàr-al'-is-is) ⇒ poliomyelitis.

infan·tilism (in-fant'-il-izm) *n* general retardation of development with persistence of child-like characteristics into adolescence and adult life.

in·farct (in'-fàr-kt) *n* area of tissue affected when the end artery supplying it is occluded, e.g. in kidney or heart. Common complication of subacute endocarditis.

infarc·tion (in-fàrk'-shun) *n* death of a section of tissue because the blood supply has been cut off. ⇒ myocardial infarction.

infec·tion (in-fek'-shun) *n* the successful invasion, establishment and growth of microorganisms in the tissues of the host. It may be of an acute or chronic nature—**infectious** *adj*. *autoinfection* infection resulting from commensals* becoming pathogenic, or when commensals or pathogens* are transferred from one part of the body to another, for example by finger. *cross infection* occurs when pathogens are transferred from one person to another. *hospital-acquired (nosocomial) infection (HAI)* one which occurs in a patient who has been in hospital for at least 72 h and did not have signs and symptoms of such infection on admission: 10%–12% of hospital patients develop a hospital-acquired infection. Urinary tract infection is the most comon type. *opportunistic infection* a serious infection with a microorganism which normally has little or no pathogenic activity but which has been activated by a serious disease or by a modern method of treatment.

infec·tious dis·ease (in-fek'-shus) a dis-ease caused by a specific, pathogenic organism and capable of being transmitted to another individual by direct or indirect contact.

infec·tious mono·nucleosis (in-fek'-shus mon'-ō-nōō-klē-ōs'-is) (*syn* glandular fever) a contagious self-limiting disease due to the Epstein-Barr virus. Characterized by fever, sore throat, enlargement of superficial lymph nodes and appearance of atypical lymphocytes resembling monocytes. Specific antibodies to Epstein-Barr virus are present in the blood as well as an abnormal antibody which has 'heterophile' activity directed against sheep's red blood cells—the basis of the Paul*-Bunnell test—which is positive in infectious mononucleosis. One attack confers complete immunity and also lifelong harboring of virus particles in the lymphocytes and in the saliva, hence the synonym 'kissing disease'.

infec·tive (in-fek'-tiv) *adj* infectious. Disease transmissible from one host to another. *infective hepatitis* ⇒ hepatitis.

in·ferior (in-fēr'-ē-or) *adj* lower; beneath.

inferi·ority com·plex (in-fēr-ē-ōr'-i-tē kom'-pleks) term first used by Adler to describe a basic feeling of inadequacy and insecurity which usually originates in childhood, and which may result in compensatory, competitive or aggressive behavior.

infer·tility (in-fėr-til'-it-ē) *n* lack of ability to reproduce. Psychological and physical causes play their part. The abnormality can be in the husband and/or wife. Special clinics exist to investigate this condition.

infes·tation (in-fes-tā'-shun) *n* the presence of animal parasites in or on the human body—**infest** *vt*.

infibul·ation (in-fib-ū-lā'-shun) *n* ⇒ circumcision.

infil·tration (in-fil-trā'-shun) *n* penetration of the surrounding tissues, the oozing or leaking of fluid into the tissues. *infiltration anesthesia* analgesia produced by infiltrating the tissues with a local anesthetic.

inflam·mation (in-flam-ā'-shun) *n* the reaction of living tissues to injury, infection, or irritation; characterized by pain, swelling, redness and heat. The degree of redness can be measured by a tintometer*—**inflammatory** *adj*.

influ·enza (in-flōō-en'-zà) *n* an acute viral infection of the nasopharynx and respiratory tract which occurs in epidemic or pandemic form—**influenzal** *adj*.

infra·red rays (in-frà-red'-rāz) long wavelength, invisible rays of the electromagnetic spectrum.

infra·spinatus muscle (in-fra spin-à'-tus) ⇒ Figure 5.

infun·dibulum (in-fun-dib'-ū-lum) *n* any funnel-shaped passage—**infundibula** *pl*. **infundibular** *adj*. *infundibulum with fimbriae* ⇒ Figure 17.

in·fusion (in-fū'-zhun) *n* **1** fluid flowing by gravity into the body. **2** an aqueous solution containing the active principle of a drug, made by pouring boiling water on the crude drug. **3** amniotic* fluid infusion.

inges·tion (in-jes'-chun) *n* **1** the act of taking food or medicine into the stomach. **2** the means by which a phagocytic cell takes in surrounding solid material such as microorganisms.

ingrow·ing toe·nail (in'-grō-ing tō'-nāl) spreading of the nail into the lateral tissue, causing inflammation.

ingui·nal (ing'-gwi-nàl) *adj* pertaining to the groin. *inguinal canal* a tubular opening through the lower part of the anterior abdominal wall, parallel to and a little above the inguinal (Poupart's) ligament. It measures 38 mm. In the male it contains spermatic cord; in the female the uterine round ligaments. *inguinal hernia* ⇒ hernia.

INH *abbr* isoniazid*.

inha·lation (in-hal-ā'-shun) *n* **1** the breathing in of air, or other vapor, etc. **2** a medicinal substance which is inhaled.

in·herent (in-hēr'-ent) *adj* innate; inborn.

inhi·bition (in-hi-bi'-shun) *n* the process of restraining one's impulses or behavior as a result of mental (psychic) influences.

in·jected (in-jek'-ted) *adj* congested, with full vessels.

injec·tion (in-jek'-shun) *n* **1** the act of introducing a fluid (under pressure) into the tissues, a vessel, cavity or hollow organ. (Air can be injected into a cavity. ⇒ pneumothorax.) **2** the substance injected.

inject·or (in-jek'-tor) *n* a device in which a high flow of fluid (gas or liquid) flows through a jet and sucks other fluid in fixed proportions from a side limb.

in·nate (in-āt') *adj* inborn, dependent on genetic constitution.

inner·vation (in-nėr-vā'-shun) *n* the nerve supply to a part.

inno·cent (in'-ō-sent) *adj* benign; not malignant.

innocu·ous (in-ok'-ū-us) *adj* harmless.

innomi·nate (in-nom'-in-āt) *adj* unnamed ⇒ hip bone.

inocu·lation (in-ok-ū-lā'-shun) *n* **1** the injection of substances, especially vaccine, into the body. **2** introduction of microorganisms into culture medium for propagation.

inor·ganic (in-ōr-gan'-ik) *adj* neither animal nor vegetable in origin.

inositol nicotin·ate (in-os'-i-tol nik-ō-tin'-āt) a vasodilator which is used in peripheral vascular disease.

ino·tropic (ī-nō-trō'-pik) *adj* affecting the force of muscle contraction, applied particularly to cardiac muscle. An inotrope is a drug which increases the contractile force of the heart.

in·quest (in'-kwest) *n* a legal enquiry, held by a coroner into the cause of sudden or unexpected death.

insec·ticide (in-sek'-ti-sīd) *n* an agent which kills insects—**insecticidal** *adj*.

insemi·nation (in-sem-in-ā'-shun) *n* introduction of semen into the vagina, normally by sexual intercourse. *artificial insemination* instrumental injection of semen into the vagina ⇒ AID. AIH.

insen·sible (in-sens'-i-bl) *adj* without sensation or consciousness. Too small or gradual to be perceived, as insensible perspiration.

inser·tion (in-sėr'-shun) *n* **1** the act of setting or placing in. **2** the attachment of a muscle to the bone it moves.

inservice education an ongoing educational program for nursing and other staff development set up within the facility in which the staff work.

insidi·ous (in-sid'-ē-us) *adj* having an imperceptible commencement, as of a disease with a late manifestation of definite symptoms.

in·sight (in'-sīt) *n* ability to accept one's limitations but at the same time to develop one's potentialities. In psychiatry means: (a) knowing that one is ill (b) a developing knowledge of one's present attitudes and past experiences and the connection between them.

in situ (in sī'-tū) in the correct position, undisturbed. Also describes a cancer which has not invaded adjoining tissue.

insom·nia (in-som'-nē-à) *n* sleeplessness.

inspi·ration (in-spir-ā'-shun) *n* the drawing of air into the lungs; inhalation—**inspiratory** *adj,* **inspire** *vt.*

inspiss·ated (in'-spis-āt-ed) *adj* thickened, as by evaporation or withdrawal of water, applied to sputum and culture media used in the laboratory.

in·step (in'-step) *n* the arch of the foot on the dorsal surface.

instil·lation (in-stil-ā'-shun) *n* insertion of drops into a cavity, e.g. conjunctival sac, external auditory meatus.

in·stinct (in'-stingkt) *n* an inborn tendency to act in a certain way in a given situation, e.g. *maternal/paternal instinct* to protect children—**instinctive** *adj,* **instinctively** *adv.*

insti·tutional·ization (in-sti-tū'-shun-ál-īz-ā'-shun) *n* a condition of apathy resulting from lack of motivation characterizing people in institutions who have been subjected to a rigid routine with deprivation of decision-making. ⇒ neurosis.

insuf·flation (in-suf-lā'-shun) *n* the blowing of air along a tube (eustachian, fallopian) to establish patency. The blowing of powder into a body cavity.

insu·lin (in'-sul-in) *n* a pancreatic hormone, made in the islet cells of Langerhans, secreted into the blood and having a profound influence on carbohydrate metabolism by stimulating the transport of glucose into cells. The hormone is prepared commercially in various forms and strengths which vary in their speed, length and potency of action and which are used in the treatment of diabetes mellitus. The U100 insulin means 100 units of insulin per ml. It is not a new type of insulin but it standardizes the strength. *insulin dependent diabetes mellitus (IDDM)* ⇒ diabetes. *insulin pump* a 250 g, 20 mm thick apparatus made of titanium, powered by a fluid called freon which is used in refrigerators. It is inserted usually into the abdomen and delivers insulin as needed; it is refilled every 4–8 weeks via a self-sealing valve under the skin. *insulin test* for determining the completeness or otherwise of surgical vagotomy. When the vagus nerve is intact hypoglycemia, in response to an intravenous injection of insulin, produces secretion of acid from the stomach. Complete vagotomy abolishes this response.

insulin·oma (in-sul-in-ō'-má) *n* adenoma of the islets of Langerhans in the pancreas.

Intal (in'-tal) *n* proprietary name for cromolyn sodium.

integu·ment (in-teg'-ū-ment) *n* a covering, especially the skin.

intel·lect (in'-tel-ekt) *n* reasoning power, thinking faculty.

intel·ligence (in-tel'-lij-ens) *n* inborn mental ability. *intelligence tests* designed to determine the level of intelligence. *intelligence quotient (IQ)* the ratio of mental age to chronological (actual) age.

inten·sive ther·apy unit (ITU) (in-ten'-siv thér'-a-pē) a unit in which highly specialized monitoring, resuscitation and therapeutic techniques are used.

inten·tion tremor (in-ten'-shun trem'-or) ⇒ tremor.

inter·action (in-tėr-ak'-shun) when two or more things or people have a reciprocal influence on each other ⇒ drug interaction.

inter·articular (in-tėr-ár-tik'-ū-lår) *adj* between joints.

inter·atrial (in-tėr-ā'-trē-ál) *adj* between the two atria of the heart.

inter·cellular (in-tėr-sel'-ū-lår) *adj* between cells.

inter·costal (in-tėr-kos'-tal) *adj* between the ribs.

inter·course (in'-tėr-kōrs) *n* **1** human communication. **2** coitus*.

inter·current (in-tėr-kur'-ent) *adj* describes a second disease arising in a person already suffering from one disease.

inter·feron (in-tėr-fēr'-on) *n* a protein effective against some viruses. When a virus infects a cell, it triggers off the cell's production of interferon. This then interacts with surrounding cells and renders them resistant to virus attack. Interferon has caused regression of tumor in some cases of multiple myclomatosis. Two human types are available, one prepared from cultured leukocytes and the other prepared from cultured fibroblasts.

inter·lobar (in-tėr-lō'-bår) *adj* between the lobes, e.g. interlobar pleurisy.

inter·lobular (in-tėr-lob'-ū-lår) *adj* between the lobules.

inter·menstrual (in-tėr-mens'-trū-ál) *adj* between the menstrual periods.

inter·mittent (in-tėr-mit'-tent) *adj* occurring at intervals. *intermittent claudication* ⇒ claudication. *intermittent peritoneal dialysis* ⇒ dialysis. *intermittent positive pressure* ⇒ positive pressure ventilation. *intermittent self catheterization* ⇒ self catheterization.

in·ternal (in-tėr'-nál) *adj* inside. *internal*

ear that part of the ear which comprises the vestibule, semicircular canals and the cochlea. *internal respiration* ⇒ respiration. *internal secretions* those produced by the ductless or endocrine glands and passed directly into the blood stream; hormones. *internal version* ⇒ version.

inter·osseous (in-tèr-os′-sē-us) *adj* between bones.

inter·phalangeal (in-tèr-fal-an′-jē-àl) *adj* between the phalanges*.

inter·position oper·ation surgical replacement of part or all of the chain of ossicles.

inter·serosal (in-tèr-sèr-ōs′-àl) *adj* between serous membrane, as in the pleural peritoneal and pericardial cavities—**interserosally** *adv*.

inter·sexuality (in-tèr-seks-ū-al′-it-ē) *n* the possession of both male and female characteristics ⇒ Turner syndrome, Klinefelter syndrome.

inter·spinous (in-tèr-spīn′-us) *adj* between spinous processes, especially those of the vertebrae.

inter·stices (in-tèr′-sti-sēz) *n* spaces.

inter·stitial (in-tèr-stish′-ē-àl) *adj* situated in the interstices of a part; distributed through the connective structures. *interstitial part of uterine tube* ⇒ Figure 17. *interstitial-cell stimulation hormone (ICSH)* a hormone released from the anterior lobe of the pituitary gland; causes production of testosterone* in the male.

inter·trigo (in-tèr-trī′-gō) *n* superficial inflammation occurring in most skin folds—**intertrigenous** *adj*.

inter·trochanteric (in-tèr-trō-kan-tèr′-ik) *adj* between trochanters, usually referring to those on the proximal femur.

inter·ventricular (in-tèr-ven-trik′-ū-làr) *adj* between ventricles, as those of the brain or heart.

inter·vertebral (in-tèr-vèr-tē′-bràl) *adj* between the vertebrae, as discs and foramina. ⇒ nucleus, prolapse.

intes·tine (in-tes′-tin) *n* a part of the alimentary canal extending from the stomach to the anus (⇒ Figure 18). It comprises the small intestine (gut) and the large intestine (bowel)—**intestinal** *adj*.

in·tima (in′-tim-à) *n* the internal coat of a blood vessel—**intimal** *adj*.

intol·erance (in-tol′-èr-ans) *n* the manifestation of various unusual reactions to particular substances such as nutrients or medications.

intra·abdominal (in-trà-ab-dom′-in-àl) *adj* inside the abdomen.

intra·amniotic (in-trà-am-nē-ot′-ik) *adj* within, or into the amniotic fluid.

intra·arterial (in-trà-àr-tēr′-ē-àl) *adj* within an artery—**intraarterially** *adv*.

intra·articular (in-trà-àr-tik′-ū-làr) *adj* within a joint.

intra·bronchial (in-trà-brong′-kē-àl) *adj* within a bronchus.

intra·canalicular (in-trà-kan-al-ik′-ū-làr) *adj* within a canaliculus.

intra·capillary (in-trà-kap′-il-ār-ē) *adj* within a capillary.

intra·capsular (in-trà-kap′-sū-làr) *adj* within a capsule, e.g. that of the lens or a joint ⇒ extracapsular *opp*.

intra·cardiac (in-trà-kàr′-dē-ak) *adj* within the heart.

intra·caval (in-trà-kā′-vàl) *adj* within the vena cava, by custom referring to the inferior one—**intracavally** *adv*.

intra·cellular (in-trà-sel′-ū-lar) *adj* within cells ⇒ extracellular *opp*.

intra·cerebral (in-trà-sèr-ē′-bral) *adj* within the cerebrum.

intra·corpuscular (in-trà-kōr-pus′-kū-lar) *adj* within a corpuscle.

intra·cranial (in-trà-krā′-nē-àl) *adj* within the skull.

intra·cranial pres·sure (ICP) maintained at a normal level by brain tissue, intracellular and extracellular fluid, cerebrospinal* fluid and blood. A change in any of these compartments can increase the pressure.

intra·cutaneous (in-trà-kū-tā′-nē-us) *adj* within the skin tissues—**intracutaneously** *adv*.

intra·dermal (in-trà-dèr′-màl) *adj* within the skin—**intradermally** *adv*.

intra·dural (in-trà-dū′-ral) *adj* inside the dura mater.

intra·gastric (in-trà-gas′-trik) *adj* within the stomach.

intra·gluteal (in-trà-glū′-te-àl) *adj* within the gluteal muscle comprising the buttock—**intragluteally** *adv*.

intra·hepatic (in-trà-hep-at′-ik) *adj* within the liver.

Intra·lipid (in-trà-lip′-id) *n* a proprietary emulsion of soy bean oil which is suitable for intravenous drip infusion. Half a liter of 20% solution contains 1000 kcal. Antibiotics or other drugs must not be added to the infusion.

intra·lobular (in-trȧ-lob′-ū-lar) *adj* within the lobule, as the vein draining a hepatic lobule.

intra·luminal (in-trȧ-lū′-min-ȧl) *adj* within the hollow of a tube-like structure—**intraluminally** *adv*.

intra·lymphatic (in-trȧ-lim-fat′-ik) *adj* within a lymphatic gland or vessel.

intra·medullary (in-trȧ-med′-ū-lā-rē) *adj* within the bone marrow.

intra·mural (in-trȧ-mūr′-ȧl) *adj* within the layers of the wall of a hollow tube or organ—**intramurally** *adv*.

intra·muscular (in-trȧ-mus′-kū-lar) *adj* within a muscle—**intramuscularly** *adv*.

intra·nasal (in-trȧ-nā′-zȧl) *adj* within the nasal cavity—**intranasally** *adv*.

intra·natal (in-trȧ-nā′-tal) *adj* ⇒ intrapartum—**intranatally** *adv*.

intra·ocular (in-trȧ-ok′-ū-lar) *adj* within the globe of the eye.

intra·oral (in-trȧ-ōr′-al) *adj* within the mouth as an intraoral appliance—**intraorally** *adv*.

intra·orbital (in-trȧ-ōr′-bit-ȧl) *adj* within the orbit.

intra·osseous (in-trȧ-os′-ē-us) *adj* inside a bone.

intra·partum (in-trȧ-pȧr′-tum) *adj* (*syn* intranatal) at the time of birth; during labor, as asphyxia, hemorrhage or infection.

intra·peritoneal (in-trȧ-pėr-it-on-ē′-ȧl) *adj* within the peritoneal cavity—**intraperitoneally** *adv*.

intra·pharyngeal (in-trȧ-fār-in-jē′-ȧl) *adj* within the pharynx—**intrapharyngeally** *adv*.

intra·placental (in-trȧ-plȧ-sen′-tȧl) *adj* within the placenta—**intraplacentally** *adv*.

intra·pleural (in-trȧ-plo͞o′-rȧl) *adj* within the pleural cavity—**intrapleurally** *adv*.

intra·pulmonary (in-trȧ-pul′-mon-ār-ē) *adj* within the lungs, as intrapulmonary pressure.

intra·punitive (in-trȧ-pūn′-it-iv) *adj* tending to blame oneself.

intra·retinal (in-trȧ-ret′-in-ȧl) *adj* within the retina.

intraserosal (in-trȧ-sėr-ōs′-ȧl) *adj* within a serous membrane—**intraserosally** *adv*.

intra·spinal (in-trȧ-spī′-nȧl) *adj* within the spinal canal—**intraspinally** *adv*.

intra·splenic (in-trȧ-splen′-ik) *adj* within the spleen.

intra·synovial (in-trȧ-sin-ō′-vē-ȧl) *adj* within a synovial membrane or cavity—**intrasynovially** *adv*.

intra·thecal (in-trȧ-thē′-kȧl) *adj* within the meninges; into the subarachnoid space—**intrathecally** *adv*.

intra·thoracic (in-trȧ-thōr-as′-ik) *adj* within the cavity of the thorax.

intra·tracheal (in-trȧ-trā′-kē-ȧl) *adj* within the trachea—**intratracheally** *adv*.

intratumor (in-tra-tū′-mor) *adj* within a tumor.

intra·uterine (in-trȧ-ū′-tėr-in) *adj* within the uterus. *intrauterine contraceptive device (IUCD, IUD)* a device which is implanted in the cavity of the uterus to prevent conception. Its exact mode of action is not known. There are over 60 different forms known by the International Planned Parenthood Federation. *intrauterine growth retardation (IUGR)* associated with a poor delivery of maternal blood to the placental bed, diminished placental exchange or a poor fetal transfer from the placental area. Serial ultrasonography is beneficial in high-risk mothers.

intra·vaginal (in-trȧ-vag′-in-ȧl) *adj* within the vagina—**intravaginally** *adv*.

intra·vascular (in-trȧ-vas′-kū-lar) *adj* within the blood vessels—**intravascularly** *adv*.

intra·venous (in-trȧ-vē′-nus) *adj* within or into a vein—**intravenously** *adv*. *intravenous infusion* commonly referred to as a 'drip'; the closed administration of fluids from a containing vessel into a vein for such purposes as hydrating the body, correcting electrolytic imbalance or introducing nutrients, *intravenous injection* the introduction of drugs, including anesthetics, into a vein. It is not a continuous procedure.

intra·ventricular (in-trȧ-ven-trik′-ū-lar) *adj* within a ventricle, especially a cerebral ventricle.

intrin·sic (in-trin′-sik) *adj* inherent or inside; from within, real; natural. *intrinsic factor* a protein released by gastric glands, essential for the satisfactory absorption of the extrinsic factor vitamin B_{12}.

in·troitus (in-trō′-it-us) *n* any opening in the body; an entrance to a cavity, particuarly the vagina.

intro·jection (in-trō-jek′-shun) *n* a mental process whereby a person incorporates another person's or group's standards and values into his own personality.

intro·spection (in-trō-spek'-shun) *n* study by a person of his own mental processes. Seen in an exaggerated form in schizophrenia*.

intro·version (in'-trō-vèr-shun) *n* the direction of thoughts and interest inwards to the world of ideas, instead of outwards to the external world.

intro·vert (in'-trō-vèrt) *n* an individual whose characteristic interests and modes of behavior are directed inwards to the self. ⇒ extravert *opp.*

intu·bation (in-tū-bā'-shun) *n* insertion of a tube into a hollow organ. Tracheal intubation is used during anesthesia to maintain an airway and to permit suction of the respiratory tract. *duodenal intubation* a double tube is passed as far as the pyloric antrum under fluoroscopy. The inner tube is then passed along to the duodenojejunal flexure. Barium sulfate suspension can then be passed to outline the small bowel.

intussus·ception (in-tus-sus-sep'-shun) *n* a condition in which one part of the bowel telescopes into another, causing severe colic and intestinal obstruction. It occurs most commonly in infants around the time of weaning.

intussus·ceptum (in-tus-sus-sep'-tum) *n* the invaginated portion of an intussusception.

intussus·cipiens (in-tus-sus-sip'-ē-ens) *n* the receiving portion of an intussusception.

inunc·tion (in-ungk'-shun) *n* the act of rubbing an oily or fatty substance into the skin.

invagin·ation (in-vaj-in-ā'-shun) *n* the act or condition of being ensheathed; a pushing inward, forming a pouch—**invaginate** *vt.*

in·vasion (in-vā'-zhun) *n* the entry of bacteria into the body.

Inversine (in'-vèr-sēn) *n* proprietary name for mecamylamine*.

inver·sion (in-vèr'-shun) *n* turning inside out, as inversion of the uterus. ⇒ procidentia.

inver·tase (in'-vèr-tās) *n* (*syn* β-fructofuranosidase) a sugar-splitting enzyme in intestinal juice.

in vitro (in vē'-trō) in glass, as in a test tube. *in vitro fertilization* (*IVF*) human ova are fertilized in test tubes in laboratories which are specialized in this technique.

in vivo (in vē'-vo) in living tissue.

invo·lucrum (in-vol-ū'-krum) *n* a sheath of new bone, which forms around necrosed bone, in such conditions as osteomyelitis. ⇒ cloaca.

invol·untary (in-vol'-un-tàr-ē) *adj* independent of the will, as muscle of the thoracic and abdominal organs.

invol·ution (in-vol-ū'-shun) *n* **1** the normal shrinkage of an organ after fulfilling its functional purpose, e.g. uterus after labor. **2** in psychiatry, the period of decline after middle life. ⇒ subinvolution—**involutional** *adj.*

iod·ides (ī'-ō-dīdz) *npl* compounds of iodine and a base. Potassium* iodide and sodium* iodide are the most common medicinal iodides.

iod·ine (ī'-ō-dīn) *n* powerful antiseptic used as a tincture for skin preparation and emergency treatment of small wounds. The solution must be fresh as it can become contaminated with *Pseudomonas aeruginosa.* Orally it is antithyroid, i.e. it decreases release of the hormones from the thyroid gland. *povidone iodine* ⇒ povidone. *radioactive iodine* ⇒ radioactive.

iod·ism (ī'-ō-dizm) *n* poisoning by iodine* or iodides*; the symptoms are those of a common cold and the appearance of a rash.

iod·ized oil (ī'-ō-dīzed) poppy-seed oil containing 40% of organically combined iodine. Should be colorless or pale yellow; darker solutions have decomposed. Used as contrast agent in X-ray examination of bronchial tract, sinuses and other cavities.

iodo·form (ī-ō'-dō-fōrm) *n* an antiseptic iodine compound of yellow color and characteristic odor. Now used chiefly as BIPP*.

iodop·sin (ī-ō-dop'-sin) *n* a protein substance which, within vitamin A, is a constituent of visual purple present in the rods in the retina of the eye.

ion (ī'-on) *n* a charged atom or radical. In electrolysis, ions in solution pass to one or the other pole, or electrode—**ionic** *adj. ion exchange resins* high molecular weight insoluble polymers with the ability to exchange its attached ions for other ions in the surrounding solution. When administered orally: (a) cation exchange resins restrict intestinal absorption (b) anion exchange resins are used as antacids in the treatment of ulcers.

ionamin (ī-ō'-nȧ-min) *n* proprietary name for phentermine*.

ionto·phoresis (ī-on-tō-fōr-ēs′-is) *n* (*syn* iontherapy) treatment whereby ions of various soluble salts (e.g. zinc, chlorine, iodine, histamine) are introduced into the tissues by means of a constant electrical current; a form of electro-osmosis.

ioniza·tion (ī-on-īz-ā′-shun) *n* 1 the dissociation of a substance in solution into ions. 2 iontophoresis*.

iopan·oic acid (ī-ō-pan-ō′-ik as′-id) a complex iodine derivative of butyric acid, used as a contrast agent in cholecystography. Side reactions are few. (Telepaque.).

IPD *abbr* intermittent peritoneal dialysis.

ipecac (ip′-i-kak) *n* dried root of the ipecacuanha plant from Brazil and other South American countries. Principal alkaloid is emetine*. Has expectorant properties and is widely used in acute branchitis and relief of dry cough. A safe emetic in larger doses.

IPPB *abbr* intermittent positive pressure breathing ⇒ positive pressure ventilation.

ipron·iazid (īp-rō-nī′-à-zid) *n* antidepressant.

ipsi·lateral (ip-si-lat′-èr-al) *adj* on the same side—**ipsilaterally** *adv.*

IQ *abbr* intelligence* quotient.

iridec·tomy (ir-id-ek′-to-mē) *n* excision of a part of the iris, thus forming an artificial pupil.

iriden-cleisis (ir-id-en-klī′-sis) *n* an older type of filtering operation. Scleral incision made at angle of anterior chamber; meridian cut in iris; either one or both pillars are left in scleral wound to contract as scar tissue. Decreases intraocular tension in glaucoma*.

irid·ium (ir-id′-ē-um) *n* implants of this metallic element are being tried as treatment for early breast cancer.

irido·cele (ir-id′-ō-sēl) *n* (*syn* iridoptosis) protrusion of part of the iris through a corneal wound (prolapsed iris).

irido·cyclitis (ir-id-ō-sī-klī′-tis) *n* inflammation of the iris* and ciliary* body.

irido·dialysis (ir-id-ō-dī-al′-is-is) *n* a separation of the iris from its ciliary attachment.

irido·plegia (ir-id-ō-plē′-jē-à) *n* paralysis of the iris.

iridop·tosis (ir-id-op-tō′-sis) *n* ⇒ iridocele.

iri·dotomy (ir-id-ot′-o-mē) *n* an incision into the iris.

iris (ī′-ris) *n* the circular colored membrane forming the anterior one-sixth of the middle coat of the eyeball (⇒ Figure 15). It is perforated in the center by an opening, the pupil. Contraction of its muscle fibers regulates the amount of light entering the eyes. *iris bombe* bulging forward of the iris due to pressure of the aqueous* behind, when posterior synechiae are present around the pupil.

iritis (ī-rī′-tis) *n* inflammation of the iris.

iron glu·conate (ī′-ron gloo̅′-kon-āt) an organic salt of iron, less irritant and better tolerated than ferrous sulfate.

irre·ducible (ir-rē-du′-si-bl) *adj* unable to be brought to desired condition. *irreducible hernia* ⇒ hernia.

irri·table (ir′-it-à-bl) *adj* capable of being excited to activity; responding easily to stimuli—**irritability** *n. irritable bowel syndrome* unusual motility of both small and large bowel which produces discomfort and intermittent pain, for which no organic cause can be found.

irri·tant (ir′-it-ant) *adj, n* describes any agent which causes irritation.

is·chemia (is-kē′-mē-à) *n* deficient blood supply to any part of the body. ⇒ angine. Volkmann—**ischemic** *adj.*

is·chemic heart dis·ease (is-kē′-mik) deficient blood supply to cardiac muscle causes central chest pain of varying intensity which may radiate to arms and jaws. The lumen of the blood vessels is usually narrowed by atheromatous plaques. If treatment with vasodilator drugs is unsuccessful, by-pass surgery may be considered. ⇒ angina pectoris, myocardial infarction.

is·chiorectal (is-kē-ō-rek′-tàl) *adj* pertaining to the ischium and the rectum, as an ischiorectal abscess which occurs between these two structures.

is·chium (is′-kē-um) *n* the lower part of the innominate bone of the pelvis; the bone on which the body rests when sitting—**ischial** *adj.*

Islands of Langer·hans (ī′-lands of lǎng′-ėr-hanz) collections of special cells scattered throughout the pancreas. They secrete insulin which is absorbed directly into the blood stream.

Ismelin (is′-mel-in) *n* proprietary name for guanethidine.

iso·carboxazid (ī-sō-kär-boks′-à-zid) *n* an antidepressant. (Marplan.)

isoetharine (ī-sō-eth′-à-rēn) *n* a smooth muscle relaxant used as a bronchodilator. (Bronkosol.)

iso·immunization (ī-sō-im-mū-nī-zā′-

shun) *n* development of anti-Rh agglutins in the blood of an Rh-negative person who has been given an Rh-positive transfusion or who is carrying an Rh-positive fetus.

iso·lation (ī-sol-ā′-shun) *n* separation of a patient from others for a variety of reasons. ⇒ containment isolation, exclusion isolation, protective isolation, source isolation.

iso·lator (ī′-sol-ā-tor) *n* apparatus ranging from what is virtually a large plastic bag in which a patient can be nursed to that in which an operation can be performed. It aims to prevent bacterial entry to or exit from the enclosed space.

iso·leucine (ī-sō-lū′-sēn) *n* one of the essential amino acids.

iso·metric (ī-sō-met′-rik) of equal proportions, *isometric exercises* carried out without movement; maintain muscle tone.

ison·iazid (ī-so-nī′-à-zid) *n* a derivative of isonicotinic acid. It has a specific action against the tubercle bacillus and is widely employed in the treatment of tuberculosis. Combined treatment with other tuberculostatic drugs such as streptomycin* and PAS* is not only more effective than any drug alone, but the risk of bacterial resistance is also reduced. Can be neurotoxic, and some preparations include pyridoxine* to counteract this tendency. (Rimifon.)

iso·propamide (ī-sō--prōp′-à-mīd) *n* a drug which prevents spasm in the digestive tract and helps to reduce acid secretion in the stomach.

iso·propanal (ī-sō-prō′-pan-àl) *n* 0.5 ml of a 70% solution is used as a chemical disinfectant for hands.

isoproterenol hydrochloride (ī-sō-prō-tēr′-en-ol) an epinephrine derivative that acts on beta-adrenergic receptors to relax bronchial smooth muscle; also acts as a cardiac stimulant. (Isuprel.)

iso·tonic (ī-sō-ton′-ik) *adj* equal tension; applied to any solution which has the same osmotic pressure as blood. Also refers to muscle contraction at constant tension. *isotonic saline* (*syn* normal saline, physiological saline), 0.9% solution of salt in water.

iso·topes (ī′-sō-tōps) *npl* two or more forms of the same element having identical chemical properties and the same atomic number but different mass numbers. Those isotopes with radiative properties are used in medicine for re-

search, diagnosis and treatment of disease.

isoxu·prine (is-oks′-ū-prēn) *n* peripheral vasodilator and spasmolyic. Acts on myometrium, preventing contractions; thus useful in premature labor. (Vasodilan.)

isth·mus (is′-thmus) *n* a narrowed part of an organ or tissue such as that connecting the two lobes of the thyroid gland. *isthmus of the uterine tube* ⇒ Figure 17.

Isuprel (ī′-sū-prel) *n* proprietary name for isoproterenol hydrochloride*.

itch a sensation on the skin which makes one want to scratch. ⇒ scabies. *itch mite Sarcoptes scabiei*.

IUCD *abbr* intrauterine* contraceptive device.

IUD *abbr* intrauterine* (contraceptive) device.

IUGR *abbr* ⇒ intrauterine growth retardation.

IV *abbr* intravenous*.

IVC *abbr* inferior vena cava*.

IVF *abbr* in* vitro fertilization.

IVP *abbr* intravenous pyelography ⇒ urography.

IV push the quick injection of medication intravenously.

J

Jacksonian epi·lepsy (jak-sōn′-ē-an) ⇒ epilepsy.

Jacquemier's sign (zhak′-mē-ās) blueness of the vaginal mucosa seen in early pregnancy.

Jakob-Creutzfeldt dis·ease (jā′-kob krutz′-feld) a recognized form of presenile dementia*.

Janimine (jan′-i-mīn) *n* proprietary name for imipramine hydrochloride*.

jaun·dice (jawn′-dis) *n* (*syn* icterus) a condition characterized by a raised bilirubin level in the blood (hyperbilirubinemia). Minor degrees are only detectable chemically. *latent jaundice*, major degrees are visible in the yellow skin, sclerae and mucosae. *overt* or *clinical jaundice*. Jaundice may be due to (a) obstruction anywhere in the biliary tract (*obstructive jaundice*) (b) excessive hemoloysis of red blood cells (*hemolytic jaundice*) (c) toxic or infective damage of liver cells (*hepatocellular jaundice*) (d) bile stasis (*cholestatic jaundice*). *acholuric jaun-*

dice (*syn* spherocytosis*) jaundice without bile in the urine. *infective jaundice* most commonly due to a virus; infective hepatitis*. *leptospiral jaundice* ⇒ Weil's disease. *malignant jaundice* acute diffuse necrosis of the liver *jaundice of the newborn* icterus* gravis neonatorum.

jaw·bone (jaw'-bōn) *n* either the maxilla (upper jaw) or mandible (lower jaw).

je·junal bi·opsy (je-jōō'-nal bī'-op-sē) *n* a test used in the diagnosis of celiac disease, a tube is passed through the child's mouth and into the jejunum. At the end of the tube is a small capsule—a Crosby capsule—which contains a blade. The small piece of jejunal mucosa which is removed is then sent for histological and enzyme examinations.

jejun·ostomy (je-jōōn-os'-to-mē) *n* a surgically made fistula between the jejunum and the anterior abdominal wall; used temporarily for feeding in cases where passage of food through the stomach is impossible or undesirable.

je·junum (je-jōō'-num) *n* that part of the small intestine between the duodenum* and the ileum*. It is about 2.44 m in length—**jejunal** *adj*.

jig·ger (jig'-ger) *n* a flea. *Tunga penetrans*, prevalent in the tropics. It burrows under the skin to lay its eggs, causing intense irritation. Secondary infection is usual.

joint *n* the articulation of two or more bones (arthrosis). There are three main classes: (a) fibrous (synarthrosis), e.g. the sutures of the skull (b) cartilaginous (*syn* chondrosis), e.g. between the manubrium and the body of the sternum and (c) synovial, e.g. elbow or hip. ⇒ Charcot's joint.

joint-breaker fever o'nyong-nyong* fever.

joule (jūl) *n* the SI unit for measuring energy, work and quantity of heat. The unit (J) is the energy expended when 1 kg (kilogram) is moved 1 m (meter) by a force of 1 N (newton). The kilojoule (kJ = 10^3 J) and the megajoule (MJ = 10^6 J) are used by physiologists and nutritionists for measuring large amounts of energy.

jugu·lar (jug'-ū-lar) *adj* pertaining to the throat. *jugular veins* two veins passing down either side of the neck (⇒ Figure 10).

junk food a term used to describe convenience foods with added chemicals, e.g. monosodium* glutamate.

junket (jun'-ket) *n* milk predigested by the addition of rennet*; curds and whey.

juxta·pose (juks-tà-pōz') *vt* to place side by side.

K

Kahn test (kan) a serological test for the diagnosis of syphilis*. The patient's serum reacts with a heterologous antigen prepared from mammalian tissue; flocculation occurs if syphilitic antibodies are present.

kala·azar (kà-là-az'-ar) *n* a generalized form of leishmaniasis* occurring in the tropics. There is anemia, fever, splenomegaly and wasting. It is caused by the parasite *Leishmania donovani* and is spread by sandflies.

kan·amycin (kan-à-mī'-sin) *n* a streptomycin*-like antibiotic with basically similar actions and neurotoxic properties.

Kanner's syn·drome (kan'-erz) autism*.

kao·lin (kā'-ō-lin) *n* natural aluminum silicate. When given orally it absorbs toxic substances, hence useful in diarrhea, colitis and food poisoning. Also used as a dusting powder; when mixed with glycerin* boric* acid, etc. it is used as a poultice.

Kaopectate (kā-ō-pek'-tāt) *n* an antidiarrhea compound containing kaolin and pectin.

Kaposi's dis·ease (kà-pō'-sēz) ⇒ xeroderma.

Kaposi's sar·coma (kà-pō'-sēz sàr-kō'-mà) *n* a malignant, multifocal neoplasm of reticuloendothelial cells. It first appears as brown or purple patches on the feet and spreads on the skin, metastasizing on the lymph nodes and viscera. Currently of interest because it can complicate acquired* immune deficiency syndrome.

Kaposi's varicelli·form erup·tion (kà-pō'-sēz vàr-i-sel'-i-fōrm ē-rup'-shun) occurs in eczematous children. Generalized bullous eczema; formerly fatal.

karyo·type (kār'-ē-ō-tīp) *n* creation of an orderly array of chromosomes, usually derived from the study of cultured cells. This is usually done for diagnostic purposes on abnormal persons, or persons prone to produce chromosomally abnormal children, or for the prenatal detection of fetal abnormality in women at risk of producing chromosomally abnormal fetuses, for example because of advancing age.

katab·olism (kà-tab'-o-lizm) *n* ⇒ catabolism.

Kay Ciel (kā-sēl) proprietary name for for potassium chloride*.

Keflex (kef'-leks) *n* proprietary name for cephalexin* monohydrate.

Kegel exercises (ke'-gel) exercises for strengthening the female pelvic floor muscles.

Keller's opera·tion (kel'-lèrz) for hallux* valgus or rigidus. Excision of the proximal half of the proximal phalanx, plus any osteophytes and exostoses on the metatarsal head. The toe is fixed in the corrected position; after healing a pseudarthrosis results.

Kell factor a blood group factor found in about 10% of caucasians; inherited according to Mendelian laws of inheritance. Anti-Kell antibodies can cross the placenta.

Kelly-Paterson syn·drome (kel'-lē pat'-èr-son) ⇒ Plummer-Vinson syndrome.

kel·oid (kē'-loyd) *n* an overgrowth of scar tissue, which may produce a contraction deformity. Keloid scarring occurs in some black skins; it tends to get progressively worse.

Kema·drin (kem'-à-drin) *n* proprietary name for procyclidine*.

Kenalog (ken'-à-log) *n* proprietary name for triamcinolone*.

kera·tectomy (ke-rà-tek'-to-mē) *n* surgical excision of a portion of the cornea.

kera·tin (kèr'-à-tin) *n* a protein found in all horny tissue. Once used to coat pills given for their intestinal effect, since keratin can withstand gastric juice.

keratiniz·ation (ker-àt-in-īz-ā'-shun) *n* conversion into horny tissue. Occurs as a pathological process in vitamin A deficiency.

kera·titic precipi·tates (KP) (ke-rà-ti'-tik prē-sip'-i-tates) large cells adherent to the posterior surface of the cornea*; present in inflammation of iris, ciliary body and choroid.

kera·titis (ker-àt-ī'-tis) *n* inflammation of the cornea*.

kerato·conjuncti·vitis (ker'-à-tō-kon-jungk-tiv-ī'-tis) *n* inflammation of the cornea and conjunctiva. *epidemic keratoconjunctivitis* due to an adenovirus. Present as an acute follicular conjunctivitis with pre-auricular and submaxillary

adenitis. *keratoconjunctivitis sicca* ⇒ Sjogren syndrome.

kerato·conus (ker-à-tō-kō'-nus) *n* a cone-like protrusion of the cornea, usually due to a non-inflammatory thinning.

kerato·iritis (ker-à-tō-ī-rī'-tis) *n* inflammation of the cornea and iris.

kerato·lytic (ker-à-tō-li'-tik) *adj* having the property of breaking down keratinized epidermis.

kera·toma (ker-à-tō'-mà) *n* ⇒ callosity*—**keratomata** *pl*.

kerato·malacia (ker-à-tō-mal-ā'-sē-à) *n* softening of the cornea; ulceration may occur; frequently caused by lack of vitamin A.

kera·tome (ker'-à-tōm) *n* a special knife with a trowel-like blade for incising the cornea.

kera·topathy (ker-à-top'-à-thē) *n* any disease of the cornea—**keratopathic** *adj*.

kerato·phakia (ker-à-tō-fāk'-ē-à) *n* surgical introduction of a biological 'lens' into the cornea to correct hypermetropia.

kerato·plasty (ker-à-tō-plas'-tē) *n* ⇒ corneal graft—**keratoplastic** *adj*.

kera·tosis (ker-à-tō'-sis) *n* thickening of the horny layer of the skin. Also referred to as hyperkeratosis. Has the appearance of warty excrescences. *keratosis palmaris et plantaris* (*syn* tylosis) a congenital thickening of the horny layer of the palms and soles.

ker·ion (kē'-rē-on) *n* a boggy suppurative mass of the scalp associated with ringworm* of the hair.

kernic·terus (kèr-nik'-tèr-us) *n* bile staining of the basal ganglia in the brain which may result in mental deficiency; it occurs in icterus* gravis neonatorum.

Kernig's sign (ker'-nigs) inability to straighten the leg at the knee joint when the thigh is flexed at right angles to the trunk. Occurs in meningitis.

Ket·alar (ket'-à-lar) *n* proprietary name for ketamine*.

keta·mine (ket'-à-mēn) *n* intravenous or intramuscular analgesic-anesthetic agent. Initial dose determined by patient's weight. Does not have muscular relaxation properties and is therefore unsuitable for intra-abdominal procedures. May cause hallucinations; postoperative absence of disturbance is important. (Ketalar.)

keto·acidosis (kē-tō-as-id-ōs'-is) *n* acidosis due to accumulation of ketones, in-

161

termediary products in the metabolism of fat—**ketoacidotic** *adj*.

ketoconazole (kē-tō-kon′-à-zōl) *n* an antifungal agent. (Nizoral.)

keto·genic diet (kē-tō-jen′-ik) a high fat content producing ketosis (acidosis).

keto·nemia (kē-tŏn-ē′-mē-à) *n* ketone bodies in the blood—**ketonemic** *adj*.

ke·tones (kē′-tōns) *n* organic compounds (e.g. ketosteroids) containing the carbonyl group. C = 0, whose carbon atom occurs within a carbon chain. *ketone bodies* (*syn* acetone bodies) a term which includes acetone, acetoacetic acid and β-hydroxybutyric acid. ⇒ diabetes mellitus.

keto·nuria (kē-tō-nū′-rē-à) *n* ketone bodies in the urine—**ketonuric** *adj*.

keto·profen (kē-tō-prō′-fen) *n* an analgesic anti-inflammatory drug which is useful in arthritic and rheumatoid conditions. (Orudis.)

ket·osis (kē-tō′-sis) *n* clinical picture arises from accumulation in blood stream of ketone bodies, β-hydroxybutyric acid, acetoacetic acid and acetone. Syndrome includes drowsiness, headache and deep respiration—**ketotic** *adj*.

keto·steroids (kē-tō-ste′-royds) *npl* steroid hormones which contain a keto group, formed by the addition of an oxygen molecule to the basic ring structure. The 17-ketosteroids (which have this oxygen at carbon-17) are excreted in normal urine and are present in excess in overactivity of the adrenal glands and the gonads.

kid·ney (kid′-nē) *n* a gland situated one on either side of the vertebral column in the upper posterior abdominal cavity (⇒ Figures 19, 20). Its main function is secretion of urine* which flows into the ureters*. It secretes renin* and renal* erythropoietic factor. *horseshoe kidney* an anatomical variation in which the inner lower border of each kidney is joined to give a horseshoe shape. Usually symptomless and only rarely interferes with drainage of urine into ureters. *kidney failure* ⇒ renal failure. *kidney machine* ⇒ dialyzer. *kidney transplant* surgical transplantation of a kidney from a previously tested suitable live donor or one who has recently died. Kidneys may also be transplanted from the renal bed to other sites in the same individual in cases of ureteric disease or trauma. *kidney function tests* various tests are available for measuring renal function. All require careful collection of urine

specimens. Those in common use are para-aminohippuric acid clearance test for measuring renal blood flow; creatinine clearance test for measuring glomerular filtration rate; ammonium chloride test for measuring tubular ability to excrete hydrogen ions; urinary concentration and dilution tests for measuring tubular function. ⇒ indigocarmine, idigocarmine.

Kielland forceps (kē′-land fŏr′-seps) obstetrical forceps with a short handle that has a sliding joint to allow one blade to move over the other.

Killian's oper·ation (kil′-lē-anz) curetting of the mucosa of the frontal sinus, leaving the supraorbital ridge intact to reduce deformity.

Kimmelstiel-Wilson syn·drome (Kim′-el-stēl wil′-son) intercapillary glomerulosclerosis* develops in diabetics, who have hypertension, albuminuria and edema.

kin·ase (kī′-nās) *n* an enzyme activator which converts a zymogen to its active form; enzymes which catalyze the transfer of a high-energy group of a donor, usually adenosine triphosphate, to some acceptor, usually named after the acceptor (e.g. fructokinase).

kine·plastic surgery (kī-nē-plas′-tik) operative measures, whereby certain muscle groups are isolated and utilized to work certain modified prostheses.

kinesthesis (kin-es-thē′-sis) *n* muscle sense; perception of movement—**kinesthetic**, *adj*.

kin·etic (kin-et′-ik) *adj* pertaining to or producing motion.

Kirschner wire (kirsch′-nèr) a wire drilled into a bone to apply skeletal traction. A hand or electric drill is used, a stirrup is attached and the wire is rendered taut by means of a special wire-tightener.

kiss of life ⇒ resuscitation.

Klebcil (kleb′-sil) *n* proprietary name for kanamycin*.

Klebsiella (kleb-sē-el′-à) *n* genus of bacteria. *Klebsiella pneumoniae* is the cause of a rare form of severe pneumonia resulting in tissue necrosis and abscess formation.

Klebs-Loeffler bacil·lus (klebs lef′-lèr) *Corynebacterium* diphtheriae.

klepto·mania (klep-tō-mā′-nē-à) *n* compulsive stealing due to mental disturbance, usually of the obsessional neurosis type—**kleptomaniac** *n. adj*.

Klinefelter syn·drome (klīn′-fel-tèr) a

chromosomal abnormality affecting boys, usually with 47 chromosomes including XXY sex chromosomes. Puberty is frequently delayed, with small firm testes, often with gynecomastia. Associated with sterility, which may be the only symptom.

Klumpke's paral·ysis (kloomp'-kēz) paralysis and atrophy of muscles of the forearm and hand, with sensory and pupillary disturbances due to injury to lower roots of brachial plexus and cervical sympathetic nerves. Clawhand results.

knee (nē) *n* the hinge joint formed by the lower end of the femur and the head of the tibia. *kneecap* the patella*. *knee jerk* a reflex contraction of the relaxed quadriceps muscle elicited by a tap on the patellar tendon; usually performed with the lower femur supported behind, the knee bent and the leg limp. Persistent variation from normal usually signifies organic nervous disorder.

knee-chest position ⇒ genupectoral position, *syn*.

knuckles (nuk'-ls) *npl* the dorsal aspect of any of the joints between the phalanges and the metacarpal bones, or between the phalanges.

Koch's bacil·lus (kōks) *Mycobacterium* *tuberculosis*.

Koch·Weeks bacil·lus (kōk-wēks) *Haemophilus* *aegyptius*.

Köhler's dis·ease (ka'-lerz) osteochondritis* of the havicular bone. Confined to children of 3–5 years.

koil·onychia (koyl-o-nik'-ē-à) *n* spoon-shaped nails, characteristic of iron deficiency anemia.

Konakion (ko-nak'-ē-on) *n* proprietary name for phytonadione*.

Koplik's spots (kop'-liks) small white spots inside the mouth, during the first few days of the invasion (prodromal) stage of measles.

Korsakoff psy·chosis, syn·drome (kōr'-sà-kof sī-kō'-sis) alcoholic dementia; polyneuritic psychosis. A condition which follows delirium and toxic states. Often due to alcoholism. The consciousness is clear and alert, but the patient is disorientated for time and place. His memory is grossly impaired, especially for recent events. Often he confabulates to fill the gaps in his memory; afflicts more men than women in the 45–55 age group.

kosher (kō'-shèr) *adj* food handled in compliance with Jewish dietary laws.

KP *abbr* keratitic* precipitates.

Krabbe disease (krab) genetically determined degenerative disease of the central nervous system associated with mental subnormality.

kraurosis vulvae (kraw-rō'-sis vul'-vē) a degenerative condition of the vaginal introitus associated with postmenopausal lack of estrogen.

Kreb's cycle (krebs) citric acid cycle. A series of reactions in which a two carbon substance is oxidized to form carbon dioxide and water; the end product of the metabolism of carbohydrates, fats and proteins, producing energy as an end result.

Kreiselman bed (krī'-sel-man) a receiving bed used for newborns in delivery rooms. Allows for lowering of the infant's head, contains suction apparatus, oxygen, and provides heat.

Krukenberg tu·mor (Kruk'-en-berg) a secondary malignant tumor of the ovary. The primary growth is usually in the stomach.

Küntscher nail (kunt'-sker) used for intramedullary fixation of fractured long bones, especially the femur. The nail has a 'clover-leaf' cross-section.

kuru (koo'-roo) *n* slow virus disease of central nervous system. Probably transmitted by cannibalism. Rare and declining in incidence. Occurred exclusively among New Guinea highlanders.

kwashi·orkor (kwash-ē-ōr'-kor) *n* a nutritional disorder of infants and young children when the diet is persistently deficient in essential protein; commonest where maize is the staple diet. Characteristic features are anemia, wasting, dependent edema and a fatty liver. Untreated, it progresses to death. Aflatoxin* has been found at postmortem in people who died from kwashiorkor.

Kwell (kwel) *n* proprietary name for gammabenzene hexachloride*.

KY jelly a proprietary mucilaginous lubricating jelly.

kymo·graph (kī'-mō-graf) *n* an apparatus for recording movements, e.g. of muscles, columns of blood. Used in physiological experiments—**kymographic** *adj*, **kymographically** *adv*.

kyphol·ordosis (kī-fō-lor-dō'-sis) *n* coexistence of kyphosis* and lordosis*.

kypho·scoliosis (kī-fō-skō-lē-ō'-sis) *n* co-existence of kyphosis* and scoliosis*.

ky·phosis (kī-fō'-sis) *n* as in Pott's* disease, an excessive backward curvature of the dorsal spine—**kyphotic** *adj*.

L

labet·alol (la-bet'ȧ-lol) *n* a combined alpha-beta-blocking drug given by i.v. infusion in the control of acute severe hypertension*. Also given orally in hypertension.

labia (lā'-bē-ȧ) *npl* lips. *labia majora* two large liplike folds extending from the mons veneris to encircle the vagina *labia minora* two smaller folds lying within the labia majora—**labium** *sing,* **labial** *adj.*

labile (lā'-bīl) *adj* unstable; readily changed, as many drugs when in solution; and blood pressure.

la·bility (la-bil'-it-ē) *n* instability. *emotional lability* rapid change in mood. Occurs especially in the mental disorders of old age.

labio·glosso·laryngeal (lā'-bē-ō-glos-ō-lār-in'-jē-al) *adj* relating to the lips, tongue and larynx. *labioglossolaryngeal paralysis* a nervous disease characterized by progressive paralysis of the lips, tongue and larynx.

labio·glosso·pharyngeal (lā'-bē-ō-glos-ō-far-in'-jē-al) *adj* relating to the lips, tongue and pharynx.

labor (lā'-bor) *n* (*syn* parturition) the act of giving birth to a child. The first stage lasts from onset until there is full dilation of the cervical os; the second stage lasts until the baby is delivered; the third stage until the placenta is expelled.

labyr·inth (lab'-i-rinth) *n* the tortuous cavities of the internal ear. *bony labyrinth* that part which is directly hollowed out of the temporal bone. *membranous labyrinth* the membrane which loosely lines the bony labyrinth—**labyrinthine** *adj.*

labyrin·thectomy (lab-i-rinth-ek'-to-mē) *n* surgical removal of part or the whole of the membranous labyrinth of the internal ear. Sometimes carried out for Ménière's disease.

labyrin·thitis (lab-i-rinth-ī'-tis) *n* inflammation of the internal ear.

lacer·ated wound (las'-er-ā-ted) one in which the tissues are torn usually by a blunt instrument or pressure: likely to become infected and to heal by second intention. ⇒ healing.

lachry·mal (lak'-ri-mal) *adj* ⇒ lacrimal.

lacri·mal, lachry·mal, lacry·mal (lak'-ri-mal) *adj* pertaining to tears. *lacrimal bone* a tiny bone at the inner side of the orbital cavity. *lacrimal duct* connects lacrimal gland to upper conjunctival sac.

lacrimal gland situated above the upper, outer canthus of the eye. ⇒ dacryocyst.

lacri·mation (lak-ri-mā'-shun) *n* an outflow of tears; weeping.

lacrimo·nasal (lak-ri-mō-nā'-zal) *adj* pertaining to the lacrimal and nasal bones and ducts.

lacry·mal (lak'-ri-mal) *n* ⇒ lacrimal.

lacta·gogue (lak'-tȧ-gog) *n* any substance given to stimulate lactation.

lact·albumin (lak-tal-bū'-min) *n* the more easily digested of the two milk proteins. ⇒ caseinogen.

lac·tase (lak'-tās) *n* (*syn* β-galactosidase) a saccharolytic enzyme of intestinal juice; it splits lactose* into glucose* (dextrose) and galactose*. *lactase deficiency* the clinical syndrome of milk sugar intolerance. In severe congenital intolerance the infant may pass a liter or more of fluid stool per day. Temporary intolerance can follow neonatal alimentary tract obstructions, but rarely gives long-term problems. In non-Caucasian races a degree of intolerance develops at weaning.

lac·tate de·hydrogenase (LDH) (lak'-tāt dē-hī-dro'-jen-ās) *n* (*syn* lactic dehydrogenase) an enzyme, of which there are five versions (isozymes), that catalyzes the interconversion of lactate and pyruvate. LDH-1 is the one found in the heart; its blood level rises rapidly when heart tissues die, e.g. after a myocardial infarction. After heart transplant, rejection is imminent when the LDH-1 activity is greater than that of its isozyme LDH-2 during the first four postoperative weeks. After 6 months this diagnostic indicator disappears. *lactate dehydrogenase test* when tissue of high metabolic activity dies the ensuing tissue necrosis is quickly reflected by an increase of the serum enzyme lactate dehydrogenase.

lac·tation (lak-tā'-shun) *n* **1** secretion of milk. **2** the period during which the child is nourished from the breast.

lac·teals (lak'-tē-als) *npl* the commencing lymphatic ducts in the intestinal villi; they absorb split fats and convey them to the receptaculum chyli.

lac·tic acid (lak'-tik as'-id) the acid that causes the souring of milk. It is obtained by the fermentation of lactose*; used as a vaginal douche, 1%. Sometimes added to milk to produce fine curds for the treatment of gastroenteritis in infants.

lactifer·ous (lak-tif'-ėr-us) *adj* conveying or secreting milk.

lactifuge (lak'-ti-fūj) *n* any agent which suppresses milk secretion.

Lacto·bacillus (lak'-tō-bà-sil'-us) *n* a genus of bacteria. A large Gram-positive rod which is active in fermenting carbohydrates, producing acid. No members are pathogenic.

lactoflavin (lak'-tō-flā-vin) *n* riboflavin*.

lacto·genic (lak-tō-jen'-ik) *adj* stimulating milk production.

lac·tometer (lak-to'-me-tèr) *n* an instrument for measuring the specific gravity of milk.

lac·tose (lak'-tōs) *n* milk sugar, a disaccharide of glucose* and galactose*. Less soluble and less sweet than ordinary sugar. Used in infant feeding to increase the carbohydrate content of diluted cow's milk. In some infants the gut is intolerant to lactose. ⇒ lactase.

lact·osuria (lak-tō-sū'-rē-à) *n* lactose in the urine—**lactosuric** *adj*.

lac·tulose (lak'-tū-lōs) *n* a sugar which is not metabolized so that it reaches the colon unchanged. Sugar-splitting bacteria then act on it, promoting a softer stool. (Cephulac, Chronulac.)

lac·una (là-kū'-nà) *n* a space between cells; usually used in the description of bone—**lacunae** *pl, lacunar adj.*

Laetrile (Lā'-e-tril) *n* amygdalin, a glycoside, vitamin B-17, with no known therapeutic benefit. Contains cyanide so can be poisonous.

laked blood (lākd) ⇒ blood.

Lamaze method of childbirth (la-maz') psychoprophylactic method of childbirth preparation. The woman and her partner are taught physical and mental techniques to help deal with childbirth.

lam·bliasis (lam-blī'-à-sis) *n* ⇒ giardiasis.

la·mella (là-mel'-à) *n* **1** a thin plate-like scale or partition. **2** a gelatin-coated disc containing a drug; it is inserted under the eyelid—**lamellae** *pl, lamellar adj.*

lam·ina (lam'-in-à) *n* a thin plate or layer, usually of bone—**laminae** *pl.*

lamin·ectomy (lam-in-ek'-to-mē) *n* removal of vertebral laminae—to expose the spinal cord nerve roots and meninges. Most often performed in the lumbar region, for removal of degenerated invertebral disc.

Lance·field's groups (lans'-fēlds) subdivision of the genus *Streptococcus* on the basis of antigenic structure. The members of each group have a characteristic capsular polysaccharide. The most dangerous streptococci of epidemiological importance to man belong to Group A.

Landry's paral·ysis (lan'-drēz) an acute ascending condition accompanied by fever; it may terminate in respiratory stasis and death. ⇒ paralysis.

lano·lin (lan'-ō-lin) *n* (*syn* adeps lanae hydrosus) wool fat containing 30% water. *Anhydrous lanolin* is that fat obtained from sheep's wool. Used in ointment bases, as such bases can form water-in-oil emulsions with aqueous constituents, and are readily absorbed by the skin. Contact sensitivity to lanolin products may occur.

Lanoxin (lan-oks'-in) *n* proprietary name for digoxin*.

la·nugo (lan-ū'-gō) *n* the soft, downy hair sometimes present on newborn infants, especially when they are premature. Usually replaced before birth by vellus hair.

lapar·oscopy (lap-ar-os'-ko-pē) *n* (*syn* peritoneoscopy) endoscopic examination of the pelvic organs by the transperitoneal route. A laparoscope is introduced through the abdominal wall after induction of a pneumoperitoneum*. It is done for biopsy, aspiration of cysts and division of adhesions. Tubal ligation for sterilization and even ventrosuspension can be performed via the laparoscope—**laparoscopic** *adj,* **laparoscopically** *adv.*

lapar·otomy (lap-ar-ot'-o-mē) *n* incision of the abdominal wall. Usually reserved for exploratory operation.

Larodopa (lār-ō-dō'-pà) *n* proprietary name for levodopa*.

larva (lar'-và) *n* an embryo which is independent before it has assumed the characteristic features of its parents. *larva migrans* itching tracks in the skin with formation of blisters; caused by the burrowing of larvae of some species of fly, and the normally animal-infesting *Ancylostoma*—**larvae** *pl, larval adj.*

larvi·cide (lar'-vi-sīd) *n* any agent which destroys larvae—**larvicidal** *adj.*

lar·yngeal (lār-in-jē'-àl) *adj* pertaining to the larynx.

lar·yngectomy (lār-in-jek'-to-mē) *n* surgical removal of the larynx.

laryn·gismus stridulus (lār-in-jis'-mus strī'-dū-lus) momentary sudden attack of laryngeal spasm with a crowing sound on inspiration. It occurs in inflammation of the larynx, in connection with rickets, and as an independent disease.

laryn·gitis (lār-in-jī'-tis) *n* inflammation of the larynx.

laryngofissure (lār-in'-gō-fish'-ūr) *n* the operation of opening the larynx in midline.

laryn·gologist (lār-in-gol'-o-jist) *n* a specialist in diseases of the larynx.

laryn·gology (lār-in-gol'-o-jē) *n* the study of diseases affecting the larynx.

laryngo·paralysis (lār-in'-gō-par-al'-is-is) *n* paralysis of the larynx.

laryngo·pharyngectomy (lār-in'-gō-fār-in-jek'-to-mē) *n* excision of the larynx and lower part of pharynx.

laryngo·pharynx (lār-in-gō-fār'-ingks) *n* the lower portion of the pharynx—**laryngopharyngeal** *adj*.

laryngo·scope (lār-in'-gō-skōp) *n* instrument for exposure and visualization of larynx, for diagnostic or therapeutic purposes or during the procedure of tracheal intubation*—**larnygoscopy** *n*. **laryngoscopic** *adj*.

laryngo·spasm (lār-in'-gō-spazm) *n* convulsive involuntary muscular contraction of the larynx, usually accompanied by spasmodic closure of the glottis.

laryngo·stenosis (lar-in'-gō-sten-ōs'-is) *n* narrowing of the glottic aperture.

laryn·gotomy (lar-in-got'-o-mē) *n* the operation of opening the larynx.

laryngo·tracheal (lar-in-gō-trāk'-ē-al) *adj* pertaining to the larynx* and trachea*.

laryngo·tracheitis (lar-in-gō-trāk-ē-ī'-tis) *n* inflammation of the larynx* and trachea*.

laryngo·tracheo·bronchitis (lar-in-gō-trāk'-ē-ō-brongk-ī'-tis) *n* inflammation of the larynx*, trachea* and bronchi*.

laryngo·tracheo·plasty (lar-in'-gō-trāk'-ē-ō-plas'-tē) *n* an operation to widen a stenosed airway—**laryngotracheoplastic** *adj*.

lar·ynx (lar'-ingks) *n* the organ of voice situated below and in front of the pharynx* and at the upper end of the trachea* (⇒ Figure 6)—**laryngeal** *adj*.

Lasen syn·drome (las'-en) multiple joint dislocations.

laser (lā'-zer) *n* acronym for Light Amplification by Stimulated Emission of Radiation. Energy is transmitted as heat which can coagulate tissue. Has been used for detached retina and cancer. Precautions must be taken by those using lasers as blindness can be an occupational hazard if precautions are neglected.

Lassa fever (las'-sà) one of the viral*hemorrhagic fevers. The incubation period is 3–16 days; early symptoms resemble typhoid* and septicemia*. By the sixth day ulcers develop in the mouth and throat; fever is variable, sometimes being very high. Fatality rate in some areas is as high as 67%. Infected people must be nursed in strict isolation.

Lassar's paste (las'-sàrz) contains zinc oxide, starch and salicylic acid in soft paraffin. Used in eczema and similar conditions as an antiseptic protective.

lassitude (las'-it-ūd) *n* fatigue, exhaustion.

latent heat (lā'-tent) that heat which is used to bring about a change in state, not in temperature.

lat·eral (lat'-ér-àl) *adj* at or belonging to the side; away from the median line—**laterally** *adv*.

latissimus dorsi (lat-is'-i-mus dōr'-sī) ⇒ Figures 4, 5.

lauda·num (lawd'-a-num) *n* old name for tincture of opium*.

laugh·ing gas (laf'-ing) ⇒ nitrous oxide.

lav·age (làv-àzh') *n* irrigation of or washing out a body cavity.

laxatives (laks'-à-tivs) *n* (*syn* aperients) drugs which produce peristalsis and promote evacuation of the bowel, usually to relieve constipation. The more powerful laxatives are known as purgatives, and drastic purgatives are termed cathartics. Laxatives are further classified, either relating to the constituents or to the function, as saline, vegetable, synthetic, bulk-increasers (bulking), or lubricators (lubricants).

LDH *abbr* lactate* dehydrogenase.

L-dopa *abbr* levodopa*.

LE *abbr* lupus* erythematosus. *LE* cells characteristic cells found in patients with lupus* erythematosus.

lead (led) *n* a soft metal with toxic salts. *lead and opium* applied as a compress to relieve bruises, pain and swelling. *lead colic* ⇒ colic. *lead lotion* a weak solution of lead subacetate used as a soothing astringent lotion for sprains and bruises. *lead poisoning* (*syn* plumbism) acute poisoning is unusual, but chronic poisoning due to absorption of small amounts over a period is less uncommon. This can occur in young children by sucking articles made of lead alloys, or painted with lead paint. Where the water supply is soft, lead poisoning may occur because drinking water picks up lead from water pipes. In spite of legislation and safety precautions, industrial poisoning is still the commonest cause. Anemia, loss of appetite, and the formation of a blue line round the gums are characteristic. Nervous symptoms, including convulsions* are seen in severe cases.

Leadbetter·Politano oper·ation (led'-bet-ėr pol-it-an'-ō) an anti-reflux measure by tunnel reimplantation of ureter into urinary bladder.

leci·thins (les'-i-thins) *npl* a group of phosphoglycerides esterified with the alcohol group of choline*. Found in animal tissues, mainly in cell membranes. They are present in surfactant*. *lecithin-sphingomyelin ratio* a test which assesses fetal lung maturity. Below 2·0 is indicative of a higher risk of respiratory* distress syndrome. Cortisone can be given to stimulate maturity of the fetal lungs and so reduce the risk of respiratory distress syndrome.

leci·thinase (les'-i-thin-ās) *n* (*syn* phospholipase D) an enzyme which catalyzes the decomposition of lecithin (phosphatidylcholine) and occurs in the toxin of *Clostridium perfringens*.

leech (lēch) *n* *Hirudo medicinalis*. An aquatic worm which can be applied to the human body to suck blood. Its saliva contains hirudin*, an anticoagulant.

Lee-white clotting time a blood coagulation test, used to detect severe bleeding disorders.

Legionella haemophila (le-jun-el'-à hē-mof'-il-à) a small Gram-negative non-acid-fast bacillus which causes legionnaire's* disease and Pontiac* fever.

legion·naires' dis·ease (lē-jun-ārz') a severe and often fatal disease caused by *Legionella* *haemophilia*: there is pneumonia, dry cough, myalgia and sometimes gastrointestinal symptoms. There can be renal impairment and eventual cardiovascular collapse ⇒ Pontiac fever.

legumen (leg-ū'-men) *n* the protein present in pulses—peas, beans and lentils.

legumes (leg-ūms') *npl* pulse vegetables—e.g. peas, beans, lentils.

Leishman-Donovan bodies (lēsh'-man-don'-o-van) the rounded forms of the protozoa *Leishmania* found in the endothelial cells and macrophages of patients suffering from leishmaniasis*.

Leish·mania (lēsh-mā'-nē-à) *n* genus of flagellated protozoon. *Leishmania donovani* responsible for disease of kala-azar* or leishmaniasis*.

leishman·iasis (lēsh-man-ī'-à-sis) *n* infestation by *Leishmania*, spread by sandflies. Generalized manifestation is kala-azar*. Cutaneous manifestation is such as oriental* sore; nasopharyngeal manifestation is espundia*.

lens (lenz) *n* the small biconvex crystalline body which is supported in the suspensory ligament immediately behind the iris of the eye (⇒ Figure 15). On account of its elasticity, the lens can alter in shape, enabling light rays to focus exactly on the retina.

len·ticular (len-tik'-ū-lar) *adj* pertaining to or resembling a lens*.

len·tigo (len-tī'-gō) *n* a freckle with an increased number of pigment cells. ⇒ epiphelides—**lentigines** *pl*.

len·til (len'-til) an inexpensive and nutritious legume containing a large amount of protein.

leon·tiasis (lē-on-tī'-à-sis) *n* enlargement of the face and head giving a lion-like appearance; most often caused by fibrous dysplasia of bone.

Leopold's maneuvers (lē'-o-polds) a series of systematic maneuvers in abdominal palpation of pregnant women to determine presentation and position of the fetus.

leprol·ogist (lep-rol'-o-jist) *n* one who specializes in the study and treatment of leprosy*.

leprol·ogy (lep-rol'-o-jē) *n* the study of leprosy* and its treatment.

lep·romata (le-prō'-mà-tà) *npl* the granulomatous cutaneous eruption of leprosy—**leproma** *sing,* **lepromatous** *adj*.

lep·rosy (lep'-ros-ē) *n* a progressive and contagious disease, endemic in warmer climates and characterized by granulomatous formation in the nerves or on the skin. Caused by *Mycobacterium leprae* (Hansen's bacillus). BCG* vaccination conferred variable protection in different trials. Leprosy can be controlled but not cured by long-term treatment with sulfone drugs—**leprous** *adj*.

lepto·cytosis (lep-tō-sī-tō'-sis) *n* thin, flattened, circulating red blood cells (leptocytes). Characteristic of thalassemia*. Also seen in jaundice, hepatic disease and sometimes after splenectomy.

lepto·meningitis (lep-tō-men-in-jī'-tis) *n* inflammation of the inner covering membranes (arachnoid* and pia* mater) of brain or spinal cord.

Lepto·spira (lep-tō-spī'-rà) *n* a genus of bacteria. Very thin, finely coiled bacteria which require dark ground microscopy for visualization. Common in water as saprophytes; pathogenic species are numerous in many animals and may infect man. *Leptospira interrogans* serotype *icterohaemorrhagiae* causes Weil's* disease in man; *Leptospira interrogans* serotype *canicola* 'yellows' in dogs and pigs, transmissible to man ⇒ leptospirosis.

lepto·spiral agglutin·ation tests (lep-tō-spī'-ral ag-loo'-tin-ā'-shun) serological tests used in the diagnosis of specific leptospiral infections e.g. Weil's* disease.

lepto·spirosis (lep-tō-spī-rō'-sis) *n* infection of man by *Leptospira* from rats, dogs, pigs, foxes, mice, and possibly cats. There is high fever, headache, conjunctival congestion, jaundice, severe muscular pains, and vomiting. As the fever abates in about a week, the jaundice disappears. ⇒ Weil's disease.

Lepto·thrix (lep'-tō-thriks) *n* a genus of bacteria. Gram-negative; found in water; non-pathogenic. A term also used in medical bacteriology to describe filamentous bacteria resembling actinomycetes*.

lesbian·ism (les'-bi-an-izm) *n* sexual attraction of one woman to another.

Lesch-Nyhan dis·ease (lesk-nī'-han) X-linked recessive genetic disorder. Overproduction of uric acid, associated with brain damage resulting in cerebral palsy and mental retardation. Victims are compelled, by a self-destructive urge, to bite away the sides of their mouth, lips and fingers.

lesion (lē'-zhun) *n* pathological change in a bodily tissue.

leu·cine (lōō'-sēn) *n* one of the essential amino* acids. Leucine-induced hypoglycemia is a genetic metabolic disorder due to a person's sensitivity to leucine.

Leucovorin (lū-kō-vōr'-in) *n* folinic acid which is given by mouth, I.M. or I.V. as an antidote to methotrexate*. Used to 'rescue' patients from high dose methotrexate therapy for malignant disease.

leu·kemia (lōō-kē'-mē-à) *n* a malignant proliferation of the leukopoietic tissues usually producing an abnormal increase in leukocytes in the blood. If immature cells proliferate it is acute leukemia which is either myeloblastic or lymphoblastic. *acute myeloblastic leukemia* is rapidly fatal if not treated; it requires intensive in-patient chemotherapy in a protected environment. The average duration of the first remission is 14 months.

acute lymphoblastic leukemia has a more favorable outlook and many children can expect to be cured after a 2-year course of treatment. If mature cells proliferate then it is chronic leukemia, which is either myelocytic (granulocytic) or lymphocytic. *chronic myelocytic leukemia* may run a static course over several years but eventually an acute phase supervenes (blast crisis). *chronic lymphocytic leukemia* occurs mainly in the elderly. Little active treatment is necessary and patients may live comfortably for many years—**leukemic** *adj*.

Leukeran (lōō'-ker-an) *n* proprietary name for chlorambucil*.

leuko·cidin (lōō-kō-sī'-din) *n* a bacterial exotoxin* which selectively destroys white blood cells.

leuko·cytes (lōō'-kō-sīts) *npl* the white corpuscles of the blood, some of which are granular and some nongranular. In the blood stream they are colorless, nucleated masses, and some are motile and phagocytic. ⇒ basophil, eosinophil, lymphocyte, mononuclear, polymorphonuclear—**leukocytic** *adj*.

leuko·cytolysis (lōō-kō-sī-tol'-is-is) *n* destruction and disintegration of white blood cells—**leukocytolytic** *adj*.

leuko·cytosis (lōō-kō-sī-tō'-sis) *n* increased number of leukocytes* in the blood. Often a response to infection—**leukocytotic** *adj*.

leuko·derma (lōō-kō-dèr'-mà) *n* defective skin pigmentation, especially when it occurs in patches or bands.

leu·koma (lōō-kō'-mà) *n* white opaque spot on the cornea—**leukomata** *pl*, **leukomatous** *adj*.

leu·konychia (lōō-kon-ik'-ē-à) *n* white spots on the nails.

leuko·penia (lōō-kō-pē'-nē-à) *n* decreased number of white blood cells in the blood—**leukopenic** *adj*.

leuko·plakia (lōō-kō-plā'-kē-à) *n* white, thickened patch occurring on mucous membranes. Occurs on lips, inside mouth or on genitalia. Sometimes denotes precancerous change. Sometimes due to syphilis. ⇒ kraurosis vulvae.

leuko·poiesis (lōō-kō-pī-ēs'-is) *n* the formation of white blood cells—**leukopoietic** *adj*.

leukor·rhoea (lōō-kō-rē'-à) *n* a sticky, whitish vaginal discharge—**leukorrhoeal** *adj*.

leu·kotomy (lōō-ko'-to-mē) (*syn* lobotomy) *n* a psychosurgical operation to sever the white pathways in the brain.

The original operations had serious side-effects. Currently stereotactic* surgery is carried out and side-effects are uncommon. It is used only infrequently in cases of obsessional neurosis and when chronic anxiety has not responded to other treatments.

leval·lorphan (lev-al'-ōr-fan) *n* narcotic antagonist. (Lorfan.)

lev·ator (lev-ā'-tor) *adj* 1 a muscle which acts by raising a part. *levator ani* a muscle which helps form the pelvic floor. *levator scapulae* ⇒ Figure 5. 2 an instrument for lifting a depressed part.

Levin tube (le-vin') a French plastic catheter used for gastric intubation; it has a closed weighted tip and an opening on the side.

levo·dopa (L-dopa) (le-vō-do'-på) *n* a synthetic anti-Parkinson drug. In Parkinson's disease there is inadequate dopamine* (a transmitter substance) in the basal ganglia. In these ganglia levodopa is converted into dopamine and replenishes the stores. Unlike dopamine levodopa can cross the blood-brain barrier. (Larodopa.) ⇒ carbidopa.

Levo Dromoran (le'-vō drom'-ōr-an) *n* proprietary name for levorphanol*.

levon·orgestrel (le-vō-nōr-jes'-trel) *n* a hormone widely used in oral contraceptives. There has been research into a preparation of six small rubber capsules containing levonorgestrel. They are inserted under the skin of a woman's forearm; the implants release small amounts of the drug; the effect is achieved in 24 h and lasts for 5 years. (Norplant.)

Levo·phed (lev'-ō-fed) *n* proprietary name for norepinephrine*.

levor·phanol (le-vōr'-fan-ol) *n* a synthetic substitute for morphine*. It is less hypnotic than morphine but has a more extended action. Almost as effective by mouth as by injection. (Levo Dromoran.)

Levoprome (lev'-ō-prōm) *n* proprietary name for methotrimeprazine*.

levothyroxine (lev-ō-thī-roks'-in) *n* synthetic thyroxine, the main hormone secreted by the thyroid gland. Used for thyroxine replacement therapy.

levu·lose (lev'-ū-lōs) *n* fructose or fruit sugar, a monosaccharide found in many sweet fruits. It is the sugar in honey and, combined with glucose, is the major constituent of cane sugar. Sweeter and more easily digested than ordinary sugar; it is useful for diabetics. *levulose test* for hepatic function. A measured amount of levulose does not normally increase the level of blood sugar, except in hepatic damage.

LGA *abbr* large for gestational age.

LGVCFT *abbr* lymphogranuloma* venereum complement fixation test.

LH *abbr* luteinizing hormone.

LHBI *abbr* lower hemi-body irradiation*.

libido (li-bi'-dō) *n* Freud's name for the urge to obtain sensual satisfaction which he believed to be the mainspring of human behavior. Sometimes more loosely used with the meaning of sexual urge. Freud's meaning was satisfaction through all the senses.

Librium (lib'-rē-um) *n* ⇒ chlordiazepoxide.

lice (līs) ⇒ pediculus.

li·chen (lī'-ken) *n* aggregations of papular skin lesions—**lichenoid** *adj*. *lichen nitidus* characterized by minute, shiny, flat-topped, pink papules of pinhead size. *lichen planus* an eruption of unknown cause showing purple, angulated, shiny, flat-topped papules. *lichen scrofulosorum* a form of tuberculide. *lichen simplex* ⇒ neurodermatitis. *lichen spinulosus* a disease of children characterized by very small spines protruding from the follicular openings of the skin and resulting from vitamin A deficiency. *lichen urticatus* papular urticaria*.

licheni·fication (lī-ken'-i-fi-kā'-shun) *n* thickening of the skin, usually secondary to scratching. Skin markings become more prominent and the area affected appears to be composed of small, shiny rhomboids. ⇒ neurodermatitis.

licorice (lik'-ōr-ish) *n* ⇒ glycyrrhiza.

Lido·caine (lī'-dō-kān) *n* a local anesthetic with a more powerful and prolonged action than procaine. The strength of solution varies from 0.5% for infiltration anesthesia to 2% for nerve block. Adrenalin* is usually added to delay absorption. Also effective for surface anesthesia as ointment (2%) and for urethral anesthesia as a 2% gel. Now widely accepted as an antiarrhythmic agent, especially in the management of ventricular tachycardia and ventricular ectopic beats occurring as complications of acute myocardial infarction. (Xylocaine.)

lien (li'-en) *n* the spleen*.

lien·culus (li-en'-kū-lus) *n* a small accessory spleen.

lien·itis (li-en-ī'-tis) *n* inflammation of the spleen*.

lieno·renal (li-en-ō-rē'-nal) *adj* pertaining to the spleen* and kidney*. In *lienorenal shunt*, the splenic vein is anastomosed to the left renal vein to relieve portal hypertension.

life expectancy the average age at which death occurs. It is not only affected by health/illness but also by social factors such as education and industry; and environmental factors such as housing and sanitation.

liga·ment (lig'-à-ment) *n* a strong band of fibrous tissue serving to bind bones or other parts together, or to support an organ—**ligamentous** *adj*. *ligament of ovary* ⇒ Figure 17.

lig·ate (lī'-gāt) *vt* to tie off blood vessels etc at operation—**ligation** *n*.

lig·ation (lī-gā'-shun) tying off; usually reserved for *ligation of the fallopian tubes*, a method of sterilization.

liga·ture (lī'-gà-chūr) *n* the material used for tying vessels or sewing the tissues. Silk, horsehair, catgut, kangaroo tendon, silver wire, nylon, linen and fascia can be used.

lighten·ing (līt'-en-ing) *n* a word used to denote the relief of pressure on the diaphragm by the abdominal viscera, when the presenting part of the fetus descends into the pelvis in the last 3 weeks of a primigravida's* pregnancy.

lightn·ing pains (līt'-ning) symptomatic of tabes dorsalis. Occur as paroxysms of swift-cutting (lightning) stabs in the lower limbs.

lime water (līm) solution of calcium hydroxide (about 0–15%). It is used in a number of skin lotions, and with an equal volume of linseed or olive oil it forms a soothing application.

lim·inal (lim'-in-àl) *adj* of a stimulus, of the lowest intensity which can be perceived by the human senses. ⇒ subliminal.

Lincocin (lin-kō'-sin) *n* proprietary name for lincomycin*.

linco·mycin (lin-kō-mī'-sin) *n* an antibiotic for serious infections caused by Grampositive pathogens. It can induce severe colitis as a side-effect. (Lincocin.)

linc·tus (link'-tus) *n* a sweet, syrupy liquid; it should be slowly sipped.

linea (lin'-ē-à) *n* a line. *linea alba* the white line visible after removal of the skin in the center of the abdomen, stretching from the ensiform cartilage to the pubis, its position on the surface being indicated by a slight depression. *linea nigra* pigmented line from umbilicus to pubis which appears in pregnancy. *lineae albicantes* white lines which appear on the abdomen after reduction of tension as after childbirth, tapping of the abdomen, etc.

lingua (ling'-gwà) *n* the tongue—**lingual** *adj*.

lini·ment (lin'-i-ment) *n* a liquid to be applied to the skin by gentle friction.

lino·lenic acid (lin-ō-lē'-nik) an unsaturated, essential fatty acid found in vegetable fats.

Lio·resal (lī-ōr'-es-al) *n* proprietary name for baclofen*.

lio·thyronine (lī-ō-thī'-ron-ēn) *n* a secretion of thyroid gland, also known as triiodothyronine. Together with thyroxine* stimulates metabolism in body tissues. (Cyomel.)

li·pase (lī'-pās) *n* any fat-splitting enzyme. *pancreatic lipase* steapsin*.

lip·emia (li-pēm'-ē-à) *n* increased lipoids (especially cholesterol) in the blood—**lipemic** *adj*.

lipid (lip'-id) *n* any water-insoluble fat or fat-like substance extractable by nonpolar solvents such as alcohol. Lipids serve as a source of fuel and are an important constituent of cell membranes.

lip·oid (lī'-poyd) *adj*, *n* a substance resembling fats or oil. Serum lipoids are raised in thyroid deficiency.

lipoid·osis (lī-poyd-ōs'-is) *n* disease due to disorder of fat metabolism—**lipoidoses** *pl*.

lipoly·sis (lī-pol'-is-is) *n* the chemical breakdown of fat by lipolytic enzymes—**lipolytic** *adj*.

lip·oma (lī-pō'-mà) *n* a benign tumor containing fatty tissue—**lipomata** *pl*, **lipomatous** *adj*.

lipo·protein (lī-pō-prō'-tē-in) *n* ⇒ high density lipoprotein.

lipo·trophic sub·stances (lī-pō-trō'-fik) factors which cause the removal of fat from the liver by transmethylation.

lip·uria (lī-pū'-rē-à) *n* (*syn* adiposuria) fat in the urine—**lipuric** *adj*.

liquor (lik'-ėr) *n* a solution. *liquor amnii* the fluid surrounding the fetus. *liquor epispasticus* a blistering fluid. *liquor folliculi* the fluid surrounding a developing ovum in a graafian follicle. *liquor picis carb* an alcoholic extract of coal tar. Used in eczema and other conditions requiring mild tar treatment. *liquor sanguinis* the fluid part of blood (plasma*).

liter (lē'-tėr) *n* in metric fluid measure, equals 1000 milliliters (ml.).

Lithane (li'-thān) *n* proprietary name for lithium carbonate*.

lith·iasis (lith-ī'-à-sis) *n* any condition in which there are calculi.

lith·ium carbon·ate (lith'-ē-um-kàr'-bon-āt) used in manic depressive illness. Possible side effects include diarrhea, vomiting, drowsiness, ataxia, coarse tremor. Contraindicated in cardiac or renal disease. Regular blood serum levels of lithium are necessary and thyroid function should be assessed before and at regular intervals during treatment. (Eskalith, Lithane.)

lithol·apaxy (lith-ol-à-paks'-ē) *n* (*syn* lithopaxy) crushing a stone within the urinary bladder and removing the fragments by irrigation.

litho·pedion (lith-ō-pē'-dē-on) *n* a dead fetus retained in the uterus, e.g. one of a pair of twins which dies and becomes mummified and sometimes impregnated with lime salts.

lith·otomy (lith-ot'-o-mē) *n* surgical incision of the bladder for the removal of calculi; achieved mainly by the abdominal route but there is a resurgence of using the perineal route. *lithotomy position* with the patient lying down, the buttocks are drawn to the end of the table to which a stirrup is attached on either side. Each foot is placed in a sling attached to the top of the stirrup so that the peritoneum is exposed for genitourinary purposes.

litho·triptor (lith-ō-trip'-tor) *n* a machine which sends shock waves through renal calculi causing them to crumble and leave the body naturally in the urine.

litho·trite (lith'-ō-trīt) *n* an instrument for crushing a stone in the urinary bladder.

lith·uresis (lith-ūr-ēs'-is) *n* voiding of gravel* in the urine.

lit·mus (lit'-mus) *n* a vegetable pigment used as an indicator of acidity (red) or alkalinity (blue). Often stored as paper strips impregnated with blue or red litmus; blue litmus paper turns red when in contact with an acid; red litmus paper turns blue when in contact with an alkali.

Little's disease (lit'-tlz) diplegia* of spastic type causing 'scissor leg' deformity. A congenital disease in which there is cerebral atrophy or agenesis.

liver (liv'-ėr) *n* the largest organ in the body, varying in weight in the adult from 13.6–18.1 kg or about one-thirtieth of

body weight. It is relatively much larger in the fetus. It is situated in the right upper section of the abdominal cavity (⇒ Figure 18). It secretes bile*, forms and stores glycogen* and plays an important part in the metabolism of proteins and fats. *liver transplant* surgical transplantation of a liver from a suitable donor who has recently died.

livid (liv'-id) *adj* showing blue discoloration due to bruising, congestion or insufficient oxygenation.

living will a statement prepared by a well person stating that in the event of terminal illness, he or she does not want extraordinary measures taken to prolong life.

LMP *abbr* last menstrual period.

LOA *abbr* left occipitoanterior; used to describe the position of the fetus in the uterus.

lobe (lōb) *n* a rounded section of an organ, separated from neighboring sections by a fissure or septum etc. ⇒ Figure 13—**lobar** *adj*.

lobec·tomy (lō-bek'-to-mē) *n* removal of a lobe, e.g. of the lung for lung abscess or localized bronchiectasis.

lobeline (lōb'-el-ēn) *n* one of the components of lobelia inflata, used to stimulate respirations.

lo·botomy (lō-bo'-to-mē) *n* a word previously used for leukotomy*.

lob·ule (lōb'-ūl) *n* a small lobe or a subdivision of a lobe—**lobular, lobulated** *adj*.

local·ize (lō'-kàl-īz) *vt* **1** to limit the spread. **2** to determine the site of a lesion—**localization** *n*.

lochia (lō'-kē-à) *n* the vaginal discharge which occurs during the puerperium*. At first pure blood, it later becomes paler, diminishes in quantity and finally ceases—**lochial** *adj*.

lock·jaw (lok'-jaw) *n* ⇒ tetanus.

loco·motor (lō-kō-mō'-tor) *adj* can be applied to any tissue or system used in human movement. Most usually refers to nerves and muscles. Sometimes includes the bones and joints. *locomotor ataxia* the disordered gait and loss of sense of position in the lower limbs, which occurs in tabes* dorsalis. Tabes dorsalis is still sometimes called 'locomotor ataxia'.

locu·lated (lok'-ū-lā-ted) *adj* divided into numerous cavities.

Logan bow (lō'-gan bō) a thin metal device, shaped like a bow; it is used after cleft lip surgery to reduce tension on the suture line.

loi·asis (lō-ī'-a-sis) *n* special form of filariasis (caused by the worm *Filaria Loa loa*) which occurs in West Africa, Nigeria and the Cameroons. The vector, a large horsefly. *Chrysops*, bites in the daytime. Larvae take 3 years to develop and may live in a man for 17 years. They creep about and cause intense itching. Accompanied by eosinophilia*.

loin (loyn) *n* that part of the back between the lower ribs and the iliac crest; the area immediately above the buttocks.

Lomo·til (lō-mō'-til) *n* proprietary mixture of diphenoxylate* hydrochloride and atropine* sulfate. Useful for loose colostomy and postvagotomy diarrhea. Reduces motility of gut and allows time for absorption of water from feces. A single dose lessens desire to defecate after 1 h, and is effective for 6 hours.

lomul·izer (lom'-ū-lī-zer) *n* device which disperses fine powder (contained in a tiny plastic cartridge) through a mouthpiece.

lomust·ine (lō-mus'-tēn) *n* an alkylating cytotoxic agent.

longsighted (long'-sīt-ed) *adj* hypermetropic. ⇒ hypermetropia.

Loni·ten (lon'-i-ten) *n* proprietary name for minoxidil.

LOP *abbr* left occiput posterior presentation of fetus.

loper·amide (lō-pėr'-à-mīd) *n* an antidiarrheal agent which is especially useful in acute cases. (lmodium.)

lopressor (lō-pres'-or) *n* proprietary name for metoprolol*.

lor·azepam (lōr-az'-ė-pam) *n* a tranquilizer similar to diazepam*. (Ativan.)

lordo·scoliosis (lōr'-dō-skō-lē-ōs'-is) *n* lordosis* complicated by the presence of scoliosis*.

lor·dosis (lōr-dō'-sis) *n* an exaggerated forward, convex curve of the lumbar spine—**lordotic** *adj*.

Lor·fan (lōr'-fan) *n* proprietary name for levallorphan*.

lotio rubra (lō'-tē-ō-rū'-brà) red* lotion.

loupe (lōōp) *n* a magnifying lens used in ophthalmology.

loup·ing ill (lōōp'-ing il) tick-borne virus meningoencephalitis in sheep. Antibodies have been found in human serum.

louse (lows) *n* ⇒ Pediculus—**lice** *pl*.

low back pain the commonest cause seems to be posteriolateral prolapse of the intervertebral disc putting pressure on the dura and cauda equina and causing the localized pain of lumbago. It can progress to trap the spinal nerve root causing the nerve distribution pain of sciatica.

low birthweight term used to indicate a weight of 2.5 kg or less at birth, whether or not gestation was below 37 weeks—'small for dates'.

lower respir·atory tract infec·tion (LRTI) ⇒ pneumonia.

LP *abbr* lumbar* puncture.

LPN *abbr* licensed practical nurse.

LRTI *abbr* lower respiratory tract infection. ⇒ pneumonia.

LSD *abbr* lysergic* acid diethylamide.

lubb-dupp (lub-dup') *n* words descriptive of the heart sounds as appreciated in auscultation.

lubri·cants (lōō'-brik-ants) *npl* drugs which are emollient in nature and facilitate the easy and painless evacuation of feces. ⇒ laxatives.

lu·cid (lōō'-sid) *adj* clear; describing mental clarity. *lucid interval* a period of mental clarity which can be of variable length, occurring in people with organic mental disorder such as dementia.

Ludwig's angina (lōōd'-vigz an-jī'-nà) ⇒ cellulitis.

lues (lōō'-ēz) *n* syphilis*—**luetic** *adj*.

Lugol's solution (lōō'-golz) an aqueous solution of iodine* and potassium* iodide. Used in the preoperative stabilization of thyrotoxic patients. It has been given by slow intravenous injection in thyrotoxic crisis.

lum·bago (lum-bā'-gō) *n* incapacitating pain low down in the back.

lum·bar (lum'-bàr) *adj* pertaining to the loin. *lumbar nerve* ⇒ Figure 11. *lumbar puncture (LP)* the withdrawal of cerebrospinal fluid through a hollow needle inserted into the subarachnoid space in the lumbar region. The fluid can be examined for its chemical, cellular and bacterial content; its pressure can be measured by the attachment of a manometer. The procedure is hazardous if the pressure is high, but the pressure for an adult has a wide range—50–200 mm water, so a better guide is examination of the optic fundi for papilledema. *lumbar sympathectomy* surgical removal of the sympathetic chain in the lumbar region; used to improve the blood supply to the lower limbs by allowing the blood vessels to dilate. *lumbar vertebrae* ⇒ Figure 3.

lumbo·costal (lum-bō-kos'-tàl) *adj* pertaining to the loin and ribs.

lumbo·sacral (lum-bō-sā'-kràl) *adj* pertaining to the loin or lumbar vertebrae and the sacrum.

Lumbri·cus (lum'-bri-kus) *n* a genus of earthworms. ⇒ ascarides, ascariasis.

lumen (loo'-men) *n* the space inside a tubular structure—**lumina** *pl*, **luminal** *adj*.

Luminal (lū'-min-al) *n* proprietary name for phenobarbital*.

lump·ectomy (lump-ek'-to-mē) *n* the surgical excision of a tumor with removal of minimal surrounding tissue.

lungs (lungz) *npl* the two main organs of respiration which occupy the greater part of the thoracic cavity; they are separated from each other by the heart and other contents of the mediastinum (⇒ Figures 6, 7). Together they weigh about 11.88 kg and they are concerned with the oxygenation of blood.

lu·nula (loo'-nū-là) *n* the semilunar pale area at the root of the nail.

lu·pus (loo'-pus) *n* several destructive skin conditions, with different causes. ⇒ collagen. *lupus erythematosus* (*LE*) an autoimmune process. The discoid variety is characterized by patulous follicles, adherent scales, telangiectasis and atrophy; commonest on nose, malar regions, scalp and fingers. The disseminated or systemic variety is characterized by large areas of erythema on the skin, pyrexia, toxemia, involvement of serous membranes (pleurisy, pericarditis) and renal damage. *lupus pernio* a form of sarcoidosis. *lupus vulgaris* the commonest variety of skin tuberculosis; ulceration occurs over cartilage (nose or ear) with necrosis and facial disfigurement.

luteo·trophin (loo'-tē-ō-trō'-fin) *n* secreted by the anterior pituitary gland; it assists the formation of the corpus luteum in the ovary. In the male it acts on Leydig cells in the testis which produce androgens.

luteum (loo'-tē-um) *n* yellow. *corpus luteum* a yellow mass which forms in the ovary after rupture of a graafian follicle. It secretes progesterone* and persists and enlarges if pregnancy supervenes.

lux·ation (luks-ā'-shun) *n* partial dislocation.

lyco·podium (lī-kō-pō'-dē-um) *n* a light, dry fungal spore; it is adsorbent and has been used for dusting the skin and excoriated surfaces. It was once used as a coating for pills.

lying-in period early post partum period.

lymph (limf) *n* the fluid contained in the lymphatic vessels. It is transparent, colorless or slightly yellow. Unlike blood, lymph contains only one type of cell, the lymphocyte*. *lymph circulation* that of lymph collected from the tissue spaces; it then passes via capillaries, vessels, glands and ducts to be poured back into the blood stream. *lymph nodes* accumulations of lymphatic tissue at intervals along lymphatic vessels. They mainly act as filters.

lymph·adenectomy (limf-ad-en-ek'-to-mē) *n* excision of one or more lymph nodes.

lymph·adenitis (limf-ad-en-ī'-tis) *n* inflammation of a lymph node.

lymph·adenopathy (limf-ad-en-op'-à-thē) *n* any disease of the lymph nodes—**lymphadenopathic** *adj*.

lymph·angi·ectasis (limf-an-jē-ek'-tà-sis) *n* dilation of the lymph vessels—**lymphangiectatic** *adj*.

lymph·angiography (limf-an-jē-og'-raf-ē) *n* ⇒ lymphography.

lymph·angioma (limf-an-jē-ōm'-à) *n* a simple tumor of lymph vessels frequently associated with similar formations of blood vessels—**lymphangiomata** *pl*, **lymphangiomatous** *adj*.

lymph·angio·plasty (limf-an'-jē-ō-plas-tē) *n* replacement of lymphatics by artificial channels (buried silk threads) to drain the tissues. Relieves the 'brawny arm' after radical mastectomy—**lymphangioplastic** *adj*.

lymph·angitis (limf-an-jī'-tis) *n* inflammation of a lymph vessel.

lym·phatic (limf-at'-ik) *adj* pertaining to, conveying or containing lymph*.

lymphatico·venous (limf-at-ik-ō-vē'-nus) *adj* implies the presence of both lymphatic vessels and veins to increase drainage from an area.

lymphedema (limf-e-dē'-mà) *n* excess of fluid in the tissues from obstruction of lymph vessels ⇒ elephantiasis, filariasis.

lympho·blast (limf'-ō-blast) *n* an abnormal cell circulating in the blood in acute lymphoblastic leukemia*. At one time it was thought to be a precursor of the lymphocyte.

lympho·blastoma (limf-ō-blast-ō'-mà) *n* malignant lymphoma in which single or multiple tumors arise from lymphoblasts* in lymph nodes. Sometimes associated with acute lymphatic leukemia.

lymphoblastoma malignum Hodgkin's* disease.

lympho·cyte (limf'-ō-sīt) *n* one variety of white blood cell. The lymphocytic stem cells undergo transformation to T lymphocytes (in the thymus) which provide cellular immunity involved in graft or organ acceptance/rejection; and B lymphocytes which form antibodies and provide humoral immunity. The transformation is usually complete a few months after birth—**lymphocytic** *adj*.

lymphocythemia (limf-ō-sī-thē'-mē-à) *n* excess of lymphocytes in the blood.

lympho·cytosis (limf-ō-sī-tō'-sis) *n* an increase in lymphocytes in the blood.

lympho·epithelioma (limf-ō-ep-ith-ēl-ē-ōm'-à) *n* rapidly growing malignant pharyngeal tumor. May involve the tonsil. Often has metastases in cervical lymph nodes—**lymphoepitheliomata** *pl*.

lympho·granuloma venereum (limf-ō-gran-ū-lō'-mà-ven-ēr'-ē-um) a tropical venereal disease caused by a virus. Primary lesion on the genitalia may be an ulcer or herpetiform eruption. Soon buboes appear in regional lymph nodes. They form a painful mass called poradenitis* and commonly produce sinuses. Further spread by lymphatics may cause severe periproctitis or rectal stricture in women. Patch skin test (lygranum) and a complement-fixation test of patient's serum are used in diagnosis.

lymph·ography (limf-og'-ràf-ē) *n* X-ray examination of the lymphatic system after it has been rendered radioopaque—**lymphographical** *adj*, **lymphogram** *n*, **lymphograph** *n*, **lymphographically** *adv*.

lymph·old (limf'-oyd) *adj* pertaining to lymph*.

lympho·kines (limf'-ō-kīnz) *npl* chemical substances derived from stimulated T lymphocytes.

lym·phoma (limf-ō'-mà) *n* a benign tumor of lymphatic tissue. *malignant lymphoma* malignant tumors arising in lymph nodes—**lymphomata** *pl*, **lymphomatous** *adj*.

lymphor·rhagia (limf-ōr-āj'-ē-à) *n* outpouring of lymph from a severed lymphatic vessel.

lympho·sarcoma (limf-ō-sàr-kō'-mà) *n* a malignant tumor arising from lymphatic tissue—**lymphosarcomata** *pl*, **lymphosarcomatous** *adj*.

lyophil·ization (lī-ō-fil-īz-ā'-shun) *n* a special method of preserving such biological substances as plasma, sera, bacteria and tissue.

lyophil·ized skin (lī'-ō-fil-īzed) skin which has been subjected to lyophilization. It is reconstituted and used for temporary skin replacement.

lypressin (lī-press'-in) *n* antidiuretic ⇒ vasopressin.

ly·sergic acid di·ethylamide (LSD) (lī-sėr'-jik as'-id dī-eth'-yl-à-mēn) a potent hallucinogenic agent. An amino oxidase inhibitor.

ly·sin (lī'-sin) *n* a cell dissolving substance in blood. ⇒ bacteriolysin, hemolysin.

ly·sine (lī'-sēn) *n* an essential amino* acid necessary for growth. Deficiency may cause nausea, dizziness and anemia. It is destroyed by dry heating, e.g. toasted bread and cereals such as Puffed Wheat.

ly·sis (lī'-sis) *n* 1 a gradual return to normal, used especially in relation to pyrexia. ⇒ crisis *opp*. 2 disintegration of the membrane of cells or bacteria.

Ly·sol (lī'-sol) *n* well known proprietary disinfectant containing 50% cresol in soap solution. It has a wide range of activity, but the preparation is caustic and this limits its use.

lyso·zyme (lī'-sō-zīm) *n* a basic enzyme which acts as an antibacterial agent and is present in various body fluids such as tears and saliva.

lytic cock·tail (lī'-tik-kok'-tāl) consists of promethazine* (Phenergan), meperidine* (Demerol) and chlorpromazine* (Thorazine) diluted in normal saline solution. Used during the induction and maintenance of hypothermia. Abolishes shivering and convulsions.

M

Maalox (mā'-loks) *n* proprietary name for aluminum hydroxide and magnesium hydroxide; an antacid.

macer·ation (mas-e-rā'-shun) *n* softening of the horny layer of the skin by moisture, e.g. in and below the toes (in tinea pedis), or in perianal area (in pruritus ani). Maceration reduces the protective quality of the integument and so predisposes to penetration by bacteria or fungi.

Mackenrodt's liga·ments (mak'-en-rod's) the transverse cervical or cardinal ligaments which are the chief uterine supports.

macri·salb (mak'-ri-salb) *n* suspension of

iodinated human albumin in the form of insoluble aggregates. After i.v. injection these aggregates are normally trapped by blood capillaries in lungs, thus their presence can be detected by their radioactivity. Absence of such activity is an indication of reduced blood supply.

macro·cephaly (mak-rō-sef'-à-lē) *n* excessive size of the head, not caused by hydrocephalus*—**macrocephalic** *adj*.

macro·cheilia (mak-rō-kil'-ē-à) *n* excessive development of the lips.

macro·cyte (mak'-rō-sīt) *n* a large red blood cell, found in association with a megaloblastic anemia, e.g. in pernicious anemia—**macrocytic** *adj, macrocytosis* an increased number of macrocytes.

macro·dactyly (mak-rō-dak'-ti-lē) *n* excessive development of the fingers or toes.

Macrodantin (mak-rō-dan'-tin) *n* proprietary name for microfurantoin*.

Macro·dex (mak'-rō-deks) *n* proprietary high molecular weight dextran* for plasma volume replacement in hypovolemic shock. Can be used as an anticoagulant when patients have to assume a particular position which increases the risk of deep vein thrombosis.

macro·glossia (mak-rō-glos'-ē-à) *n* an abnormally large tongue.

macro·mastia (mak-rō-mas'-tē-à) *n* an abnormally large breast.

macro·phages (mak'-rō-fāj-es) *npl* mononuclear cells, which scavenge foreign bodies and cell debris. Part of the reticuloendothelial* system. ⇒ histiocytes.

macro·scopic (mak-rō-skop'-ik) *adj* visible to the naked eye; gross. ⇒ microscopic *opp*.

mac·ula (mak'-ū-là) a spot—**macular** *adj, macula lutea* the yellow spot on the retina, the area of clearest central vision.

mac·ule (mak'-ūl) *n* a non-palpable localized area of change in skin color—**macular** *adj*.

maculo·papular (mak-ū-lō-pap'-ū-lar) *adj* the presence of macules and raised palpable spots (papules) on the skin.

ma·dura foot (ma-dū'-ra) (*syn* mycetoma) fungus disease of the foot found in India and the tropics. Characterized by swelling and the development of nodules and sinuses. May terminate in death from sepsis.

mafenide acetate (maf'-en-īd as'-e-tāt) *n* antiseptic dermatological cream used to treat burns.

mag·nesium carbon·ate (mag-nē'-zē-um kar'-bon-āt) a powder widely used as an antacid in peptic ulcer and as a laxative.

magn·esium hydrox·ide (mag-nē'-zē-um hī-droks'-īd) a valuable antacid and laxative. It is sometimes preferred to magnesium and other carbonates, as it does not liberate carbon dioxide in the stomach. Also used as an antidote in poisoning by mineral acids.

mag·nesium sulfate (mag-nē'-zē-um sul'-fāt) (*syn* Epsom salts) an effective rapid-acting laxative, especially when given in dilute solution on an empty stomach. It is used as a 25% solution as a wet dressing for inflamed conditions of the skin, and as a paste with glycerin for the treatment of boils and carbuncles. It has been given by injection for magnesium deficiency.

mag·nesium tri·silicate (mag-nē'-zē-um tri-sil'-i-kāt) tasteless white powder with a mild but prolonged antacid action. It is therefore used extensively in peptic ulcer, often combined with more rapidly acting antacids. It does not cause alkalosis, and large doses can be given without side-effects.

magnetic resonance imaging (MRI) (mag-net'-ik rez'-on-ans im'-a-jing) (*syn* nuclear magnetic resonance (NMR)) a technique of imaging by computer using a strong magnetic field and radiofrequency signals to examine thin slices through the body. Has the advantage over computed* tomography that no X-rays are used, thus no biological harm is thought to be caused to the subject.

mag·num (mag'-num) *adj* large or great, as foramen magnum in occipital bone.

mal (mal) *n* disease. *mal de mer* seasickness. *grand mal* major epilepsy*. *petit mal* minor epilepsy*.

mal·absorption (mal-ab-sorb'-shun) *n* poor or disordered absorption of nutrients from the digestive tract. *malabsorption syndrome* loss of weight and steatorrhea*, varying from mild to severe. Caused by: (a) lesions of the small intestine (b) lack of digestive enzymes or bile salts (c) surgical operations.

ma·lacia (mal-ā'-sē-à) *n* softening of a part. ⇒ keratomalacia, osteomalacia.

maladjust·ment (mal-ad-just'-ment) *n* bad or poor adaptation to environment, socially, mentally or physically.

mal·aise (mal-āz') *n* a feeling of illness and discomfort.

malalign·ment (mal-al-īn'-ment) *n* faulty

alignment—as of the teeth, or bones after a fracture.

malar (mā'-lăr) *adj* relating to the cheek.

ma·laria (mà-lār'-ē-à) *n* a tropical disease caused by one of the genus *Plasmodium* and carried by infected mosquitoes of the genus Anopheles. *Plasmodium falciparum* causes *malignant tertian malaria*. *Plasmodium vivax* causes *benign tertian malaria* and *Plasmodium malariae* causes *quartan malaria*. Signs and symptoms are caused by the presence in the blood cells of the erythrocyte (E) stages of the parasite. In the falciparum malaria *only* the blood-forms of the parasite exist. There is an additional persistent infection in the liver (the extraerythrocytic or EE form) in vivax malaria, it is the factor responsible for relapses. Clinical picture is one of recurring rigors, anemia, toxemia and splenomegaly—**malarial** *adj*.

malari·ologist (ma-lār-ē-ol'-o-jist) *n* an expert in the study of malaria.

malassimi·lation (mal-as-im-il-ā'-shun) *n* poor or disordered assimilation.

mal·athion (mal-ath-ī'-on) *n* organophosphorus compound, used as an insecticide in agriculture. Powerful and irreversible anticholinesterase action follows excessive inhalation. Potentially dangerous to man for this reason.

male fern ⇒ filix mas.

mal·formation (mal-för-mā'-shun) *n* abnormal shape or structure; deformity.

malig·nant (mal-ig'-nant) *adj* virulent and dangerous; that which is likely to have a fatal termination—**malignancy** *n*. *malignant growth or tumor* ⇒ cancer, sarcoma, *malignant pustule* ⇒ anthrax.

malinger·ing (mal-ing'-ėr-ing) *n* deliberate (volitional) production of symptoms to evade an unpleasant situation.

mal·leolus (mal-lē'-o-lus) *n* a part or process of a bone shaped like a hammer. *external malleolus* at the lower end of the fibula*. *internal malleolus* situated at the lower end of the tibia*—**malleoli** *pl*, **malleolar** *adj*.

mal·leus (mal'-ē-us) *n* the hammer-shaped lateral bone of the middle ear (⇒ Figure 13).

malnu·trition (mal-nū-tri'-shun) *n* the state of being poorly nourished. May be caused by inadequate intake of one or more of the essential nutrients or by malassimilation.

mal·occlusion (mal-ok-klū'-shun) *n* failure of the upper and lower teeth to meet properly when the jaws are closed.

mal·position (mal-pō-zi'-shun) *n* any abnormal position of a part.

mal·practice (mal-prak'-tis) *n* unethical professional behavior; improper or injurious medical or nursing treatment.

mal·presentation (mal-prez-en-tā'-shun) *n* any unusual presentation of the fetus in the pelvis.

Malta fever (mawl'-ta) ⇒ brucellosis.

malt·ase (mawl'-tās) *n* (*syn* α-glucosidase) a sugar splitting (saccharolytic) enzyme found especially in intestinal juice.

malt·ose (mawl'-tōs) *n* malt sugar. A disaccharide produced by the hydrolysis of starch by amylase during digestion. Used as a nutrient and sweetener.

mal·union (mal-ūn'-yon) *n* the union of a fracture in a bad position.

mamma (ma'-mà) *n* the breast—**mammae** *pl*, **mammary** *adj*.

mamma·plasty (ma'-mà-plas-tē) *n* any plastic operation on the breast—**mammaplastic** *adj*.

mam·milla (mam-il'-à) *n* **1** the nipple **2** a small papilla—**mammillae** *pl*.

mam·mography (mam-og'-raf-ē) radiographic demonstration of the breast by use of specially low-penetration (long wavelength) X-rays—**mammographic** *adj*, **mammographically** *adv*.

mammo·trophic (mam-ō-trōf'-ik) *adj* having an effect upon the breast.

Manchester oper·ation (man'-chest-er) ⇒ Fothergill's operation.

Mandel·amine (man-del'-a-mēn) *n* proprietary name for methenamine* mandelate.

mania (mā'-nē-à) *n* one phase of manic depressive psychoses in which the prevailing mood is one of undue elation and there is pronounced psychomotor overactivity and often pathological excitement. Flight of ideas and grandiose delusions are common—**maniac** *adj*.

manic depress·ive psy·chosis (man'-ik dē-pres'-iv-sī-kō'-sis) a type of mental disorder which alternates between phases of excitement and phases of depression. Often between these phases there are periods of complete normality.

manipu·lation (man-ip-u-lā'-shun) *n* using the hands skillfully as in reducing a fracture or hernia, or changing the fetal position.

man·nitol (man'-it-ol) *n* a natural sugar that is not metabolized in the body and acts as an osmotic diuretic. Especially useful in some cases of drug overdose and in cerebral edema.

mannitol hexanitrate (man'-i-tol heks-à-nī'-trāt) a long-acting vasodilator, used mainly for the prophylactic treatment of angina pectoris. Prolonged administration may cause methemoglobinemia.

mannose (man'-ōs) *n* a fermentable monosaccharide.

man·ometer (man-om'-et-èr) *n* an instrument for measuring the pressure exerted by liquids or gases.

Mantoux react·ion (man'-tōo) intradermal injection of old tuberculin or PPD (purified protein derivative, a purified type of tuberculin) into the anterior aspect of forearm. Inspection after 48–72 h. If positive, there will be an area of induration and inflammation greater than 5 mm in diameter.

ma·nubrium (ma-nū'-brē-um) *n* a handle-shaped structure; the upper part of the breast bone or sternum.

MAOI *abbr* monoamine* oxidase inhibitor.

maple syrup urine dis·ease genetic disorder of recessive familial type. Leucine*, isoleucine* and valine* are excreted in excess in urine giving the smell of maple syrup. Symptoms include spasticity, poor feeding and respiratory difficulties; severe damage to the CNS may occur. A diet low in the three amino acids may be effective if started sufficiently early, otherwise the disorder is rapidly fatal. Genetic counseling may be indicated. In the pregnant woman, investigation may reveal evidence of the disorder and in such cases it may be wise to advise termination of pregnancy.

maras·mus (mar-az'-mus) *n* wasting away of the body, especially that of a baby, usually as a result of malnutrition. The currently preferred term is failure* to thrive—**marasmic** *adj*.

marble bones ⇒ osteopetrosis.

Marburg disease (mar'-berg) (*syn* green monkey disease) a highly infectious viral disease characterized by a sudden onset of fever, malaise, headache and myalgia. Between days 5 and 7 a rash appears. Treatment is symptomatic. Virus can persist in the body for 2–3 months after the initial attack. Cross infection probably occurs by the aerosol route. Incubation period believed to be 4–9 days and mortality rate in previous outbreaks has been around 30%.

Mar·cain (màr'-kān) *n* proprietary name for bupivacaine*.

Marezine (mār'-uh-zēn) *n* proprietary name for cyclizine.

Mar·fan's syn·drome (mar'-fanz) a he-reditary genetic disorder of unknown cause. There is dislocation of the lens, congenital heart disease and arachnodactyly with hypotonic musculature and lax ligaments, occasionally excessive height and abnormalities of the iris.

mari·huana (mar-i-wa'-nà) *n* ⇒ cannabis indica.

Marion's dis·ease (mār'-ē-onz) hypertrophic stenosis of the internal urinary meatus at the neck of the bladder.

Mar·plan (màr'-plan) *n* proprietary name of isocarboxozid*.

mar·row (mār'-ōw) *n* ⇒ bone marrow.

Marshall-Marchetti-Krantz oper·ation (mar'-shal mar-ket'-ē krantz) for stress incontinence. A form of abdominal cysto-urethropexy usually undertaken in patients who have not been controlled by a colporrphaphy. 85% success rate.

marsupial·ization (màr-sū-pē-àl-īz-ā'-shun) *n* an operation for cystic abdominal swellings, which entails stitching the margins of an opening made into the cyst to the edges of the abdominal wound, thus forming a pouch.

maso·chism (mas'-ō-kizm) *n* the deriving of pleasure from pain inflicted by others or occasionally by oneself. It may be a conscious or unconscious process and is frequently of a sexual nature. ⇒ sadism *opp*.

mass·age (mas-azh') *n* the soft tissues are kneaded, rubbed, stroked or tapped for the purpose of improving circulation, metabolism and muscle tone, breaking down adhesions and generally relaxing the patient. *cardiac* massage* done for cardiac arrest. With the patient on his back on a firm surface, the lower portion of sternum is depressed 37–50 mm each second to massage the heart. ⇒ resuscitation.

mas·talgia (mas-tal'-jē-à) *n* pain in the breast.

mastec·tomy (mas-tek'-to-mē) *n* surgical removal of the breast. ⇒ lumpectomy. *simple mastectomy* removal of the breast with the overlying skin. Combined with radiotherapy this operation is a treatment for carcinoma of the breast. *radical mastectomy* removal of the breast with the skin and underlying pectoral muscle together with all the lymphatic tissue of the axilla: carried out for carcinoma when there has been spread to the glands.

masti·cation (mas-ti-kā'-shun) *n* the act of chewing.

mas·titis (mas-tī'-tis) *n* inflammation of

the breast. *chronic mastitis* the name formerly applied to the nodular changes in the breasts now usually called fibrocystic* disease.

mas·toid (mas'-toyd) *adj* nipple-shaped. *mastoid air cells* extend in a backward and downward direction from the antrum. *mastoid antrum* the air space within the mastoid process, lined by mucous membrane continuous with that of the tympanum and mastoid cells. *mastoid process* the prominence of the mastoid portion of the temporal bone just behind the ear.

mastoid·ectomy (mas-toyd-ek'-to-mē) *n* drainage of the mastoid air-cells and excision of diseased tissue. *cortical mastoidectomy* all the mastoid cells are removed making one cavity which drains through an opening (aditus) into the middle ear. The external meatus and middle ear are untouched. *radical mastoidectomy* the mastoid antrum, and middle ear are made into one continuous cavity for drainage of infection. Loss of hearing is inevitable.

mastoid·itis (mas-toyd-ī'-tis) *n* inflammation of the mastoid air-cells.

mastoidotomy (mas-toyd-o'-to-mē) *n* incision into the mastoid process of the temporal bone.

mastur·bation (mas-tur-bā'-shun) *n* the production of sexual excitement by friction of the genitals.

match test a rough test of respiratory function. If a person is unable to blow out a lighted match held 10 cm from a fully open mouth there is a significant reduction in expiratory airflow.

materia medica (mat-ēr'-ē-a med'-i-ka) (*syn*, pharmacology) the science dealing with the origin, action and dosage of drugs.

matrix (mā'-triks) *n* the foundation substance in which the tissue cells are embedded.

matter (gray and white) (mat'-ter) ⇒ Figure 1.

Matulane (mat'-ū-lān) *n* proprietary name for procarbazine*.

matur·ation (mat-ūr-ā'-shun) *n* the process of attaining full development.

Maurice Lee tube (mōr'-is lē) a double-bored tube which combines nasogastric aspiration and jejunal feeding.

Maxi·dex (maks'-i-deks) *n* proprietary steroid drops for eyes to counteract inflammatory condition.

max·illa (maks-il'-à) *n* the jawbone; in particular the upper jaw—**maxillary** *adj*.

maxillo·facial (maks-il-ō-fā'-shal) *adj* pertaining to the maxilla and face. A subdivision in plastic surgery.

Mazanor (maz'-a-nōr) *n* proprietary name for mazindol*.

maz·indol (maz'-in-dol) *n* an appetite depressant. (Mazanor, Sanorex.)

MBC *abbr* maximal breathing capacity. ⇒ respiratory function tests.

McBurney's point (mak-ber'-nēz) a point one-third of the way between the anterior superior iliac spine and the umbilicus, the site of maximum tenderness in cases of acute appendicitis.

McMurray's oste·ostomy (mak-mur'-ēz os'-tē-ot'-o-mē) division of femur between lesser and greater trochanter. Shaft displaced inwards beneath the head and abducted. This position maintained by a nail plate. Restores painless weight bearing. In congenital dislocation of hip, deliberate pelvic osteotomy renders the outer part of the socket (acetabulum) more horizontal.

measles (mēz'-lz) *n* (*syn* morbilli) an acute infectious disease caused by a virus. Characterized by fever, a blotchy rash and catarrh of mucous membranes. Endemic and worldwide in distribution.

me·atotomy (mē-a-to'-to-mē) *n* surgery to the urinary meatus for meatal ulcer and stricture in men.

me·atus (mē-ā'-tus) *n* an opening or channel—**meatal** *adj*.

mebendazole (me-ben'-da-zōl) *n* drug used to treat hookworm. (Vermox.)

mecamylamine (mek-am-il'-a-mēn) *n* an orally effective ganglionic blocking agent used in the treatment of hypertension. (Inversine.)

mech·anism of labor the forces which extrude the fetus through the birth canal together with the opposing, resisting forces which affect its position.

mechlorethamine (me-klōr-eth'-à-mēn) *n* cytotoxic agent. (Mustargen.)

Meckel's diver·ticulum (mek'-elz dī-ver-tik'-ū-lum) a blind, pouchlike sac sometimes arising from the free border of the lower ileum. Occurs in 2% of population; usually symptomless. May cause gastrointestinal bleeding; may intussuscept or obstruct.

mecli·zine (mek'-li-zēn) *n* an antihistamine*. (Sca Legs.)

mecon·ium (me-kō'-nē-um) *n* the discharge from the bowel of a newly born baby. It is a greenish-black, viscid substance. *meconium ileus* impaction of meconium in bowel. It is one presentation of cystic* fibrosis.

Mede·tron (me'-de-tron) *n* a brand of stethoscope* which can be used over clothing.

media (mē'-dē-à) **1** *n* the middle coat of a vessel. **2** *npl* nutritive jellies used for culturing bacteria. ⇒ medium.

me·dial (mē'-dē-àl) *adj* pertaining to or near the middle—**medially** *adv*.

me·dian (mē'-dē-an) *adj* the middle. *median line* an imaginary line passing through the center of the body from a point between the eyes to between the closed feet. *median nerve* ⇒ Figure 11. *median vein* ⇒ Figure 10.

medias·tinum (mē-dē-as-tī'-num) *n* the space between the lungs—**mediastinal** *adj*.

mediastin·oscopy (mē-dē-as'-tin-os'-ko-pē) *n* a minor surgical procedure for visual inspection of the mediastinum. May be combined with biopsy of lymph nodes for histological examination.

mediate (mē'-dē-āt) *v* to go between two sides.

medical juris·prudence (med'-i-kal jūr-is-proo'-dens) ⇒ forensic medicine.

medic·ament (med-ik'-a-ment) *n* a remedy or medicine. ⇒ drug.

medi·cated (med'-i-kā-ted) *adj* impregnated with a drug or medicine.

med·icinal (med-is'-in-al) *adj* pertaining to a medicine.

medi·cine (med'-is-in) *n* **1** science or art of healing, especially as distinguished from surgery* and obstetrics*. **2** a therapeutic substance. ⇒ drug.

medico·chirurgical (med-ik-ō-kī-rur'-ji-kal) *adj* pertaining to both medicine and surgery.

medico·social (med-i-kō-sō'-shal) *adj* pertaining to medicine and sociology.

medio·lateral (mē-dē-ō-lat'-er-al) *adj* pertaining to the middle and one side.

Mediter·ranean anemia (med-it-er-ān'-ē-um) thalessemia*.

Mediter·ranean fever a genetically inherited disease characterized by polyserositis*.

me·dium (mēd'-ē-um) *n* a substance used in bacteriology for the growth of organisms—**media** *pl*.

MEDLARS *abbr* Medical Literature Analysis and Retrieval System, the computerized bibliography service of the U.S. Library of Medicine.

medroges·tone (med-rō-jest'-ōn) *n* a female hormone, given orally or by injection. Shrinks diseased prostate gland.

Med·rol (med'-rol) *n* proprietary name for methyl* prednisolone.

medroxy·progesterone (med-roks-ē-prō-jest'-er-ōn) *n* a hormone product useful for threatened and recurrent abortion, functional uterine bleeding, secondary amenorrhea, endometrial carcinoma, endometriosis and short-term contraception.

medroxy·progesterone ace·tate (med-roks-ē-prō-jest'-er-ōn as'-e-tāt) long-acting (90 days) contraceptive given by injection. (Depo-Provera, Provera.)

med·ulla (me-dul'-là) *n* **1** the marrow in the center of a long bone. **2** the soft internal portion of glands, e.g. kidneys, adrenals, lymph nodes, etc. *medulla oblongata* the upper part of the spinal cord between the foramen magnum of the occipital bone and the pons cerebri (Figure 1)—**medullary** *adj*.

medul·lated (med'-ū-lā-ted) *adj* containing or surrounded by a medulla* or marrow, particularly referring to nerve fibers.

medullo·blastoma (med-ū-lō-blas-tō'-mà) *n* malignant, rapidly growing tumor occurring in children; appears in the midline of the cerebellum.

mefen·amic acid (mef-en-am'-ik as'-id) an analgesic. Also has anti-inflammatory and antipyretic actions. As a prostaglandin inhibitor it is effective in dysmenorrhea and menorrhagia in some women using intrauterine* contraceptive devices. (Ponstel.)

mega·cephalic (meg-à-sef-al'-ik) *adj* (*syn* macrocephalic, megalocephalic) large headed.

mega·colon (meg-à-kō'-lon) *n* dilatation and hypertrophy of the colon. *aganglionic megacolon* due to congenital absence of ganglionic cells in a distant segment of the large bowel with loss of motor function resulting in hypertrophic dilatation of the normal proximal colon. *acquired megacolon* associated with chronic constipation in the presence of normal ganglion cell innervation: it can accompany amoebic or ulcerative colitis.

mega·karyocyte (meg-à-kār'-ē-ō-sīt) *n* large multinucleated cells of the marrow which produce the blood platelets.

179

megalo·blast (meg'-à-lō-blast) *n* a large, nucleated, primitive red blood cell formed where there is a deficiency of vitamin B_{12} or folic acid—**megaloblastic** *adj.*

megalo·cephalic (meg-à-lō-sef-al'-ik) *adj* ⇒ megacephalic.

megalo·mania (meg-à-lō-mā'-nē-à) *n* delusion of grandeur, characteristic of general* paralysis of the insane.

meibom·ian cyst (mī-bō'-mē-an sist) a cyst* on the edge of the eyelid from retained secretion of the meibomian glands.

meibom·ian glands (mī-bō'-mē-an glands) sebaceous glands lying in grooves on the inner surface of the eyelids, their ducts opening on the free margins of the lids.

Meigs syn·drome (mīgs) a benign, solid ovarian tumor associated with ascites* and hydrothorax*.

mei·osis (mī-ōs'-is) *n* the process which, through two successive cell divisions, leads to the formation of mature gametes—ova* and sperm*. The process starts by the pairing of the partner chromosomes, which then separate from each other at the meiotic divisions, so that the diploid* chromosome number (i.e. 23 pairs in man) is halved to 23 chromosomes, only one member of each original pair; this set constitutes the haploid complement) ⇒ mitosis, germ cells.

melan·cholia (mel-an-kō'-lē-à) *n* term reserved in psychiatry to mean severe forms of depression—**melancholic** *adj.*

mel·anin (mel'-an-in) *n* a black pigment found in hair, skin and the choroid of the eye.

mela·noma (mel-an-ō'-mà) *n* a tumor arising from the pigment-producing cells of the deeper layers in the skin, or of the eye—**melanomata** *pl*, **melanomatous** *adj.*

melano·sarcoma (mel'-an-ō-sar-kō'-mà) *n* one form of malignant melanoma—**melanosarcomata** *pl*, **melanosarcomatous** *adj.*

melan·osis (mel-an-ōs'-is) *n* dark pigmentation of surfaces as in sunburn, Addison's disease etc—**melanotic** *adj.*

melan·uria (mel-an-ūr'-ē-à) *n* melanin* in the urine—**melanuric** *adj.*

mela·tonin (mel-à-tōn'-in) *n* a catecholamine hormone produced by the pineal gland. It appears to inhibit numerous endocrine functions. Recent research shows that sunlight treatment stops its secretion; in depressed patients it resulted in mood improvement.

melena (mel'-e-nà, mel-ē'-nà) *n* black, tarlike stools, evidence of gastrointestinal bleeding.

meli·tensis (mel-i-ten'-sis) *n* ⇒ brucellosis.

Mel·laril (mel'-a-ril) *n* proprietary name for thioridazine*.

mel·phalan (mel'-fa-lan) *n* an alkylating cytotoxic agent of the nitrogen* mustard group. It is effective orally for multiple myelomatosis. It can be given intravenously, and in the treatment of malignant melanoma it is perfused via the intra-arterial route. (Alkaran.)

mem·brane (mem'-brān) *n* a thin lining or covering substance—**membranous** *adj.* *basement membrane* a thin layer beneath the epithelium of mucous surfaces. *hyaloid membrane* the transparent capsule surrounding the vitreous humor of the eye. *mucous membrane* contains glands which secrete mucus. It lines the cavities and passages that communicate with the exterior of the body. *serous membrane* a lubricating membrane lining the closed cavities, and reflected over their enclosed organs. *synovial membrane* the membrane lining the intra-articular parts of bones and ligaments. It does not cover the articular surfaces. *tympanic membrane* the eardrum (⇒ Figure 13).

men·adiol (men-à-dī'-ol) *n* a water soluble analogue of vitamin* K. It is given orally or by injection in hypothrombinemia and neonatal hemorrhage. (Synkavite.)

men·arche (men-ar'-kē) *n* when the menstrual periods commence and other bodily changes occur.

Men·del's law (men'-dels) the fundamental theory of heredity and its laws, evolved by an Austrian monk, Gregor Mendel. The laws determine the inheritance of different characters, and particularly the interaction of dominant and recessive traits in cross-breeding, the maintenance of the purity of such characters during hereditary transmission and the independent segregation of genetically different characteristics, such as the size of pea plants and the characters of their pollen grains.

Mendel·son syn·drome (men'-del-son) inhalation of regurgitated stomach contents, which can cause immediate death from anoxia, or it may produce extensive lung damage or pulmonary edema with severe bronchospasm.

Meniere's dis·ease (man'-ē-ārz') distention of membranous labyrinth of inner ear from excess fluid. Pressure causes failure of function of nerve of hearing and balance, thus there is fluctuating deafness, tinnitus and repeated attacks of vertigo.

men·inges (men-in'-jēz) *n* the surrounding membranes of the brain and spinal cord. They are three in number: (a) the dura mater (outer) (b) arachnoid membrane (middle) (c) pia mater (inner)—**meninx** *sing*, **meningeal** *adj*.

meningi·oma (men-in-jē-ō'-mȧ) *n* a slowly growing fibrous tumor arising in the meninges—**meningiomata** *pl*, **meningiomatous** *adj*.

meningism (men'-in-jism) *n* (*syn* meningismus) a condition presenting with signs and symptoms of meningitis (e.g. neck stiffness); meningitis does not develop.

menin·gitis (men-in-jī'-tis) *n* inflammation of the meninges. An epidemic form is known as cerebrospinal fever, the infecting organism is *Neisseria* meningitidis* (meningococcus). The term *meningococcal meningitis* is now preferred. ⇒ leptomeningitis, pachymeningitis—**meningitides** *pl*.

meningo·cele (men-ing'-gō-sēl) *n* protrusion of the meninges through a bony defect. It forms a cyst filled with cerebrospinal fluid. ⇒ spina bifida.

meningo·coccus (men-ing-go-kok'-us) *n* *Neisseria* meningitidis*—**meningococcal** *adj*.

meningo·encephal·itis (men-ing'-gō-en-sef-ȧ-lī'-tis) *n* inflammation of the brain and the meninges—**meningoencephalitic** *adj*.

meningo·myelo·cele (men-ing'-gō-mī'-el-ō-sēl) *n* (*syn* myelomeningocele) protrusion of a portion of the spinal cord and its enclosing membranes through a bony defect in the spinal canal. It differs from a meningocele* in being covered with a thin, transparent membrane which may be granular and moist.

meniscec·tomy (men-is-ek'-to-mē) *n* the removal of a semilunar* cartilage of the knee joint, following injury and displacement. The medial cartilage is damaged most commonly.

menis·cus (men-is'-kus) *n* **1** semilunar* cartilage, particularly in the knee joint. **2** the curved upper surface of a column of liquid—**menisci** *pl*.

meno·pause (men'-ō-pawz) *n* the end of the period of possible sexual reproduction, as evidenced by the cessation of menstrual periods, normally between the ages of 45 and 50 years. Other bodily and mental changes may occur. *artificial menopause* an earlier menopause induced by radiotherapy or surgery for some pathological condition—**menopausal** *adj*.

menor·rhagia (men-ōr-ā'-jē-ȧ) *n* an excessive regular menstrual flow.

menorrhea (men-ōr-ē'-ȧ) *n* normal menstrual flow.

menotropins (men-ō-trō'-pins) *n* gonadotropin used to stimulate follicle growth and maturation for inducing ovulation in anovulatory women. (Pergonal.)

menses (men'-sēz) *n* the sanguineous fluid discharged from the uterus during menstruation; menstrual flow.

men·strual (men'-str$\overline{oo}$-ȧl) *adj* relating to the menses*. *menstrual cycle* the cyclical chain of events that occurs in the uterus in which a flow of blood (menstrual flow) occurs for 4–5 days every 28 days. The cycle is governed by hormones from the anterior pituitary gland and the ovaries.

men·struation (men-str$\overline{oo}$-ā'-shun) *n* the flow of blood from the uterus once a month in the female. It commences about the age of 13 years and ceases about 45 years.

men·tal (men'-tȧl) *adj* pertaining to the mind. *mental aberration* a pathological deviation from normal thinking. *mental age n* the age of a person with regard to his intellectual development which can be determined by intelligence tests. If a person of 30 years can only pass the tests for a child of 12 years the mental age is 12 years. *mental disorder* mental illness, arrested or incomplete development of mind, psychopathic disorder and any other disorder or disability of mind, and 'mentally disordered' shall be construed accordingly. *mental subnormality* ⇒ subnormality.

men·thol (men'-thol) *n* mild analgesic obtained from oil of peppermint. Used in liniments and ointments for rheumatism, and as an inhalation or drops for nasal catarrh.

mento·anterior (men-tō-an-tē'-rē-or) *adj* forward position of the fetal chin in the maternal pelvis in a face presentation.

mento·posterior (men-tō-post-ē'-rē-or) *adj* backward position of the fetal chin in the maternal pelvis in a face presentation.

meperidine hydrochloride (me-pèr'-i-dēn) *n* a synthetic analgesic and spasmolytic. Widely used for pre- and postoperative and obstetrical anesthesia instead of morphine. May produce physical and/or psychological dependence. (Demerol.)

mepivacaine (me-piv'-à-kān) *n* a local anesthetic. More potent and less toxic than procaine. Used for nerve block.

meprob·amate (mep-rō-bam'-āt) *n* a mild tranquilizer which, by central nervous action, produces mental relaxation. (Miltown.)

mercapto·purine (mer-kap'-tō-pū'-rēn) *n* used in the treatment of acute leukemia in children. Prevents synthesis of nucleic acid. (Puri-nethol.)

mercurial·ism (mer-kūr'-ē-al-izm) *n* toxic effects on human body of mercury—the ancient cure for syphilis. May result from use of calomel-containing teething powders or calomel (as an abortifacient). Symptomatology includes stomatitis, loosening of teeth, gastroenteritis and skin eruptions.

mer·curic oxide (mer-kūr'-ik oks'-īd) *n* a bright yellow powder, once used mainly as oculent hydrarg, ox, flav (golden eye ointment). It is antiseptic and is occasionally used in conjunctivitis and other eye conditions.

mercuro·chrome (mer-kūr'-ō-krōm) *n* a red dye containing mercury in combination. Has antiseptic properties.

mercury (mer'-kū-rē) *n* the only common metal that is liquid at room temperature. Used in measuring instruments such as thermometers and sphygmomanometers. Forms two series of salts: mercurous ones are univalent, and mercuric* ones are bivalent. ⇒ mercurialism.

Merthiolate (mer-thī'-ō-lāt) *n* proprietary name for thimerosal*, organic iodine solution.

mes·arteritis (mes-art-er-ī'-tis) *n* inflammation of the middle coat of an artery.

mesca·line (mes'-ka-lin) *n* a hallucinogenic agent; it can be used to produce the abreaction*.

mesen·cephalon (mes-en-sef'-a-lon) *n* the midbrain *.

mesen·tery (mes'-en-ter-ē) *n* a large sling-like fold of peritoneum passing between a portion of the intestine and the posterior abdominal wall—**mesenteric** *adj*.

mesoderm (mes'-ō-dèrm) *n* the middle layer of cells which form during the early development of the embryo. The other two layers are the ectoderm and the endoderm—**mesodermal** *adj*.

meso·thelioma (mes-ō-thēl-ē-ōm'-a) *n* a rapidly fatal tumor that spreads over the mesothelium of the pleura, pericardium or peritoneum. Of current interest because of its association with the absestos industry.

Mes·tinon (mes'-tin-on) *n* proprietary name for pyridostigmine*.

meta·bolic (met-a-bol'-ik) *adj* pertaining to metabolism. *basal metabolic rate* (*BMR*) the expression of basal metabolism in terms of kJ per sq m of body surface per hour—**metabolically** *adj*.

metab·olism (met-ab'-ol-izm) *n* the continuous series of chemical changes in the living body by which life is maintained. Food and tissues are broken down (catabolism), new substances are created for growth and rebuilding (anabolism) and energy is released in anabolism and utilized in catabolism and heat production ⇒ adenosine diphosphate, adenosine triphosphate—**metabolic** *adj*. *basal metabolism* the minimum energy expended in the maintenance of respiration, circulation, peristalsis, muscle tonus, body temperature and other vegetative functions of the body.

metab·olite (met-ab'-ol-īt) *n* any product of or substance taking part in metabolism. An *essential metabolite* is a substance which is necessary for normal metabolism e.g. vitamins.

metacarpo·phalangeal (met-a-kar'-pō-fal-an'-jē-al) *adj* pertaining to the metacarpus* and the phalanges*.

meta·carpus (met-a-kar'-pus) *n* the five bones which form that part of the hand between the wrist and fingers (⇒ Figures 2, 3)—**metacarpal** *adj*.

Metamucil (met-à-mū'-sil) *n* proprietary name for psyllium*.

metaproterenol sulfate (met-a-prō-ter'-en-ol sul'-fāt) *n* a bronchodilator for relief of bronchospasm. A derivative of epinephrine*. Available as tablets or aerosol. (Alupent.)

metar·aminol (met-ar-am'-in-ol) *n* vasopressor agent used in hypotensive shock. (Aramine.)

met·astasis (met-as'-tas-is) *n* the spread of tumor cells from one part of the body to another, usually by blood or lymph. A secondary growth—**metastases** *pl*, **metastatic** *adj*, **metastasize** *vi*.

metatar·salgia (met-a-tar-sal'-jē-a) *n* pain under the metatarsal heads. *Morton's metatarsalgic* neuralgia caused by a neuroma on the digital nerve, most commonly that supplying the third toe cleft.

metatarso·phalangeal (met-a-tar'-sō-fal-an'-jē-al) *adj* pertaining to the metatarsus and the phalanges.

meta·tarsus (met-a-tar'-sus) *n* the five bones of the foot between the ankle and the toes (⇨ Figure 2)—**metatarsal** *adj*.

metazoa (met-à-zō'-à) *n* multicellular animal organisms with differentiation of cells to form tissues—**metazoal** *adj*.

meteor·ism (mē'-tē-ōr-izm) *n* ⇨ tympanites.

metha·cycline (meth-a-sī'-klin) *n* an antibiotic particularly useful in exacerbations of chronic bronchitis.

metha·done (meth'-a-dōn) *n* a synthetic morphine*-like analgesic, but with a reduced sedative action. Can be given orally or by injection. Particularly valuable in visceral pain and useful in the treatment of unproductive cough. May cause addiction if treatment is prolonged. Can be used in withdrawal programs for heroin addicts. (Dolophine.)

methandrostenolone (meth-an-drō-sten'-o-lōn) *n* an anticatabolic agent, useful in muscle wasting occurring as a result of the body's attempt to restore nitrogen balance, as when protein nitrogen is lost in serum from a large wound or pressure sore, and in senile debility.

meth·ane (meth'-ān) *n* CH_4 a colorless, odorless, inflammable gas produced as a result of putrefaction and fermentation of organic matter.

methantheline (meth-an'-thel-ēn) *n* an anticholinergic* used in peptic ulcer and gastritis. (Banthine.)

meth·aqualone (meth-a-kwal'-ōn) *n* oral hypnotic, because of illegal use, no longer available in the U.S.

met·hem·albumin (meth-ēm-al-bū'-min) *n* abnormal compound in blood from combination of hem with plasma albumen.

methemo·globin (meth-ēm'-ō-glō-bin) *n* a form of hemoglobin consisting of a combination of globin with an oxidized hem, containing ferric iron. This pigment is unable to transport oxygen. It may be formed following the administration of a wide variety of drugs, including the sulfonamides*. It may be present in the blood as a result of a congenital abnormality.

methemo·globinemia (meth-ēm'-ō-glō-bin-ēm'-ē-a) *n* methemoglobin in the blood. If large quantities are present, individuals may show cyanosis, but otherwise no abnormality except, in severe cases, breathlessness on exertion, because the methemoglobin cannot transport oxygen—**methemoglobinemic** *adj*.

methemo·globinuria (meth-ēm'-ō-glō-bin-ūr'-ē-a) *n* methemoglobin in the urine—**methemoglobinuric** *adj*.

methenamine mandelate (meth-en'-a-mēn man'-del-āt) *n* a urinary antiseptic. (Mandelamine.)

methi·cillin (meth-i-sil'-in) *n* a semisynthetic penicillin given by injection and active against pencillin-resistant staphylococci. The emergence of resistant strains of staphylococci has led to the decline of methicillin and more potent derivatives such as cloxacillin* are now preferred. (Staphcillin.)

meth·ionine (meth-ī'-on-ēn) *n* one of the essential sulfur-containing amino* acids. Occasionally used in hepatitis, paracetamol overdose and other conditions associated with liver damage.

methixene (me-thiks'-ēn) *n* an atropine-like drug useful in parkinsonism. It relieves tremor more than rigidity.

metho·carbamol (meth-ō-kàr'-bà-mol) *n* skeletal muscle relaxant useful in muscle injury. (Robaxin.)

methohexital sodium (meth-ō-heks'-i-tol) *n* an ultrashort-acting barbiturate given i.v. pre-operatively as induction agent for anesthesia. (Brevital.)

metho·trexate (meth-ō-treks'-āt) *n* a folic acid antagonist, useful in the treatment of acute lymphoblastic leukemia, some lymphomas and sometimes resistant psoriasis.

methotrim·eprazine (meth-ō-trī-mep'-ra-zēn) *n* a chlorpromazine*-like drug with tranquilizing and analgesic properties useful in schizophrenia and terminal illness. (Levoprome.)

methox·amine (meth-oks'-à-mēn) *n* a pressor drug used to restore blood pressure during anesthesia. It has few side effects on the heart or central nervous system. Given intravenously or intramuscularly. (Vasoxyl.)

meth·oxyflurane (meth-oks-i-flūr'-ān) *n* a liquid whose vapor is an inhalational anesthetic. Used in self-administered obstetric anesthesia but otherwise superseded. (Penthrane.)

methsuximide (meth-suks'-i-mīd) *n* an anticonvulsant used for control of temporal lobe epilepsy and petit mal. (Celontin.)

methyl·ated spirit (meth'-yl-āt-ed) alcohol containing 5% of wood naphtha to make it non-potable. The methylated spirit used for spirit stoves etc. is less pure, and is colored to distinguish it from the above.

methyl·cellulose (meth-il-sel'-ū-lōs) *n* a compound which absorbs water and gives bulk to intestinal contents thus encouraging peristalsis. (Cologel.)

methyl·dopa (meth-il-dō'-på) *n* inhibitor of dopa decarboxylase. Hypotensive agent. Action increased with thiazide diuretics*. (Aldomet.)

methyl·ene blue (meth'-il-ēn blōo) antiseptic dye formerly used in urinary infections, often with hexamine*. The intramuscular injection of a 2.5% solution has been used as a renal function test.

methylphenidate (meth-il-fen'-i-dāt) *n* a cerebral stimulant, chemically similar to amphetamine. It has a paradoxical calming effect on hyperkinetic children. (Ritalin.)

methyl·prednisolone (meth-il-pred-ni-so-lōn) *n* steroid suitable for rheumatoid arthritis, inflammatory and allergic conditions. Sometimes injected locally for exophthalmos. (Medrol.)

methyl·salicylate (meth-il-sal-is'-il-āt) *n* (oil of Wintergreen) used externally as a mild counterirritant and analgesic in rheumatic and similar conditions. Supplied as ointment or liniment.

methyl·testosterone (meth-il-tes-tos'-tėr-ōn) *n* an orally active form of testosterone*. Given as sublingual tablets.

methyl·thiouracil (meth-il-thī-ō-ū'-rà-sil) *n* an antithyroid compound used in thyrotoxicosis. It inhibits the formation of thyroxine*.

methy·prylon (meth-il-prī'-lon) *n* a non-barbiturate hypnosedative. (Noludar.)

methy·sergide (meth-il-sėr'-jīd) *n* a drug which is of value in the long-term prophylaxis of migraine. Can cause retroperitoneal fibrosis, requiring immediate withdrawal, especially in patients with cardiovascular disease, hypertension, and liver or renal dysfunction. (Sansert.)

Meti·nex (met'-in-eks) *n* proprietary name for metolazone*.

meto·clopramide (me-tō-klō'-prà-mīd) *n* a gastric sedative and antiemetic; can be given orally or by injection. Given in high doses to control vomiting due to cytotoxic drugs. Not so effective in vomiting of labyrinthine origin. (Reglan.)

metola·zone (met-ol'-a-zōn) *n* a diuretic.

Meto·pirone (met-ō-pī'-rōn) *n* proprietary name for metyrapone*. *Metopirone test* a test of pituitary and adrenal function. The urinary excretion of 17 hydroxy-corticosteroids is estimated before and after the oral administration of Metopirone. Disease of the pituitary or adrenal cortex causes an abnormal result.

meto·prolol (met-ō-prō'-lol) *n* a beta-adrenergic blocking agent for treatment of hypertension. By reducing the rate and force of cardiac contraction and decreasing the rate of conduction of impulses through the conducting system, it reduces the response to stress and exercise. (Lopressor.)

me·tritis (me-trī'-tis) *n* inflammation of the uterus.

metroni·dazole (me-trō-ni'-da-zōl) *n* an antimicrobial agent especially useful for treating anaerobic bacterial pathogens. Can be given intravenously and orally. Also drug of choice for amoebiasis, trichomonas and Vincent's infection. (Flagyl.)

metro·pathia hemor·rhagica (met-rō-path'-ē-à hem-ō-ra'-jik-à) irregular episodes of anovular uterine bleeding due to excessive and unopposed estrogens* in the blood stream. Usually associated with a follicular cyst in the ovary.

metror·rhagia (met-rō-rā'-jē-à) *n* uterine bleeding between the menstrual periods.

metyra·pone (me-tēr'-à-pōn) *n* a drug which has an indirect diuretic action by inhibiting the secretion of aldosterone in the adrenal cortex. Usually given in conjunction with spironolactone* or a thiazide* drug (Metopirone.) ⇒ Metopirone test.

metyro·sine (met-ir'-ō-sēn) *n* an inhibitor of catecholamine* synthesis. Used in preoperative control of phetochromocytoma. (Demser.)

mexil·etine (meks-il'-e-tēn) *n* an antiarrhythmic agent. Controls ventricular arrhythmia occurring after myocardial infarction and can be used as a prophylactic. (Mexitil.)

Mexitil (meks'-i-til) *n* proprietary name for mexiletine*.

Mezlin (mez'-lin) *n* proprietary name for mezlocillin*.

mezlo·cillin (mez-lō-sil'-lin) *n* a broad spectrum antibiotic similar to ampicillin*. (Mezlin.)

Michel's clips (mī'-kels) small metal clips used instead of sutures for the closure of a wound.

micona·zole (mī-kon'-à-zōl) *n* an antifungal agent used as a pessary and cream for treatment of vulvovaginal candidiasis. (Monistat Cream.)

micro·angiopathy (mī-krō-an-jē-op′-ath-ē) *n* thickening and reduplication of the basement membrane in blood vessels. It occurs in diabetes mellitus, the collagen diseases, infections and cancer. Common manifestations are kidney failure and purpura.

mi·crobe (mī′-krōb) *n* ⇒ microorganism—**microbial, microbic** *adj*.

micro·biology (mī-krō-bī-ol′-o-jē) *n* the science of microorganisms—**microbiological** *adj*, **microbiologically** *adv*.

micro·cephalic (mī-krō-sef-al′-ik) *adj* pertaining to an abnormally small head.

micro·circulation (mī-krō-sir-kū-lā′-shun) *n* arterioles, blood capillaries and venules involved in tissue respiration. Of current interest as the site of trauma in pressure sores.

Micro·coccus (mī-krō-kok′-us) *n* a genus of bacteria. Gram-positive spherical bacteria occurring in irregular masses. They comprise saprophytes, parasites and pathogens.

micro·cyte (mī′-krō-sīt) *n* an undersized red blood cell found especially in iron deficiency anemia. *microcytosis* an increased number of microcytes—**microcytic** *adj*.

microcytosis (mī-krō-sī-tō′-sis) *n* an increased number of microcytes in the circulating blood.

micro·environment (mī-krō-en-vī′-ron-ment) *n* the environment at the microscopic or cellular level immediately surrounding the body.

microfilaria (mī-krō-fil-ār′-ē-à) *n* a genus of tiny worms which cause filariasis*.

micro·gnathia (mī-krō-nath′-ē-à) *n* small jaw, especially the lower one.

mi·cron (mī′-kron) *n* a millionth part of a meter represented by the Greek letter mu (μ).

micronor (mī′-krō-nōr) *n* a mini-pill or progestin-only oral contraceptive containing low dose of norethindrone*.

micronutrients (mī-krō-noō′-tre-ents) *npl* trace* elements.

micro·organism (mī-krō-ōr′-gan-izm) *n* (*syn* microbe) a microscopic cell. Often synonymous with bacterium but includes virus, protozoon, rickettsia, fungus, alga and lichen.

micro·scopic (mī-krō-skop′-ik) *adj* extremely small; visible only with the aid of a microscope. ⇒ macroscopic *opp*.

Micro·sporum (mī-krō-spōr′-um) *n* a genus of fungi. Parasitic, living in kera-

tin-containing tissues of man and animals. *Microsporum audouini* is the commonest cause of scalp ringworm*.

micro·surgery (mī-krō-sur′-je-rē) *n* use of the binocular operating microscope during the performance of operations—**microsurgical** *adj*.

microvascular surgery (mī-krō-vas′-kū-lar) surgery carried out on blood vessels using a binocular operating microscope.

micro·villi (mī-krō-vil′-lī) *npl* microscopic projections from the free surface of cell membranes whose purpose is to increase the exposed surface of the cell.

mictur·ition (mik-tur-i′-shun) *n* (*syn* urination) the act of passing urine.

Midamor (mīd′-a-mōr) proprietary name for amiloride*.

mid·brain *n* ⇒ Figure 1.

Midol (mī′-dol) *n* a combination of aspirin and ephedrine, used for relief of symptoms of dysmenorrhea.

mid·riff (mid′-rif) *n* the diaphragm*.

Midrinn (mī′-drin) *n* proprietary name for dichloralphenazone*.

midwife (mid′-wīf) *n* a person (usually female) who aids in delivering babies.

MIE *abbr* meconium* ileus equivalent.

migraine (mī′-grān) *n* recurrent localized headaches which are often associated with vomiting and visual and sensory disturbances (the aura); caused, it is thought, by intracranial vasoconstriction—**migrainous** *adj*.

Mig·ral (mī′-gral) *n* proprietary preparation containing ergotamine*, cyclizine* and caffeine*. Useful in early treatment of migraine.

Milkulicz disease (mik′-ū-lich) chronic hypertrophic enlargement of the lacrimal and salivary glands. Now thought to be an autoimmune process.

mili·aria (mil-i-ār′-ē-à) *n* (*syn* strophulus) prickly heat common in the tropics, and affects waistline, cubital fossae and chest. Vesicular and erythematous eruption, caused by blocking of sweat ducts and their subsequent rupture, or their infection by fungi or bacteria.

miliary (mil′-i-ār-ē) *adj* resembling a millet seed. *miliary tuberculosis* ⇒ tuberculosis.

milium (mil′-i-um) *n* condition in which tiny, white, cystic excrescences appear on the face, especially about the eyelids; associated with seborrhea*.

milk *n* provided that the mother is taking an adequate diet, human milk contains all the essential nutrients for a newborn in the correct proportions. It contains IgA and lactoferrin which increases the newborn infant's resistance to infection. *milk sugar* lactose*. *milk of magnesia* (M.O.M., *abbr*) magnesium hydroxide, an antacid.

Miller-Abbot tube (mil'-ler ab'-ot) *n* a double lumen rubber tube used for intestinal suction. The second channel leads to a balloon near the tip of the tube. This balloon is inflated when the tube reaches the duodenum and it is then carried down the intestine by peristaltic activity.

Milontin (mil-on'-tin) *n* proprietary name for phensuximide*.

Miltown (mil'-town) *n* proprietary name for meprobamate*.

Milwaukee brace (mil-waw'-kē) a body splint which is worn at all times during the treatment period for correction of spinal curvature (scoliosis). It applies fixed traction between the occiput and the pelvis.

mineralo·corticoid (min-ėr-al'-ō-kōr'-ti-koyd) *n* ⇒ aldosterone.

miner's anemia (mī'-nerz a-nē'-mē-a) hookworm disease ⇒ ankylostomiasis.

miner's elbow (mī'-nerz el'-bō) olecranon bursitis*.

miner's lung (mī'-nerz lung) ⇒ hematite.

Min·ims (min'-ims) *n* a proprietary range of ophthalmic drugs presented in single-use eyedroppers.

Minipress (min'-i-pres) *n* proprietary name for prazosin*.

Mino·cin (min-ō'-sin) *n* proprietary name for minocycline*.

mino·cycline (min-ō-sī'-klēn) *n* one of the tetracyclines which is absorbed from the stomach in the presence of food and so can be taken at a time convenient to the patient; it rarely causes skin sensitivity to sunlight. (Minocin.)

Min·ovral (min-ōv'-ral) *n* a proprietary oral contraceptive containing both estrogen and progestogen.

minoxi·dil (min-oks'-i-dil) *n* used in severe hypertension resistant to other drugs.

Min·tezol (min'-ta-zol) *n* proprietary name for thiabendazole*.

mi·osis (myosis) (mī-ōs'-is) *n* excessive contraction of the pupil of the eye.

Miostat (mī'-ō-stat) *n* proprietary name for carbachol*.

mi·otic (myotic) (mī-ot'-ik) *adj* pertaining to or producing miosis*.

mis·carriage (mis'-kār-aj) *n* termination of pregnancy before the fetus has reached viability.

missed abortion ⇒ abortion.

mistura (mis-tū'-ra) *n* a fluid for oral administration in which there may be soluble or suspended insoluble substances. They are not chemically united. Should always be well shaken before use.

Mithra·cin (mith-rā'-sin) *n* proprietary name for mithramycin*.

mithra·mycin (mith-rȧ-mī'-sin) *n* an antibiotic with cytotoxic activity. It is now used mainly in the hypercalcemia associated with malignant disease. Given intravenously. (Mithracin.)

mito·chondrion (mī-tō-kon'-drē-on) *n* a highly specialized structure within cell cytoplasm. It is an important site of ATP synthesis: it contains enzymes which are essential for many biochemical processes.

mito·mycin (mī-tō-mī'-sin) *n* a cytotoxic antibiotic which is used in cancer of the breast and upper gastrointestinal tract. May cause lung damage and delayed bone marrow toxicity.

mi·tosis (mī-tō'-sis) *n* the ordinary type of nuclear (cell) division, preceded by the faithful replication of chromosomes. Through this process, daughter cells, derived from division of a mother cell, retain the diploid chromosome number, 46 in man. ⇒ meiosis—**mitotic** *adj*.

mitral (mī'-tràl) *adj* miter-shaped, as the valve between the left atrium and ventricle of the heart (bicuspid valve). *mitral incompetence* a defect in the closure of the mitral valve whereby blood tends to flow backwards into the left artium from the left ventricle. *mitral stenosis* narrowing of the mitral orifice, usually due to rheumatic fever. *mitral valvulotomy (valvotomy)* an operation for splitting the cusps of a stenosed mitral valve.

mittelschmerz (mit'-el-shmärts) *n* abdominal pain midway between menstrual periods, at time of ovulation.

MLNS *abbr* mucocutaneous* lymph node syndrome.

Modur·etic (mod-ūr-et'-ik) *n* a proprietary mixture of amiloride* and hydrochlorothiazide*.

moist wound healing achieved by application of an occlusive, semipermeable dressing which permits the exudate to collect under the film to carry out its bactericidal functions. ⇒ OpSite.

molar teeth (mō'-lar) the teeth fourth and

mold (mōld) *n* multicellular fungus.

molding (mōld'-ing) *n* the compression of the fetal head during its passage through the birth canal in labor.

mole (mōl) *n* a pigmented area on the skin, usually brown. Some moles are flat, some are raised and occasionally have hairs growing from them. Malignant changes can occur in them.

molecule (mol'-e-kūl) *n* a combination of two or more atoms to form a specific chemical substance—**molecular** *adj*.

mollities (mol'-it-ēz) *n* softness. *mollities ossium* osteomalacia*.

mol·luscum (mo-lus'-kum) *n* a soft tumor. *molluscum contagiosum* an infectious condition common in infants caused by a virus. Tiny translucent papules with a central depression are formed. *molluscum fibrosum* the superficial tumors of von* Recklinghausen's disease.

MOM *abbr* milk* of magnesia.

mon·articular (mon-àr-tik'-ū-lar) *adj* relating to one joint.

Mönckeberg's sclerosis (menk'-ē-bergz skler-ōs'-is) senile degenerative change resulting in calcification of the median muscular layer in arteries, especially of the limbs; leads to intermittent claudication and rarely to gangrene, if atherosclerosis coexists.

mon·gol (mon'-gol) *n* a person afflicted with Down* syndrome.

mongolism (mong'-gol-izm) *n* ⇒ Down syndrome.

Monilia (mon-il'-ē-à) *n* ⇒ Candida.

moniliasis (mon-il-ī'-à-sis) *n* ⇒ candidiasis.

Monistat Cream (mon'-i-stat) *n* proprietary name for miconazole.*

moni·toring (mon'-i-tor-ing) *n* sequential recording. Term usually reserved for automatic visual display of such measurements as temperature, pulse, respiration and blood pressure. *fetal monitoring* use of a fetal monitor to detect heart beat and uterine contractions.

mono·amine oxi·dase (mon'-ō-à-mēn oks'-i-dās) an enzyme which inhibits the breakdown of serotonin* and catecholamines* in the brain. *monoamine oxidase inhibitor (MAOI)* a substance which, by inhibiting the action of monoamine oxidase, increases the level of serotonin and catecholamines in the brain; useful for relief of exogenous or reactive depression. Increases the effects of many drugs; alcohol, and barbiturates in particular; patients re advised to abstain from cheese, Marmite, Bovril, broadbeans (because of episodic hypertension and possibility of subarachnoid hemorrhage) and any drug not ordered by the doctor. (Eutonyl.)

mono·cular (mon-ok'-ū-lar) *adj* pertaining to one eye.

mono·cyte (mon'-ō-sīt) *n* a mononuclear* cell—**monocytic** *adj*.

mono·mania (mon-ō-mā'-nē-à) *n* obsession with a single idea.

mono·nuclear (mon-ō-noo'-klē-ar) *adj* with a single nucleus. Usually refers to a type of blood cell (monocyte), the largest of the cells in the normal blood with a round, oval or indented nucleus.

mono·nucleosis (mon-ō-noo-klē-ō'-sis) *n* an increase in the number of circulating monocytes (mononuclear* cells) in the blood. *infectious mononucleosis* ⇒ infectious*.

mono·plegia (mon-ō-plē'-jē-à) *n* paralysis of only one limb—**monoplegic** *adj*.

monorchidism, monorchism (mon-ōr'-kid-izm, mon'-ōr-kizm) *n* a condition in which only one testis is descended, the other may be absent or undescended.

mono·saccharide (mon-ō-sak'-à-rīd) *n* a simple sugar carbohydrate with the general formula CH_2O. Examples are glucose*, fructose* and galactose*.

mono·sodium gluta·mate (mon-ō-sō'-dēum glū'-tà-māt) a chemical which can be added to food as a flavor-enhancer. It can cause Chinese* restaurant syndrome.

mono·somy (mon-ō-sō'-mē) *n* state resulting from the absence of a chromosome from an otherwise diploid* chromosome complement (e.g. monosomy for chromosome 21).

mon·ovular (mon-ō'-vū-lar) *adj* ⇒ uniovular.

mons veneris (mons ven-èr'-is) the eminence formed by the pad of fat which lies over the pubic bone in the female.

Mooren's ul·cer (moor'-enz) a gutter-like excoriation of the peripheral cornea with a tendency to spread.

mor·bidity (mōr-bid'-it-ē) *n* the state of being diseased.

mor·billi (mōr-bil'-lī) *n* ⇒ measles.

morbilli·form (mōr-bil'-i-fôrm) *adj* describes a rash resembling that of measles*.

187

mori·bund (mōr′-i-bund) *adj* in a dying state.

morning after pill series of pills begun 24–72 hours after sexual intercourse to prevent pregnancy. Contains high doses of estrogens, progesterone, or a combination of both. If pregnancy does occur, the use of these pills may cause birth defects.

Moro reflex (mō′-rō) on being startled a baby throws out his arms, then brings them together in an embracing movement.

mor·phine (mōr′-fēn) *n* the active principle of opium* and a most valuable analgesic. Widely used in pain due to spasm, in hemorrhage and shock. May cause some respiratory depression, especially in full doses.

mor·phea (mōr′-fē-à) *n* ⇒ scleroderma.

mor·phology (mōr-fol′-o-jē) *n* the science which deals with the form and structure of living things—**morphological** *adj*, **morphologically** *adv*.

mor·tality (mōr-tal′-i-tē) *n* number or frequency of deaths. *mortality rate* the death-rate; the ratio of the total number of deaths to the total population.

morti·fication (mōr-tif-i-kā′-shun) *n* death of tissue. ⇒ gangrene.

Morton's metatar·salgia (mōr′-tonz met-a-tar-sal′-jē-a) ⇒ metatarsalgia.

mosquito-trans·mitted hemor·rhagic fevers infections which occur mainly in a tropical climate: they result in bleeding particularly into joints, muscles and the skin. The important ones are chikungunya, dengue, Rift valley fever and yellow fever.

mo·tile (mō′-til) *adj* capable of spontaneous movement—**motility** *n*.

mo·tion (mō′-shun) *n* an evacuation of the bowel.

motor (mō′-tor) *adj* pertaining to action. ⇒ neuron.

motor nerve (mō′-tor) ⇒ Figure 1. *motor neuron disease* a progressive degenerative disease of the motor part of the nervous system. It occurs in middle age and results in increasing muscle weakness and wasting.

Motrin (mō′-trin) *n* proprietary name for ibuprofen*.

mottling (mot′-ling) *n* discoloration of the skin.

moun·tain sick·ness symtoms of sickness, tachycardia and dyspnea caused by low oxygen content of rarefied air at high altitude.

mouth-to-mouth resuscitation ⇒ resuscitation.

MRSA *abbr* methicillin-resistant staphylococcus aureus.

MS *abbr* multiple sclerosis.

Mucaine (mū′-kān) *n* proprietary name for oxethazaine*.

muci·lage (mū′-si-laj) *n* the solution of a gum in water—**mucilaginous** *adj*.

mu·cin (mū′-sin) *n* a mixture of glycoproteins found in and secreted by many cells and glands—**mucinous** *adj*.

mucin·ase (mū′-sin-ās) *n* a specific mucin-dissolving substance contained in some aerosols. Useful in cystic fibrosis.

mucin·olysis (mū-sin-ol′-is-is) *n* dissolution of mucin*—**mucinolytic** *adj*.

muco·cele (mū′-kō-sēl) *n* distension of a cavity with mucus*.

muco·cutaneous (mū-kō-kū-tān′-ē-us) *adj* pertaining to mucous membrane* and skin. *mucocutaneous lymph node syndrome (MLNS)* a disease affecting mainly babies and children first noticed in Japan in the late 1960s. Characterized by fever, dry lips, red mouth and strawberry-like tongue. A rash in a glove-and-stocking distribution is followed by desquamation. There is cervical adenitis, polymorphonuclear leukocytosis and a raised ESR.

mu·coid (mū′-koyd) *adj* resembling mucus*.

muco·lytics (mū-kō-li′-tiks) *npl* drugs which reduce viscosity of secretion from the respiratory tract.

muco·polysacchari·doses (mū′-kō-pol-ē-sak′-à-rīd-ōs′-ez) *npl* a group of inherited neurometabolic conditions in which genetically determined specific enzyme defects lead to accumulation of abnormal amounts of mucopolysaccharides. ⇒ gargoylism, Hunter syndrome.

muco·purulent (mū-kō-pū′-ru-lent) *adj* containing mucus and pus.

muco·pus (mū′-kō-pus) *n* mucus containing pus.

mu·cosa (mū-kō′-sà) *n* a mucous membrane*—**mucosae** *pl*, **mucosal** *adj*.

muco·sitis (mū-kō-sī′-tis) *n* inflammation of a mucous membrane*.

mu·cous (mū′-kus) *adj* pertaining to or containing mucus*. *mucous colitis* also called mucomembranous colitis. Possibly a functional disorder, manifested by passage of mucus in the stool, obstinate constipation and occasional colic. *mucous polypus* a growth (adenoma) of mucous membrane which becomes pedunculated. *mucous membrane* ⇒ membrane.

muco·viscidosis (mū-kō-vis-i-dō'-sis) *n* cystic* fibrosis.

mu·cus (mū'-kus) *n* the viscid fluid secreted by mucous glands—**mucous, mucoid** *adj*.

multi·cellular (mul-ti-sel'-ū-lar) *adj* constructed of many cells.

multi·gravida (mul-ti-grav'-id-à) *n* (*syn* multipara) a woman who has had more than one pregnancy—**multigravidae** *pl*.

multi·lobular (mul-ti-lōb'-ū-lar) *adj* possessing many lobes.

multi·locular (mul-ti-lok'-ū-lar) *adj* possessing many small cysts, loculi or pockets.

multi·nuclear (mul-ti-noo'-klē-ar) *adj* possessing many nuclei—**multinucleate** *adj*.

multi·para (mul-tip'-a-rà) ⇒ multigravida—**multiparae** *pl*.

mul·tiple scler·osis (MS) (mul'-tip-l skler-ōs'-is) (*syn* disseminated sclerosis) now considered as one of the muscular dystrophies. It is a variably progressive disease of the nervous system, most commonly first affecting young adults in which patchy, degenerative changes occur in nerve sheaths in the brain, spinal cord and optic nerves, followed by sclerosis*. The presenting symptoms can be diverse, ranging from diplopia to weakness or unsteadiness of a limb; disturbances of micturition are common.

Multi·vite (mul'-ti-vīt) *n* proprietary tablets containing vitamin A, aneurine hydrochloride, ascorbic acid and calciferol.

mumps (mumps) *n* (*syn* infectious parotitis) an acute, specific inflammation of the parotid* glands, caused by a virus.

Munchausen syn·drome (men-chow'-zen) patients consistently produce false stories so they receive needless medical investigations, operations and treatments. *Munchausen syndrome by proxy* is the term used when the mother produces false stories for her child.

mu·ral (mū'-ral) *adj* pertaining to the wall of a cavity, organ or vessel.

mur·mur (mur'-mur) *n* (*syn* bruit) abnormal sound heard on auscultation of heart or great vessels. *presystolic murmur* characteristic of mitral stenosis in regular rhythm.

Musca (mus'-ka) *n* genus of the common house-fly, capable of transmitting many enteric infections.

muscle (mus'-l) *n* strong, contractile tissue which produces movement in the body (⇒ Figures 2, 3)—**muscular** *adj*. *cardiac muscle* makes up the middle wall of the heart; it is involuntary, striated and innervated by autonomic nerves. *skeletal muscle* surrounds the skeleton; it is voluntary, striated and innervated by the peripheral nerves of the central nervous system. *visceral (internal) muscle* is nonstriated and involuntary and is innervated by the autonomic nerves. *muscle relaxants* a group of drugs which is widely used in surgery, in tetanus to prevent spasm, in mechanically aided respiration and in the convulsive shock therapy for mental disorder. There are two types, depolarizing and non-depolarizing; the latter are reversed by anticholinesterases, e.g. neostigmine*. Muscle relaxants paralyze all skeletal muscles, including those of breathing. They have no sedative action.

mus·cular dys·trophies (mus'-kū-lar dis'-trō-fēz) a group of genetically transmitted diseases; they are all characterized by progressive atrophy of different groups of muscles with loss of strength and increasing disability and deformity. Pseudohypertrophic or Duchenne type is the most severe. Presents in early childhood. Runs a malignant course. A clue to future treatment lies in recent advances in biochemical knowledge of the condition. ⇒ Duchenne muscular dystrophy.

mus·cular rheum·atism (mus'-kū-lar roo'-mà-tism) ⇒ fibrositis.

muscu·lature (mus'-kū-là-chur) *n* the muscular system, or any part of it.

musculo·cutaneous (mus-kū-lō-kū-tā'-nē-us) *adj* pertaining to muscle and skin.

musculo·skeletal (mus-kū-lō-skėl'-e-tal) *adj* pertaining to the muscular and skeletal systems.

mus·tard (mus'-tàrd) *n* crushed seeds of the mustard plant which have been used orally as an emetic or externally as a counterirritant.

mustargen (mus'-tar-jen) *n* a nitrogen* mustard, mechlorethamine.

mut·agen (mū'-tà-jen) *n* an agent which induces gene or chromosome mutation.

muta·genesis (mū-tà-jen'-es-is) *n* the production of mutations—**mutagenic, mutagenetic** *adj*, **mutagenetically** *adv*.

muta·genicity (mū-tà-jen-is'-it-ē) *n* the capacity to produce gene mutations or chromosome aberrations.

189

mu·tant (mū´-tant) *n* a cell (or individual) which carries a genetic change or mutation.

mu·tation (mū-tā´-shun) *n* an alteration in genes or chromosomes of a living cell gives rise to genetic change, as a result of which the characters of the cell alter. The change is heritable. *induced mutation* a gene mutation or change produced by known agents outside the cell that interact with and affect the chromosomal DNA and may alter chromosome structure or number, e.g. ionizing radiation and mutagenic chemicals, ultraviolet radiation, etc. *spontaneous mutation* a genetic mutation taking place without apparent influence from outside the cell.

mute (mūt) **1** *adj* unable to speak. **2** *n* a person who is unable to speak.

mutilat·ion (mū-til-ā´-shun) *n* the condition resulting from the removal of a limb or other part of the body. It results in a change of body image, to which there has to be considerable physical, psychological and social adjustment for a successful outcome.

mu·tism (mū´-tizm) *n* (*syn* dumbness) inability or refusal to speak. It may be due to congenital causes, the most common being deafness; it may be the result of physical disease, the most common being a stroke, and it can be a manifestation of mental disease.

my·algia (mī-al´-jē-à) *n* pain in the muscles—**myalgic** *adj*. *epidemic myalgia* ⇒ Bornholm disease.

My·ambutol (mī-am´-bū-tol) *n* proprietary name for ethambutol*.

myas·thenia (mī-as-thē´-nē-à) *n* muscular weakness—**myasthenic** *adj*. *myasthenia gravis* a disorder characterized by marked fatiguability of voluntary muscles, especially those of the eye. Due to a biochemical defect associated with abnormal behavior of acetylcholine* at neuromuscular junctions. There is considerable evidence for an autoimmune process. It is thought that the patient forms antibody (to his own striated muscle fibers) which competes with actylcholine and prevents it from carrying out its transmission functions especially when only small quantities are available. Research on twins suggests that a rare recessive trait may be instrumental in causing the disease.

myas·thenic crisis (mī-as-thēn´-ik krī´-sis) a sudden deterioration with weakness of respiratory muscles due to an increase in severity of myasthenia. It is distinguished from cholinergic* crisis by giving edrophonium chloride 10 mg intravenously. Marked improvement confirms myasthenic crisis. ⇒ edrophonium test.

myatonia (mī-à-tō´-nē-à) *n* absence of muscle tone. *myatonia congenita* a form of congenital muscular dystropathy in infancy. Child is unable to bear the weight of his head on his shoulders—**myatonic**, *adj*.

my·celium (mī-sēl´-ē-um) *n* a mass of branching filaments (hyphae) of molds or fungi—**mycelial** *adj*.

my·cetoma (mī-se-tō´-mà) *n* ⇒ Madura foot.

Mycifra·din (mī-sif´-ra-din) proprietary name for neomycin*.

Myco·bacterium (mī-kō-bak-tēr´-ē-um) *n* a genus of rod-shaped acid-fast bacteria. *Mycobacterium avium* ⇒ avian. *Mycobacterium leprae* causes leprosy and *Mycobacterium tuberculosis* causes tuberculosis.

mycol·ogist (mī-kol´-o-jist) *n* a person who has expert knowledge of mycology* and the methods used to study it.

my·cology (mī-kol´-o-jē) *n* the study of fungi—**mycological** *adj*, **mycologically** *adv*.

Myco·plasma (mī-kō-plaz´-mà) *n* a genus of microscopic organisms considered as the smallest free-living organisms. Some are parasites, some are saprophytes and others are pathogens. *Mycoplasma pneumoniae* causes primary atypical pneumonia, previously called viral pneumonia. *Mycoplasma hominis* is associated with inflammatory disease of the female upper genital tract and *Ureaplasma* with non-gonococcal urethritis.

my·cosis (mī-kō´-sis) *n* disease caused by any fungus—**mycotic** *adj*. *mycosis fungoides* is a chronic and usually fatal lymphomatous disease, not fungal in origin. It is manifested by generalized pruritus, followed by skin eruptions of diverse character which become infiltrated and finally develop into granulomatous ulcerating tumors.

Mycostatin (mī´-kō-stat-in) *n* proprietary name for nystatin*.

myco·toxins (mī-kō-toks´-ins) *npl* the secondary metabolites of molds or microfungi. About 100 chemical substances have been identified as mycotoxins, many capable of causing cancer as well as other diseases—**mycotoxic** *adj*.

My·driacyl (mi´-drē-ak-l) *n* proprietary name for tropicamide*.

my·driasis (mid-rī'-à-sis) *n* abnormal dilation of the pupil of the eye.

my·driatics (mid-rē-at'-iks) *npl* drugs which cause mydriasis*.

my·elin (mī'-e-lin) *n* the white, fatty substance constituting the medullary sheath of a nerve.

myel·itis (mī-el-ī'-tis) *n* inflammation of the spinal cord.

myelo·blasts (mī'-el-ō-blasts) *npl* the earliest identifiable cells which after several stages become granulocytic white blood cells—**myeloblastic** *adj*.

myelo·cele (mī'-el-ō-sēl) *n* an accompaniment of spina* bifida wherein development of the spinal cord itself has been arrested, and the central canal of the cord opens on the skin surface discharging cerebrospinal fluid.

myelo·cytes (mī'-el-ō-sīts) *npl* precursor cells of granulocytic white blood cells normally present only in bone marrow—**myelocytic** *adj*.

myelo·fibrosis (mī'-el-ō-fī-brō'-sis) *n* formation of fibrous tissue within the bone marrow cavity. Interferes with the formation of blood cells.

myelo·genous (mī-el-o'-jen-us) *adj* produced in or by the bone marrow.

myel·ography (mī-el-og'-raf-ē) *n* radiographic examination of the spinal canal by injection of a contrast medium into the subarachnoid space—**myelographic** *adj*, **myelogram** *n*, **myelograph** *n*, **myelographically** *adv*.

my·eloid (mī'-el-oyd) *adj* pertaining to the granulocyte precursor cells in the bone marrow.

myel·oma (mī-el-ō'-mà) *n* malignant condition arising from plasma cells, usually in the bone marrow—**myelomata** *pl*, **myelomatous** *adj*. *multiple myeloma* the formation of a number of myelomata in bones.

myelo·matosis (mī'-el-ō-mà-tō'-sis) *n* plasma cell neoplasia. Crowding of the bone marrow by abnormal plasma cells, suppression of normal blood cells leading to anemia, thrombocytopenia and neutropenia. Consequently the patient is immunosuppressed and is therefore susceptible to infection. May produce changes in serum globulins and Bence-Jones proteinuria.

myelo·meningocele (mī-el-ō-men-in'-gō-sēl) *n* ⇒ meningomyelocele.

myel·opathy (mī-el-op'-à-thē) *n* disease of the spinal cord. Can be a serious complication of cervical spondylosis—**myelopathic** *adj*.

Mylanta (mī-lan'-tà) *n* aluminum hydroxide and magnesium hydroxide suspension, an antacid.

Myleran (mī'-lèr-an) *n* proprietary name for busulfan*.

myo·cardial infarc·tion (mī-ō-kàr'-dē-al in-fàrk'-shun) death of a part of the myocardium* from deprivation of blood. The deprived tissue becomes necrotic and requires time for healing. The patient experiences a 'heart attack' with sudden intense chest pain which may radiate to arms and jaws. Because of the danger of ventricular fibrillation many patients are nursed in a coronary care or intensive care unit. ⇒ angina (pectoris), ischemic heart disease.

myo·carditis (mī-ō-kàr-dī'-tis) *n* inflammation of the myocardium*.

myo·cardium (mī-ō-kar'-dē-um) *n* the middle layer of the heart wall. ⇒ muscle—**myocardial** *adj*.

myo·cele (mī'-ō-sēl) *n* protrusion of a muscle through its ruptured sheath.

myo·clonus (mī-ō-klō'-nus) *n* clonic contractions of individual or groups of muscles.

Myochrysine (mī-ō-kris'-ēn) *n* proprietary name for aurothiomalate*.

myo·electric (mī-ō-ē-lek'-trik) *adj* pertaining to the electrical properties of muscle.

myofibril (mī-ō-fī'-bril) *n* a small fibril of muscular tissue.

myo·fibrosis (mī-ō-fī-brō'-sis) *n* excessive connective tissue in muscle. Leads to inadequate functioning of part—**myofibroses** *pl*.

myo·genic (mī-ō-jen'-ik) *adj* originating in or starting from muscle.

myo·globin (mī-ō-glō'-bin) ⇒ myohemoglobin.

myo·globinuria (mī-ō-glō-bin-ūr'-ē-a) *n* ⇒ myohemoglobinuria.

myo·hemoglobin (mī-ō-hē'-mō-glō-bin) *n* (*syn* myoglobin) a muscle protein resembling a single subunit of hemoglobin and thus of much lower molecular weight than blood hemoglobin. It combines with the oxygen released by the erythrocytes, stores it and transports it to the muscle cell mitochondria where energy is generated for synthesis and heat production. It is liberated from muscle and appears in the urine in the 'crush syndrome'.

myo·hemoglobin·uria (mī-ō-hē-mō-glo-bin-ūr′-ē-à) *n* (*syn* myoglobinuria) excretion of myohemoglobin in the urine as in crush syndrome.

myo·kymia (mī-ō-kī′-mē-à) *n* muscle twitching. In the lower eyelid it is benign. *facial myokymia* may result from long use of phenothiazine* drugs; has also been observed in patients with multiple sclerosis.

my·oma (mī-ō′-mà) *n* a tumor of muscle tissue—**myomata** *pl*, **myomatous** *adj*.

myo·malacia (mī-ō-mal-ā′-sē-à) *n* softening of muscle, as occurs in the myocardium after infarction.

myo·mectomy (mī-ō-mek′-to-mē) *n* enucleation of uterine fibroid(s)*.

myo·metrium (mī-ō-mē′-trē-um) *n* the thick muscular wall of the uterus.

myo·neural (mī-ō-noo͞o′-ral) *adj* pertaining to muscle and nerve.

my·opathy (mī-op′-à-thē) *n* any disease of the muscles. ⇒ glycogenosis—**myopathic** *adj*.

myope (mī′-ōp) *n* a shortsighted person—**myopic** *adj*.

my·opia (mī-ōp′-ē-à) *n* shortsightedness. The light rays come to a focus in front of, instead of on, the retina—**myopic** *adj*.

myo·plasty (mī′-ō-plas-tē) *n* plastic surgery of muscles—**myoplastic** *adj*.

myo·sarcoma (mī-ō-sàr-kō′-mà) *n* a malignant tumor derived from muscle—**myosarcomata** *pl*, **myosarcomatous** *adj*.

myo·sin (mī′-ō-sin) *n* one of the main proteins of muscle; reacts with actin in the muscle cell to cause contraction.

my·osis (mī-ōs′-is) *n* ⇒ miosis—**myotic** *adj*.

myo·sitis (mī-ō-sī′-tis) *n* inflammation of a muscle. *myositis ossificans* deposition of active bone cells in muscle, resulting in hard swellings.

my·otomy (mī-ot′-o-mē) *n* cutting or dissection of muscle tissue.

Myotonachol (mī-ō-tō′-nak-ol) *n* proprietary name for bethanecol*.

myo·tonia (mī-ō-tō′-nē-à) *n* an increase in muscle tone at test—**myotonic** *adj. myotonia congenita* a genetically-determined form of congenital muscular weakness, usually presenting in infancy and due to degeneration of anterior horn cells in the spinal cord. Fibrillation of affected muscles is characteristic.

myringa (mī-ring′-à) *n* the eardrum or tympanic membrane.

myrin·gitis (mī-ring-ī′-tis) *n* inflammation of the eardrum* (tympanic membrane).

myringo·plasty (mī-ring′-ō-plas′-tē) *n* this operation is designed to close a defect in the tympanic membrane. Grafts are frequently used—**myringoplastic** *adj*.

myringo·tome (mī-ring′-ō-tōm) *n* a delicate instrument for incising the eardrum* (tympanic membrane).

myrin·gotomy (mī-ring-ot′-o-mē) *n* incision into the eardrum* (tympanic membrane). Performed for the drainage of pus or fluid from the middle ear. Middle ear ventilation maintained by insertion of a grommet or Teflon tube.

My·soline (mī′-sō-lēn) *n* proprietary name for primidone*.

Mystec·lin F (mis-tek′-lin-ef) *n* a proprietary combination of tetracycline* and an antifungal powder.

myx·edema (miks-e-dē′-mà) *n* clinical syndrome of hypothyroidism*. Patient becomes slow in movement and dull mentally; there is bradycardia, low temperature, dry skin and swelling of limbs and face. Associated with low serum thyroxine and raised thyrotrophin levels—**myxedematous** *adj. pretibial myxederma* violaceous indurated areas of skin, usually on foreleg, in some cases of thyrotoxicosis*. May be associated with exophthalmos and clubbing of fingers. *myxedema coma* impaired level of consciousness in severe myxedema. Mortality rate high from hypothermia, heart failure, cardiac arrhythmias or bronchopneumonia.

myx·oma (miks-ō′-mà) *n* a connective tissue tumor composed largely of mucoid material—**myxomata** *pl*, **myxomatous** *adj*.

myxo·sarcoma (miks-ō-sàr-kō′-mà) *n* a malignant tumor of connective tissue with a soft, mucoid consistency—**myxosarcomata** *pl*, **myxosarcomatous** *adj*.

myxo·viruses (miks-ò-vī′-rus-es) *npl* name for the influenza group of viruses.

N

naboth·ian fol·licles (na-both′-ē-an) cystic distension of chronically inflamed cervical glands of uterus, where the duct of the gland has become obliterated by a healing epithelial covering and the normal mucus cannot escape.

Naegele's ob·liquity (na′-ge-lēz ob-lik′-wit-ē) (*syn* asynclitism) tilting of the fetal head to one or other side to decrease the transverse diameter presented to the pelvic brim.

Nafcil (naf'-sil) *n* proprietary name for nafcillin sodium*.

nafcillin sodium (naf-sil'-in) *n* a penicillin used for treating infections caused by penicillinase-producing staphylococci. (Nafcil.)

NAI *abbr* non-accidental injury. ⇒ battered baby syndrome.

nali·dixic acid (nal-i-diks'-ik as'-id) a chemotherapeutic agent which is especially useful for urinary infections. (Negram.)

nal·oxone (nà-loks'-ōn) *n* a narcotic antagonist; it reverses all actions of narcotics and has no analgesic action itself. Lasts about half an hour. (Narcan.)

nan·drolone phenyl·propionate (nan'-dro-lōn fen'-il-prō'-pē-on-āt) an agent which has similar protein-forming and tissue building functions to testosterone but without the masculinizing effects on women. It is used for patients who have extensive tissue damage from any cause, or wasting diseases. (Durabolin.)

nape (nāp) *n* the back of the neck; the nucha.

naphazo·line (naf-az'-ō-lēn) *n* decongestive substance used in allergic nasal conditions, and in rhinitis; 1 in 2000 to 1 in 1000 solution as spray or drops.

Napro·syn (nap'-rō-sin) *n* proprietary name for naproxen*.

naproxen (nà-proks'-en) *n* relieves pain, reduces inflammation and eases joint stiffness without causing gastric bleeding. (Naprosyn.)

Nar·can (nar'-kan) *n* proprietary naloxone*.

narciss·ism (nar-sis'-izm) *n* self-love. In psychiatry the narcissistic type of personality is one where the sexual love-object is the self.

narco·analysis (nar-kō-an-al'-is-is) *n* analysis of mental content under light anesthesia, usually an intravenous barbiturate—**narcoanalytic** *adj.* **narcoanalytically** *adv.*

narco·lepsy (nar'-kō-lep-sē) *n* an irresistible tendency to go to sleep. It is more usual to speak of the narcolepsies rather than of narcolepsy, for sudden, repetitive attacks of sleep occurring in the daytime arise in diverse clinical conditions—**narcoleptic** *adj.*

nar·cosis (nar-kō'-sis) *n* unconsciousness produced by a drug. *carbon dioxide narcosis* full bounding pulse, muscular twitchings, mental confusion and eventual coma due to increased CO_2 in the blood. *continuous narcosis* treatment by prolonged sleep by spaced administration of narcotics. Used occasionally in mental illness to cut short attacks of excitement or for severe emotional upset.

narco·synthesis (nar-kō-sin'-the-sis) *n* the building up of a clearer mental picture of an incident involving the patient by reviving memories of it, under light anesthesia, so that both he and the therapist can examine the incident in clearer perspective.

nar·cotic (nar-kot'-ik) *n, adj* describes a drug which produces abnormally deep sleep. Strong analgesic narcotics, morphine and opiates, cause profound respiratory depression which is reversible by the use of narcotic antagonists*.

Narcotic Control Act controls manufacture, sale, prescribing and dispensing of narcotics and marijuana.

Nardil (nar'-dil) *n* proprietary name for phenelzine*.

nares (när'-ēz) *npl* (*syn* choanae) the nostrils—**naris** *singl. anterior nares* the pair of openings from the exterior into the nasal cavities. *posterior nares* the pair of openings from the nasal cavities into the nasopharynx*.

nasal (nā'-zl) *adj* pertaining to the nose.

naso·esophageal (nā-zō-ē-sof-à-jē'-al) *adj* pertaining to the nose and the esophagus, as passing a tube via this route.

naso·gastric (nā-zō-gas'-trik) *adj* pertaining to the nose and stomach, as passing a *nasogastric tube* via this route, usually for suction, lavage or feeding. ⇒ enteral.

naso·jejunal (nā-zō-je-jū'-nal) *adj* pertaining to the nose and jejunum, usually referring to a tube passed via the nose into the jejunum. ⇒ gavage feeding.

naso·lacrimal (nā-zō-lak'-ri-mal) *adj* pertaining to the nose and lacrimal apparatus.

naso·pharyn·gitis (nā-zō-fār-in-jī'-tis) *n* inflammation of the nasopharynx*.

nasop·haryngo·scope (nā-zō-fār-ing'-gō-skōp) *n* an endoscope for viewing the nasal passages and postnasal space—**nasopharyngoscopic** *adj.*

naso·pharynx (nā-zō-fār'-inks) *n* the portion of the pharynx above the soft palate—**nasopharyngeal** *adj.*

naso·sinusitis (nā-zō-sī'-nus-ī'-tis) *n* inflammation of the nose and adjacent sinuses.

nata·mycin (nat-a-mī′-sin) *n* antifungal antibiotic, active against candidal infection. (Natacyn.)

Naturetin (nă-tūr-ē′-tin) *n* proprietary name for bendroflumethazide*.

natur·opathy (nă-tūr-o′-path-ē) *n* a system of therapeutics based on natural foods grown without chemical fertilizers, and medicines which are prepared from herbs, spices and plants. Advocates believe that these procedures enable the natural body processes an optimal environment for healing—**naturopathic** *adj*.

nausea (naw′-sē-à) *n* a feeling of impending vomiting—**nauseate** *vt*.

Navane (nă′-văn) *n* proprietary name for thiothixene*.

navel (nă′-vl) *n* ⇒ umbilicus.

navicu·lar (na-vik′-ū-lar) *adj* shaped like a canoe.

Neb·cin (neb′-sin) *n* proprietary name for tobramycin*.

neb·ula (neb′-ū-la) *n* a greyish, corneal opacity.

nebu·lizer (neb′-ū-lī-zer) *n* an apparatus for converting a liquid into a fine spray. It can contain medicaments for application to the skin, or nose, or throat.

NEC *abbr* necrotizing* enterocolitis.

Nec·ator (nĕk-ā′-tor) *n* a genus of hookworms*.

nec·ropsy (ne-krop′-sē) *n* the examination of a dead body.

ne·crosis (ne-krō′-sis) *n* localized death of tissue—**necrotic** *adj*.

necro·tizing entero·colitis (NEC) (ne′-krŏ-tī-zing en′-ter-ō-kō-lī′-tis) a condition occurring primarily in preterm or low birth-weight neonates. Parts of the gut wall become necrotic, leading to intestinal obstruction and peritonitis. Probably caused by a combination of ischemia and infection.

need·ling (nēd′-ling) *n* ⇒ discission.

negativ·ism (neg′-à-tiv-izm) *n* active refusal to co-operate, usually shown by the patient consistently doing the exact opposite of what he is asked. Common in schizophrenia*.

neg·ligence (neg′-li-jens) *n* in law, want of proper care or attention resulting in damage to another person. Medical negligence is failure by a doctor or nurse to treat a patient with that standard of care and skill commensurate with his/her training, qualifications and experience. It is a professional duty to avoid patient injury or suffering caused in this way. It can become the basis of litigation for damages.

Neg·ram (neg′-ram) *n* proprietary name for nalidixic acid*.

Neis·seria (nī-sē′-rē-à) *n* a genus of bacteria. Gram-negative cocci, usually arranged in pairs, which are found as commensals of man and animals, e.g. *Neisseria catarrhalis*, or pathogens to man. *Neisseria gonorrheae* causes gonorrhea and *Neisseria meningitidis* causes meningitis.

Nel·aton's line (nel′-a-tonz) an imaginary line joining the anterior superior iliac spine to the ischial tuberosity. The greater trochanter of the femur normally lies on or below this line.

Nelson syn·drome (nel′-son) associated with a pituitary tumor. The skin changes color, that is white becomes black and black becomes white.

nema·todes (nē′-mà-tōdz) *npl* wormlike creatures that have two sexes and an intestinal canal. Various species are parasitic to man and can be divided into two groups: (a) those that mainly live in the intestine, e.g. hookworms, and whipworm (b) those that are mainly tissue parasites, e.g. guinea worms, filiarial worms.

Nem·butal (nem′-bū-tal) *n* proprietary name for pentobarbital*.

neoarthrosis (nē-ō-àr-thrō′-sis) *n* abnormal articulation; a false joint, as at the site of a fracture.

neol·ogism (nē-ŏl′-oj-izm) *n* a specially coined word, often nonsensical; may express a thought disorder.

neo·mycin (nē-ō-mī′-sin) *n* an antibiotic frequently used with corticosteroids in the treatment of inflamed and infected skin conditions. Sometimes given orally for intestinal infections. (Mycifradin.)

neonatal intensive care unit (NICU) usually reserved for preterm and small-for-dates infants between 700–2000 grams in weight but also used for other newborns requiring the use of high technology available in these units.

neo·natal per·iod (nē-ō-nă′-tal) the first 28 days of life in a baby. *neonatal mortality* the death rate of babies in the first month of life. *neonatal herpes* a comparatively rare disease acquired during vaginal delivery from a mother actively shedding herpes simplex virus. It is a devastating illness with a 75% mortality rate and a high incidence of severe neurological sequelae among survivors.

neo·nate (nē'-ō-nāt) *n* a newborn baby up to 4 weeks old.

neonat·ology (nē-ō-nă-tol'-o-jē) *n* the scientific study of the newborn.

neonat·orum (nē-ō-nă-tōr'-um) *adj* pertaining to the newborn.

neo·plasia (nē-ō-plā'-zē-ă) *n* literally, the formation of new tissue. By custom refers to the pathological process in tumor formation—**neoplastic** *adj*.

neo·plasm (nē'-ō-plazm) *n* a new growth; a tumor which is either cancerous or non-cancerous—**neoplastic** *adj*.

Neo·sporin (nē-ō-spōr'-in) *n* proprietary ophthalmic drops containing polymyxin*, neomycin* and gramicidin*.

neo·stigmine (nē-ō-stig'-mēn) *n* a synthetic compound used in myasthenia gravis; as a curarine antagonist; and in postoperative ileus and urinary retention. Given orally and by injection. Can cause excess bronchial secretion. (Prostigmin.)

neph·ralgia (nef-ral'-jē-ă) *n* pain in the kidney. ⇒ Dietl's crisis.

nephrec·tomy (nef-rek'-to-mē) *n* surgical removal of a kidney.

neph·ritis (nef-rī'-tis) *n* a term embracing a group of conditions in which there is either an inflammatory or an inflammatory-like reaction, focal or diffuse, in the kidneys. ⇒ glomerulonephritis, glomerulosclerosis, nephrotic syndrome, renal failure—**nephritic** *adj*.

nephro·calcinosis (nef-rō-kal-sin-ō'-sis) *n* multiple areas of calcification within the kidney.

nephro·capsulectomy (nef-rō-kap-sōo-lek'-to-mē) *n* surgical removal of the kidney capsule. Occasionally done for polycystic* renal disease.

nephro·genic (nef-rō-jen'-ik) *adj* arising in or produced by the kidney.

nephro·graphy (nef-ro'-gra-fē) the technique of imaging renal shadow following injection of opaque medium, demonstrated in aortograph series—**nephrographical** *adj*, **nephrogram** *n*, **nephrograph** *n*, **nephrographically** *adv*.

nephro·lithiasis (nef-rō-lith-ī'-ă-sis) *n* the presence of stones in the kidney.

nephro·lithotomy (nef-rō-lith-ot'-o-mē) *n* removal of a stone from the kidney by an incision through the kidney substance.

nephro·logy (nef-rol'-o-jē) *n* special study of the kidneys and the diseases which afflict them.

neph·ron (nef'-ron) *n* the basic unit of the kidney, comprising a glomerulus*, Bowman's capsule, proximal and distal convoluted tubules, with the loop of Henle connecting them; a straight collecting tubule follows via which urine is conveyed to the renal pelvis.

neph·ropathy (nef-ro'-pă-thē) *n* kidney disease. May be of vasomotor origin, when it is often reversible—**nephropathic** *adj*.

neph·ropexy (nef'-rō-peks-ē) *n* surgical fixation of a floating* kidney.

neph·roplasty (nef-rō-plas'-tē) *n* any plastic operation on the kidney, especially for large aberrant renal vessels that are dissected off the urinary tract and the kidney folded laterally upon itself. ⇒ hydronephrosis.

neph·roptosis (nef-rop-tō'-sis) *n* downward displacement of the kidney. The word is sometimes used for a floating* kidney.

nephro·pyosis (nef-rō-pī-ōs'-is) *n* pus formation in the kidney.

nephro·sclerosis (nef-rō-sklēr-ōs'-is) renal insufficiency from hypertensive vascular disease, developing into a clinical picture identical with that of chronic nephritis. ⇒ renal failure—**nephrosclerotic** *adj*.

nephro·scope (nef'-rō-skōp) *n* an endoscope* for viewing kidney tissue. It can be designed to create a continuous flow of irrigating fluid and provide an exit for the fluid and accompanying debris—**nephroscopic** *adj*.

neph·rosis (nef-rō'-sis) *n* any degenerative, non-inflammatory change in the kidney—**nephrotic** *adj*.

neph·rostomy (nef-ros'-to-mē) *n* a surgically established fistula from the pelvis of the kidney to the body surface.

neph·rotic syn·drome (nef-rot'-ik) characterized by reduction in blood plasma albumen, albuminuria and edema, usually with hyperlipemia. There are minimal histological changes in the kidneys. It may occur in other conditions such as amyloid disease and glomerulosclerosis* complicating diabetes.

neph·rotomogram (nef-rō-tō'-mō-gram) *n* a tomograph* of the kidney.

neph·rotomy (nef-rot'-o-mē) *n* an incision into the kidney substance.

neph·rotoxic (nef-rō-toks'-ik) *adj* any substance which inhibits or prevents the functions of kidney cells, or causes their destruction—**nephrotoxin** *n*.

nephro·ureterectomy (nef-rō-ūr-ē′-tèr-ek′-to-mē) *n* removal of the kidney along with a part or the whole of the ureter.

nerve (nèrv) *n* an elongated bundle of fibers which serves for the transmission of impulses between the periphery and the nerve centers. *afferent nerve* one conveying impulses from the tissues to the nerve centers; also known as 'receptor' and 'sensory' nerves. *efferent nerve* one which conveys impulses outwards from the nerve centers; also known as 'effector', 'motor', 'secretory', 'trophic', vasoconstrictor', 'vasodilator' etc according to function and location.

ner·vous (nèr′-vus) *adj* 1 relating to nerves or nerve tissue. 2 referring to a state of restlessness or timidity. *nervous system* the structures controlling the actions and functions of the body; it comprises the brain and spinal cord and their nerves (central nervous system), and the ganglia and fibers forming the autonomic* system (⇒ Figure 11, peripheral, sympathetic).

nettle rash (net′-tl) (*syn.* hives) urticaria; weals of the skin.

network (net′-wèrk) *n* a netlike structure of fibers, a reticulum.

neur·al (nōō′-ral) *adj* pertaining to nerves. *neural canal* ⇒ vertebral canal. *neural tube* formed from fusion of the neural folds from which the brain and spinal cord arise. *neural tube defect* any of a group of congenital malformations involving the neural tube including anencephaly*, hydrocephalous* and spina* bifida.

neur·algia (nōō-ral′-jē-à) *n* pain in the distribution of a nerve—**neuralgic** *adj*.

neur·apraxia (nōō-rà-praks′-ē-à) *n* temporary loss of function in peripheral nerve fibers. Most commonly due to crushing or prolonged pressure. ⇒ axonotmesis.

neur·asthenia (nōō-ras-thē′-nē-à) *n* a frequently misused term, the precise meaning of which is an uncommon nervous condition consisting of lassitude, inertia, fatigue and loss of initiative. Restless fidgeting, over-senstivity, undue irritability and often an asthenic physique are also present—**neurasthenic** *adj*.

neur·ectomy (nōō-rek′-to-mē) *n* excision of part of a nerve.

neuril·emma (nōō-ri-lem′-à) *n* the thin membranous outer covering of a nerve fiber surrounding the myelin sheath.

neur·itis (nōō-rī′-tis) *n* inflammation of a nerve—**neuritic** *adj*.

neuro·blast (nōō′-rō-blast) *n* a primitive nerve cell.

neuro·blastoma (nōō-rō-blas-tō′-mà) *n* malignant tumor arising in adrenal medulla from tissue of sympathetic origin. Most cases show a raised urinary catecholamine excretion—**neuroblastomata** *pl*, **neuroblastomatous** *adj*.

neuro·dermatitis (nōō-rō-dèr-mà-tī′-tis) *n* (*syn* lichen simplex) leathery, thickened patches of skin secondary to pruritus and scratching. As the skin thickens, irritation increases, scratching causes further thickening and so a vicious circle is set up. The appearance of the patch develops characteristically as a thickened sheet dissected into small, shiny, flat-topped papules. Common manifestations of atopic* dermatitis.

neuro·fibroma (nōō-rō-fī-brō′-mà) *n* a tumor arising from the connective tissue of nerves—**neurofibromata** *pl*, **neurofibromatous** *adj*.

neuro·fibromat·osis (nōō-rō-fī-brō-mà-tō′-sis) *n* a genetically determined condition in which there are many fibromata. ⇒ von Recklinghausen's disease.

neuro·genic (nōō-rō-jen′-ik) *adj* originating within or forming nervous tissue. *neurogenic bladder* interference with the nerve control of the urinary bladder causing either retention of urine, which presents as incontinence, or continuous dribbling without retention. When necessary the bladder is emptied by exerting manual pressure on the anterior abdominal wall.

neurog·lia (nōō-rō′-glē-à) *n* (*syn* glia) the supporting tissue of the brain and cord—**neuroglial** *adj*.

neuro·glycopenia (nōō-rō-glī-kō-pē′-nē-à) *n* shortage of glucose in nerve cells, which is the immediate cause of brain dysfunction when it occurs in hypoglycemia—**neuroglycopenic** *adj*.

neuro·leptics (nōō-rō-lep′-tiks) *npl* drugs acting on the nervous system. Includes the major antipsychotic tranquilizers.

neurol·ogist (nōō-rol′-o-jist) *n* a specialist in neurology*.

neurol·ogy (nōō-rol′-o-jē) *n* 1 the science and study of nerves—their structure, function and pathology. 2 the branch of medicine dealing with diseases of the nervous system—**neurological** *adj*.

neuro·muscular (nōō-ro-mus′-kū-lar) *adj* pertaining to nerves and muscles.

neur·on (nōō′-ron) *n* the basic structural unit of the nervous system comprising fibers (dendrites) which convey impulses to the nerve cell; the nerve cell itself, and the fibers (axons) which convey impulses from the cell. ⇒ motor neuron disease—**neuronal, neural** *adj. lower motor neutron* the cell is in the spinal cord and the axon passes to skeletal muscle. *upper motor neuron* the cell is in the cerebral cortex and the axon passes down the spinal cord to arborize with a lower motor neuron.

neur·onotmesis (noo-ron-ot-mē'-sis) *n* ⇒ axonotmesis.

neuro·pathic (noo-rō-path'ik) *adj* relating to disease of the nervous system—**neuropathy** *n*.

neuro·pathology (noo-rō-path-ol'-o-jē) *n* a branch of medicine dealing with diseases of the nervous system—**neuropathological** *adj.*

neuro·peptides (noo-rō-pep'-tīds) *npl* chemical substances secreted continually in the brain, and currently associated with moods and states. They include the endorphins*.

neuro·pharma·cology (noo-rō-fàr-màkol'-o-jē) *n* the branch of pharmacology dealing with drugs which affect the nervous system—**neuropharmacological** *adj.*

neuro·plasticity (noo-rō-plas-tis'-it-ē) *n* the capacity of nerve cells to regenerate.

neuro·plasty (noo'-rō-plas-tē) *n* surgical repair of nerves—**neuroplastic** *adj.*

neuro·psychiatry (noo-rō-sī-kī'-à-trē) *n* the combination of neurology and psychiatry. Specialty dealing with organic and functional disease—**neuropsychiatric** *adj.*

neuror·rhaphy (noo-ror'-à-fē) *n* suturing the ends of a divided nerve.

neur·osis (noo-rō'-sis) *n* (*syn* psychoneurosis) a functional (i.e. psychogenic*) disorder consisting of a symptom or symptoms, caused, though usually unknown to the patient, by mental disorder. The four commonest are anxiety state, reactive depression, hysteria and obsessional neurosis. Distinguished from a psychosis* by the fact that a neurosis arises as a result of stresses and anxieties in the patient's environment—**neurotic** *adj. institutional neurosis* apathy, withdrawal and non-participation occurring in long-stay patients as a result of the environment. May be indistinguishable from the signs and symptoms for which the patient was admitted to the institution. ⇒ institutionalization.

neuro·surgery (noo-rō-sèr'-jèr-ē) *n* surgery of the nervous system—**neurosurgical** *adj.*

neuro·syphilis (noo-rō-sif'-il-is) *n* infection of brain or spinal cord, or both, by *Treponema pallidum*. The variety of clinical pictures produced is large, but the two common syndromes encountered are tabes* dorsalis and general* paralysis of the insane (GPI). The basic pathology is disease of the blood vessels, with later development of pathological changes in the meninges and the underlying nervous tissue. Very often symptoms of the disease do not arise until 20 years or more after the date of primary infection. ⇒ Argyll Robertson pupil—**neurosyphilitic** *adj.*

neuro·tmesis (noo-rot-mē-sis) *n* ⇒ axonotmesis.

neur·otomy (noo-rot'-o-mē) *n* surgical cutting of a nerve.

neuro·toxic (noo-rō-toks'-ik) *adj* poisonous or destructive to nervous tissue—**neurotoxin** *n.*

neuro·tropic (noo-rō-trō'-pik) *adj* with predilection for the nervous system. *Treponema pallidum* often produces neurosyphilitic complications. Neurotropic viruses (rabies, poliomyelitis, etc.) make their major attack on the cells of the nervous system.

neutro·penia (noo-trō-pē'-nē-à) *n* shortage of neutrophils, i.e. less than 500 circulating neutrophils per µl blood, but not sufficient to warrant the description agranulocytosis*—**neutropenic** *adj.*

neutro·phil (noo'-trō-fil) *n* the most common form of granulocyte in the blood, in which the granules are neither strongly basophilic nor strongly eosinophilic.

nevoid amentia (nē'-voyd ā-men'-shē-a) ⇒ Sturge-Weber syndrome.

nevus (nē'-vus) *n* a mole; a circumscribed lesion of the skin arising from pigment-producing cells (melanoma) or due to a developmental abnormality of blood vessels (angioma)—**nevi** *pl,* **nevoid** *adj.*

NGU *abbr* non*-gonococcal urethritis.

niacin (nī'-à-sin) *n* ⇒ nicotinic acid.

niclos·amide (ni-klō'-sa-mīd) *n* causes expulsion of adult tapeworm. Given in a single dose of 2 g. No starvation or purgation necessary. (Yomesan.)

nicotina·mide (ni-ko-tin'-à-mīd) *n* a derivative of nicotinic* acid useful when the vasodilator action of that drug is not desired as in treatment of pellegra.

nic·otinic acid (ni-kō-tin'-ik as'-id) one of

the essential food factors of the vitamin B complex. The vasodilator action of the compound is useful in chilblains, migraine etc. (*Syn* niacin.)

nicti·tation (nik-ti-tā'-shun) *n* rapid and involuntary blinking of the eyelids.

NICU *abbr* neonatal intensive care unit.

ni·dation (nī-dā'-shun) *n* implantation of the early embryo in the uterine mucosa.

ni·dus (nī'-dus) *n* the focus of an infection. A septic focus.

Niemann·Pick dis·ease (nē'-man pik) a lipoid metabolic disturbance, chiefly in female Jewish infants. Now thought to be due to absence or inadequacy of enzyme sphingomyelinase. There is enlargement of the liver, spleen and lymph nodes with mental subnormality. Now classified as a lipid reticulosis.

night blind·ness (*syn* nyctalopia) sometimes occurs in vitamin A deficiency and is a maladaptation of vision to darkness.

night cry a shrill noise, uttered during sleep. May be of significance in hip disease when pain occurs in the relaxed joint.

night sweat profuse sweating, usually during sleep; typical of tuberculosis*.

nihil·istic (nī-hil-is'-tik) *adj* involving delusions and ideas of unreality; of not existing.

niketh·amide (ni-keth'-à-mīd) *n* a central nervous system stimulant used in respiratory depression and collapse. Given intravenously or intramuscularly. (Coramine.)

Nikolsky's sign (ni-kol'-skēz) slight pressure on the skin causes 'slipping' of apparently normal epidermis, in the way that a rubber glove can be moved on a wet hand. Characteristic of pemphigus*.

nipple (nip'-pl) *n* the conical eminence in the center of each breast, containing the outlets of the milk ducts.

Nisentil (nis'-en-til) *n* proprietary name for alphaprodine hydrochloride*.

nit (nit) *n* the egg of the head louse (*Pediculus* capitis). It is firmly cemented to the hair.

ni·tric acid (nī'-trik) a dangerous caustic. Occasionally used in testing urine for albumen.

nitro·furantoin (nī-trō-fūr'-an-tō-in) *n* a urinary antiseptic, of value in Gram-positive and Gram-negative infections. Unrelated to sulfonamides or antibiotics. (Furadantin.)

nitro·furazone (nī-trō-fūr'-à-zōn) *n* an an-tibacterial agent for local use. Available as ointment and solution for topical application. (Furacin.)

nitro·gen (nī'-trō-jen) *n* 1 an almost inert gaseous element: the chief constituent of the atmosphere, but it cannot be utilized directly by man. However, certain organisms in the soil and roots of legumes are capable of nitrogen fixation. It is an important constituent of many complements of living cells, e.g. proteins. 2 the essential constituent of protein foods—**nitrogenous** *adj*. *nitrogen balance* is when a person's daily intake of nitrogen from proteins equals the daily excretion of nitrogen: a negative balance occurs when excretion of nitrogen exceeds the daily intake. Nitrogen is excreted mainly as urea in the urine; ammonia, creatinine and uric acid account for a further small amount. Less than 10% total nitrogen excreted in feces. *nitrogen mustards* a group of cytotoxic drugs, derivatives of mustard gas.

nitroglycerin (nī-tro-gli'-sèr-in) *n* a vasodilator used mainly in angina pectoris. Given mainly as tablets which should be chewed, or dissolved under the tongue; or transdermally by application as a gel to the skin.

ni·trous oxide (nī'-trus oks'-īd) (*syn* laughing gas) widely used inhalation gaseous anesthetic. Supplied in blue cylinders.

Nizoral (nī'-zōr-al) *n* proprietary name for ketoconazole*.

NMR *abbr* ⇒ magnetic resonance imaging.

noc·turia (nok-tū'-rē-à) *n* passing urine at night.

noc·turnal (nok-tur'-nal) *adj* nightly; during the night.

node (nōd) *n* a protuberance or swelling. A constriction. *atrioventricular node* the commencement of the bundle of His in the right atrium of the heart. *node of Ranvier* the construction in the neurilemma of a nerve fiber. *sinoatrial node* situated at the opening of the superior vena cava into the right atrium; the wave of contraction begins here, then spreads over the heart.

nod·ule (nod'-ūl) *n* a small node—**nodular** *adj*.

Noludar (nol'-ū-dar) *n* proprietary name for methyprylon*.

non·acci·dental in·jury (non-ak-si-dent'-al) ⇒ battered baby syndrome.

non·com·pliance (non-kom-plī'-ans) *n* a term used when patients who understand their drug regime do not comply with it.

non compos mentis (non kom'-pōs men'-tis) of unsound mind.

non·compre·hension (non-kom-prē-hen'-shun) *n* a term used when patients do not understand their drug regime: it may result in non*-compliance, but not necessarily.

non·gono·coccal ureth·ritis (NGU) (non-gon-ō-kok'-al ū-rē-thrī'-tis) (*syn* non-specific urethritis—NSU) a common sexually transmitted disease. About half the cases are caused by *Chlamydia*; other causatory organisms are *Ureaplasma* and *Mycoplasma genitalium*.

non-Hodgkin's lymph·oma (non-hoj'-kinz) a disease of lymphoid tissue, which can infiltrate into any organ or tissue. Cytotoxic drugs are effective but eventual prognosis is not good.

non·insulin depen·dent diabetes mellitus (NIDDM) (non-in'-su-lin dē-pen'-dent dī-a-bē'-tēz) ⇒ diabetes.

non·invasive (non-in-vās'-iv) *adj* describes any diagnostic or therapeutic technique which does not require penetration of the skin or of any cavity or organ.

non·protein nitro·gen (NPN) (non-prō'-tē-in nī'-trō-jen) nitrogen derived from all nitrogenous substances other than protein, i.e. urea, uric acid, creatinine, creatine and ammonia.

nonsense syn·drome Ganser* syndrome.

non·specific ureth·ritis (NSU) (non-spes-if'-ik ū-rē-thrī'-tis) non*-gonococcal urethritis.

non-steroidal anti-inflammatory drugs (NSAID) (non-ster-oyd'-al an'-tī-in-flam'-a-tōr'-ē) the name implies the function. Useful in the rheumatological diseases but they can produce gastric ulceration and bleeding from the alimentary mucous membrane.

non-stress test (*abbr* NST) a test of fetal well-being performed by applying the external fetal monitor to a pregnant woman and recording the fetal heart baseline and variability.

Noonan syn·drome (noo'-nan) (*syn* Bonnevie-Ullrich syndrome) in either males or females, with eyes set apart (hypertelorism) and other ocular and facial abnormalities; short stature, sometimes with neck webbing (and other Turner*-like features). The commonest and most characteristic cardiac abnormality is congenital pulmonary stenosis. Generally not chromosomal, most cases sporadic; a few either dominantly or recessively inherited.

Norcuron (nōr'-kūr-on) *n* proprietary name for vecuronium*.

nor·epinephrine (nor-ep-in-ef'-rin) *n* endogenous norepinephrine is a neuruhumoral transmitter which is released from adrenergic nerve endings. Although small amounts are associated with epinephrine in the adrenal medulla, its role as a hormone is a secondary one. It has an intense peripheral vasoconstrictor action, and is given by slow intravenous injection in shock and peripheral failure. (Levophed.)

norethindrone (nōr-eth-in'-drōn) *n* progestogen; said to suppress the gonadotropin production by the pituitary; used in oral contraceptives.

Norflex (nōr'-fleks) proprietary name for orphenadrine*.

normo·blast (nōr'-mō-blast) *n* a normal sized nucleated red blood cell, the precursor of the erythrocyte—**normoblastic** *adj*.

normo·cyte (nōr'-mō-sīt) *n* a red blood cell of normal size—**normocytic** *adj*.

normo·glycemic (nōr-mō-glī-sē'-mik) *adj* a normal amount of glucose in the blood—**normoglycemia** *n*.

normo·tension (nōr-mō-ten'-shun) *n* normal tension, by current custom alluding to blood pressure—**normotensive** *adj*.

normo·thermia (nōr-mō-ther'-mē-a) *n* normal body temperature, as opposed to hyperthermia* and hypothermia*—**normothermic** *adj*.

normo·tonic (nōr-mō-ton'-ik) *adj* normal strength, tension, tone, by current custom referring to muscle tissue. Spasmolytic drugs induce normotonicity in muscle, and can be used before radiography—**normotonicity** *n*.

Norpace (nōr'-pās) *n* proprietary name for disopyramide*.

Norplant (nōr'-plant) *n* a proprietary preparation of levonorgestrel*.

nor·triptyline (nōr-trip'-tl-in) *n* an antidepressant similar to amitriptyline*. (Pamelor.)

nose (nōz) ⇒ Figure 6, 14.

noso·comial (nō-sō-kō'-mē-al) *adj* pertaining to a hospital. ⇒ infection.

nostal·gia (nos-tal'-jē-à) *n* homesickness; a longing to return to a 'place' to which, and where, one may be emotionally bound—**nostalgic** *adj*.

nos·trils (nos'-trils) *n* the anterior openings in the nose; the anterior nares. choanac.

Novo·cain (nō'-vō-kān) *n* proprietary name for procaine*.

NRDS *abbr* neonatal respiratory* distress syndrome.

NSAID *abbr* non-steroidal anti-inflammatory drugs. An abbreviation used to differentiate them from corticosteroids*.

NSU *abbr* ⇒ non-gonococcal urethritis.

nucha (nū'-kà) *n* the nape* of the neck—**nuchal** *adj*.

nu·clear mag·netic reson·ance (NMR) (nū'-klē-ar mag-net'-ik) ⇒ magnetic resonance imaging.

nu·cleated (nū'-klē-ā-ted) *adj* possessing one or more nuclei.

nucleo·proteins (nū'-klē-ō-prō'-tēns) *n* proteins found especially in the nuclei of cells. They consist of a protein conjugated with nucleic acid and are broken down during digestion. Among the products are the purine and pyrimidine bases. An end product of nucleoprotein metabolism is uric acid which is excreted in the urine.

nucleo·toxic (nū-klē-ō-toks'ik) *adj* poisonous to cell nuclei. The term may be applied to chemicals and viruses—**nucleotoxin** *n*.

nu·cleus (nū'-klē-us) *n* **1** the inner part of a cell which contains the chromosomes. The genes which are located in the chromosomes control the activity and function of the cell by specifying the nature of the enzymes and structural proteins for that cell. **2** a circumscribed accumulation of nerve cells in the central nervous system associated with a particular function—**nuclei** *pl*, **nuclear** *adj*. *nucleus pulposus* the soft core of an intervertebral disc which can prolapse into the spinal cord and cause sciatica.

nul·lipara (nul-ip'-a-rà) *n* a women who has not borne a child—**nulliparous** *adj*, **nulliparity** *n*.

num·mular (num'-ū-lar) *adj* coin shaped; resembling rolls of coins, as the sputum in phthisis.

Nuper·caine (nū'-per-kān) *n* proprietary name for dibucaine*.

nu·tation (nū-tā'-shun) *n* nodding; applied to uncontrollable head shaking.

Nutrasweet (nū'-trà swēt) *n* proprietary name for aspartame*.

nu·trient (nū'-trē-ent) *n*, *adj* a substance serving as or providing nourishment. *nu-*

trient artery one which enters a long bone. *nutrient foramen* hole in a long bone which admits the nutrient artery.

nu·trition (nū-tri'-shun) *n* the sum total of the processes by which the living organism receives and utilizes materials necessary for survival, growth and repair of worn-out tissues.

nux vomica (nuks vom'-ik-à) *n* the nuts from which strychnine* is obtained. Occasionally used with other bitters as a gastric stimulant.

nyc·talgia (nik-tal'-jē-à) *n* pain occurring during the night.

nycta·lopia (nik-tà-lō'-pē-à) *n* night blindness.

nycto·phobia (nik-tō-fō'-bē-à) *n* abnormal fear of the night and darkness.

nyct·uria (nik-tū'-rē-à) *n* incontinence of urine at night.

nymphae (nim'-fē) *n* the labia* minora.

nympho·mania (nim-fō-mā'-nē-à) *n* excessive sexual desire in a female—**nymphomaniac** *adj*.

nystag·mus (nis-tag'-mus) *n* involuntary and jerky repetitive movement of the eyeballs.

nys·tatin (nī-stat'-in) *n* an antifungal antibiotic effective in the treatment of candidiasis. Prevents intestinal fungal overgrowth during broad spectrum antibiotic treatment. (Mycostatin.)

O

OA *abbr* occipito-anterior*.

oat cell carci·noma a malignant epithelial bronchogenic neoplasm which spreads along submucosal lymphatics. One-third of all long tumors are of this type. The prognosis is poor as surgical resection has no influence on the prognosis. Similarly, chemotherapy and radiotherapy, although very effective, have little influence on prognosis because the tumor is usually widespread by the time treatment begins.

OB *abbr* obstetrics.

obe·sity (ō-bē'-sit-ē) *n* the deposition of excessive fat around the body, particularly in the subcutaneous tissue. The intake of food is in excess of the body's energy requirements. Obesity can be measured by weighing and measuring height and calculating the weight/height ratio, and by measuring the thickness of skin folds.

Obetrol (ō'-bet-rol) *n* proprietary preparation of amphetamine and dextroamphetamine*.

objec·tive (ob-jek'-tiv) *adj* pertaining to things external to one's self. ⇒ subjective *opp. objective signs* those which the observer notes, as distinct from the symptoms of which the patient complains.

obli·gate (ob'-lig-āt) *adj* characterized by the ability to survive only in a particular set of environmental conditions, e.g. an obligate parasite cannot exist other than as a parasite.

oblique (ō-blēk') external and internal muscles. ⇒ Figures 4,5.

OBS *abbr* organic brain syndrome. ⇒ dementia.

ob·sessional neur·osis (ob-sesh'-un-al nū-rō'-sis) two types are recognized: (a) obsessive compulsive thoughts; constant preoccupation with a constantly recurring morbid thought which cannot be kept out of the mind, and enters against the wishes of the patient who tries to eliminate it. The thought is almost always painful and out of keeping with the person's normal personality (b) obsessive compulsive actions; consists of a feeling of compulsion to perform repeatedly a simple act, e.g. handwashing, touching door knobs, etc. Ideas of guilt frequently form the basis of an obsessional state.

obste·trician (ob-stet-rish'-un) *n* a qualified doctor who practices the science and art of obstetrics.

obstet·rics (ob-stet'-riks) *n* the science dealing with the care of the pregnant woman during the antenatal, parturient and puerperal stages; midwifery.

obtu·rator (ob'-tū-rā-tor) *n* that which closes an aperture. *obturator foramen* the opening in the innominate bone which is closed by muscles and fascia *obturator infernus* ⇒ Figure 5. *obturator nerve* ⇒ Figure 11.

occipi·tal (ok-sip'-it-al) *adj* pertaining to the back of the head. *occipital bone* characterized by a large hole through which the spinal cord passes.

occipito·anterior (ok-sip'-it-ō-an-tē'-rē-or) *adj* describes a presentation when the fetal occiput lies in the anterior half of the maternal pelvis.

occipito·frontal (ok-sip'-it-ō-front'-al) *adj* pertaining to the occiput* and forehead.

occipito·posterior (ok-sip'-it-ō-pōst-ēr'-ē-or) *adj* describes a presentation when the fetal occiput is in the posterior half of the maternal pelvis.

occiput (ok'-sip-ut) *n* the posterior region of the skull.

oc·clusion (ok-klōō'-zhun) *n* the closure of an opening, especially of ducts or blood vessels. In dentistry, the fit of the teeth as the two jaws meet—**occlusal** *adj*.

occult blood (ō-kult') ⇒ blood.

occu·pational dis·ease (ok-ū-pā'-shun-al) ⇒ industrial disease.

occu·pational health (ok-ū-pā'-shun-al helth) ⇒ hygiene.

occu·pational ther·apy (ok-ū-pā'-shun-al ther'-a-pē) teaching/learning crafts to exercise particular sets of muscles as therapy and prevention of boredom; also includes assessment of and helping with a patient's activities of daily living (ADLs).

OCT *abbr* oxytocin challenge test ⇒ stress test.

ocu·lar (ok'-ū-lar) *adj* pertaining to the eye.

ocu·lentum (ok-ū-len'-tum) *n* eye ointment—**oculenta** *pl*.

ocu·list (ok'-ū-list) *n* a medically qualified person who refracts and treats eye disease.

oculo·genital (ok-ū-lō-jen'-it-al) *adj* pertaining to the eye and genital region, as the virus TRIC*, which is found in the male and female genital canals and in the conjunctival sacs of the newborn.

oculo·gyric (ok-ū-lō-jī'-rik) *adj* referring to movements of the eyeball.

oculo·motor (ok-ū-lō-mō'-tor) *n* the third cranial nerve which moves the eye and supplies the upper eye lid.

OD *abbr* oculus dexter, right eye.

odon·talgia (ō-don-tal'-jē-à) *n* toothache.

odon·tic (ō-don'-tik) *adj* pertaining to the teeth.

odontitis (ō-don-tī'-tis) *n* inflammation of the teeth.

odon·toid (ō-don'-toyd) *adj* resembling a tooth.

odontolith (ō-don'-tō-lith) tartar; the concretions which are deposited around teeth.

odon·tology (ō-don-tol'-o-jē) *n* dentistry.

odon·toma (ō-don-tō'-ma) *n* a tumor developing from or containing tooth structures—**odontomatous** *adj*.

odontoprisis (ō-don-tō-prī'-is) *n* grinding of the teeth.

odonto·therapy (ō-don-tō-thér′-à-pē) *n* the treatment given for diseases of the teeth.

Oedi·pus com·plex (ed′-i-pus kom′-pleks) an unconscious attachment of a son to his mother resulting in a feeling of jealousy towards the father and then guilt, producing emotional conflict. This process was described by Freud as part of his theory of infantile sexuality and he considered it to be normal in male infants.

OL *abbr* oculus laevus, left eye.

ole·cranon pro·cess (ō-lek′rā-non) the large process at the upper end of the ulna; it forms the tip of the elbow when the arm is flexed. *olecranon bursitis* ⇒ bursitis.

oleum ricini (ō′-lē-um ri-sin′-ī) castor* oil.

olfact·ory (ōl-fak′-tō-rē) *adj* pertaining to the sense of smell—olfaction *n*. *olfactory bulb* ⇒ Figure 14. *olfactory nerve* the nerve supplying the olfactory region of the nose; the first cranial nerve. *olfactory organ* the nose (⇒ Figure 14).

oli·gemia (ō-lig-ē′-mē-à) *n* (*syn* hypovolemia) diminished total quantity of blood—**oligemic** *adj*.

oligo·hydramnios (ō-lig-ō-hī-dram′-nē-ōs) *n* deficient amniotic fluid.

oligomenorrhea (ō-lig-ō-men-ōr-rē′-à) *n* infrequent menstruation; normal cycle is prolonged beyond 35 days.

oligo·phrenia (ol-ig-ō-frē′-nē-à) *n* mental deficiency.—**oligophrenic** *adj*.

oligo·spermia (ol-ig-ō-spér′-mē-à) *n* reduction in number of spermatozoa in the semen.

oli·guria (ol-ig-ō-ūr′-ē-à) *n* deficient urine secretion—**oliguric** *adj*.

olive oil (ol′-iv oyl) *n* used in gastric ulcer and as a laxative. Useful externally as an emollient.

omen·tum (ō-men′-tum) *n* a sling-like fold of peritoneum—**omental** *adj*. *gastrosplenic omentum* connects the stomach and spleen. The functions of the omentum are protection, repair and fat storage. *greater omentum* the fold which hangs from the lower border of the stomach and covers the front of the intestines. *lesser omentum* a smaller fold, passing between the transverse fissure of the liver and the lesser curvature of the stomach.

omphal·itis (omf-al-īt′-is) *n* inflammation of the umbilicus*.

omphalo·cele (omf-al′-ō-sēl) *n* ⇒ hernia.

Oncho·cerca (ong-kō-sèr′-kà) *n* a genus of filarial worms.

oncho·cerciasis (ong-kō-sèr-kī′-à-sis) *n* infestation of man with *Onchocerca*. Adult worms encapsulated in subcutaneous connective tissue. Can cause 'river blindness' if the larvae migrate to the eyes.

oncogenes (on′-kō-gēns) *n* genes thought to be made active by a chemical when they become capable of making 'forged' chemical keys and locks that can trick cells into uncontrollable cancerous growth.

onco·genic (on-kō-jen′-ik) *adj* capable of tumor production.

on·cology (on-kol′-o-jē) *n* the scientific and medical study of neoplasms—**oncological** *adj*, **oncologically** *adv*.

on·colysis (on-kol′-is-is) *n* destruction of a neoplasm. Sometimes used to describe reduction in size of tumor—**oncolytic** *adj*.

On·covin (on′-kō-vin) *n* proprietary name for vincristine*.

onychia (on-ik′-ē-à) *n* acute inflammation of the nail matrix; suppuration may spread beneath the nail, causing it to become detached and fall off.

onycho·cryptosis (on-kō-krip-tō′-sis) *n* ingrowing of the nail.

onycho·gryphosis, oncogryposis (on-kō-grī-fō′-sis, on-kō-grī-pō′-sis) *n* a ridged, thickened deformity of the nails, common in the elderly.

onycho·lysis (on-ik-ol′-is-is) *n* loosening of toe or finger nail from the nail bed—**onycholytic** *adj*.

onycho·mycosis (on-ik-ō-mī-kō′-sis) *n* a fungal infection of the nails.

o'nyong·nyong fever (on-i′-ong-ni′-ong) (*syn* joint-breaker fever) caused by a virus transmitted by mosquitoes in East Africa. First noted in 1959 in north-west Uganda.

oocyte (ō′-ō-sīt) *n* an immature ovum.

oogenesis (ō-ō-jen′-e-sis) *n* the production and formation of ova* in the ovary—**oogenetic** *adj*.

oophor·ectomy (o-ō-fōr-ek′-to-mē) *n* (*syn* ovariectomy, ovariotomy) excision of an ovary*.

oophor·itis (ō-ō-fōr-ī′-tis) *n* (*syn* ovaritis) inflammation of an ovary*.

oophoron (ō-ō′-fōr-on) *n* an ovary*.

oophoro·salpingectomy (ō′-ō-fōr-ō-salping-ek′-to-mē) *n* excision of an ovary and its associated fallopian tube.

oosperm (ō'-ō-spėrm) *n* a fertilized ovum.

OP *abbr* occipito-posterior.

opacity (ō-păs'-it-ē) *n* non-transparency, cloudiness; an opaque spot, as on the cornea or lens.

open frac·ture ⇒ fracture.

operant condition·ing (op'-er-ant) ⇒ conditioning.

opera·ting micro·scope an illuminated binocular microscope enabling surgery to be carried out on delicate tissues such as nerves and blood vessels. Some models incorporate a beam splitter and a second set of eyepieces to enable a second person to view the operation site.

ophthal·mia (of-thal'-mē-à) *n* (*syn* ophthalmitis) inflammation of the eye. *ophthalmia neonatorum* defined by law in 1914 as a purulent discharge from the eyes of an infant commencing within 21 days of birth. Only 6% of total cases are gonorrheal, but all are notifiable. **sympathetic ophthalmia** iridocyclitis of one eye secondary to injury or disease of the other.

ophthal·mic (of-thal'-mik) *adj* pertaining to the eye.

ophthal·mitis (of-thal-mī'-tis) *n* ⇒ ophthalmia.

ophthal·mologist (of-thal-mol'-o-jist) *n* a person who studies ophthalmology.

ophthal·mology (of-thal-mol'-o-jē) *n* the science which deals with the structure, function and diseases of the eye—**ophthalmological** *adj*, **ophthalmologically** *adv*.

ophthalmo·plegia (of-thal-mō-plē'-jē-à) *n* paralysis of one or more muscles which move the eye—**ophthalmoplegic** *adj*.

ophthalmo·scope (of-thal'-mo-skōp) *n* an instrument fitted with a lens and illumination for examining the interior of the eye—**ophthalmoscopic** *adj*.

ophthalmo·tonometer (of-thal'-mō-ton-o'-me-tėr) *n* an instrument for determining the intraocular pressure.

opioid (ō'-pē-oyd) *adj* like opium* or an opiate* in pharmacological action.

opistho·tonos (op-is-tho-tō'-nus) *n* extreme extension of the body occurring in tetanic spasm. Patient may be supported on his heels and his head alone—**opisthotonic** *adj*.

opium (ō'-pē-um) *n* the dried juice of opium poppy capsules. Contains morphine*, codeine* and other alkaloids. Valuable analgesic, but more constipating than morphine. Also used as tincture of opium and as paregoric (camphorated tincture of opium). Its use is not permitted in the U.S.

opportunistic infection (op-por-tōō-nis'-tik) ⇒ infection.

op·sonic index (op-son'-ik in'-deks) a figure obtained by experiment which indicates the ability of phagocytes to ingest foreign bodies such as bacteria.

op·sonin (op-son'-in) *n* an antibody which unites with an antigen, usually part of intact cells, and renders the cells more susceptible to phagocytosis*. ⇒ immunoglobulins—**opsonic** *adj*.

op·tic (op'-tik) *adj* pertaining to sight. *optic chiasma* ⇒ chiasma. *optic disc* the point where the optic nerve enters the eyeball. *optic nerve* ⇒ Figure 15.

op·tical aber·ration (op'ti-kal, ab-er-ā'-shun) imperfect focus of light rays by a lens.

op·tician (op-tish'-un) *n* one who prescribes glasses to correct refractive errors.

op·tics (op'-tiks) *n* the branch of physics which deals with light rays and their relation to vision.

opti·mum (op'-tim-um) *adj* most favorable *optimum position* that which will be least awkward and most useful should a limb remain permanently paralyzed.

op·tometry (op-to'-me-trē) *n* measurement of visual acuity.

ora·base (ōr'-à-bās) *n* a proprietary gel product which protects lesions on mucous membranes.

oral (ōr'-àl) *adj* pertaining to the mouth—**orally** *adj*.

Orap (ōr'-ap) *n* proprietary name for pimozide*.

Oratrol (ōr'-à-trol) *n* proprietary name for dichlorphenamide*.

orbic·ular (ōr-bik'-ū-lar) *adj* resembling a globe; spherical or circular.

or·bit (ōr'-bit) *n* the bony socket containing the eyeball and its appendages—**orbital** *adj*.

orchi·dectomy (ōr-kid-ek'-to-mē) *n* excision of a testis*.

orchido·pexy (ōr-kid-ō-peks'-ē) *n* the operation of bringing an undescended testis* into the scrotum*, and fixing it in this position.

orchis (ōr'-kis) *n* the testis.

or·chitis (ōr-kī'-tis) *n* inflammation of a testis.

orf (ōrf) *n* skin lesions caused by a virus normally affecting sheep.

organic (ōr-gan′-ik) *adj* pertaining to an organ. Associated with life, *organic brain syndrome* ⇒ dementia. *organic disease* one in which there is structural change.

organ·ism (ōr′-gan-izm) *n* a living cell or group of cells differentiated into functionally distinct parts which are interdependent.

or·gasm (ōr′-gazm) *n* the climax of sexual excitement.

orien·tal sore (ōr-ē-en′-tal) (*syn* Delhi boil) a form of cutaneous leishmaniasis* producing papular, crusted, granulomatous eruptions of the skin. A disease of the tropics and subtropics.

orien·tation (ōr-ē-en-tā′-shun) *n* clear awareness of one's position relative to the environment. In mental conditions orientation 'in space and time' means that the patient knows where he is and recognizes the passage of time, i.e. can give the correct date. Disorientation means the reverse.

ori·fice (ōr′-if-is) *n* a mouth or opening.

ori·gin (ōr′-i-gin) *n* the commencement or source of anything. *origin of a muscle* the end that remains relatively fixed during contraction of the muscle.

Orinase (ōr′-in-ās) *n* proprietary name for tolbutamide*.

orni·thine (ōr′-ni-thēn) *n* an amino acid, obtained from arginine* by splitting off urea*.

orni·thosis (ōr-ni-thō′-sis) *n* human illness resulting from disease of birds. ⇒ Chlamydia.

oro·genital (ōr-ō-jen′-i-tal) *adj* pertaining to the mouth and the external genital area.

oro·pharynx (ōr-ō-făr′-inks) *n* that portion of the pharynx which is below the level of the soft palate and above the level of the hyoid bone.

oro·pharyngeal (ōr-ō-făr-in-jē′-al) *adj* pertaining to the mouth and pharynx.

orphen·adrine (ōr-fen′-à-drēn) *n* an anticholinergic agent used in Parkinson's disease. May reduce drug-induced parkinsonism caused by tranquilizers. (Norflex.)

ortho·dontics (ōr-thō-don′-tiks) *n* a branch of dentistry dealing with prevention and correction of irregularities of the teeth.

ortho·dox sleep (ōr′-thō-doks slēp) *n* lasts approximately one hour in each sleep* cycle. The metabolic rate and

therefore oxygen consumption is lowered.

Ortho-Novum (ōr′-thō nō′-vum) *n* a proprietary name for oral contraceptive containing estrogen combined with progestogen.

ortho·pedics (ōr-thō-pēd′-iks) *n* formerly a specialty devoted to the correction of deformities in children. It is now a branch of surgery dealing with all conditions affecting the locomotor system.

orthop·nea (ōr-thop′-nē-à) *n* breathlessness necessitating an upright, sitting position for its relief—**orthopneic** *adj*.

orthop·tics (ōr-thop′-tiks) *n* the study and treatment of muscle imbalances of eye (squint*).

or·thosis (ōr-thō′-sis) *n* a device which can be applied to or around the body in the care of physical impairment or disability. ⇒ prosthesis—**orthoses** *pl*, **orthotic** *adj*.

ortho·static (ōr-thō-stat′-ik) *adj* caused by the upright stance. *orthostatic albuminuria* occurs in some healthy subjects only when they take the upright position. When lying in bed the urine is normal.

or·thotics (ōr-tho′-tiks) *n* the scientific study and manufacture of devices which can be applied to or around the body in the care of physical impairment or disability.

orthot·ist (ōr-tho′-tist) *n* a person who practices orthotics*.

Ortolani's sign (ōr-to-la′-nēz sīn) a test performed shortly after birth to discern dislocation of the hip.

Orudis (ōr′-u-dis) *n* proprietary name for ketoproten*.

os (os) *n* a mouth *external os* the opening of the cervix into the vagina (⇒ Figure 17). *internal os* the opening of the cervix into the uterine cavity—**ora** *pl*.

oscil·lation (os-il-ā′-shun) *n* a swinging or moving to and fro; a vibration.

oscil·lometry (os-il-om′-e-trē) *n* measurement of vibration, using a special apparatus (oscillometer). Measures the magnitude of the pulse wave more precisely than palpation.

Osgood-Schlatter's disease (oz′-good shlat′-erz) ⇒ Schlatter's disease.

Osler's nodes (oz′-lerz) small painful areas in pulp of fingers or toes, or palms and soles, caused by emboli and occurring in subacute bacterial endocarditis.

osmol·ality (os-mō-lal′-it-ē) *n* the number of osmoles per kilogram of solution.

osmol·arity (os-mō-lăr′-it-ē) *n* the osmotic pressure exerted by a given concentration of osmotically active solute in aqueous solution, defined in terms of the number of active particles per unit volume.

os·mole (os′-mōl) *n* the standard unit of osmotic pressure which is equal to the gram molecular weight of a solute divided by the number of particles or ions into which it dissociates in solution.

os·mosis (os-mō′-sis) *n* the passage of pure solvent across a semi-permeable membrane under the influence of osmotic* pressure.

os·motic pres·sure (os-mot′-ik) the pressure with which solvent molecules are drawn across a semi-permeable membrane separating two concentrations of solute (such as sodium chloride, sugars, urea) dissolved in the same solvent, when the membrane is impermeable to the solute but permeable to the solvent.

oss·eous (os′-ē-us) *adj* pertaining to or resembling bone.

oss·icles (os′-ik-ls) *n* small bones, particularly those contained in the middle ear; the malleus, incus and stapes.

ossifi·cation (os-if-ik-ā′-shun) *n* the conversion of cartilage, etc. into bone—**ossify** *vt, vi.*

oste·itis (os-tē-ī′-tis) *n* inflammation of bone *osteitis deformans* ⇒ Paget's disease *osteitis fibrosa* cavities form in the interior of bone. The cysts may be solitary or the disease may be generalized. This second condition may be the result of excessive parathyroid secretion and absorption of calcium from bone.

osteo·arthritis (os′-tē-ō-àrth-rī′-tis) *n* degenerative arthritis, may be primary, or may follow injury or disease involving the articular surfaces of synovial joints. The articular cartilage becomes worn, osteophytes form at the periphery of the joint surface and loose bodies may result. ⇒ arthropathy, spondylosis deformans—**osteoarthritic** *adj.*

osteo·blast (os′-tē-ō-blast) *n* a bone-forming cell—**osteoblastic** *adj.*

osteo·chondritis (os-tē-ō-kon-drī′-tis) *n* originally an inflammation of bone cartilage. Usually applied to non-septic conditions, especially avascular necrosis involving joint surfaces, e.g. osteochondritis dissecans in which a portion of joint surface may separate to form a loose body in the joint. ⇒ Scheuermann's disease. Köhler's disease.

osteo·chondroma (os-tē-ō-kon-drō′-mà) *n* a benign bony and cartilaginous tumor.

osteo·clasis (os-tē-ō-klā′-sis) *n* the therapeutic fracture of a bone.

osteo·clast (os′-tē-ō-klast) *n* bone destroyer, the cell which dissolves or removes unwanted bone.

osteo·clastoma (os-tē-ō-klas-tō′-mà) *n* a tumor of the osteoclasts. May be benign, locally recurrent, or frankly malignant. The usual site is near the end of a long bone. ⇒ myeloma.

osteo·cyte (os′-tē-ō-sīt) *n* a bone cell.

osteo·dystrophy (os′-tē-ō-dis′-tro-fē) *n* faulty growth of bone.

osteo·genic (os-tē-ō-jen′-ik) *adj* bone-producing *osteogenic sarcoma* malignant tumor originating in cells which normally produce bone.

Osteo·gene·sis imper·fecta (os-tē-ō-jen′-es-is im-pèr-fek′-tà) a hereditary disorder usually transmitted by an autosomal dominant gene. The disorder may be congenital or develop during childhood. The congenital form is much more severe and may lead to early death. The affected child's bones are extremely fragile and may fracture after the mildest trauma.

osteo·lytic (os-tē-ō-li′-tik) *adj* destructive of bone, e.g. osteolytic malignant deposits in bone.

oste·oma (os-tē-ōm′-à) *n* a benign tumor of bone which may arise in the compact tissue (*ivory osteoma*) or in the cancellous tissue. May be single or multiple.

osteo·malacia (os-tē-ō-mal-ā′-sē-à) *n* demineralization of the mature skeleton, with softening and bone pain. It is commonly caused by insufficient dietary intake of vitamin D or lack of sunshine, or both.

osteo·myelitis (os-tē-ō-mī-el-ī′-tis) *n* inflammation commencing in the marrow of bone—**osteomyelitic** *adj.*

oste·opath (os′-tē-ō-path) *n* one who practices osteopathy.

oste·opathy (os-tē-op′-à-thē) *n* a theory which attributes a wide range of disorders to mechanical derangements of the skeletal system, which it is claimed can be rectified by suitable manipulations—**osteopathic** *adj.*

osteo·petrosis (os-tē-ō-pet-rō′-sis) (*syn* Albers-Schönberg disease, marble bones) a congenital abnormality giving rise to very dense bones which fracture easily.

oste·ophony (os-tē-of'-ō-nē) *n* the conduction of sound waves to the inner ear by bone.

osteo·phyte (os'-tē-ō-fīt) *n* a bony outgrowth or spur, usually at the margins of joint surfaces, e.g. in osteoarthritis—**osteophytic** *adj.*

osteo·plasty (os-tē-ō-plas'-tē) *n* reconstructive operation on bone—**osteoplastic** *adj.*

osteo·porosis (os-tē-ō-por-ōs'-is) *n* loss of bone density caused by excessive absorption of calcium and phosphorus from the bone, due to progressive loss of the protein matrix of bone which normally carries the calcium deposits—**osteoporotic** *adj.*

osteo·sarcoma (os-tē-ō-sàr-kō'-mà) *n* a sarcomatous tumor growing from bone—**osteosarcomata** *pl,* **osteosarcomatous** *adj.*

osteo·sclerosis (os-tē-ō-sklėr-ōs'-is) *n* increased density or hardness of bone—**osteosclerotic** *adj.*

osteo·tome (os'-tē-o-tōm) *n* an instrument for cutting bone; it is similar to a chisel, but it is bevelled on both sides of its cutting edge.

oste·otomy (os-tē-ot'-o-mē) *n* division of bone followed by realignment of the ends to encourage union by healing. *McMurray's osteotomy* ⇒ McMurray's.

os·tium (os'-tē-um) *n* the opening or mouth of any tubular passage—**ostia** *pl,* **ostial** *adj.*

OT *abbr* occupational therapist.

otal·gia (ō-tal'-jē-a) *n* earache.

OTC *abbr* over the counter, refers to medicines sold without a prescription.

otitis (ō-tī'-tis) *n* inflammation of the ear. *otitis externa* inflammation of the skin of the external auditory canal. *otitis media* inflammation of the middle ear cavity. The effusion tends to be serous, mucoid or purulent. Non-purulent effusions in children are often called glue* ear. ⇒ grommet.

oto·laryn·gology (ot-ō-lār-in-gol'-o-jē) *n* the science which deals with the structure, function and diseases of the ear and larynx, each of which can be a separate speciality. ⇒ otology, laryngology.

oto·liths (ot'-ō-liths) *npl* tiny calcareous deposits within the membranous labyrinth of the internal ear.

otol·ogist (o-tol'-o-jist) *n* a person who specializes in otology.

otol·ogy (o-tol'-o-jē) *n* the science which deals with the structure, function and diseases of the ear.

oto·mycosis (o-tō-mī-kō'-sis) *n* a fungal (*Aspergillus, Candida*) infection of the external auditory meatus—**otomycotic** *adj.*

otorhino·laryngology (ō-tō-rī-nō-lār-in-gol'-o-jē) *n* the science which deals with the structure, function and diseases of the ear, nose and throat; each of these three may be considered a specialty. ⇒ laryngoly, otology, rhinology.

otorrhea (ō-tō-rē'-à) *n* a discharge from the external auditory meatus.

oto·sclerosis (ō-tō-sklėr-ōs'-is) *n* new bone formation affecting primarily the footplate of the stapes* and a common cause of progressive deafness—**otosclerotic** *adj.*

otoscope (ō'-tō-skōp) *n* instrument used for examination of the ear.

oto·toxic (ō-tō-toks'-ik) *adj* having a toxic action on the ear.

ouabaine (oo̅-à-bān) *n* a cardiac glycoside. Like digoxin*, it has a steadying effect on the heart.

ova (ō'-và) *npl* the female reproductive cells—**ovum** *sing.*

ovar·ian (ō-vā'-rē-àn) *adj* pertaining to the ovaries. *ovarian cyst* a tumor of the ovary, usually containing fluid—may be benign or malignant. It may reach a large size and can twist on its stalk creating an acute emergency surgical condition.

ovari·ectomy (ō-vā-rē-ek'-to-mē) *n* ⇒ oophorectomy.

ovari·otomy (ō-vā-rē-ot'-o-mē) *n* literally means incision of an ovary, but is the term usually applied to the removal of an ovary (oophorectomy).

ovar·itis (ō-var-ī'-tis) *n* ⇒ oophoritis.

ovary (ō'-var-ē) *n* one of two small oval bodies situated on either side of the uterus on the posterior surface of the broad ligament (⇒ Figure 17). The structures in which the ova* are developed—**ovarian** *adj. cystic ovary* retention cysts in ovarian follicles. Cysts contain estrogen-rich fluid which causes menorrhagia.

overbite (ō'-ver bīt) *n* the overriding of the upper front teeth over the lower teeth when the jaw is closed.

overcompen·sation (ō'-ver kom-pen-sā'-shun) *n* name given to any type of behavior which a person adopts in order to cover up a deficiency. Thus a person who is afraid may react by becoming arrogant or boastful or quarrelsome.

ovi·duct (ō'-vi-dukt) *n* ⇒ fallopian tubes.

ovu·lation (ō-vū-lā'-shun) *n* the maturation and rupture of a graafian* follicle with the discharge of an ovum.

oxacillin (oks-à-sil'-in) *n* an isoxazole penicillin active against penicillinase-producing strains of staphylococcus aureus.

oxa·luria (oks-à-lū'-rē-à) *n* excretion of urine containing calcium oxalate crystals; associated often with dyspepsia.

ox·azepam (oks-az'-e-pam) *n* a mild tranquilizer; one of the benzodiazepines*. (Serax.)

oxi·dase (oks'-i-dās) *n* any enzyme which promotes oxidation.

oxi·dation (oks-i-dā'-shun) *n* the act of oxidizing or state of being oxidized. It involves an increase of positive charges on an atom or the loss of a pair of hydrogen atoms or the addition of oxygen. Oxidation must be accompanied by reduction of an acceptor molecule. Part of the process of metabolism, resulting in the release of energy.

oxi·meter (oks-i'-me-tèr) *n* an instrument attached to the ear to 'sense' the oxygen saturation of arterial blood. An accurate non-invasive technique.

oxpren·olol hydro·chloride (oks-pren'-o-lol) a beta-adrenergic blocking agent used in the treatment of hypertension. (Trasicor.)

Oxy·cel (oks'-i-sel) *n* a proprietary preparation of oxidized cellulose; used to achieve hemostasis when conventional methods of ligature, sutures or diathermy have failed. The material is subsequently absorbed by the tissues.

oxycodone (oks-i-kō'-dōn) *n* a narcotic analgesic obtained from an opium alkaloid, can produce drug dependency. (Percodan.)

oxy·gen (oks'-i-jen) *n* a colorless, odorless, gaseous element, necessary for life and combustion. Constitutes 20% by weight of atmospheric air. Used medicinally as an inhalation. Supplied in cylinders (black with a white top) in which the gas is at a high pressure. ⇒ hyperbaric oxygen treatment *oxygen concentrator* a device for removing nitrogen from the air to provide a high concentration of oxygen.

oxygen·ation (oks-i-jen-ā'-shun) *n* the saturation of a substance (particularly blood) with oxygen. Arterial oxygen tension* indicates degree of oxygenation; reference range 90–100 mmHg (*c* 13·0 kPa)—**oxygenated** *adj.*

oxygen·ator (oks'-i-jen-ā-tor) *n* artificial 'lung' as used in heart surgery.

oxy·hemo·globin (oks-i-hē'-mō-glō-bin) *n* oxygenated hemoglobin, an unstable compound formed from hemoglobin on exposure to alveolar gas in the lungs.

oxy·metazoline (oks-i-met-a-zōl'-ēn) *n* nasal vasoconstrictor; gives quick relief but the action is short-lived; there is a danger of rebound congestion after repeated use.

oxy·metholone (oks-i-meth'-o-lōn) *n* an anabolic steroid. ⇒ anabolic compound.

oxy·ntic (oks-in'-tik) *adj* producing acid. *oxyntic cells* the cells in the gastric mucosa which produce hydrochloric acid.

oxy·phenbutazone (oks-i-fen-bū'-ta-zōn) *n* an anti-inflammatory, analgesic, antiarthritic drug. Because of toxicity no longer used except as an eye ointment. (Tanderil.)

oxyphenonium (oks-i-fen-ōn'-ē-um) *n* an antispasmodic used to treat peptic ulcer.

oxy·tetracycline (oks-i-tet-ri-sī'-klin) *n* an orally effective antibiotic with a wide range of activity. May be given by slow intravenous injection in severe infections. Prolonged use may cause candidal overgrowth in the intestinal tract. (Terramycin.)

oxy·tocic (oks-i-tō'-sik) *adj, n* hastening parturition; an agent promoting uterine contractions.

oxy·tocin (oks-i-tō'-sin) *n* one of the posterior pituitary hormones. Contracts muscle in milk ducts and hence causes milk ejection. There is a preparation of pituitary extract (Syntocinon, Pitocin) that can cause uterine contractions, and so it is useful in postpartum hemorrhage. Given intramuscularly, subcutaneously, orally, nasally, or intravenously in titration method with a positive pressure peristaltic pump. *oxytocin* challenge test (OCT) ⇒ stress test.

Oxy·uris (oks-i-ūr'-is) *n* a genus of nematodes, commonly called threadworms.

ozena (ō-zē'-na) *n* atrophic* rhinitis.

ozone (ō'-zōn) *n* an allotropic form of oxygen. O_3. Has powerful oxidizing properties and is therefore antiseptic and disinfectant. It is both irritating and toxic in the pulmonary system.

P

³²P *abbr* radioactive phosphorus.

pace·maker (pās'-mā-kèr) *n* the region of the heart which initiates atrial contraction and thus controls heart rate. The natural pacemaker is the sinoatrial node which is situated at the opening of the superior vena cava into the right atrium; the wave of contraction begins here, then spreads over the heart. *artificial pacemaker* ⇒ cardiac.

pachy·blepharon (pak-i-blef'-à-ron) *n* thick eyelids.

pachy·cephalia (pak-i-sef-al'-ē-à) *n* a thick skull.

pachy·chilia (pak-i-kī'-lē-à) *n* thick lip(s).

pachy·dermia (pak-i-dèr'-mē-à) *n* thick skin. ⇒ elephantiasis.

pachy·meningitis (pak-i-men-in-jī'-tis) *n* inflammation of the dura mater (pachymeninx).

Paget·Schroetter syn·drome (pa'-jet shrō'-der) axillary or subclavian vein thrombosis, often associated with effort in fit young persons.

Paget's dis·ease (pa'-jets) **1** (*syn* osteitis deformans) excess of the enzyme alkaline phosphatase causes too rapid bone formation; consequently bone is thin. There is loss of stature, crippling deformity, enlarged head, collapse of vertebrae and neurological complications can result. Sufferers are particularly susceptible to sarcoma of bone. If the auditory nerve is involved, there is impairment of hearing. Calcitonin* is the drug of choice. **2** erosion of the nipple caused by invasion of the dermis by intraduct carcinoma of the breast.

painter's colic (pǎn'-ters kol'-ik) ⇒ colic.

pal·ate (pal'-at) *n* the roof of the mouth (⇒ Figure 14)—**palatal, palatine** *adj. cleft palate* ⇒ cleft palate. *hard palate* the front part of the roof of the mouth formed by the two palatal bones. *soft palate* situated at the posterior end of the palate and consisting of muscle covered by mucous membrane.

pala·tine (pal'-à-tīn) *adj* pertaining to the palate. *palatine arches* the bilateral double pillars or arch-like folds formed by the descent of the soft palate as it meets the pharynx.

palato·plegia (pal-à-tō-plē'-jē-à) *n* paralysis of the soft palate—**palatoplegic** *adj.*

palli·ative (pal'-ē-à-tiv) *adj, n* describes anything which serves to alleviate but cannot cure a disease—**palliation** *n*.

palli·dectomy (pal-id-ek'-to-mē) *n* destruction of a predetermined section of globus pallidus. ⇒ chemopallidectomy, stereotactic surgery.

palli·dotomy (pal-id-ot'-o-mē) *n* surgical severance of the fibers from the cerebral cortex to the corpus striatum. Used to be carried out to relieve the tremor in Parkinson's disease.

palm *n* the anterior or flexor surface of the hand.

pal·mar (pal'-mar) *adj* pertaining to the palm* of the hand. *palmar arches* superficial and deep, are formed by the anastomosis of the radial and ulnar arteries (⇒ Figure 9).

pal·maris longus (pal-mar'-is long'us) ⇒ Figure 4.

pal·pable (pal'-pà-bl) *adj* capable of being palpated.

pal·pation (pal-pā'-shun) *n* the act of manual examination—**palpate** *vt.*

pal·pebra (pal-pē'-brà) *n* an eyelid—**palpebrae** *pl*, **palpebral** *adj.*

palpi·tation (pal-pi-tā'-shun) *n* rapid forceful beating of the heart of which the patient is conscious.

palsy (pal'-sē) *n* paralysis*. A word which is only retained in compound forms— Bell's* palsy, cerebral* palsy and Erb's* palsy.

Pamelor (pam'-e-lor) *n* proprietary name for nortriptyline*.

panacea (pan-à-sē'-à) *n* a treatment claimed to cure all diseases.

Pan·adol (pan'-a-dol) *n* proprietary name for acetaminophen*.

pan·arthritis (pan-àrth-rī'-tis) *n* inflammation of all the structures of a joint.

pan·carditis (pan-kàr-dī'-tis) *n* inflammation of all the structures of the heart.

pan·creas (pan'-krē-as) *n* a tongue-shaped glandular organ lying below and behind the stomach (⇒ Figure 18). Its head is encircled by the duodenum and its tail touches the spleen. It is about 18 cm long and weighs about 100 g. It secretes the hormone insulin*, and also pancreatic juice which contains enzymes involved in the digestion of fats and proteins in the small intestine.

pancreatec·tomy (pan-krē-à-tek'-to-mē) *n* excision of part or the whole of the pancreas.

pan·creatic func·tion test (pan-krē-at'-ik) Levin's tubes are positioned in the stomach and second part of duodenum. The response of the pancreatic gland to various hormonal stimuli can be measured by analyzing the duodenal aspirate. ⇒ selenomethionine.

pan·creatin (pan'-krē-à-tin) *n* a mixture of enzymes obtained from the pancreas. Used in pancreatic diseases and deficiency. Standard and triple-strength products are available.

pancrea·titis (pan-krē-à-tī'-tis) *n* inflammation of the pancreas*. The lipase level of blood and urine is used as an indicator of pancreatitis. ⇒ diastase.

pancreas·trophic (pan-krē-à-trō'-fik) *adj* having an affinity for or an influence on the pancreas. Some of the anterior pituitary hormones have a pancreatrophic action.

pancreo·zymin (pan-krē-ō-zī'-min) *n* a hormone secreted by the duodenal mucosa; it stimulates the flow of pancreatic enzymes, especially amylase.

pan·curonium bromide (pan-kū-rō'-nē-um brō'-mīd) non-depolarizing muscle relaxant. Produces neuromuscular block by competing with acetylcholine at the neuromuscular junction. Complete paralysis is induced but there is no alteration in the level of consciousness. (Pavulon.)

pan·cytopenia (pan-sī-tō-pē'-nē-à) *n* describes peripheral blood picture when red cells, granular white cells and platelets are reduced as occurs in suppression of bone marrow function.

pan·demic (pan-dem'-ik) *n* an infection spreading over a whole country or the world.

panhysterectomy (pan-his-tèr-ek'-to-mē) *n* an old term for the removal of the uterus and adnexa; more accurately described as a total hysterectomy* with bilateral salpingo-oophorectomy*.

pan·nus (pan'-us) *n* corneal vascularization, often associated with conjunctival irritation.

pan·ophthal·mitis (pan-of-thal-mī'-tis) *n* inflammation of all the tissues of the eyeball.

pan·osteitis (pan-os-tē-ī'-tis) *n* inflammation of all constituents of a bone—medulla, bony tissue and periosteum.

panto·thenic acid (pan-tō-then'-ik) a constituent of the vitamin B complex.

PAO *abbr* peak acid output. ⇒ pentagastrin test.

PaO₂ *abbr* pulmonary arterial oxygen saturation and tension.

Pap test (Papanicolaou) a smear of epithelial cells taken from the cervix is stained and examined under the microscope for detection of the early stages of cancer.

papaver·ine (pa-pà-vèr'-ēn) *n* one of the less important alkaloids of opium*, used mainly as a relaxant in spasm, asthma and peripheral vascular disorders.

pa·pilla (pa-pil'-là) *n* a minute nipple-shaped eminence—**papillae** *pl*, **papillary** *adj*. *renal papilla* ⇒ Figure 20.

papilledema (pap-il-e-dē'-mà) *n* (*syn* choked disc) edema of the optic disc; suggestive of increased intracranial pressure.

papil·litis (pap-il-ī'-tis) *n* **1** inflammation of the optic disc. **2** inflammation of a papilla. Can arise in the kidney after excessive phenacetin* intake.

papil·loma (pap-il-ō'-mà) *n* a simple tumor arising from a non-glandular epithelial surface—**papillomata** *pl*, **papillomatous** *adj*.

papilloma·tosis (pap-il-ō-mà-tō'-sis) *n* the growth of benign papillomata on the skin or a mucous membrane. Removal by laser means fewer recurrences.

pap·ule (pap'-ūl) *n* (*syn* pimple) a small circumscribed elevation of the skin—**papular** *adj*.

papulo·pustular (pap-ū-lō-pus'-tū-lar) *adj* pertaining to both papules* and pustules*.

para·amino·benzoic acid (pàr-a-a-mēn'-ō-benz-ō'-ik) filters the ultraviolet rays from the sun and in a cream or lotion protects the skin from sunburn.

para·amino·salicyclic acid (PAS) (pàr-a-a-mēn'-ō-sal-i-sil'-ik) formerly widely used antitubercular drug, in association with isoniazid* or streptomycin*.

para·aortic (pàr-à-ā-ōr'-tik) *adj* near the aorta*.

para·casein (pàr-à-kās'-ēn) *n* ⇒ casein.

para·centesis (pàr-à-sen-tē'-sis) *n* ⇒ aspiration—**paracenteses** *pl*.

Paradione (pàr-à-dī'-ōn) *n* proprietary name for paramethadione*.

para·doxical respiration (pàr-a-doks'-i-kal) ⇒ respiration.

para·doxical sleep *n* (*syn* REM sleep) constitutes about a quarter of sleeping time. Characterized by rapid eye movements during which dreaming occurs.

paraesophageal (pàr-à-ē-sof-à-jē'-al) *adj* near the esophagus.

paraf·fin (păr′-à-fin) *n* medicinal paraffins are: *liquid paraffin*, used as a laxative; *soft paraffin*, the familiar ointment base; and *hard paraffin*, used in wax baths for rheumatic conditions.

para·formal·dehyde (păr-à-fŏrm-al′-de-hīd) *n* a solid modification of formaldehyde used for sterilizing catheters and disinfecting rooms.

para·ganglioma (păr-à-gang-lē-ō′-mà) *n* ⇒ pheochromocytoma.

para·influenza·virus (păr-à-in-flū-en′-zà vi′-rus) *n* causes acute upper respiratory infection. One of the myxoviruses.

paral·dehyde (păr-al′-de-hīd) *n* a liquid with a characteristic odor. Has sedative properties similar to chloral*. Given orally, intramuscular injection or rectally as a solution in olive oil. Now rarely used.

paral·ysis (par-al′-is-is) *n* complete or incomplete loss of nervous function to a part of the body. This may be sensory or motor or both. *paralysis agitans* ⇒ parkinsonism.

paral·ytic (păr-à-lit′-ik) *adj* pertaining to paralysis. *paralytic ileus* paralysis of the intestinal muscle so that the bowel content cannot pass onwards even though there is no mechanical obstruction. ⇒ aperistalsis.

para·median (păr-à-mēd′-ē-an) *adj* near the middle.

paramedic (păr-à-med′-ik) *n* a non-physician trained to do rescue work or to be a physician's assistant.

para·medical (păr-à-mēd′-i-kal) *adj* associated with the medical profession. The paramedical services include occupational, physical and speech therapy and medical social work.

para·menstruum (păr-à-men′-strū-um) *n* the four days before the start of menstruation and the first four days of the period itself.

paramethadione (păr-à-meth-à-dī′-ōn) *n* an anticonvulsant compound, useful in petit mal seizures. (Paradione.)

paramethasone (păr-à-meth′-à-zōn) *n* one of the corticosteroids.

para·metritis (păr-à-mē-trī′-tis) *n* ⇒ cellulitis.

para·metrium (păr-à-mē′-trē-um) *n* the connective tissues immediately surrounding the uterus—**parametrial** *adj*.

para·nasal (para-à-nā′-zal) *adj* near the nasal cavities, as the various sinuses.

paraneo·plastic (păr-à-nē-ō-plas′-tik) *adj* describes syndromes associated with malignancy but not caused by the primary growth or its metastases.

para·noia (păr-à-noy′-à) *n* a mental disorder characterized by the insidious onset of delusions of persecution—**paranoid** *adj*.

para·noid behav·ior (păr′-à-noyd) acts denoting suspicion of others.

paranoid schizophrenia (păr′-à-noyd skiz′-o-frē′-nē-à) a form of schizophrenia dominated by delusions and, to a lesser extent, hallucinations.

para·phimosis (păr-à-fī-mō′-sis) *n* retraction of the prepuce* behind the glans* penis so that the tight ring of skin interferes with the blood flow in the glans.

para·phrenia (păr-à-frē′-nē-à) *n* a psychiatric illness in the elderly characterized by well-circumscribed delusions, usually of a persecutory nature—**paraphrenic** *adj*.

para·plegia (păr-à-plē′-jē-à) *n* paralysis of the lower limbs, usually including the bladder and rectum—**paraplegic** *adj*.

para·psychology (păr-à-sī-kol′-o-jē) *n* the study of extrasensory perception, telepathy, and other psychic phenomena.

para·quat (păr′-à-kwat) *n* widely used as a weed killer. If ingested it causes delayed toxic effects in the lungs, liver and kidneys. Poisoning may cause death from progressive pneumonia.

para·rectal (păr-à-rek′-tal) *adj* near the rectum.

para·site (păr′-à-sīt) *n* an organism which obtains food or shelter from another organism, the 'host'—**parasitic** *adj*.

para·sitemia (păr-à-sīt-ēm′-ē-a) *n* parasites in the blood—**parasitemic** *adj*.

parasiti·cide (păr-à-sīt′-i-sīd) *n* an agent which will kill parasites.

para·suicide (păr-à-sū′-is-īd) *n* a suicidal gesture; a self-multilating act which may or may not be motivated by a genuine desire to die. It is common in young people who are distressed but not mentally ill.

para·sympathetic (păr-à-sim-path-et′-ik) *adj* describes a portion of the autonomic nervous system derived from some of the cranial and sacral nerves belonging to the central nervous system.

para·sympatholytic (păr-à-sim-path-ō-lit′-ik) *adj* capable of neutralizing the effect of parasympathetic stimulation, e.g. atropine* and scopolamine*.

para·thion (păr-à-thī′-on) *n* an organic phosphate used as insecticide in agriculture. Has a powerful and irreversible, anticholinesterase action. Potentionally dangerous to man for this reason.

para·thormone (păr-àth-ōr'-mōn) *n* a hormone secreted by the parathyroid* glands, which controls the level of calcium in the blood, partly by its effect on calcium content of bone. Excess hormone causes mobilization of calcium from the bones, which become rarefied.

para·thyroid glands (păr-à-thī'-royd) *npl* four small endocrine glands lying close to or embedded in the posterior surface of the thyroid* gland. They secrete a hormone, parathormone.

para·thyroid·ectomy (păr-à-thī-royd-ek'-to-mē) *n* excision of one or more parathyroid* glands.

para·tracheal (păr-à-trā'-kē-al) *adj* near the trachea.

para·typhoid fever (păr-à-tī'-foyd) a variety of enteric fever, less severe and prolonged than typhoid* fever. Caused by *Salmonella paratyphi A* and *B*, and more rarely *C*. ⇒ TAB.

para·urethral (păr-à-ū-rē'-thral) *adj* near the urethra.

para·vaginal (păr-à-vaj'-in-al) *adj* near the vagina.

para·vertebral (păr-à-vėr-tē'-bral) *adj* near the spinal column. *paravertebral block anesthesia* (more correctly, 'analgesia') is induced by infiltration of local anesthetic around the spinal nerve roots as they emerge from the intervertebral foramina. *paravertebral injection* of local anesthetic into sympathetic chain, can be used as a test in ischemic limbs to see if sympathectomy will be of value.

paregoric (păr-e-gōr'-ik) *n* camphorated tincture of opium used for diarrhea. Only treats symptoms, may mask signs of underlying disease.

paren·chyma (păr-eng-kī'-mà) *n* the parts of an organ which, in contradistinction to its interstitial tissue, are concerned with its function—**parenchymal, parenchymatous** *adj*.

par·enteral (păr-en'-tėr-al) *adj* not via the alimentary tract. *parenteral feeding* is necessary when it is impossible to provide adequate nutrition via the gastrointestinal tract. A sterile solution of nutrients is infused into a silicone catheter inserted into a large peripheral or, more usually, a large central vein (e.g. the vena cava). An infusion pump regulates the number of drops per minute. Patients and their families can learn to manage parenteral feeding at home. Mouth hygiene needs special attention—**parenterally** *adv*.

par·esis (pa-rē'-sis) *n* partial or slight paralysis; weakness of a limb—**paretic** *adj*.

paresthesia (păr-es-thēz'-ē-a) *n* any abnormality of sensation.

par·eunia (par-ūn'-ē-à) *n* coitus*.

par·ietal (par-ī'-et-al) *adj* pertaining to a wall. *parietal bones* the two bones which form the sides and vault of the skull.

par·ity (păr'-i-tē) *n* status of a woman with regard to the number of children she has borne.

parkinson·ism (păr'-kin-son-izm) *n* syndrome of mask-like expression, shuffling gait, tremor of the limbs and pill-rolling movements of the fingers. Can be drug-induced. The postencephalitic type comes on in the 30–40 age group and there may or may not be a clear history of encephalitis (sporadic type). Degenerative type of parkinsonism (paralysis agitans) comes on during middle life; arteriosclerotic type comes on in the elderly. Characterized by a distinctive clinical pattern of tremor and rigidity. Some people differentiate between Parkinson's disease, which is a degenerative process associated with aging, and parkinsonism, the causes of which are multiple and include such factors as injury, stroke, atherosclerosis, various toxic agents and the viral infection encephalitis lethargica.

Parlodel (par'-lō-del) *n* proprietary name for bromocriptine*.

Par·nate (par'-nāt) *n* proprietary name for tranylcypromine*.

paromomycin (păr-ō-mō-mī'-sin) *n* an amebicide only administered orally. Useful for temporary or long-term suppression of bowel flora; treatment of various forms of acute enteritis. (Humatin.)

paron·ychia (păr-on-ik'-ē-à) *n* (*syn* whitlow) inflammation around a fingernail which may be bacterial or fungal. The virus of herpes simplex may also cause multiple vesicles over inflamed skin—*herpetic paronychia*.

par·osmia (par-os'-mē-à) *n* perverted sense of smell, usually of halucinatory nature.

parotid·ectomy (par-ot'-id-ek'-to-mē) *n* excision of a parotid* gland.

par·otid gland (par-ot'-id) the salivary gland situated in front of and below the ear on either side.

211

par·otitis (par-ō-tī′-tis) *n* inflammation of a parotid* gland *infectious parotitis* mumps*. *septic parotitis* refers to ascending infection from the mouth via the parotid duct, when a parotid abscess may result.

par·ous (pār′us) *adj* having borne a child or children.

par·oxysm (pār′-oks-izm) *n* a sudden, temporary attack.

par·oxysmal (pār-oks-iz′-mal) *adj* coming on in attacks or paroxysms. *paroxysmal dyspnea* occurs mostly at night in patients with cardiac disease. *paroxysmal fibrillation* occurs in the atrium of the heart and is associated with a ventricular tachycardia and total irregularity of the pulse rhythm. *paroxysmal tachycardia* may result from ectopic impulses arising in the atrium or in the ventricle itself.

par·rot dis·ease (pār′-rot) ⇒ psittacosis*.

Par·rot's nodes (pār′-rots) bossing of frontal bones in the congenital syphilitic ⇒ pseudoparalysis.

partial pressure (par′-shal presh′-ur) pressure exerted by gas in a mixture of gases in proportion to concentration.

par·turient (par-tū′-rē-ent) *adj* pertaining to childbirth.

partur·ition (par-tū-ri′-shun) *n* ⇒ labor.

PAS *abbr* 1 para-aminosalicylic acid. ⇒ aminosalicyclic acid. 2 periodic acid-Schiff reaction, used to test for glycogen, epithelial mucins, ventral polysaccharides and glycoproteins.

pass·ive (pas′-siv) *adj* inactive. ⇒ active *opp*. *passive hyperemia* ⇒ hyperemia. *passive immunity* ⇒ immunity. *passive movement* performed by the physiotherapist, the patient being relaxed.

Pasteur·ella (pas-te-rel′-a) *n* a genus of bacteria. Short Gram-negative rods, staining more deeply at the poles (bipolar staining). Pathogenic in man and animals.

pasteur·ization (pas-tūr-ī-zā′-shun) *n* a process whereby pathogenic organisms in fluid (especially milk) are killed by heat. *flash method of pasteurization* (HT, ST—high temperature short time), the fluid is heated to 72° C, maintained at this temperature for 15 s, then rapidly cooled. *holder method of pasteurization* the fluid is heated to 63–65.5° C maintained at this temperature for 30 min then rapidly cooled.

Patau's syn·drome (pa-tōz′) autosomal trisomy of chromosome 13. Closely associated with mental subnormality.

There are accompanying physical defects.

patch test a skin test for identifying reaction to allergens which are incorporated in an adhesive patch applied to the skin. Another patch with nothing on it is used as a control. Allergy is apparent by redness and swelling.

pa·tella (pà-tel′-à) *n* a triangular, sesamoid bone; the kneecap (⇒ Figure 2)—**patel·lae** *pl*, **patellar** *adj*.

patell·ectomy (pa-tel-ek′-to-mē) *n* excision of the patella*.

patent (pā′-tent) *adj* open; not closed or occluded—**patency** *n*. *patent ductus arteriosus* failure of ductus arteriosus to close soon after birth, so that the abnormal shunt between the pulmonary artery and the aorta is preserved. *patent interventricular septum* a congenital defect in the dividing wall between the right and left ventricle of the heart.

patho·gen (path′-ō-jen) *n* a disease-producing agent, usually restricted to a living agent—**pathogenic** *adj*, **pathogenicity** *n*.

patho·genesis (path-ō-jen′-e-sis) *n* the origin and development of disease—**pathogenetic** *adj*.

pathogen·icity (path-ō-jen-is′-it-ē) *n* the capacity to produce disease.

patho·gnomonic (path-og-nō-mon′-ik) *adj* characteristic of or peculiar to a disease.

patho·logical frac·ture (path-ol-oj′-i-kal) ⇒ fracture.

path·ology (path-ol′-o-jē) *n* the science which deals with the cause and nature of disease—**pathological** *adj*, **pathologically** *adv*.

patho·phobia (path-ō-fō′-bē-à) *n* a morbid dread of disease—**pathophobic** *adj*.

patho·physiology (path-ō-fiz′-ē-ol′-o-jē) *n* the science which deals with abnormal functioning of the human being—**pathophysiological** *adj*, **pathophysiologically** *adv*.

patient com·pliance (pā′-shent kom-plī′-ans) a term used when a patient introduces into his body the prescribed drug, in the prescribed dose, at the prescribed time and by the prescribed route ⇒ patient non-compliance *opp*.

patu·lous (pat′-ū-lus) *adj* opened out; expanded.

Paul-Bunnell test (pawl bun-el′) a serological test used in the diagnosis of infectious mononucleosis. Antibodies which occur in patients with this disease agglutinate sheep's erythrocytes.

Paul-Mikulicz operation (pawl mik'-u-liz) a method for excision of a portion of the colon whereby the two cut ends of the bowel are kept out on the surface of the abdomen, and are joined at a later date without entering the peritoneal cavity. The method was designed to lessen the risk of peritonitis from leakage at the suture line.

Paul tube a flanged glass tube used to collect the contents after the bowel has been opened on the surface of the abdomen.

Pav·ulon (pav'-ū-lon) n proprietary name for pancuronium* bromide.

Pawlik's grip (paw'-liks) a method of determining the engagement or otherwise of the fetal head in the maternal pelvic brim.

PBI abbr protein bound iodine. Iodine combined with protein as part of the thyroid hormone. Low in thyroid deficiency.

PCB's abbr polychlorinated byphenyls, industrial compounds now widely dispersed.

PCM abbr protein* caloric malnutrition.

PDR abbr Physician's* Desk Reference.

peak-expiratory flow rate the measured amount of air in a forced exhalation over one second.

Pearson bed (pēr'-son) a special type of hospital bed used for fractures. It is higher and narrower than the usual type. Instead of springs there are light strips of webbing. The mattress is in three or four sections. A Balkan* beam is attached to the bed frame.

peau d'orange (pō-dōr-ongzh') term applied to the appearance of the skin over the breast in acute inflammation or in advanced carcinoma, when lymphedema causes the orifices of the hair follicles to appear as dimples, resembling the pits in the skin of an orange.

pectineus muscle (pek-tin-ē'-us) ⇒ Figure 4.

pec·toral (pek'-tor-al) adj pertaining to the breast.

pec·tus (pek'-tus) the chest. *pectus carinatum* ⇒ pigeon chest. *pectus excavatum* ⇒ funnel chest.

pedal (pē'-dal) adj pertaining to the foot.

peda·scope (pē'-dà-skōp) n allows shoe fitting under fluoroscopy.

pedia·trician (pē-dē-à-tri'-shun) a specialist in children's medicine.

pedi·atrics (pē-dē-at'-riks) n the branch of medicine dealing with children and their diseases—**pediatric**, adj.

ped·icle (ped'-i-kl) n a stalk, e.g. the narrow part by which a tumor is attached to the surrounding structures.

pedicu·losis (ped-ik-ū-lō'-sis) n infestation with lice (pediculi).

Pedi·culus (ped-ik'-ū-lus) n a genus of parasitic insects (lice) important as vectors of disease. *Pediculus capitis* the head louse. *Pediculus corporis* the body louse. *Pediculis* (more correctly, *Phthirius*) *pubis* the pubic or crab louse. In some parts of the world body lice are involved in transmitting relapsing fever and typhus.

Ped·o·jet (pēd'-ō-jet) n proprietary apparatus for introduction of vaccines under pressure into the skin. Avoids the use of a needle with consequent danger of spreading serum hepatitis.

pedo·pompholyx (pē-dō-pom'-fol-iks) n ⇒ cheiropompholyx.

ped·uncle (ped-ungk'-l) n a stalk-like structure, often acting as a support—**peduncular, pedunculated** adj.

peel·ing (pēl'-ing) n desquamation*.

Peganone (peg'-a-nōn) n proprietary name for ethotoin*.

Pel-Ebstein fever (pel eb'-stīn) recurring bouts of pyrexia in regular sequence found in lymphadenoma (Hodgkin's disease). A less frequent manifestation with improving treatment.

Pelizaeus-Merzbacher dis·ease (pel-ēz'-ē-us merz'-bak-er) genetically determined degenerative disease associated with mental subnormality.

pel·lagra (pel-ā'-grà) n a deficiency disease caused by lack of vitamin B complex and protein. Syndrome includes glossitis, dermatitis, peripheral neuritis and spinal cord changes (even producing ataxia), anemia and mental confusion.

pel·let (pel'-et) n a little pill. ⇒ implant.

pel·vic floor (pel'-vik flōr) a mainly muscular partition with the pelvic cavity above and the perineum below. In the female, weakening of these muscles can contribute to urinary incontinence and uterine prolapse.

pel·vic floor repair ⇒ Fothergill's operation.

pel·vic girdle (pel'-vik ger'-dl) the bony

pelvis comprising two innominate bones, the sacrum and coccyx.

pelvic inflammatory disease (PID) an inflammatory process that results from other pelvic diseases; may result from gonorrhea, tuberculosis, or post-partal infection.

pel·vic pain syn·drome (PPS) pelvic pain which occurs in women but for which no pathological cause is evident, consequently there is no effective treatment.

pelvim·eter (pel-vim′-et-ėr) *n* an instrument especially devised to measure the pelvic diameters for obstetric purposes.

pelvim·etry (pel-vim′-et-rē) *n* the measurement of the dimension of the pelvis—**pelvimetric** *adj.*

pel·vis (pel′-vis) *n* 1 a basin-shaped cavity, e.g. pelvis of the kidney (⇒ Figure 20). 2 the large bony basin-shaped cavity formed by the innominate bones and sacrum, containing and protecting the bladder, rectum and, in the female, the organs of generation—**pelvic** *adj. contracted pelvis* one in which one or more diameters are smaller than normal; this may result in difficulties in childbirth. *false pelvis* the wide expanded part of the pelvis above the brim. *true pelvis* that part of the pelvis below the brim.

pemphi·goid (pem′-fi-goyd) *n* allied to pemphigus*. A bullous eruption in the latter half of life which is of autoimmune cause. Histological examination of the base of a blister differentiates it from pemphigus.

pemphi·gus (pem′-fig-us) *n* skin conditions with bullous (blister) eruptions, but more correctly used of a group of dangerous diseases called pemphigus vulgaris, pemphigus vegetans and pemphigus erythematosus. The latter two are rare. *pemphigus neonatorum* (a) a dangerous form of impetigo* occurring as an epidemic in the hospital nursery (b) bullous eruption in congenital syphilis of the newborn. *pemphigus vulgaris* a bullous disease of middle-age and later, of autoimmune etiology. Edema of the skin results in blister formation in the epidermis, with resulting secondary infection and rupture, so that large raw areas develop. Bullae develop also on mucous membranes. Death is from malnutrition or intercurrent disease.

Pen·britin (pen-brit′-in) *n* proprietary name for ampicillin*.

pendu·lous (pen′-dū-lus) *adj* hanging down. *pendulous abdomen* a relaxed condition of the anterior wall, allowing it to hang down over the pubis.

penetrating ulcer (pen′-e-trāt-ing) an ulcer* which is locally invasive and may erode a blood vessel causing hematemesis or melena in the case of gastric or duodenal ulcer respectively.

penetrat·ing wound (pen′-e-trāt-ing) (*syn* puncture wound) caused by a sharp, usually slim object, or a missile, which passes through the skin into the tissues beneath.

penicil·lamine (pen-is-il′-ā-mēn) *n* a degradation product of penicillin* used in the treatment of heavy metal intoxication. Wilson's disease and lead poisoning. It is occasionally useful in rheumatoid arthritis when the symptoms are not relieved by other drugs.

peni·cillin (pen-is-il′-in) *n* the first antibiotic, also known as 'penicillin G' or 'benzyl penicillin'. Widely used by injection in many infections due to Gram-positive bacteria, some cocci and spirochetes. High blood levels are obtained rapidly, and can be supplemented by injections of the slower acting procaine-penicillin or the longer acting benethamine penicillin. The dose of penicillin varies widely according to the severity of infection, the largest being given in bacterial endocarditis (2 000 000 units).

penicillinase (pen-is-il′-in-ās) *n* an enzyme which destroys penicillin*.

Penicil·lium (pen-is-il′-ē-um) *n* a genus of molds. The hyphae bear spores characteristically arranged like a brush. A common contaminant of food. *Penicilllium chrysogenum* is now used for the commercial production of the antibiotic. *Penicillium notatum* is a species shown by Fleming (1928) to produce penicillin.

penis the male organ of copulation (⇒ Figure 16)—**penile** *adj.*

penta·erythritol tetra·nitrate (pen-tà-er-ith′-rit-ol tet-rà-nī′-trāt) a coronary vasodilator in tablet form. (Peritrate.)

penta·gastrin (pen-tà-gas′-trin) *n* a synthetic hormone which has largely replaced histamine as the stimulant of choice for evoking maximal acid secretion in gastric function tests. *pentagastrin test* when injected, pentagastrin causes parietal cells in the stomach to secrete acid to their utmost capacity, expressed as mEq H + in 1 h, for the peak 30 min after injection—PAO (peak acid output).

pent·amidine (pen-tam′-i-dēn) *n* synthetic

compound used in trypanosomiasis, kala-azar and leishmaniasis.

pent·azocine (pen-taz′-ō-sēn) *n* used for the relief of moderate pain. In the presence of bradycardia or hypertension pentazocine is better than morphine*. Can be given orally, intramuscularly, intravenously. (Talwin.)

Pen·thrane (pen′-thrān) *n* methoxyflurane*.

pento·barbital (pen-tō-bar′-bi-tol) *n* one of the short-acting barbiturates*. Often used for premedication in children. (Nembutal.)

pen·tose (pen′-tōs) *n* a class of monosaccharides with five carbon atoms in their molecule.

pento·suria (pen-tō-sū′-rē-à) *n* pentose* in the urine. Can be due to a metabolic disorder—**pentosuric** *adj*.

Pento·thal (pen′-tō-thal) *n* proprietary name for thiopental*.

pepper·mint (pep′-ėr-mint) *n* an aromatic carminative and stimulant. Also used as a flavoring agent.

pep·sin (pep′-sin) *n* a proteolytic enzyme of the gastric juice which hydrolyzes proteins to polypeptides. It has an optimum pH of $1·5-2·0$ and a specificity for peptide bonds involving the aromatic amino acids although other bonds are split.

pepsin·ogen (pep-sin′-ō-jen) *n* a zymogen secreted mainly by the chief cells in the gastric mucosa and converted into pepsin by contact with hydrochloric acid (gastric acid) or pepsin itself.

pep·tic (pep′-tik) *adj* pertaining to pepsin or to digestion generally. *peptic ulcer* a non-malignant ulcer* in those parts of the digestive tract which are exposed to the gastric secretions; hence usually in the stomach or duodenum but sometimes in the lower esophagus or with a Meckel's diverticulum.

pep·tides (pep′-tīdz) *npl* low molecular weight compounds which yield two or more amino acids on hydrolysis; e.g. dipeptides, tripeptides and polypeptides.

pep·tones (pep′-tōnz) *npl* substances produced when a proteolytic enzyme (e.g. pepsin) or an acid acts upon a native protein during the first stage of protein digestion.

pepto·nuria (pep-tōn-ūr′-ē-à) *n* peptones in the urine—**peptonuric** *adj*.

per·cept (pėr′-sept) *n* the mental product of a sensation; a sensation plus memories of similar sensations and their relationships.

percep·tion (pėr-sep′-shun) *n* the reception of a conscious impression through the senses by which we distinguish objects one from another and recognize their qualities according to the different sensations they produce.

Percodan (pėrk′-ō-dan) *n* proprietary name for oxycodone* plus aspirin.

percol·ation (pėr-kō-lā′-shun) *n* the process by which fluid slowly passes through a hard but porous substance.

Per·corten (per-kōr′-ten) *n* proprietary name for desoxycorticosterone*.

per·cussion (pėr-kush′-un) *n* tapping to determine the resonance or dullness of the area examined. Normally a finger of the left hand is laid on the patient's skin and the middle finger of the right hand (plexor) is used to strike the left finger.

percu·taneous (pėr-kū-tā′-nē-us) *adj* through the skin. $\Rightarrow$ cholangiography.

perfor·ation (pėr-fōr-ā′-shun) *n* a hole in an intact sheet of tissue. Used in reference to perforation of the tympanic membrane, or the wall of the stomach or gut, (perforating ulcer*) constituting a surgical emergency.

Pergonal (pėr′-gon-al) *n* proprietary name for menotropins*.

Periactin (pār-ē-ak′-tin) *n* proprietary name for cyproheptadine* hydrochloride.

peri·adenitis (pėr-ē-ad-en-ī′-tis) *n* inflammation in soft tissues surrounding glands. Responsible for the 'bull' neck in rubella.

peri·anal (pėr-ē-ā′-nal) *adj* surrounding the anus.

peri·arterial (pėr-ē-ȧr-tēr′-ē-al) *adj* surrounding an artery.

peri·arteritis (pėr-ē-ȧr-ter-ī′-tis) *n* inflammation of the outer sheath of an artery and the periarterial tissue. *periarteritis nodosa* $\Rightarrow$ polyarteritis.

peri·arthritis (pėr-ē-ȧrth-rī′-tis) *n* inflammation of the structures surrounding a joint. Sometimes applied to frozen* shoulder.

per·articular (pār-ē-ȧr-tik′-ū-lar) *adj* surrounding a joint.

peri·cardectomy (pār-ē-kȧr-dek′-to-mē) *n* surgical removal of the pericardium*, thickened from chronic inflammation (pericarditis) and embarrassing the heart's action.

peri·cardio·centesis (păr-i-kȧr-dē-ō-sen-tē′-sis) *n* aspiration of the pericardial sac.

peri·carditis (păr-i-kȧr-dī′-tis) *n* inflammation of the outer, serous covering of the heart. It may or may not be accompanied by an effusion and formation of adhesions between the two layers. ⇒ Broadbent's sign, pericardectomy.

peri·cardium (păr-i-kȧr-dē-um) *n* the double membranous sac which envelops the heart. The layer in contact with the heart is called 'visceral'; that reflected from the sac is called 'parietal'. Between the two is the pericardial cavity, which normally contains a small amount of serous fluid—**pericardial** *adj*.

peri·chondrium (păr-i-kon′-drē-um) *n* the membranous covering of cartilage—**perichondrial** *adj*.

peri·colic (păr-i-kōl′-ik) *adj* around the colon.

peri·cranium (păr-i-krā′-nē-um) *n* the periosteal covering of the cranium—**pericranial** *adj*.

peri·follicular (păr-i-fol-ik′-ū-lar) *adj* around a follicle.

peri·lymph (păr′-i-limf) *n* the fluid contained in the internal ear, between the bony and membranous labyrinth.

peri·metrium (păr′-i-mē′-trē-um) *n* the peritoneal covering of the uterus—**perimetrial** *adj*.

peri·natal (păr-ē-nā′-tal) *adj* currently used to describe the weeks before a birth, the birth and the succeeding few weeks.

perinatology (păr-ē-nă-tol′-o-jē) *n* the medical specialty which includes the time before, during and immediately after the birth of an infant.

perine·ometer (păr-in-ē-om′-e-tėr) *n* a pressure gauge inserted into the vagina to register the strength of contraction in the pelvic floor muscles.

perineor·raphy (păr-in-ē-ȯr′-af-ē) *n* an operation for the repair of a torn perineum.

peri·neotomy (păr-in-ē-ot′-o-mē) *n* episiotomy*.

peri·nephric (păr-i-nef′-rik) *adj* surrounding the kidney.

peri·neum (păr-in-ē′-um) *n* the portion of the body included in the outlet of the pelvis—**perineal** *adj*.

per·iodic breath·ing (pĕr-ē-od′-ik) a period of apnea in a newborn baby of 5–10 seconds followed by a period of hyperventilation at a rate of 50–60 breaths a minute, for a period of 10–15 seconds. The overall respiratory rate remains between 30 and 40 breaths per minute.

periodontal disease (păr-è-o-don′-tal dis-ēz′) commonly an inflammatory disease of the periodontal tissues resulting in the gradual loss of the supporting membrane and bone around the root of the tooth and a deepened gingival sulcus* or periodontal pocket. ⇒ pyorrhea.

peri·onychia (păr-i-on-ik′-ē-à) *n* red and painful swelling around nail fold. Common in hands that are much in water or have poor circulation. Due to infection from the fungus *Candida*. More common now because of the use of antibiotics which subdue organisms that previously curtailed the activity of *Candida*. Secondary infection can occur.

peri·operative (păr-i-op′-ėr-à-tiv) *adj* refers to the period during which a surgical operation is carried out, as well as to the pre- and postoperative periods.

peri·oral (păr-ē-ōr′-al) *adj* around the mouth. *perioral dermatitis* a red scaly or papular eruption around the mouth. Common in young adult females. Thought to be due to the use of corticosteroids* on the face.

peri·osteum (păr-ē-os′-te-um) *n* the membrane which covers a bone. In long bones only the shaft as far as the epiphysis is covered. It is protective and essential for regeneration—**periosteal** *adj*.

peri·ostitis (păr-ē-os-tī′-tis) *n* inflammation of the periosteum*. *diffuse periostitis* that involving the periosteum of long bones. *hemorrhagic periostitis* that accompanied by bleeding between the periosteum and the bone.

periostosis (per-ē-os-tō′-sis) *n* inflammatory hypertrophy of bone.

peri·partum (păr-ē-păr′-tum) *n* at the time of delivery. A precise word for what is more commonly called perinatal.

periph·eral (per-if′-ėr-al) *adj* pertaining to the outer parts of an organ or of the body. *peripheral nervous system* a term usually reserved for those nerves which supply the musculoskeletal system and surrounding tissues to differentiate from the autonomic nervous* system. *peripheral resistance* the force exerted by the arteriolar walls which is an important factor in the control of normal blood pressure. *peripheral vascular disease (PVD)* any abnormal condition arising in the blood vessels outside the heart, the main one being atherosclerosis*, which can lead to thrombosis and occlusion of the vessel resulting in gangrene. *peripheral vision* that surrounding the central field of vision.

peri·portal (păr-ē-pōr′-tal) *adj* surrounding the portal vein.

peri·proctitis (păr-ē-prok-tī′-tis) *n* inflammation around the rectum and anus.

peri·renal (păr-ē-rē′-nal) *adj* around the kidney.

peri·splenitis (păr-ē-splen-ī′-tis) *n* inflammation of the peritoneal coat of the spleen and of the adjacent structures.

peri·stalsis (păr-i-stal′-sis) *n* the characteristic movement of the intestines by which the contents are moved along the lumen. It consists of a wave of contraction preceded by a wave of relaxation—**peristaltic** *adj*.

per·itomy (păr-it′-o-mē) *n* excision of a portion of conjunctiva at the edge of the cornea to prevent vascularization of a corneal ulcer.

peri·toneal dial·ysis (păr-it-on-ē′-al dī-al′-is-is) ⇒ dialysis.

peritone·oscopy (păr-it-on-ē-os′-kop-ē) ⇒ laparoscopy.

perito·neum (păr-it-on-ē′-um) *n* the delicate serous membrane which lines the abdominal and pelvic cavities and also covers the organs contained in them—**peritoneal** *adj*.

periton·itis (păr-it-on-ī′-tis) *n* inflammation of the peritoneum, usually secondary to disease of one of the abdominal organs.

peri·tonsillar abscess (quinsy) (păr-ē-ton′-sil-ar) acute inflammation of the tonsil and surrounding loose tissue, with abscess formation.

Peritrate (păr′-i-trat) *n* proprietary name for pentaerythritol* tetranitrate.

peri·trichous (păr-i-trī′-kus) *adj* applied to a bacteria which possess flagella on all sides of the cell. ⇒ Bacillus.

peri·umbilical (păr-ē-um-bil′-i-kal) *adj* surrounding the umbilicus.

peri·urethral (păr-ē-ūr-ē′-thral) *adj* surrounding the urethra, as a periurethral abscess.

peri·vascular (păr-ē-vas′-kū-lar) *adj* around a blood vessel.

perleche (pėr-lesh′) *n* lip licking. An intertrigo* at the angles of the mouth with maceration, fissuring, or crust formation. May result from use of poorly fitting dentures, bacterial infection, thrush infestation, vitamin deficiency, drooling or thumbsucking.

per·meable (pėr′-mē-a-bl) *adj* pervious; permitting passage of a substance.

per·meability (pėr-mē-à-bil′-it-ē) *n* in physiology, the extent to which substances dissolved in the body fluids are able to pass through the membranes of cells or layers of cells (e.g. the walls of capillary blood vessels, or secretory or absorptive tissues).

Permitil (per′-mit-il) *n* proprietary name for fluphenazine.*

pernic·ious (pėr-nish′-us) *adj* deadly, noxius.

pernic·ious ane·mia (pėr-nish′-us a-nē′-mē-a) ⇒ anemia.

perni·osis (pėr-nē-ōs′-is) *n* chronic chilblains. The smaller arteioles go into spasm readily from exposure to cold.

pero·melia (per-ō-mē′-lē-à) *n* a teratogenic malformation of a limb.

per·oneal nerve (păr-on-ē′-al) ⇒ Figure 11.

per·oneus muscles (păr-on-ē′-us) ⇒ Figures 4, 5.

per·oral (per-ōr′-al) *adj* through the mouth, as biopsy of the small bowel.

per·oxide (per-oks′-īd) hydrogen* peroxide.

per·phenazine (per-fen′-à-zēn) *n* a tranquilizing and antiemetic agent.

Per·santine (per-san′-tēn) proprietary name for dipyridamole.*

persever·ation (pėr-sev-ėr-ā′-shun) *n* constant repetition of a meaningless word or phrase.

person·ality (pėr-son-al′-it-ē) *n* the various mental attitudes and characteristics which distinguish a person. The sum total of the mental make-up. ⇒ psychopathic personality.

perspir·ation (pėrs-pėr-ā′-shun) *n* the excretion from the sweat glands through the skin pores. *insensible perspiration* (*syn* percutaneous water loss) that water which is lost by evaporation through the skin surface other than by sweating. It is greatly increased in inflammed skin. *sensible perspiration* the term used when there are visible drops of sweat on the skin.

Perthes' dis·ease (pėr′-tēz) (*syn* pseudocoxalgia) avascular degeneration of the upper femoral epiphysis; revascularization occurs, but residual deformity of the femoral head may subsequently lead to arthritic changes.

217

Per·tofrane (per'-tō-frān) *n* proprietary name for despiramine*.

per·tussis (pėr-tus'-sis) *n* (*syn* whooping cough) an infectious disease of children with attacks of coughing which reach a peak of violence ending in an inspiratory whoop. The basis of the condition is respiratory catarrh and the organism responsible is *Bordetella* pertussis. Prophylactic vaccination is responsible for a decrease in case incidence.

pes (pes)*n* a foot or foot-like structure. *pes cavus* ⇒ claw-foot. *pes planus* ⇒ flat-foot.

pess·ary (pes'-sar-ē) *n* 1 an instrument inserted into the vagina to correct uterine displacements. A *ring* or *shelf pressary* is used to support a prolapse. A *hodge pessary* is used to correct a retroversion. 2 a medicated suppository used to treat vaginal infections, or as a contraceptive.

pest·cides (pes'-ti-sīdz) *npl* substances which kill pests.

pet·echia (pe-tē'-kē-à) *n* a small, hemorrhagic spot—**petechiae** *pl*, **petechial** *adj*.

pethi·dine (peth'-i-din) *n* internationally used name for meperidine hydrochloride, a synthetic analgesic and spasmolytic. Widely used for both preoperative and postoperative analgesia instead of morphine*. Can be given orally or intramuscularly. Intravenous injection requires care, as it may cause a fall in blood pressure.

petit mal (pe'-tē mal) minor epilepsy. ⇒ epilepsy.

petris·sage (pa-tri-sahzh) *n* kneading; the part, usually an identified muscle or tendon, is picked up between the thumb and index finger and kneading movements with firm pressure are carried out in a centripetal direction.

pet·rous (pet'-rus) *adj* resembling stone.

Peyer's patches (pī'ėrz) flat patches of lymphatic tissue situated in the small intestine but mainly in the ileum; they are the seat of infection in typhoid fever; also known as 'aggregated lymph nodules'.

peyote (pā-ō'-tē) *n* mescaline*.

Peyronie's dis·ease (pay-ron-ēz') deformity and painful erection of penis due to fibrous tissue formation unknown cause. Often associated with Dupuytren's* contracture.

pH *abbr* the concentration of hydrogen ions expressed as a negative logarithm. A neutral solution has a pH 7.0. With increasing acidity the pH falls and with increasing alkalinity it rises.

phaco·emulsifi·cation ((fāk'-ō-ē-muls-if-i-kā'-shun) *n* ultrasonic vibration is used to liquefy mature lens fibers. The liquid lens matter is then sucked out in an action similar to that of a vacuum cleaner.

phago·cyte (fag'-ō-sīt) *n* a cell capable of engulfing bacteria and other particulate material—**phagocytic** *adj*.

phago·cytosis (fag-ō-sī-tō'-sis) *n* the engulfment by phagocytes of bacteria or other particles.

phal·anges (fal-an'-jēz) *n* the small bones of the fingers and toes (⇒ Figure 2, 3)—**phalanx** *sing*, **phalangeal** *adj*.

phal·lus (fal'-us) *n* the penis*—**phallic** *adj*.

phan·tasy (fan'-tà-sē) *n* ⇒ fantasy.

phan·tom limb (fan'-tom) the sensation that a limb is still attached to the body after it has been amputated. Pain may seem to come from the amputated limb.

phan·tom preg·nancy (fan'-tom preg'-nans-ē) (*syn* pseudocyesis) signs and symptoms simulating those of early pregnancy; it occurs in a childless person who has an overwhelming desire to have a child.

pharma·ceutical (fàr-mà-sōō'-ti-kal) *adj* relating to drugs. *pharmaceutical name* ⇒ proprietary name.

pharmacist (fàr'-mà-sist) *n* a druggist; person who dispenses drugs.

pharmaco·kinetics (fàr-mà-kō-kin-et'-iks) *n* the study of the way in which drugs are absorbed, distributed and excreted from the body. It increases knowledge of drug concentrations in different parts of the body at different times throughout each 24 hours.

pharma·cology (fàr-mà-kol'-o-jē) *n* the science dealing with drugs—**pharmacological** *adj*, **pharmacologically** *adv*.

phar·yngeal pouch (fàr-in-jē'-al) pathological dilatation of the lower part of the pharynx.

pharyn·gectomy (fàr-in-jek'-to-mē) *n* surgical removal of part of the pharynx.

pharyn·gismus (fàr-in-jis'-mus) *n* spasm of the pharynx.

pharyn·gitis (fàr-in-jī'-tis) *n* inflammation of the pharynx*.

pharyngo·laryngeal ((fàr-ing'-gō-làr-in-jē'-al) *adj* pertaining to the pharynx* and larynx*.

pharyngo·laryngectomy (fàr-ing'-gō-làr-in-jek'-to-mē) *n* surgical removal of the pharynx and larynx.

pharyngo·plasty (fār-ing'-gō-plas-tē) *n* any plastic operation to the pharynx.

pharyn·gotomy (fār-ing-got'-o-mē) *n* the operation of opening into the pharynx.

pharyngo-tympanic tube (fār-ing'-gō-tim-pan'-ik) ⇒ eustachian tube.

phar·ynx (fār'-ingks) *n* the cavity at the back of the mouth (⇒ Figures 6, 14). It is cone shaped, vanes in length (average 75 mm), and is lined with mucous membrane; at the lower end it opens into the esophagus*. The eustachian tubes pierce its lateral walls and the posterior nares pierce its anterior wall. The larynx lies immediately below it and in front of the esophagus—**pharyngeal** *adj*.

PHC *abbr* primary* health care.

phen·acetin (fen-ȧ-sē'-tin) *n* an analgesic. Prolonged use has caused kidney damge leading to necrosis and eventual renal* failure.

phenazo·pyridine hydro·chloride (fen-ȧ-zō-pī'-ri-dēn) a urinary tract sedative, especially useful in cystitis. (Pyridium.)

phenel·zine (fen'-el-zēn) *n* an antidepressant drug; a monoamine oxide inhibitor. (Nardil.)

Phener·gan (fen'-ēr-gan) *n* proprietary name for promethazine*.

pheneth·icillin (fen-eth'-is-il'-in) *n* a drug which is acid stable and can be given by mouth. Alternative to penicillin* but contraindicated in penicillin sensitivity. (Syncillin.)

phenmetrazine (fen-met'-rȧ-zēn) *n* appetite depressant; danger of addiction and psychosis of a paranoid nature. (Preludin.)

pheno·barbital (fēn-ō-barb'-it-al) *n* long-acting barbiturate and anticonvulsant. Used as a general sedative, and in epilepsy. (Luminal.)

phen·ol (fē'-nol) *n* (*syn* carbolic acid) the first disinfectant which paved the way to the current era of aseptic surgery. It has been replaced for most purposes by more active and less toxic compounds. It is still used in calamine lotion for its local anesthetic effect in relieving itching.

phe·nolic dis·infectants (fē-nol'-ik) the constituent phenols may cause jaundice; they are absorbed from the skin and lungs.

phenol·phthalein (fē-nol-thal'-ē-in) *n* a powerful non-toxic purgative, often given with liquid paraffin*.

pheno·thiazines (fē-nō-thī'-ȧ-zēnes) *npl*

powerful tranquilizing drugs, represented by chlorpromazine*.

phenotype (fēn'-ō-tīp) *n* the physical characteristics of an organism, based on the interplay between its genetic makeup (genotype) and environment.

phenoxy·benzamine (fē-noks-i-ben'-zȧ-mēn) *n* a peripheral vasodilator used in Raynaud's disease, as an antihypertensive agent and in the symptomatic relief of benign prostatic hypertrophy. (Dibenzyline.)

phenoxy·methyl·penicillin (fen-oks'-i-meth-l-pen-i-sil'-in) *n* an oral penicillin*.

phensuximide (fen-suks'-i-mīd) *n* an anticonvulsant used in treating petit mal seizures. (Mitontin.)

phenter·mine (fen'-tèr-mēn) *n* an appetite suppressant. (Ionamin.)

phen·tolamine (fen-tol'-ȧ-mēn) *n* an adrenaline antagonist, used mainly by injection in the diagnosis and surgery of pheochromocytoma, to control excessive variation of blood pressure. Occasionally used orally in vasospasm. (Regitine, Rogitine.)

phenyl·alanine (fen-l-al'-ȧ-nēn) *n* an essential amino* acid. Those unable to metabolize it develop phenylketonuria*.

phenyl·butazone (fen-l-bū'-tȧ-zōn) *n* an analgesic with powerful and prolonged action. Toxic effects are common and the drug is now used only in hospital for ankylosing spondylitis. (Butazolidin.)

phenyl·ephrine *n* a vasoconstrictor and pressor drug similar to epinephrine*, but more stable. Can be given intramuscularly or subcutaneously. Used mainly as eyedrops (0.5–10%) and as nasal spray (0.25%).

phenyl·ketonuria (PKU) (fen-l-kē-tō-nū'-rē-ȧ) *n* metabolites of phenylalanine* (the best known being the phenylketones) in urine. Occurs in hyperphenylalaninemia, owing to the lack of inactivity of the phenylalanine hydroxylase enzyme in the liver which converts dietary phenylalanine into tyrosine*. Autosomal recessive disease, resulting in mental subnormality unless discovered by screening and treated with an appropriate diet from birth—**phenylketonuric** *adj*.

phenyl·pyruvic oligo·phrenia (fen-l-pī-rōō'-vik ol-ig-ō-frē'-nē-a) ⇒ phenylketonuria.

pheny·toin (fen-i-tō'-in) *n* an anticonvulsant used in major epilepsy, sometimes in association with phenobarbital*. (Dilantin.)

pheochromocytoma (fē-ō-krō-mō-sī-tō'-ma) *n* (*syn* paraganglioma) a condition in which there is a tumor of the adrenal medulla, or of the structurally similar tissues associated with the sympathetic chain. It secretes adrenaline and allied hormones and the symptoms are due to the excess of these substances. Etiology unknown. ⇒ Rogitine test.

phi·mosis (fī-mō'-sis) *n* tightness of the prepuce so that it cannot be retracted over the glans penis.

pHiso·Hex (fī'-sō-heks) *n* an antiseptic and antibacterial skin cleansing agent combining a detergent—Entsufon. 3% hexachlorophene, lanolin, cholesterols and petrolatum, in an emulsion with the same pH as skin.

phleb·ectomy (fleb-ek'-to-mē) *n* excision of a vein. *multiple cosmetic phlebectomy (MCP)* removal of varicose veins through little stab incisions which heal without scarring.

phleb·itis (fleb-ī'-tis) *n* inflammation of a vein—phlebitic *adj*.

phleb·ography (fleb-og'-raf-ē) ⇒ venography.

phlebo·lith (fleb'-ō-lith) *n* a concretion which forms in a vein.

phlebo·thrombosis (fle-bō-throm-bō'-sis) *n* thrombosis in a vein due to sluggish flow of blood rather than to inflammation in the vein wall, occurring chiefly in bedridden patients and affecting the deep veins of the lower limbs or pelvis. The loosely attached thrombus is liable to break off and lodge in the lungs as an embolus.

phleboto·mist (fle-bo'-to-mist) *n* a technician who is trained to carry out phlebotomy.

phleb·otomy (fle-bo'-to-mē) *n* ⇒ venesection.

phlegm (flem) *n* the secretion of mucus expectorated from the bronchi.

phleg·matic (fleg-mat'-ik) *adj* describes an emotionally stable person.

phlyc·tenule (flik-ten'-ūl) *n* a minute blister (vesicle) usually occurring on the conjunctiva or cornea—phlyctenular *adj*.

pho·bia (fō'-bē-à) *n* morbid fear, e.g. cardiac phobia (fear of heart disease), cancer phobia etc—phobic *adj*.

phoco·melia (fō-kō-mē'-lē-à) *n* teratogenic malformation. Arms and feet attached directly to trunk giving a seal-like appearance. An epidemic in the 1960s was caused by pregnant women taking the sedative drug thalidomide.

phon·ation (fō-nā'-shun) *n* the production of voice by vibration of the vocal cords.

phono·cardiography (fō-nō-kàr-dē-og'-raf-ē) *n* the graphic recording of heart sounds and murmurs by electric reproduction. The fetal heart rate and its relation to uterine contraction can be measured continuously—**phonocardiographic** *adj*, **phonocardiogram** *n*, **phonocardiograph** *n*, **phonocardiographically** *adv*.

phos·phaturia (fos-fa-tū'-rē-à) *n* excess of phosphates in the urine—phosphaturic *adj*.

phos·pholine iodide (fos'-fō-lēn-ī'-ō-dīd) an anticholinesterase drug; a powerful miotic.

phospho·lipase D (fos-fō-lī'-pās dē) *n* ⇒ lecithinase.

phospho·nates (fos'-fō-nāts) *npl* when deposited in bone makes it harder for osteoclasts to reabsorb that bone. Being tried medicinally for Paget's disease.

phospho·necrosis (fos-fō-nek-rō'-sis) *n* 'fossy-jaw' occurring in workers engaged in the manufacture of matches made with white phosphorus; necrosis of the jaw with loosening of the teeth.

phos·phorus (fos'-fōr-us) *n* a non-metallic element forming an important constituent of bone and nerve tissue. *radioactive phosphorus* (^{32}P) is used in the treatment of thrombocythemia.

phosphoryl·ation (fos'-for-il-ā'-shun) *n* the metabolic process of introducing a phosphatic group into an organic molecule.

phot·algia (fō-tal'-jē-à) *n* pain in the eyes from exposure to intense light.

photo·chemical (fō-tō-kem'-i-kal) *adj* chemically reactive in the presence of light.

photo·chemotherapy (fō-tō-kē-mō-thèr'-à-pē) *n* the effect of the administered drug is enhanced by exposing the patient to ultraviolet light.

photo·coagulation (fō-tō-kō-ag'-ū-lā'-shun) *n* burning of the tissues with a powerful, focused light source.

photo·endoscope (fō-tō-en'-dō-skōp) *n* an endoscope to which a camera is attached for the purpose of making a permanent record—**photoendoscopic** *adj*, **photoendoscopy** *n*, **photoendoscopically** *adv*.

photo·phobia (fō-tō-fō'-bē-à) *n* inability to expose the eyes to light—photophobic *adj*.

photo·sensitive (fō-tō-sens'-it-iv) *adj* sensitive to light, as the pigments in the eye.

photo·therapy (fō-tō-thėr'-à-pē) *n* exposure to artificial blue light. In hyperbilirubinemia it appears to dehydrogenate the bilirubin to biliverdin. Used for mild neonatal jaundice and to prevent jaundice in premature infants.

phren (fren) *n* the diaphragm—**phrenic** adj.

phreni·cotomy (fren-i-kot'-o-mē) *n* division of the phrenic nerve to paralyze one-half of the diaphragm.

phreno·plegia (fren-ō-plē'-jē-à) *n* paralysis of the diaphragm—**phrenoplegic** *adj*.

phreno·tropic (fren-ō-trō'-pik) *adj* having an effect upon the mind, usually used to describe certain drugs.

phthalyl·sulfa·thiazole (thā-lil-sul-fa-thī'-à-zol) *n* a sulfonamide* poorly absorbed from the alimentary tract. Formerly used in intestinal infections and before abdominal surgery.

phthi·sis (thī'-sis) *n* an old term for pulmonary tuberculosis*.

physi·cal abuse (fiz'-i-kal a-būs') ⇒ battering, battered baby syndrome.

physician (fi-zish'-un) *n* a person licensed as a medical doctor.

Physician's Desk Reference (PDR, *abbr*) a yearly publication of current drugs, with descriptions and information on their usage.

physico·chemical (fiz-i-kō-kem'-i-kal) *adj* pertaining to physics and chemistry.

physio·logical (fiz-ē-ō-loj'-i-kal) *adj* in accordance with natural processes of the body. Adjective often used to describe a normal process or structure, to distinguish it from an abnormal or pathological feature (e.g. the physiological level of glucose in the blood is from 3.0–5.0 mmol per liter; higher and lower levels are pathological and indicative of disease). *physiological age* ⇒ biological age. *physiological saline* ⇒ isotonic. *physiological solution* a fluid isotonic* with the body fluids and containing similar salts.

physi·ology (fiz-ē-ol'-o-jē) *n* the science which deals with the normal functions of the body—**physiological** *adj*, **physiologically** *adv*.

physo·stigmine (fī-sō-stig'-mēn) *n* an alkaloid used in glaucoma as drops (0.5–1%) and to reverse the action of atropine*. Occasionally used in paralytic ileus.

phyto·nadione (fī-tō-nà-dī'-ōn) *n* vitamin* K_1. Used mainly in overdose and haemorrhage following synthetic anticoagulants such as warfarin*, and in vitamin K deficiency in the newborn. (Aquamephyton, Konakion.)

pia, pia mater (pē'-à mà'-tėr) the innermost of the meninges; the vascular membrane which lies in close contact with the substance of the brain and spinal cord.

pica (pī'-kà) *n* a desire for extraordinary articles of food, a feature of some pregnancies.

Pick's disease (piks) **1** syndrome of ascites, hepatic enlargement, edema and pleural effusion occurring in constrictive pericarditis. **2** a type of cerebral atrophy which produces mental changes similar to presenile dementia*.

picornavirus (pī-kōr-nà-vī'-rus) *n* from pico (very small) and RNA (ribonucleic acid). Small RNA viruses. The group includes polio, coxsackie, echo and rhinoviruses. ⇒ virus.

PID *abbr* pelvic inflammatory disease.

pigeon chest (pij'-un) (*syn* pectus carinatum) a narrow chest, bulging anteriorly in the breast bone region.

pig·ment (pig'-ment) *n* any coloring matter of the body.

pigmen·tation (pig-ment-ā'-shun) *n* the deposit of pigment, especially when abnormal or excessive.

piles *n* ⇒ hemorrhoids.

pilo·carpine (pī-lō-kàr'-pēn) *n* an alkaloid used in a 0.5–1% solution as a miotic in glaucoma. Stimulates the salivary glands and is occasionally used in high dose atropine* therapy. *pilocarpine iontophoresis* introduction of pilocarpine ions into the tissues through the skin by means of electricity. Used as a test for those suspected of having cystic fibrosis.

pilo·motor nerves (pī-lō-mō'-tor) tiny nerves attached to the hair follicle; innervation causes the hair to stand upright and give the appearance of 'goose flesh'.

pilo·nidal (pī-lō-nī'-dal) *adj* hair-containing. *pilonidal sinus* a sinus containing hairs which is usually found in hirsute people in the cleft between the buttocks. In this situation it is liable to infection.

pilo·sebaceous (pī-lō-se-bā'-shus) *adj* pertaining to the hair follicle and the sebaceous gland opening into it.

pilosis (pī-lō'-sis) *n* an abnormal growth of hair.

221

pimo·zide (pī'-mō-zīd) *n* a long-acting neuroleptic and powerful antischizophrenic drug. Often considered a first-choice drug for apathetic patients. (Orap.)

pim·ple (pim'-pl) *n* ⇒ papule.

pin·eal body (pin'-ē-al bod'-ē) a small reddish-grey conical structure on the dorsal surface of the midbrain (⇒ Figure 1). Its functions are not fully understood but there is some evidence that it secretes melatonin* which appears to inhibit secretion of the luteinizing hormone.

pin·guecula (pin-gwek'-ū-là) *n* a yellowish, slightly elevated thickening of the bulbar conjunctiva near the lid aperture. Associated with the ageing eye.

pink dis·ease ⇒ erythredema polyneuritis.

pink·eye *n* a popular name for acute contagious conjunctivitis, which spreads rapidly in closed communities such as day care centers and institutions where children mix facecloths.

pinna (pin'-à) *n* that part of the ear which is external to the head; the auricle (⇒ Figure 13).

pinta (pin'tà) *n* color changes in patches of skin due to *Treponema pinta*, identical with the spirochete of syphilis* and yaws*.

piper·acillin sodium (pī-pèr-à-sil'-in sō'-dē-um) an antibiotic with wide activity, low toxicity and high stability with less bacterial resistance. It is inactive orally. (Pipracil.)

piper·azine citrate (pī-per'-a-zēn sī'-trāt) *n* a highly effective anthelmintic against threadworms and roundworms. Piperazine therapy can be followed by incidents of unsteadiness and falling— 'worm wobble'. (Pipril.)

Pipracil (pī'-prà-sil) *n* proprietary name for piperacillin sodium*.

Pip·ril proprietary name for piperazine citrate*.

piri·formis muscle (pir'-i-fôrm-is) ⇒ Figure 5.

piroxi·cam (pir-oks'-i-kam) *n* a non-steroidal anti-inflammatory agent. (Feldene.)

Pitocin (pit-ō'-sin) *n* synthetic oxytocin*.

Pitres·sin (pi-tres'-in) *n* a synthetic preparation of vasopressin*.

pit·ting (pit'-ing) *n* **1** making an indentation in edematous tissue. **2** depressed scars left on the skin, especially after smallpox.

pitu·itary gland (pit-ū'-it-rār'-ē) (*syn* hypophysis cerebri) a small oval endocrine gland lying in the pituitary fossa of the sphenoid bone (⇒ Figure 5). The anterior lobe secretes several hormones: growth hormone, corticotrophin, thyrotrophin, luteotrophin, follicle stimulating hormone and prolactin. It is under the control of the hypothalamus*. The overall function of pituitary hormones is to regulate growth and metabolism.

Pituitrin (pit-$\overline{oo}$'-it-rin) *n* proprietary name for extract of the posterior pituitary.

pity·riasis (pit-i-rī'-à-sis) *n* scaly (branny) eruption of the skin. *pityriasis alba* a common eruption in children characterized by scaly hypopigmented macules on the cheeks and upper arms. *pityriasis capitis* dandruff. *pityriasis rosea* a slightly scaly eruption of ovoid erythematous lesions which are widespread over the trunk and proximal parts of the limbs. There may be mild itching. It is a self-limiting condition. *pityriasis rubra pilaris* a chronic skin disease characterized by tiny red papules of perifolicular distribution. *pityriasis versicolor* called also 'tinea versicolor', is a yeast infection which causes the appearance of buff-colored patches on the chest.

Pityro·sporum (pit-ē-ō-spōr'-um) *n* genus of yeasts. *P. orbiculare (Malassezia furfur)* is associated with pityriasis versicolor.

PKU *abbr* phenylketonuria*.

pla·cebo (plà-sē'-bō) *n* a harmless substance given as medicine. In experimental research an inert substance, identical in appearance with the material being tested. Neither the physician nor the patient knows which is which.

pla·centa (plà-sen'-tà) *n* the afterbirth, a vascular structure developed about the third month of pregnancy and attached to the inner wall of the uterus. Through it the fetus is supplied with nourishment and oxygen and through it the fetus gets rid of its waste products. In normal labor it is expelled within an hour of the birth of the child. When this does not occur it is termed a *retained placenta* and may be an *adherrent placenta*. The placenta is usually attached to the upper segment of the uterus; where it lies in the lower uterine segment it is called a *placenta previa* and usually causes placental* abruption—**placental** *adj*.

placen·tal abrup·tion (plà-sent'-al abrup'-shun) (*syn* antepartum hemorrhage) premature separation of the placenta from the uterine wall, accompanied by severe abdominal pain, rigid abdomen, and hemorrhage.

placen·tal insuf·ficiency (plà-sent'-al in-suf-ish'-ens-ē) inefficiency of the placenta. Can occur due to maternal disease or postmaturity of fetus giving rise to a 'small for dates' baby.

placen·tography (plà-sent-og'-raf-ē) n X-ray examination of the placenta after injection of opaque substance.

plague (plāg) n very contagious epidemic disease caused by *Yersinia pseudotuberculosis syn pestis,* and spread by infected rats. Transfer of infection from rat to man is through the agency of fleas. The main clinical types are bubonic, septicemic or pneumonic.

plan·tar (plan'-tar) *adj* pertaining to the sole of the foot. *plantar arch* the union of the plantar and dorsalis pedis arteries in the sole of the foot. *plantar flexion* downward movement of the big toe.

plan·taris muscle (plant-ār'-is) ⇒ Figure 5.

plaque (plak) n ⇒ dental plaque.

Pla·quenil (pla'-kwe-nil) n proprietary name for hydroxychloroquine*. ⇒ chloroquine.

plasma (plaz'-mà) n the fluid fraction of blood. *blood plasma* is used for infusion in cases of hemoconcentration of the patient's blood, as in severe burns. *dried plasma* is in the form of a yellow powder which must be 'reconstituted' before being used for infusion. Various plasma substitutes are available, e.g. Dextran, Plasmosan. *plasma cell* a normal cell with an eccentric nucleus produced in the bone marrow and reticuloendothelial system and concerned with the production of antibodies; abnormally produced in myelomatosis.

plasma·pheresis (plaz-mà-fèr-ēs'-is) n taking blood from a donor, removing some desired fraction then returning the red cells and repeating the whole process. It can be used in the treatment of some diseases which are caused by antibodies or immune complexes circulating in the patient's plasma. Removing the plasma and replacing it with human plasma protein fraction (PPF) or a plasma* substitute can improve the prognosis of the disease and prevent or delay the onset of renal failure.

plas·min (plaz'-min) n a fibrinolysin*.

plasmin·ogen (plaz-min'-ō-jen) n precursor of plasmin*. Release of activators from damaged tissue promotes the conversion of plasminogen into plasmin.

Plas·modium (plaz-mō'-dē-um) n a genus of protozoa. Parasites in the blood of warm-blooded animals which complete their sexual cycle in blood-sucking arthropods. Four species cause malaria* in man—**plasmodial** *adj.*

plaster of Paris (plas'ter) ⇒ gypsum.

plas·tic (plas'-tik) *adj* capable of taking a form or mold. *plastic surgery* transfer of healthy tissue to repair damaged area and to restore and create form.

plate·let (plāt'-let) n ⇒ thrombocyte. *platelet stickiness test* the stickiness of platelets is increased in multiple sclerosis and rapidly growing tumors. May be consequent on degradation of neural tissue, as it is rich in phospholipid, fractions of which have been shown to be potent aggregators of platelets in a suspension.

platy·helminth (plat-i-hel'-minth) n flat worm; fluke. ⇒ schistosomiasis.

platypelloid (plat'-i-pel-oyd) *adj* having a broad pelvis.

platysma muscle (plat-iz'-ma) ⇒ Figure 4.

play ther·apist a person who uses play constructively to help children to come to terms with emotional and/or physical trauma.

pleo·morphism (plē-ō-mōr'-fizm) n denotes a wide range in shape and size of individuals in a bacterial population—**pleomorphic** *adj.*

pleth·ora (ple'-thō-rà) n fullness; overloading—**plethoric** *adj.*

plethys·mograph (ple-this'-mō-graf) n an instrument which measures accurately the blood flow in a limb—**plethysmographic** *adj.*

pleura (ploo'-rà) n the serous membrane covering the surface of the lung (visceral pleura), the diaphragm, the mediastinum and the chest wall (parietal pleura)—**pleural** *adj.*

pleur·isy pleuritis (ploo'-ri-sē, ploo-rī'-tis) n inflammation of the pleura*. May be fibrinous (dry), be associated with an effusion (wet), or be complicated by empyema—**pleuritic** *adj.*

pleuro·desis (ploo-rō-dē'-sis) n adherence of the visceral to the parietal pleura. Can be achieved therapeutically by using iodized talc.

pleuro·dynia (ploo-rō-dī'-nē-à) n intercostal myalgia or muscular rheumatism (fibrositis). It is a feature of Bornholm disease.

pleuro·pulmonary (plōō-rō-pul'-mon-ār-ē) *adj* pertaining to the pleura and lung.

pleurothotonus (plū-rō-thot-ō'-nus) *n* a muscle spasm in which the body is curved to one side.

plexus (pleks'-us) *n* a network of vessels or nerves (⇒ Figure 11).

pli·cation (pli-kā'-shun) *n* a surgical procedure of making tucks or folds to decrease the size of an organ—**plica** *sing*, **plicae** *pl*, **plicate** *adj*, *vt*.

plom·bage (plom-bazh') *n* extrapleural compression of a tuberculous lung cavity.

plum·bism (plum'-bizm) *n* ⇒ lead poisoning.

plum·bum (plum'-bum) *n* the Latin name for the metal lead.

Plummer-Vinson syn·drome (plum'-er-vin'-son) (*syn* Kelly-Paterson syndrome) a combination of severe glossitis with dysphagia and nutritional iron deficiency anemia. Iron taken orally usually leads to complete recovery.

pluri·glandular (plū-ri-glan'-dū-lar) *adj* pertaining to several glands, as mucoviscidosis.

PMS *abbr* premenstrual* syndrome.

pneumatic (nū-mat'-ik) *adj* referring to air or gas; relating to respiration.

pneuma·turia (nū-mà-tū'-rē-à) *n* the passage of flatus with urine, usually as a result of vesico-colic (bladder-bowel) fistula.

pneumo·coccus (nū-mō-kok'-us) *n* *Strept. pneumoniae,* a coccal bacterium arranged characteristically in pairs. A common cause of lobar pneumonia and other infections—**pneumococcal** *adj*.

pneumo·coniosis (nū-mō-kon-ī'-à-sis) *n* (*syn* dust disease) fibrosis of the lung caused by long continued inhalation of dust in industrial occupations. The most important complication is the occasional superinfection with tuberculosis—**pneumoconioses** *pl*. *rheumatoid pneumoconiosis* fibrosing alveolitis occurring in patients suffering from rheumatoid arthritis. ⇒ anthracosis, asbestosis, byssinosis, siderosis, silicosis.

Pneumo·cystis carinii (nū-mō-sis'-tis kar-ēn'-ī) a microorganism which causes pneumonia. The most usual victims are infants, debilitated and immunosuppressed patients; mortality is high.

pneumo·cytes (nū'-mō-sīts) *npl* special cells which line the alveolar walls in the lungs. Type I are flat. Type II are cuboidal and secrete surfactant.

pneumo·encephalography (nū-mō-en-sef-al-og'-raf-ē) *n* radiographic examination of cerebral ventricles after injection of air by means of a lumbar or cisternal puncture—**pneumoencephalogram** *n*.

pneumo·gastric (nū-mō-gas'-trik) *adj* pertaining to the lungs and stomach. ⇒ vagus.

pneu·molysis (nū-mol'-is-is) *n* separation of the two pleural layers, or the outer pleural layer from the chest wall, to collapse the lung.

pneumo·mycosis (nū-mō-mī-kō'-sis) *n* fungus infection of the lung such as aspergillosis, actinomycosis, candidiasis—**pneumomycotic** *adj*.

pneumon·ectomy (nū-mon-ek'-to-mē) *n* excision of a lung.

pneu·monia (nū-mō'-nē-à) *n* traditionally used for inflammation of the lung; when resulting from allergic reaction it is often referred to as alveolitis; that which is due to physical agents is pneumonitis, the word 'pneumonia' being reserved for invasion by microorganisms.

pneumo·nitis (nū-mon-ī'-tis) *n* inflammation of lung tissue.

pneumo·peritoneum (nū-mō-pèr-it-on-ē'-um) *n* air or gas in the peritoneal cavity. Can be introduced for diagnostic or therapeutic purposes.

pneumo·thorax (nū-mō-thōr'-aks) air or gas in the pleural cavity separating the visceral from the parietal pleura so that lung tissue is compressed. A pneumothorax can be secondary to asthma, carcinoma of bronchus, chronic bronchitis, congenital cysts, emphysema, intermittent positive pressure ventilation, pneumonia, trauma or tuberculosis—**pneumothoraces** *pl*. *artificial pneumothorax* induced in the treatment of pulmonary tuberculosis. *spontaneous pneumothorax* occurs when an overdilated pulmonary air sac ruptures, permitting communication of respiratory passages and pleural cavity. *tension pneumothorax* occurs where a valve-like wound allows air to enter the pleural cavity at each inspiration but not to escape on expiration, thus progressively increasing intrathoracic pressure and constituting an acute medical emergency.

PNI *abbr* psychoneuroimmunology*.

poda·lic ver·sion (pod-al'-ik) ⇒ version.

podiatry (po-dī'-à-trē) *n* diagnosis and treatment of problems of the feet.

podophyllum (pod-of'-il-um) *n* powerful

purgative; a suspension in liquid paraffin is used to remove condylomata.

podopom·pholyx (po-do-pom'-fō-liks) *n* pompholyx* on the feet.

polar·ized light (pō'-lar-īzed) the whole of the visible and infra-red spectrum; currently being used in biostimulation of leg ulcers and chronic wounds to achieve healing.

polio·encephalitis (pō-lē-ō-en-sef-à-lī'-tis) *n* inflammation of the cerebral gray matter—this may or may not include the central nuclei—**polioencephalitic** *adj*.

polio·myelitis (pō-lē-ō-mī-el-ī'-tis) *n* (*syn* infantile paralysis) an epidemic virus infection which attacks the motor neurons of the anterior horns in the brain stem (*bulbar poliomyelitis*) and spinal cord. An attack may or may not lead to paralysis of the lower motor neuron type with loss of muscular power and flaccidity. Vaccination against the disease is desirable. When it occurs within two days of vaccination with any alum-containing prophylactic, the term *provocative paralytic poliomyelitis* is used. ⇒ Sabin vaccine. Salk vaccine.

polio·viruses (pō-lē-ō-vī'-rus-es) *npl* cause poliomyelitis*. ⇒ virus.

Politzer's bag (pol'-it-zèrs) a rubber bag for inflation of the eustachian tube.

pollen·osis (pol-en-ōs'-is) *n* an allergic condition arising from sensitization to pollen.

polliciz·ation (pol-is-īz-ā'-shun) *n* a surgical procedure whereby the index finger is rotated and shortened to produce apposition as a thumb.

pollution (pol-ū'-shun) *n* the condition of defiling or making impure.

Polya oper·ation (pol'-ē-a) partial gastrectomy*.

poly·arteritis (pol-ē-àr-tèr-ī'-tis) *n* inflammation of many arteries. In *polyarteritis nodosa* (*syn* periarteritis nodosa) aneurysmal swellings and thrombosis occur in the affected vessels. Further damage may lead to hemorrhage and the clinical picture presented depends upon the site affected. ⇒ collagen.

poly·arthralgia (pol-ē-àrth-ral'-jē-à) *n* pain in several joints.

poly·arthritis (pol-ē-àrth-rī'-tis) *n* inflammation of several joints at the same time. ⇒ Still's disease.

Polycillin-N (pol-ē-sil'-in) *n* proprietary name for ampicillin*.

poly·cystic (pol-ē-sis'-tik) *adj* composed of many cysts. Polycystic kidney disease comprises a number of separate conditions which may be rapidly or slowly fatal and are often associated with cysts of the liver.

poly·cythemia (pol-ē-sī-thē'-mē-à) *n* increase in the number of circulating red blood cells. This may result from dehydration or be a compensatory phenomenon to increase the oxygen carrying capacity, as in congenital heart disease. *polycythemia vera* (*syn* erythremia) is an idiopathic condition in which the red cell count is very high. The patient complains of headache and lassitude, and there is danger of thrombosis and hemorrhage.

poly·dactyly, polydactylism (pol-ē-dak'-til-ē, pol-ē-dak'-til-izm) *n* having more than the normal number of fingers or toes.

poly·dipsia (pol-ē-dip'-sē-à) *n* excessive thirst.

poly·graph (pol'-ē-graf) *n* instrument which records several variables simultaneously.

poly·hydramnios (pol-ē-hī-dram'-nē-ōs) *n* an excessive amount of amniotic fluid.

poly·morpho·nuclear (pol-ē-mōr-fō-nū'-klē-ar) *adj* having a many-shaped or lobulated nucleus, usually applied to the phagocytic neutrophil leukocytes (granulocytes) which constitute 70% of the total white blood cells.

poly·myalgia rheumatica (pol-ē-mī-al'-jē-à roo-mat'-ik-à) a syndrome occurring in elderly people comprising of a sometimes crippling ache in the shoulders, pelvic girdle muscles and spine, with pronounced morning stiffness and a raised ESR. There is an association with temporal arteritis. Clinically different from rheumatoid arthritis ⇒ arthritis.

poly·myositis (pol-ē-mī-ō-sī'-tis) *n* manifests as muscle weakness, most commonly in middle age. Microscopic examination of muscle reveals inflammatory changes; they respond to corticosteroid drugs. ⇒ dermatomyositis.

polymyxin B (pol-ē-miks'-in bē) an antibiotic occasionally used in Gram-negative infections, particularly those due to *Pseudomonas aeruginosa*. It is usually given by slow intravenous infusion as it causes pain when given intramuscularly. There are topical preparations for ear and eye infections. (Aerosporin.)

poly·neuritis (pol-ē-nū-rī'-tis) *n* multiple neuritis—**polyneuritic** *adj*.

poly·oma (pol-ē-ōm'-à) *n* one of the tumor-producing viruses.

poly·opia (pol-ē-ō'-pē-à) *n* seeing many images of a single object.

polyp, polypus (pol'-ip(-us)) *n* a pedunculated tumor arising from any mucous surface, e.g. cervical, uterine, nasal etc. Usually benign but may become malignant—**polypi** *pl*, **polypous** *adj*.

polyp·ectomy (pol-ip-ek'-to-mē) *n* surgical removal of a polyp.

poly·peptides (pol-ē-pep'-tīds) *npl* proteins which on hydrolysis yield more than two amino acids.

poly·pharmacy (pol-ē-får'-ma-sē) *n* a word used when several oral drugs are prescribed for the same patient. It increases the risk of patient non*-compliance and non*-comprehension.

polyploidy (pol'-ē-ployd-ē) *n* having a multiple of the haploid number of chromosomes.

poly·poid (pol'-ē-poyd) *adj* resembling a polyp(us).

poly·posis (pol-ē-pō'-sis) *n* a condition in which there are numerous polypi in an organ. *polyposis coli* a dominantly-inheritable condition in which polypi occur throughout the large bowel and which can often lead to carcinoma of the colon. Prevention is by removal of polyps.

poly·saccharide (pol-ē-sak'-à-rīd) *n* carbohydrates ($C_6H_{10}O_5$) containing a large number of monosaccharide groups. Starch, inulin, glycogen, dextrin and cellulose are examples.

poly·serositis (pol-ē-sér-os-ī'-tis) *n* inflammation of several serous membranes. A genetic type is called familial Mediterranean fever. ⇒ amyloidosis.

poly·thiazide (pol-ē-thī'-à-zīd) *n* a saluretic diuretic. (Renese.)

poly·uria (pol-ē-ūr'-ē-à) *n* excretion of an excessive amount of urine—**polyuric** *adj*.

pom·pholyx (pom'-fol-iks) *n* vesicular skin eruption on the skin associated with itching or burning. ⇒ cheiropompholyx.

POMR *abbr* problem-oriented medical record.

Pon·deral (pon'-dèr-al) *n* proprietary name for fenfluramine* hydrochloride.

pons (ponz) *n* a bridge; a process of tissue joining two sections of an organ. *pons varolii* the white convex mass of nerve tissue at the base of the brain which serves to connect the various lobes of the brain (⇒ Figure 1)—**pontine** *adj*.

Pon·stel (pon'-stel) *n* proprietary name for mefenamic* acid.

Pontiac fever (pon'-tē-ak) a flu-like illness with little or no pulmonary involvement and no mortality caused by *Legionella* *pneumophilia*.

Pontocaine (pon'-tō-kān) *n* proprietary name for tetracaine*.

popli·teal (pop-li-tē'-al) *adj* pertaining to the popliteus. *popliteal artery* ⇒ Figure 9. *popliteal space* the diamond-shaped depression at the back of the knee joint, bounded by the muscles and containing the popliteal nerve and vessels. *popliteal vein* ⇒ Figure 10.

poplit·eus (pop-li-tē'-us) *n* a muscle in the popliteal space which flexes the leg and aids it in rotating.

poraden·itis (pōr-ad-en-ī'-tis) *n* painful mass of iliac glands, characterized by abscess formation. Occurs in lymphogranuloma* inguinale.

pore (pōr) *n* a minute surface opening. One of the mouths of the ducts (leading from the sweat glands) on the skin surface; they are controlled by fine papillary muscles, contracting and closing in the cold and dilating in the presence of heat.

por·phyria (pōr-fī'-rē-à) *n* an inborn error in porphyrin metabolism, usually hereditary, causing pathological changes in nervous and muscular tissue in some varieties and photosensitivity in others, depending on the level of the metabolic block involved. Excess porphyrins or precursors are found in the urine or stools or both. In some cases attacks are precipitated by certain drugs.

por·phyrins (pōr-fī'-rins) *npl* light-sensitive organic compounds which form the basis of respiratory pigments, including hemoglobin. Naturally occurring porphyrins are uroporphyrin and coproporphyrin* ⇒ porphyria.

porphyrin·uria (pōr-fī-rin-ū'-rē-à) *n* excretion of porphyrins in the urine. Such pigments are produced as a result of an inborn error of metabolism.

porta (pōr'-tà) *n* the depression (hilum) of an organ at which the vessels enter and leave—**portal** *adj*. *porta hepatis* the transverse fissure through which the portal vein, hepatic artery and bile ducts pass on the under surface of the liver.

porta·caval, porto·caval (pōr-tà-kā'-val) *adj* pertaining to the portal vein and inferior vena cava. *portacaval anastomosis* a fistula made between the portal vein and the inferior vena cava with the object of reducing the pressure within the portal vein in cases of cirrhosis of the liver.

porta·hepatitis (pŏr-tà-hep-à-tī'-tis) *n* inflammation around the transverse fissure of the liver.

portal hyper·tension (pŏr'-tal hī-per-ten'-shun) increased pressure in the portal vein. Usually caused by cirrhosis of the liver; results in splenomegaly, with hypersplenism and alimentary bleeding. ⇒ esophageal varices.

portal circu·lation (pŏr'-tal ser-kū-lā'-shun) that of venous blood (collected from the intestines, pancreas, spleen and stomach) to the liver before return to the heart.

portal vein (pŏr'-tal vān) that conveying blood into the liver; it is about 75 mm long and is formed by the union of the superior mesenteric and splenic veins.

port·wine stain a purplish-red birthmark.

pos·ition (po-zish'-un) *n* posture.

pos·itive pres·sure ventilation (poz'-i-tiv presh'-ur) positive pressure inflation of lungs to produce inspiration. Exhaled air, hand bellows or more sophisticated apparatus can be used. Expiration results from elastic recoil of the lung. *intermittent positive pressure ventilation* mechanically applied ventilation of the lungs for controlled ventilation during muscular paralysis as part of general anesthesia or intensive care.

possum (pos'-um) *n* Patient-Operated Selector Mechanism. An apparatus which can be operated by a slight touch, or by suction using the mouth if no other muscle movement is possible. It may transmit messages or be adapted for typing, telephoning and other activities.

post·anesthetic (pōst-an-es-thet'-ik) *adj* after anesthesia.

post·anal (pōst-ān'-al) *adj* behind the anus.

post·coital (pōst-kō'-it-al) *adj* after sexual intercourse. The word describes the 'morning after' contraceptive.

post·concussional syn·drome (pōst-kon-kush'-un-al) the association of headaches, giddiness and a feeling of faintness, which may persist for a considerable time after a head injury.

post·diphtheritic (pōst-dif-thèr-it'-ik) *adj* following an attack of diphtheria. Refers especially to the paralysis of limbs and palate.

post·encephalitic (pōst-en-sef-al-it'-ik) *adj* following encephalitis lethargica. The adjective is commonly used to de-

scribe the syndrome of parkinsonism, which so often results from an attack of this kind of encephalitis.

post·epileptic (pōst-ep-il-ep'-tik) *adj* following on an epileptic seizure. *postepileptic automatism* is a fugue state, following on a fit, when the patient may undertake a course of action, even involving violence, without having any memory of this (amnesia).

post·erior (pōst-ē'-rē-or) *adj* situated at the back. ⇒ anterior *opp. posterior chamber of the eye* the space between the anterior surface of the lens and the posterior surface of the iris. ⇒ aqueous—**posteriorly** *adv.*

post·ganglionic (pōst-gang-lē-on'-ik) *adj* situated after a collection of nerve cells (ganglion) as a postganglionic nerve fiber.

post·gastrectomy syn·drome (pōst-gas-trek'-to-mē) covers two sets of symptoms, those of hypoglycemia when the patient is hungry, and those of a vaso-vagal attack immediately after a meal.

post·hepatic (pōst-hep-at'-ik) *adj* behind the liver.

post·herpetic (pōst-hèr-pet'-ik) *adj* after shingles*.

posth·itis (pōs-thī'-tis) *adj* inflammation of the prepuce*.

posthum·ous (pos'-tū-mus) *adj* occurring after death. *posthumous birth* **1** delivery of a baby by cesarian section after the mother's death. **2** birth occurring after the death of the father.

post·mature (pōst-mà-tūr') *adj* past the expected date of delivery. A baby is postmature when labor is delayed beyond the usual 40 weeks—**postmaturity** *n.*

post·menopausal (pōst-men-ō-pawz'-al) *adj* occurring after the menopause* has been established.

post·mortem (pōst-mŏr'-tem) *adj* after death, usually implying dissection of the body. ⇒ antemorten *opp,* autopsy. *postmortem wart* ⇒ verruca.

post·myocardial infarc·tion syn·drome (pōst-mī-ō-kàr'-dē-al in-fàrk'-shun) pyrexia and chest pain associated with inflammation of the pleura, lung or pericardium. Due to sensitivity to released products from dead muscle.

post·nasal (pōst-nā'-zal) *adj* situated behind the nose and in the nasopharynx—**postnasally** *adv.*

post·natal (pōst-nā'-tal) *adj* after delivery. ⇒ antenatal *opp. postnatal depression*

227

describes a low mood experienced by some mothers for a few days following the birth of a baby; sometimes called 'baby blues'. Less severe than puerperal* psychosis. *postnatal examination* routine examination 6 weeks after delivery—**postnatally** *adv.*

post·operative (pŏst-op´-ėr-à-tiv) *adj* after operation—**postoperatively** *adv.*

post·partum (pŏst-pår´-tum) *adj* after a birth (parturition).

post·prandial (pŏst-pran´-dĭ-al) *adj* following a meal.

pos·tural (pos´-tū-ral) *adj* pertaining to posture. *postural albuminuria* orthostatic* albuminuria. *postural drainage* usually infers drainage from the respiratory tract, by elevation of the foot of the bed or by using a special frame.

pos·ture (pos´-tūr) *n* active or passive arrangement of the whole body, or a part, in a definite position.

post·vaccinal (pŏst-vak´-sin-al) *adj* after vaccination.

post·vagotomy diar·rhea (pŏst-vă-got´-o-mē) three types: (a) transient diarrhea shortly after operation, lasting from a few hours to a day or two. These episodes disappear in 3–6 months. (b) if they recur later than this and the attacks last longer, the term 'recurrent episodic diarrhea' is used. (c) an increased daily bowel frequency; may be of disabling severity, but often acceptable in contrast to preoperative constipation.

Potaba-6 (po-ta´-ba) *n* proprietary name for potassium para-aminobenzoate.

potass·ium chlor·ate (pŏ-ta´-sē-um) a mild antiseptic used in mouthwashes and gargles. Distinguished from potassium chloride.

potass·ium chlor·ide (pŏ-ta´-sē-um klŏr´-ĭd) used in potassium replacement solutions, and as a supplement in thiazide diuretic therapy.

potass·ium citrate (pŏ-ta´-sē-um sĭ´-trāt) alkalinizes urine; still used in cystitis, etc. and during sulfonamide therapy to prevent renal complications.

potass·ium de·ficiency (pŏ-ta´-sē-um dē-fish´-ens-ē) disturbed electrolyte balance; can occur after excessive vomiting, and/or diarrhea; after prolonged use of diuretics, steroids, etc. The signs and symptoms are variable, but nausea and muscle weakness are often present. Heart failure can quickly supervene.

potass·ium hydrox·ide (pŏ-ta´-sē-um hĭ-droks´-ĭd) caustic potash; occasionally used for warts.

potass·ium iodide (pŏ-ta´-sē-um ĭ´-ō-dĭd) used as an expectorant in bronchitis and asthma; also used in the prophylaxis of simple goiter, and preoperatively in toxic goiter.

potass·ium para-amino·benzoate (pŏ-ta´-sē-um pår-à-mē´-nō-benz´-ō-āt) used in scleroderma and Peyronie's disease. Has an antifibrotic effect. 3 g capsules orally four times daily with meals for several months. (Potaba-6.)

potass·ium permanganate (pŏ-ta´-sē-um pėr-mang´-an-āt) purple crystals with powerful disinfectant and deodorizing properties. Used as lotion 1 in 1000; 1 in 5000 to 10 000 for baths.

potter's rot (pot´-ėrz rot) one of the many popular names for silicosis* arising in workers in the pottery industry.

Pott's dis·ease (pots) spondylitis; spinal caries; spinal tuberculosis. The resultant necrosis of the vertebrae causes kyphosis.

Pott's frac·ture a fracture-dislocation of the ankle joint. A fracture of the lower end of the tibia and fibula, 75 mm above the ankle joint, and a fracture of the medial malleolus of the tibia.

pouch (powch) *n* a pocket or recess. *pouch of Douglas* the rectouterine pouch.

povi·done iodine (pov´-i-dōn ĭ´-ō-dĭn) a liquid from which iodine is slowly liberated when in contact with the skin and mucous membranes. It is therefore useful for preoperative skin preparation and as a douche. (Betadine.)

PPD *abbr* purified protein derivative. ⇒ Mantoux reaction.

PPLO *abbr* pleuropneumonia-like organism, similar to the agent that causes contagious pleuropneumonia in cattle. ⇒ Mycoplasma.

PPS *abbr* pelvic* pain syndrome.

PR *abbr* per rectum; describes the route used for examination of the rectum, or introduction of substances into the body.

Prader-Willi syn·drome (prä´-dėr wil´-ĭ) a metabolic condition characterized by congenital hypotonia, hyperphagia, obesity and mental retardation. Diabetes mellitus develops in later life.

praz·osin (praz´-ō-sin) *n* an antihypertensive agent which is said to act peripherally by direct vasodilation. (Minipress.)

pre-anes·thetic (prē-an-es-thet´-ik) *adj* before an anesthetic.

pre·cancerous (prē-kan′-ser-us) *adj* occurring before cancer, with special reference to nonmalignant pathological changes which are believed to lead on to, or to be followed by, cancer.

pre·cipitin (prē-sip′-it-in) *n* an antibody which is capable of forming an immune complex with an antigen and becoming insoluble—a precipitate. This reaction forms the basis of many delicate diagnostic serological tests for the identification of antigens in serum and other fluids ⇒ immunoglobulins.

pre·conceptual (prē-kon-sep′-shū-al) *adj* before conception. Health education stresses that attention to an adequate diet, avoidance of alcohol and smoking in the months before a couple decide to have a baby reduces the risk of complications.

preconscious (prē-kon′-shus) *n* that part of the mind which is not conscious in the present but can be recalled.

pre·cordial (prē-kōr′-dē-al) *adj* pertaining to the area of the chest immediately over the heart.

precur·sor (prē′-kurs-or) *adj* forerunner.

pre·diabetes (prē-dī-ab-ē′-tēz) *n* potential predisposition to diabetes* mellitus. Preventive mass urine testing can detect the condition. Early treatment prevents ketoacidosis and may help to prevent the more serious complications such as retinopathy and neuropathy—**prediabetic** *adj, n*.

pre·digestion (prē-dī-jes′-chun) *n* artificial digestion of protein (e.g. in peptonized foods) or amylolysis (e.g. in malt extracts or dextrinized cereals) before digestion takes place in the body.

pre·disposition (prē-dis-pos-i′-shun) a natural tendency to develop or contract certain diseases.

prednis·olone (pred-nis′-o-lōn) *n* a synthetic hormone with properties similar to those of cortisone* but side effects, such as salt and water retention, are markedly reduced. Widely prescribed for connective tissue diseases, conditions involving immune reaction including autoimmune disorders.

pred·nisone (pred′-nis-ōn) converted into prednisolone* in the liver, therefore prescribed for the same conditions as prednisolone.

preeclamp·sia (prē-ē-klamp′-sē-à) *n* a condition characterized by albuminuria, hypertension and edema, arising usually in the latter part of pregnancy—**preeclamptic** *adj*.

pre·frontal (prē-front′-al) *adj* situated in the anterior portion of the frontal lobe of the cerebrum. ⇒ leukotomy.

pre·ganglionic (prē-gang-lē-on′-ik) *adj* preceding or in front of a collection of nerve cells (ganglion), as a preganglionic nerve fiber.

preg·nancy (preg′-nan-sē) *n* being with child, i.e. gestation from last menstrual period to parturition, normally 40 weeks or 280 days. ⇒ ectopic pregnancy, phantom pregnancy. *pregnancy-associated hypertension* solely a disease of pregnancy, most commonly of the primigravida. Blood pressure returns to normal and protein and urea, if present in the blood, resolve quickly after delivery in nearly all instances.

preg·nanediol (preg-nan-e-dī′-ol) *n* a urinary excretion product from progesterone*.

Preg·nyl (preg′-nil) *n* a proprietary preparation of human* chorionic gonadotrophin. It is useful for undescended and ectopic testes.

pre·hensile (prē-hen′-sīl) *adj* equipped for grasping.

Preludin (pre′-lū-din) *n* proprietary name for phenmetrazine*.

Pre·marin (prem′-à-rin) *n* a proprietary preparation of conjugated estrogens. Can be given orally. Useful for menopausal symptoms.

prema·ture (prē-mà-tūr′) *adj* occurring before the proper time. *premature baby* where the birth weight is less than 2.5 kg (5½ lb) and therefore special treatment is needed. Current synonyms are low birth-weight or dysmature baby. Not all low birthweight babies are premature, but are included in a new category 'small for dates.' ⇒ placental insufficiency. *premature beat* ⇒ extrasystole.

pre·medication (prē-med-ik-ā′-shun) *n* drugs given before the administration of another drug, e.g. those given before an anesthetic. The latter are of several types: (a) sedative or anxiolytic, e.g. morphine, meperidine, which also have sedative properties (b) drugs which inhibit the secretion of saliva and of mucus from the upper respiratory tract and cause tachycardia.

pre·menstrual (prē-men′-stroo-àl) *adj* preceding menstruation. *premenstrual (cyclical) syndrome (PMS)* a group of physical and mental changes which begin any time between 2 and 14 days before menstruation and which are relieved almost immediately once the flow starts. Recent research reveals a deficiency of essential fatty acids.

pre·molars (prē-mōl'-arz) *n* the teeth, also called bicuspids, situated fourth and fifth from the midline of the jaws, used with the molars for gripping and grinding food.

pre·natal (prē-nā'-tal) *adj* pertaining to the period between the last menstrual period and birth of the child, normally 40 weeks or 280 days—**prenatally** *adv.*

pre·operative (prē-op'-ėr-à-tiv) *adj* before operation—**preoperatively** *adv.*

pre·paralytic (prē-pàr-à-lit'-ik) *adj* before the onset of paralysis, usually referring to the early stage of poliomyelitis.

pre·patellar (prē-pà-tel'-ar) *adj* in front of the kneecap, as applied to a large bursa. ⇒ bursitis.

pre·pubertal (prē-pū'-bėr-tal) *adj* before puberty.

pre·puce (prē'-pūs) *n* the foreskin of the penis (⇒ Figure 16).

pre·renal (prē-rē'-nal) *adj* literally, before or in front of the kidney, but used to denote states in which, for instance, renal failure has arisen not within the nephrons but in the vascular fluid compartment, as in severe dehydration.

presby·opia (pres-bē-ō'-pē-à) *n* long-sightedness, due to failure of accommodation in those of 45 years and older—**presbyopic** *adj,* **presbyope** *n.*

prescrip·tion (pres-krip'-shun) *n* a written formula, signed by a physician, directing the pharmacist to supply the required drugs.

pre·senile de·mentia (prē-sēn'-īl dē-men'-shē-à) ⇒ dementia.

pre·senility (prē-sē-nil'-i-tē) *n* a condition occurring before senility is established. ⇒ dementia—**presenile** *adj.*

present·ation (prez-en-tā'-shun) *n* the part of the fetus which first enters the pelvic brim and will be felt by the examining finger through the cervix in labor. May be vertex, face, brow, shoulder or breech.

pressor (pres'-or) *n* a substance which raises the blood pressure.

press·ure areas the bony prominences of the body, over which the flesh of bed-ridden patients is denuded of its blood supply as it is compressed between the bone and an external source of pressure; the latter is usually the bed, but may be a splint, plaster, upper bedclothes, chair etc.

press·ure point (presh'-ur poynt) a place at which an artery passes over a bone, against which it can be compressed, to stop bleeding.

press·ure sore (presh'-ur sōr) (*syn* bedsore, decubitus ulcer) it is now customary to classify pressure sores as superficial or deep. *superficial pressure sores* involve destruction of the epidermis with exposure of the dermis so that microorganisms can penetrate the exposed tissue which is moist with lymph. *deep pressure sores* are caused by damage to the microcirculation in the deep tissues usually resulting from shearing force. The inflammatory and necrotic residue then tracks out to the skin surface destroying the dermis and epidermis. Deep sores are usually infected, discharging an exudate which results in protein and fluid loss from the body. Deep sores can take many weeks or months to heal and quite often require surgical closure to prevent further debility. Pressure sores can be a source of cross infection*.

pre·systole (prē-sis'-to-lē) *n* the period preceding the systole or contraction of the heart muscle—**presystolic** *adj.*

prevesical (prē-ves'-i-kal) *adj* anterior to the bladder.

pria·pism (prī'-àp-izm) *n* prolonged penile erection in the absence of sexual stimulation.

prickly heat (prik'-lē) ⇒ miliaria.

prima·quine (prī'-mà-qwin) *n* an antimalarial. Useful for eradication of *Plasmodium vivax* from the liver.

pri·mary complex (prī'-màr-ē kom'-pleks) (*syn* Ghon focus) the initial tuberculous infection in a person, usually in the lung, and manifest as a small focus of infection in the lung tissue and enlarged caseous, hilar glands. It usually heals spontaneously.

pri·mary health care (prī'-màr-ē helth kār) **1** the first level contact with the health care system. **2** a concept developed by WHO/UNICEF; 'a practical approach to making essential health care universally acceptable to individuals and families in the community in an acceptable and affordable way and with their full participation'.

primi·done (prim'-i-dōn) *n* an anticonvulsant used mainly in major epilepsy, but sometimes effective in minor epilepsy. (Mysoline.)

primi·gravida (prīm-i-grav'-i-dà) *n* a woman who is pregnant for the first time—**primigravidae** *pl.*

primi·para (prīm-ip'-ar-à) *n* a woman who has given birth to a child for the first time—**primiparous** *adj.*

primor·dial (prī-mör'-dē-al) *adj* primitive, original; applied to the ovarian follicles present at birth.

Pris·coline (pris'-kō-lēn) *n* proprietary name for tolazoline*.

pro·band (prō'-band) *n* in the genetically-inherited diseases, the first family member to present for investigation.

Pro-ban·thine (prō-ban'-thēn) *n* proprietary name for propantheline*.

proben·ecid (prō-be'-ne-sid) *n* a drug which inhibits the renal excretion of certain compounds, notably penicillin* and para-aminosalicyclic* acid, and is used to increase the blood level of such drugs. It also hinders the reabsorption of urates by the renal tubules, so increasing the excretion of uric acid, and on that account it is used in the treatment of gout. (Benemid.)

procain·amide (prō-kān'-à-mīd) *n* a derivative of procaine* used in cardiac arrhythmias such as paroxysmal tachycardia. Also helps to relax voluntary muscle and thus overcome myotonia. Given orally or by slow intravenous injection. (Pronestyl.)

pro·caine (prō'-kān) *n* a once widely-used local anesthetic of high potency and low toxicity. Used mainly for infiltration and anesthesia as a 0.5–2% solution. Now replaced by lidocaine. (Novocain.) *procaine benzylpenicillin* longer acting than benzyl* penicillin.

pro·carbazine (prō-kàr'-bà-zēn) *n* a drug of the nitrogen* mustard group useful in Hodgkin's disease. (Matulane.)

pro·cess (pro'-ses) *n* a prominence or outgrowth of any part.

prochlor·perazine (prō-klör-per'-à-zēn) *n* one of the phenothiazines. Has sedative and anti-emetic properties. Useful for vertigo, migraine, Ménière's disease, severe nausea and vomiting, schizophrenia. (Compazine.)

proci·dentia (pro-si-den'-shē-à) *n* complete prolapse of the uterus, so that it lies within the vaginal sac but outside the contour of the body.

proc·talgia (prok-tal'-jē-à) *n* pain in the rectal region.

proc·titis (prok-tī'-tis) *n* inflammation of the rectum.* *granular proctitis* acute proctitis, so called because of the granular appearance of the inflamed mucous membrane.

procto·clysis (prok-tō-klī'-sis) *n* ⇒ enterolysis.

procto·colectomy (prok-tō-kol-ek'-to-mē) *n* surgical excision of the rectum and colon.

procto·colitis (prok-tō-kol-ī'-tis) *n* inflammation of the rectum and colon; usually a type of ulcerative colitis*.

procto·scope (prok'-tō-skōp) *n* an instrument for examining the rectum. ⇒ endoscope—**proctoscopic** *adj*, **proctoscopy** *n.*

procto·sigmoiditis (prok'-tō-sig-moyd-ī'-tis) *n* inflammation of the rectum and sigmoid colon.

procycli·dine (prō-sī'-kli-dēn) *n* a spasmolytic drug similar in action to benzhexol* and used in the treatment of parkinsonism. It reduces the rigidity but has little action on the tremor. (Kemadrin.)

prod·romal (prō-drō'-mal) *adj* preceding, as the transitory rash before the true rash of an infectious disease.

pro-drug (prō'-drug) *n* a compound with reduced intrinsic activity, but which, after absorption, is metabolized to release the active components. It avoids side-effects on the gastrointestinal tract.

pro·flavine (prō-flā'-vēn) *n* an antiseptic very similar to acriflavine*.

Progest·asert (prō-jest'-à-sèrt) a brand of flexible T-shaped unit, like an IUCD; contains the natural hormone progesterone*, released at a continuous rate of 65 mg daily.

progest·ational (prō-jest-ā'-shun-al) *adj* before pregnancy. Favoring pregnancy—**progestation** *n.*

progester·one (prō-jest'-èr-ōn) *n* the hormone of the corpus luteum*. Used in the treatment of functional uterine hemorrhage, and in threatened abortion. Given by intramuscular injection.

progest·ogen (prō-jest'-ō-jen) *n* any natural or synthetic progestational hormone progesterone*.

pro·glottis (prō-glot'-is) a sexually mature segment of tapeworm—**proglottides** *pl.*

prog·nosis (prog-nō'-sis) *n* a forecast of the probable course and termination of a disease—**prognostic** *adj.*

projec·tion (prō-jek'-shun) *n* a mental mechanism occurring in normal people unconsciously, and in exaggerated form in mental illness, especially paranoia, whereby the person fails to recognize certain motives and feelings in himself but attributes them to others.

pro·lactin (prō-lak′-tin) *n* a hormone secreted by the anterior pituitary, concerned with lactation and reproduction. Increased levels found in some pituitary tumors (prolactinomas) result in amenorrhea and infertility.

pro·lapse (prō′-laps) *n* descent; the falling of a structure. *prolapse of an intervertebral disc (PID)* protrusion of the disc nucleus into the spinal canal. Most common in the lumbar region where it causes low back pain and/or sciatica. *prolapse of the iris* iridocele*. *prolapse of the rectum* the lower portion of the intestinal tract descends outside the external anal sphincter. *prolapse of the uterus* the uterus descends into the vagina and may be visible at the vaginal orifice. ⇒ procidentia.

prolifer·ate (prō-lif′-ėr-āt) *vi* increase by cell division—**proliferation** *n*, **proliferative** *adj*.

pro·lific (prō-lif′-ik) *adj* fruitful, multiplying abundantly.

Prolixin (prō-liks′-in) *n* proprietary name for fluphenazine*.

prom·azine (prō′-mȧ-zēn) *n* a tranquilizing drug similar to, but less hepatotoxic than chlorpromazine*. Also useful in obstetrics, treatment of alcoholism, senile agitation and for shivering attacks. (Sparine.)

prometh·azine (prō-meth′-ȧ-zēn) *n* an antihistamine of high potency and low toxicity. Hypnotic side effect useful in psychiatry and obstetrics. Also useful for travel sickness. Given 2 hours before a journey its effect will last for 6–12 h. (Phenergan.)

prom·ontory (prom′-on-tōr-ē) *n* a projection; a prominent part.

pro·nate (prō′-nāt) *vt* to place ventral surface downward, e.g. on the face; to turn (the palm of the hand) downwards ⇒ supinate *opp*—**pronation** *n*.

pro·nator (prō′-nā-tor) *n* that which pronates, usually applied to a muscle. ⇒ supinator *opp. pronator teres* ⇒ Figure 4.

prone (prōn) *adj* 1 lying on the anterior surface of the body with the face turned to one or other side. 2 of the hand, with the palm downwards. ⇒ supine *opp*.

Pron·estyl (prō-nes′-tl) *n* proprietary name for procainamide*.

propan·theline (prō-pan′-thel-ēn) *n* a synthetic compound with an atropine*-like action. Used for its antispasmodic effects in pylorospasm, peptic ulcer etc. Dryness of the mouth may occur in some patients. (Pro-banthine.)

prophy·laxis (prō-fil-aks′-is) *n* (attempted) prevention—**prophylactic** *adj*, **prophylactically** *adv*.

propran·olol (prō-pran′-ol-ol) *n* an effective drug in the prevention or correction of cardiac arrhythmias and dysrhythmias. It reduces frequency of anginal attacks by blocking the effects of beta-receptor activation in the heart. Bronchoconstriction may occur as a side-effect in some patients. Prepared as eye drops for glaucoma. (Inderal.)

proprietary name (prō-prī′-et-ār-ē) (*syn* brand name) the name given to a drug by the pharmaceutical firm which produced it. The name should always be spelt with a capital letter to distinguish it from the approved name (pharmaceutical name) which can be used by any manufacturer.

prop·tosis (prop-tō′-sis) *n* forward protrusion, especially of the eyeball.

propyl·thiouracil (prō-pil-thī-ūr′-ȧ-sil) *n* inhibits thyroid activity and is used occasionally in thyrotoxicosis.

pro·quanil (prō′-kwan-il) *n* an antimalarial drug.

pro·sector's wart (prō-sek′tor) ⇒ verruca.

pros·ody (prōs′-o-dē) *n* the science of versification involving inflection, stress and rhythm, absence of which makes speech dull and monotonous.

prosta·cyclin (prost-ȧ-sī′-klin) *n* a naturally occurring substance formed by endothelial cells of blood vessel walls. It inhibits platelet aggregation.

prosta·glandins (prost-ȧ-gland′-ins) *npl* share some of the properties of hormones, vitamins, enzymes and catalysts. All body tissues probably contain some prostaglandins. Used pharmaceutically to terminate early pregnancy, and for asthma and gastric hyperacidity.

pros·tate (pros′-tāt) *n* a small conical gland at the base of the male bladder and surrounding the first part of the urethra (⇒ Figure 16)—**prostatic** *adj*.

prostatec·tomy (pros-tȧ-tek′-to-mē) *n* surgical removal of the prostate* gland. *retropubic prostatectomy* the prostate is reached through a lower abdominal (suprapubic) incision, the bladder being retracted upwards to expose the prostate behind the pubis. *transurethral prostatectomy* the operation whereby chippings of prostatic tissue are cut from within the urethra using either a cold knife or electric cautery; usually restricted to small fibrous glands or to cases of prostatic carcinoma. ⇒ resectoscope. *transvesical prostatectomy* the operation in which the prostate is approached through the bladder, using a lower abdominal (suprapubic) incision.

pros·tatic acid phosphatase (prost-at'-ik as'-id fos'-fa-tās) an enzyme in seminal fluid secreted by the prostate gland. *prostatic acid phosphatase test* (PAP test) an increase in this enzyme in the blood is indicative of carcinoma of the prostate gland.

prosta·tism (pros'-tat-ism) *n* general condition produced by hypertrophy or chronic disease of the prostate gland, characterized by the obstructive symptoms of hesitancy, a poor stream and post-micturition dribbling.

prosta·titis (pros-tà-tī'-tis) *n* inflammation of the prostate* gland.

prostato·cystitis (pros-tà-tō-sis-tī'-tis) *n* inflammation of the prostate gland and male urinary bladder.

pros·thesis (pros-thē'-sis) *n* an artificial substitute for a missing part—**prostheses** *pl*, **prosthetic** *adj*.

pros·thetics (pros-thet'-iks) *n* the branch of surgery which deals with prostheses.

prostho·keratoplasty (pros-thō-ker'-à-tō-plas-tē) *n* keratoplasty in which the corneal implant is of some material other than human or animal tissue.

Prostig·min (pro-stig'-min) *n* proprietary name for neostigmine*.

Prostin (prost'-in) *n* proprietary pessaries containing prostaglandin E_2; they are given to induce labor.

pro·tamine sulfate (prō'-tà-mēn) a protein of simple structure used as an antidote to heparin* 1 ml of 1% solution will neutralize the effects of about 1000 units of heparin.

pro·tamine zinc insulin (prō'-tà-mēn) an insoluble form of insulin*, formed by combination with protamine (a simple protein) and a trace of zinc. It has an action lasting over 24 h, and in association with initial doses of soluble insulin permits a wide degree of control.

pro·tease (prō'-tē-ās) *n* any enzyme which digests protein: a proteolytic enzyme.

protec·tive isol·ation (prō-tek'-tiv ī-sō-lā'-shun) is carried out for those patients who are rendered highly susceptible to infection by disease or treatment. ⇒ barrier nursing.

pro·tein calorie mal·nutrition (PCM) (prō'-tē-in kal'-or-ē mal-nōō-tri'-shun) (protein energy malnutrition—PEM) describes a condition in which individuals have depleted body fat and protein resulting from an inadequate diet.

pro·teins (prō'-tē-inz) *npl* highly complex nitrogenous compounds found in all animal and vegetable tissues. They are built up of amino* acids and are essential for growth and repair of the body. Those from animal sources are of high biological value since they contain the essential amino acids. Those from vegetable sources contain not all, but some of the essential amino acids. Proteins are hydrolyzed in the body to produce amino acids which are then used to build up new body proteins.

protein·uria (prō-tēn-ūr'-ē-à) *n* albuminuria*.

proteol·ysis (prō-tē-ol'-is-is) *n* the hydrolysis of the peptide bonds of proteins with the formation of smaller polypeptides—**proteolytic** *adj*.

proteol·ytic en·zymes (prō-tē-ō-li'-tik en'-zīmz) enzymes that promote proteolysis; they have a limited use in liquefying slough and necrotic tissue and are enzymatic debriding agents.

pro·teose (prō'-tē-ōs) *n* a mixture of cleavage products from the breakdown of proteins, intermediate between protein and peptone.

Pro·teus (prō'-tē-us) *n* a bacterial genus. Gram-negative motile rods which swarm in culture. Found in damp surroundings. Sometimes a commensal of the intestinal tract. May be pathogenic, especially in wound and urinary tract infections as a secondary invader. Production of alkali turns infected urine alkaline.

pro·thrombin (prō-throm'-bin) *n* a precursor of thrombin formed in the liver. The *prothrombin time* is a measure of its production and concentration in the blood. It is the time taken for plasma to clot after the addition of thrombokinase. It is inversely proportional to the amount of prothrombin present, a normal person's plasma being used as a standard of comparison. Prothrombin time is lengthened in certain hemorrhagic combinations and in a patient on anticoagulant drugs. ⇒ thrombin. *prothrombin test* indirectly reveals the amount of prothrombin in blood. To a sample of oxalated blood are added all the factors needed to bring about clotting, except prothrombin. The time taken for clot to form is therefore dependent on amount of prothrombin present. Normal time is 10–12 s.

proto·pathic (prō-tō-path'-ik) *adj* the term applied to a less sensibility. ⇒ epicritic *opp.*

proto·plasm (prō'-tō-plazm) *n* ⇒ cytoplasm—**protoplasmic** *adj.*

proto·zoa (prō-tō-zō'-à) *npl* the smallest type of animal life; unicellular organisms. The phylum includes the genera *Plasmodium* (malarial parasites) and *Entamoeba*. The commonest protozoan infestation is *Trichomonas vaginalis*, classed with the intestinal flagellates—**protozoon** *sing,* **protozoal** *adj.*

protript·yline (prō-trip'-tl-in) *n* an antidepressant similar to imipramine* but the response to treatment is more rapid. It does not have a sedative effect. (Vivactil.)

proud flesh excessive granulation tissue.

Provera (prō-vėr'-à) *n* proprietary name for medroxyprogesterone*.

pro·vitamin (prō-vīt'-à-min) *n* a vitamin precursor, e.g. carotene is converted into vitamin A.

proxi·mal (proks'-i-mal) *adj* nearest to the head or source—**proximally** *adv.*

prune belly syn·drome a condition found in male infants with obstructive uropathy and atrophy of the abdominal musculature. The term is descriptive.

pru·rigo (prōō-rī'-gō) *n* a chronic, itching disease occurring most frequently in children. *prurigo estivale* hydroa* estivale. *Besnier's prurigo* ⇒ Besnier's.

pru·ritus (prōō-rī'-tis) *n* itching. *Pruritus ani* and *pruritus vulvae* are considered to be psychosomatic conditions (neurodermatitis) except in the few cases where a local cause can be found, e.g. worm infestation, vaginitis. Generalized pruritus may be a symptom of systemic disease as in diabetes, icterus, Hodgkin's disease, carcinoma etc. It may be psychogenic—**pruritic** *adj.*

prussic acid (prus'-ik) ⇒ hydrocyanic acid.

pseudo·angina (sū-dō-an-jī'-nà) *n* false angina. Sometimes referred to as 'left mammary pain', it occurs in anxious individuals. Usually there is no cardiac disease present. May be part of effort* syndrome.

pseudo·arthrosis (sū-dō-àrth-rō'-sis) *n* a false joint, e.g. due to ununited fracture; also congenital, e.g. in tibia.

pseudo·bulbar paral·ysis (sū-dō-bul'-bar par-al'-is-is) there is gross disturbance in control of tongue bilateral hem-

iplegia and mental changes following on a succession of 'strokes'.

pseudo-cholinesterase (sū-dō-kō-lin-es'-tėr-ās) an enzyme present in plasma and tissues (other than nerve tissue) and is synthesized in the liver.

pseudo·coxalgia (sū-dō-koks-al'-jē-à) *n* ⇒ Perthes' disease.

pseudo·crisis (sū-dō-krī'-sis) *n* a rapid reduction of body temperature resembling a crisis, followed by further fever.

pseudo·cyesis (sū-dō-sī-ē'-sis) *n* ⇒ phantom pregnancy.

pseudo-ephedrine (sū-dō-ef-ed'-rin) *n* an isomer of ephedrine; the hydrochloric salt is used as a nasal decongestant. May cause hallucinations in some young children.

pseudo·hermaphrodite (sū-dō-hėr-maf'-rō-dīt) *n* a person in whom the gonads of one sex are present, whilst the external genitalia comprise those of the opposite sex.

pseudol·ogia fantastica (sū-dō-log'-ē-à fan-tas'-tik-à) a tendency to tell, and defend, fantastic lies plausibly, found in some hysterics and psychopaths.

Pseudo-monas (sū-dō-mō'-nas) *n* a bacterial genus. Gram-negative motile rods. Found in water and decomposing vegetable matter. Some are pathogenic to plants and animals and *Pseudomonas aeruginosa (pyocanea)* is able to produce disease in men. Found commonly as a secondary invader in urinary tract infections and wound infections. Produces a blue pigment (pyocyanin) which colors the exudate or pus.

pseudo·mucin (sū-dō-mū'-sin) *n* a gelatinous substance (not mucin) found in some ovarian cysts.

pseudo·paralysis (sū-dō-par-al'-is-is) *n* a loss of muscular power not due to a lesion of the nervous system. *pseudoparalysis of Parrot* inability to move one or more of the extremities because of syphlitic osteochondritis: occurs in neonatal congenital syphilis.

pseudo·parkinsonism (sū-dō-pàr'-kin-son-izm) *n* the signs and symptoms of parkinsonism when they are not post-encephalitic.

pseudo-plegia (sū-dō-plē'-jē-à) *n* paralysis mimicking that of organic nervous disorder but usually hysterical in origin.

pseudo·podia (sū-dō-pō'-dē-à) *n* literally false legs; cytoplasmic projections of an amoeba or any mobile cell which help it to move. Not to be confused with cilia or microvilli which are non-retractile prejections from the cell surface—**pseudopodium** *sing.*

pseudo·polyposis (sū-dō-pol-i-pōs'-is) *n* widely scattered polypi, usually the result of previous inflammation—sometimes ulcerative colitis.

psitta·cosis (sit-à-kō'-sis) *n* disease of parrots, pigeons and other birds which is occasionally responsible for a form of pneumonia in man. Caused by *Chlamydia psittaci*. It behaves as a bacterium though multiplying intracellularly. Sensitive to sulfonamides and antibiotics.

psoas (sō'-as) *n* muscles of the loin. *psoas abscess* a cold abscess* in the psoas muscle, resulting from tuberculosis of the lower dorsal or lumbar vertebrae. Pressure in the abscess causes pus to track along the tough ligaments so that the abscess appears as a firm smooth swelling which does not show signs of inflammation—hence the adjective 'cold'.

psor·alen (sōr'-à-len) *n* a naturally occurring photosensitive compound which on exposure to ultraviolet radiation increases melanin* in the skin. Pharmaceutical psoralen has been used in psoriasis and vitiligo.

pso·riasis (sōr-ī'-à-sis) *n* a genetically-determined chronic skin disease in which erythematous areas are covered with adherent scales. Although the condition may occur on any part of the body, the characteristic sites are extensor surfaces, especially over the knees and elbows. Inpatients' skin may be colonized or infected with hospital strains of *Staphylococcus aureus*. Due to the exfoliative nature of psoriasis sensitive modification of patient management is required to protect others from infection. A common cause of erythroderma—**psoriatic** *adj.*

psori·atic arthritis (sōr-ī-at'-ik àrth-rī'-tis) articular symptoms similar to those of rheumatoid arthritis occur in 3–5% of patients with psoriasis.

PSRO *abbr* Professional Standards Review Organization.

psy·chiatry (sī-kī'-at-rē) *n* the branch of medical study devoted to the diagnosis and treatment of mental illness—**psychiatric** *adj.*

psy·chic (sī'-kik) *adj* of the mind.

psycho·analysis (sī-kō-an-al'-is'-is) *n* a specialized branch of psychiatry founded by Freud*. It is a method of diagnosis and treatment of neuroses.

Briefly the method is to revive past forgotten emotional experiences and effect a cure of the neurosis by helping the patient readjust his attitudes to those experiences—**psychoanalytic** *adj.*

psycho·chemotherapy (sī-kō-kē-mō-thèr'-à-pē) *n* the use of drugs to improve or cure pathological changes in the emotional state—**psychochemotherapeutic** *adj,* **psychochemotherapeutically** *adv.*

psycho·drama (sī'-ko-drà-mà) *n* a method of psychotherapy whereby patients act out their personal problems by taking roles in spontaneous dramatic performances. Group discussion aims at giving the patients a greater awareness of the problems presented and possible methods of dealing with them.

psycho·dynamics (sī-kō-dī-nam'-iks) *n* the science of the mental processes, especially of the causative factors in mental activity.

psycho·genesis (sī-kō-jen'-es-is) *n* the development of the mind.

psycho·genic (sī-kō-jen'-ik) *adj* arising from the psyche or mind. *psychogenic symptom* originates in the mind rather than in the body.

psycho·geriatric (sī-kō-jèr-è-at'-rik) *adj* pertaining to psychology as applied to geriatrics. *psychogeriatric dependency rating scales* construction of these scales was based on three basic dimensions—psychological deterioration, physical infirmity and psychological agitation.

psy·chology (sī-kol'-o-jē) *n* the study of the behavior of an organism in its environment. Medically, the study of human behavior.

psycho·metry (sī-kom'-e-trē) *n* the science of mental testing.

psycho·motor (sī-kō-mō'-tor) *adj* pertaining to the motor effect of psychic or cerebral activity.

psycho·neuro·immunology (PNI) (sī-kō-noō-rō-im-ūn-ol'-o-jē) *n* the study of white blood cell counts and their correlation with stressful conditions and illness. Early research shows an inverse relationship.

psycho·neurosis (sī-kō-noō-rō'-sis) *n* ⟹ neurosis.

psycho·path (sī'-kō-path) *n* one who is morally irresponsible and intent on instant gratification—**psychopathic** *adj.*

psycho·pathic person·ality (sī-kō-path'-ik per-son-al'-i-tē) a persistent disorder or disability of mind (whether or not including subnormality of intelligence) which results in abnormally aggressive or seriously irresponsible conduct that requires, or is susceptible to, medical treatment.

psycho·pathology (sī-kō-path-ol′-o-jē) *n* the pathology of abnormal mental processes—**psychopathological** *adj,* **psychopathologically** *adv.*

psycho·pathy (sī-kop′-à-thē) *n* any disease of the mind. The term is used by some people to denote a marked immaturity in emotional development—**psychopathic** *adj.*

psycho·pharmacology (sī-kō-fàr-mà-kol′-o-jē) *n* the use of drugs which influence the affective and emotional state.

psycho·physics (sī-kō-fiz′-iks) *n* a branch of experimental psychology dealing with the study of stimuli and sensations—**psychophysical** *adj.*

psycho·prophylactic (sī-kō-prō-fil-ak′-tik) *adj* that which aims at preventing mental disease.

psychoprophylactic method of childbirth (*syn* Lamaze method) physical and mental preparation of the mother and her partner for childbirth.

psy·chosis (sī-kō′-sis) *n* a major mental disorder of organic or emotional origin in which a person's ability to think, respond emotionally, remember, communicate, interpret reality and behave appropriately is impaired. Insight is usually absent—**psychoses** *pl,* **psychotic** *adj.*

psychosomatic (sī-kō-som-at′-ik) *n* mind-body illness; illness where emotional factors produce physical symptoms. These arise mainly from overactivity of the autonomic nervous system which is influenced by the emotional state, e.g. chronic blushing may be due to feelings of guilt, the skin arterioles dilate as a result of autonomic overactivity, inflammation follows, death of some skin cells results in the development of a rash. The same 'blushing' can occur in the bowel; the *psychosomatic process* is the same, resulting in ulcerative colitis. Other *psychosomatic conditions* include hyperthyroidism, asthma, migraine, urticaria, hay-fever, peptic ulcer and several skin conditions.

psycho·somimetics (sī-kō-sō-mim′-et-iks) *npl* (*syn* hallucinogens) drugs, e.g. mescaline, LSD, that produce psychosis-like symptoms.

psycho·therapy (sī-kō-thèr′-a-pē) *n* treatment of mental disorder by psychological means using discussion, explanation and reassurance—**psychotherapeutic**

adj. group psychotherapy a product of Second World War when free discussion of 'effort syndrome' produced therapeutic results. At a meeting, the anxieties of staff and patients are discussed and everyone is enlisted in the treatment program.

psycho·tropic (sī-kō-trō′-pik) *adj* that which exerts its specific effect upon the brain cells.

psyl·lium (sil′-ē-um) *n* the seeds of an African plant. They contain mucilage, which swells on contact with water; useful as a bulk-forming laxative. (Metamucil).

pteroyl·glutamic acid (tēr′-ō-il-glōō-tam′-ik) ⇒ folic acid.

ptery·gium (te-rij′-ē-um) *n* a wing-shaped degenerative condition of the conjunctiva which encroaches on the cornea—**pterygial** *adj.*

ptomaine (tō′-mān) *n* one of a group of poisonous substances formed by the decaying of protein by bacterial action.

pto·sis (tō′-sis) *n* a drooping, particularly that of the eyelid. ⇒ visceroptosis—**ptotic** *adj.*

ptya·lin (tī′-à-lin) *n* salivary amylase* which is a slightly acid medium (pH 6.8) which converts starch into dextrin* and maltose*.

ptyal·ism (tī′-à-lizm) *n* excessive salivation.

ptyal·olith (tī′-al-ō-lith) *n* a salivary calculus.

pubertas praecox (pū′-ber-tas prā′-coks) premature (precocious) sexual development.

pu·berty (pū′-bèr-tē) *n* the age at which the reproductive organs become functionally active. It is accompanied by secondary characteristics—**pubertal** *adj.*

pubes (pū′-bēz) *n* the hairy region covering the pubic bone.

pubi·otomy (pū-bē-ot′-o-mē) *n* cutting the pubic bone to facilitate delivery of a live child.

pu·bis (pū′-bis) *n* the pubic bone or os pubis, forming the center bone of the front of the pelvis—**pubic** *adj.*

PUBS *abbr* percutaneous umbilical blood sampling; samples of fetal blood taken from the umbilical cord through the abdomen of the mother.

pu·dendal block (pū-den′-dal) the rendering insensitive of the pudendum by the injection of local anesthetic. Used mainly for episiotomy and forceps delivery. ⇒ transvaginal.

pu·dendum (pū-den'-dum) *n* the external reproductive organs, especially of the female—*pudenda pl*, **pudendal** *adj*.

Pudenz-Hayer valve (pū'-denz hāy'-er) one-way valve implanted at operation for relief of hydrocephalus.

puer·peral (pū-ėr'-pe-ral) *adj* pertaining to childbirth. *puerperal psychosis* a mental illness (psychosis) occurring in the puerperium*. ⇒ baby blues and postpartum depression. *puerperal sepsis* infection of the genital tract occurring within 21 days of abortion or childbirth.

puer·perium (pū-ėr-pėr'-ē-um) *n* the period immediately following childbirth to the time when involution is completed, usually 6–8 weeks—**puerperia** *pl*.

pulmo·flator (pul'-mō-flā-tor) *n* apparatus for inflation of lungs.

pul·monary (pul'-mon-ār-ē) *adj* pertaining to the lungs. *pulmonary artery* ⇒ Figures 7, 9. *pulmonary circulation* deoxygenated blood leaves the right ventricle; flows through the lungs where it becomes oxygenated and returns to the left atrium of the heart. *pulmonary emphysema* stretching of the alveolar membrane rendering it less efficient in the diffusion of gases. It can be generalized resulting from chronic bronchitis. It can be localized, either distal to partial obstruction of a bronchiole or bronchus (obstructive emphysema), or in alveoli adjacent to a segment of collapsed lung (compensatory emphysema). *pulmonary hypertension* raised blood pressure within the blood vessels supplying the lungs, due to increased resistance to blood flow within the pulmonary circulation. It is associated with increased pressure in the right cardiac ventricle, then the atrium. It may be due to disease of the left side of the heart or in the lung. In primary pulmonary hypertension the cause is not known. It usually leads to death from congestive heart failure in 2–10 years. *pulmonary edema* a form of 'waterlogging' of the lungs because of left ventricular failure or mitral stenosis. *pulmonary vein* ⇒ Figures 7, 10.

pulp (pulp) the soft, interior part of some organs and structures. *dental pulp* found in the pulp cavity and root canals of teeth; carries blood, nerve and lymph vessels. *digital pulp* the tissue pad of the finger tip. Infection of this is referred to as 'pulp space infection'.

pul·satile (pul'-să-tīl) *adj* beating, throbbing.

pul·sation (pul-sā'-shun) *n* beating or throbbing, as of the heart or arteries.

pulse (puls) *n* the impulse transmitted to arteries by contraction of the left ventricle, and customarily palpated in the radial artery at the wrist. The *pulse rate* is the number of beats or impulses per minute and is about 130 in the newborn infant, 70–80 in the adult and 60–70 in old age. The *pulse rhythm* is its regularity—can be regular or irregular; the *pulse volume* is the amplitude of expansion of the arterial wall during the passage of the wave; the *pulse force* or tension is its strength, estimated by the force needed to obliterate it by pressure of the finger. *pulse deficit* the difference in rate of the heart (counted by stethoscope) and the pulse (counted at the wrist). It occurs when some of the ventricular contractions are too weak to open the aortic valve and hence produce a beat at the heart but not at the wrist, and occurs commonly in atrial fibrillation. *pulse pressure* is the difference between the systolic and diastolic pressures. ⇒ beat.

'pulse·less' dis·ease (puls'-les) progressive obliterative arteritis of the vessels arising from the aortic arch resulting in diminished or absent pulse in the neck and arms. Thromboendarterectomy or a bypass procedure may prevent blindness by improving the carotid blood flow at its commencement in the aortic arch.

pulsus alter·nans (pul'-sus awl'-tėr-nans) a regular pulse with alternate beats of weak and strong amplitude; a sign of left ventricular disease.

pulsus bigem·inus (pul'-sus bī-jem'-in-us) double pulse wave produced by interpolation of extrasystoles. A coupled beat. A heart rhythm often due to excessive digitalis administration of paired beats, each pair being followed by a prolonged pause. The second weaker beat of each pair may not be strong enough to open the aortic valve, in which case it does not produce a pulse beat and the type of rhythm can then only be detected by listening at the heart.

pulsus para·doxus (pul'-sus pàr-à-doks'-us) arterial pulsus paradoxus is alteration of the volume of the arterial pulse sometimes found in pericardial effusion. The volume becomes greater with expiration. Venous pulsus paradoxus (Kusman's sign) is an increase in the height of the venous pressure with inspiration, the reverse of normal. Sometimes found in pericardial or right ventricular disease.

pulvis (pul'-vis) *n* a powder.

punctate (pungk′-tāt) *adj* dotted or spotted, e.g. punctate basophilia describes the immature red cell in which there are droplets of blue-staining material in the cytoplasm—**punctum** *n*, **puncta** *pl*.

punc·ture (pungk′-tūr) *n* a stab; a wound made with a sharp pointed hollow instrument for withdrawal or injection of fluid or other substance. *cisternal puncture* insertion of a special hollow needle with stylet through the atlanto-occipital ligament between the occiput and atlas, into the cisterna magna. One method of obtaining cerebrospinal fluid. *lumbar puncture* insertion of a special hollow needle with stylet either through the space between the third and fourth lumbar vertebrae or, lower, into the subarachnoid space to obtain cerebrospinal fluid. *puncture wound* ⇒ penetrating wound.

PUO *abbr* pyrexia* of unknown origin.

pu·pil (pū′-pil) *n* the opening in the center of the iris of the eye to allow the passage of light (⇒ Figure 15)—**pupillary** *adj*.

pupil·lary (pū′-pil-ār-ē) *adj* pertaining to the pupil.

pupillary reflex constriction of the pupil when exposed to light.

pur·gative (pur′-gȧ-tiv) *n* a drug causing evacuation of fluid feces. *drastic purgative* even more severe in action, when the fluid feces may be passed involuntarily.

purines (pū′-rēnz) *npl* constituents of nucleoproteins from which uric acid is derived. Gout is thought to be associated with the disturbed metabolism and excretion of uric acid, and foods of high purine content are excluded in its treatment.

Purinethol (pūr-in-eth′-ol) *n* proprietary name for mercaptopurine*.

Purkinje fibers (poor-kin′-jēz) muscle cell fibers found beneath the endocardium of the heart; make up the impulse-conducting network of the heart.

purpura (pur′-pur-ȧ) *n* a disorder characterized by extravasation of blood from the capillaries into the skin, or into or from the mucous membranes. Manifest either by small red spots (petechiae) or large bruises (ecchymoses) or by oozing from minor wounds, the latter, in the absence of trauma, being confined to the mucous membranes. It is believed that the disorder can be due to impaired integrity of the capillary walls, or to defective quality or quantity of the blood platelets. Purpura can be caused by many different conditions, e.g. infective,

toxic, allergic, etc. ⇒ Henoch-Schönlein purpura. *anaphylactoid purpura* excessive reaction between antigen and the protein globulin IgG (antibody). Antigen often unknown, but may be derived from beta-hemolytic streptococci, or drugs such as sulfonamides which may interact chemically with body proteins. *purpura hemorrhagica* (thrombocytopenic purpura) is characterized by a greatly diminished platelet count. The clotting time is normal but the bleeding time is prolonged. The patient is usually well, but intracranial hemorrhagic can occur.

puru·lent (pū′-rū-lent) *adj* pertaining to or resembling pus.

pus *n* a liquid, usually yellowish in color, formed in certain infections and composed of tissue fluid containing bacteria and leukocytes. Various types of bacteria are associated with pus having distinctive features, e.g. the fecal smell of pus due to *Escherichia coli*; the green color of pus due to *Pseudomonas aeruginosa*.

pus·tule (pus′-tūl) *n* a small inflammatory swelling containing pus—**pustular** *adj*. *malignant pustule* ⇒ anthrax.

putre·faction (pū-tre-fak′-shun) *n* the process of rotting; the destruction of organic material by bacteria—**putrefactive** *adj*.

pu·trescible (pū-tres′-i-bl) *adj* capable of undergoing putrefaction.

PUVA *abbr* psoralen* with long wavelength ultraviolet light.

PVD *abbr* peripheral* vascular disease.

py·arthrosis (pī-ārth-rō′-sis) *n* pus in a joint cavity.

pyel·itis (pī-el-ī′-tis) *n* mild form of pyelonephritis* with pyuria but minimal involvement of renal tissue. Pyelitis on the right side is a common complication of pregnancy.

pyel·ography (pī-el-og′-ra-fē) *n* ⇒ urography—**pyelographic** *adj*, **pyelogram** *n*, **pyelographically** *adv*.

pyelolithotomy (pī-el-ō-lith-ot′-o-mē) *n* the operation for removal of a stone from the renal pelvis.

pyelo·nephritis (pī-el-ō-nef-rī′-tis) *n* a form of renal infection which spreads outwards from the pelvis to the cortex of the kidney. The origin of the infection is usually from the ureter and below, or from the blood stream—**pyelonephritic** *adj*.

pyelonephrosis (pī-el-ō-nef-rō′-sis) *n* any disease of the kidney pelvis.

pyelo·plasty (pī′-el-ō-plas-tē) *n* a plastic

operation on the kidney pelvis. ⇒ hydronephrosis.

pyel·ostomy (pī-el-os′-to-mē) *n* surgical formation of an opening into the kidney pelvis.

pyemia (pī-ēm′-ē-à) *n* a grave form of septicemia in which blood borne bacteria lodge and grow in distant organs, e.g. brain, kidneys, lungs and heart, to form multiple abscesses—**pyemic** *adj*.

pyknolepsy (pik′-nō-lep-sē) *n* a frequently recurring form of minor epilepsy seen in children. Attacks may number a hundred or more in a day.

pyle·phlebitis (pī-lē-fleb-ī′-tis) *n* inflammation of the veins of the portal system secondary to intraabdominal sepsis.

pyle·thrombosis (pī-lē-throm-bō′-sis) *n* an intravascular blood clot in the portal vein or any of its branches.

pyloric stenosis (pī-lōr′ik sten-ōs′-is) **1** narrowing of the pylorus due to scar tissue formed during the healing of a duodenal ulcer. **2** *congenital hypertrophic pyloric stenosis,* due to a thickened pyloric sphincter muscle.

pyloro·duodenal (pī-lōr-ō-dū-od′-en-al) *adj* pertaining to the pyloric sphincter and the duodenum.

pyloro·myotomy (pī-lōr-ō-mī-ot′-o-mē) *n* (*syn* Ramstedt's operation) incision of the pyloric sphincter muscle as in pyloroplasty.

pyloro·plasty (pī-lōr′-ō-plas-tē) *n* a plastic operation on the pylorus designed to widen the passage.

pyloro·spasm (pī-lōr′-ō-spazm) *n* spasm of the pylorus usually due to the presence of a duodenal ulcer.

py·lorus (pī-lōr′-us) *n* the opening of the stomach into the duodenum, encircled by a sphincter muscle—**pyloric** *adj*.

pyo·colpos (pī-ō-kol′-pus) *n* pus in the vagina.

pyo·dermia, pyo·derma (pī-ō-dėr′-mē-à) *n* chronic cellulitis of the skin, manifesting itself in granulation tissue, ulceration, colliquative necrosis or vegetative lesions—**pyodermic** *adj*.

pyo·genic (pī-ō-jen′-ik) *adj* pertaining to the formation of pus.

py·ometra (pī-ō-mē′-trà) *n* pus retained in the uterus and unable to escape through the cervix, due to malignancy or atresia—**pyometric** *adj*.

pyo·nephrosis (pī-ō-nef-rō′-sis) *n* distension of the renal pelvis with pus—**pyonephrotic** *adj*.

Pyo·pen (pī′-ō-pen) *n* proprietary name for carbenicillin*.

pyoperi·carditis (pī-ō-per-ē-kår-dī′-tis) *n* pericarditis* with purulent effusion.

pyopneumo·thorax (pī-ō-nū-mō-thōr′-aks) *n* pus and gas or air within the pleural sac.

pyor·rhea (pī-ōr-ē′-à) *n* a flow of pus, usually referring to that caused by periodontal* disease, *pyorrhea alveolaris.*

pyo·salpinx (pī-ō-sal′-pinks) *n* a fallopian tube containing pus.

pyo·thorax (pī-ō-thōr′-aks) *n* pus in the pleural cavity.

pyramid of the kidney (pir′-à-mid) ⇒ Figure 20.

pyrami·dal (pi-ram′-id-al) *adj* applied to some conical eminences in the body. *pyramidal cells* nerve cells in the pre-Rolandic area of the cerebral cortex, from which originate impulses to voluntary muscles. *pyramidal tracts* in the brain and spinal cord transmit the fibers arising from the pyramidal cells to the voluntary muscles.

pyrantel pamoate (pi-ran′-tel) *n* an antihelmintic used for treating roundworm and pinworm.

pyrazin·amide (pir-az-in′-à-mīd) *n* expensive oral antituberculosis drug. Hepatotoxicity guarded against by SGOT* tests twice weekly. Can produce gastrointestinal side effects. (Tebrazid.)

py·rexia (pī-reks′-ē-à) *n* ⇒ fever—**pyrexial** *adj*.

Pyrid·ium (pī-ri′-dē-um) *n* proprietary name for phenazopyridinc* hydrochloride.

pyrido·stigmine (pī-ri-dō-stig′-mēn) *n* a drug which inhibits the breakdown of acetylcholine at neuromuscular junctions. Used in myasthenia gravis. Less toxic and potent, and has more prolonged action than neostigmine. (Mestinon.)

pyri·doxine (pī-ri-doks′-ēn) *n* vitamin* B_6; may be connected with the utilization of unsaturated fatty acids or the synthesis of fat from proteins. Deficiency may lead to dermatitis and neuritic pains. Used in nausea of pregnancy and radiation sickness, muscular dystrophy, pellagra, the premenstrual syndrome etc.

pyri·methamine (pī-ri-meth′-à-mēn) *n* a powerful antimalarial widely used in prophylaxis. Suitable for administration to children. (Daraprim.)

pyro·gen (pī′-rō-jen) *n* a substance capable of producing fever—**pyrogenic** *adj*.

py·rosis (pī-rō′-sis) *n* (*syn* heartburn) eructation of acid gastric contents into the mouth, accompanied by a burning sensation felt behind the sternum.

pyro·therapy (pī-rō-thėr′-à-pē) *n* production of fever by artificial means. ⇒ hyperthermia.

pyrvinium pamoate (per-vin′-ē-um pam′-ō-āt) anthelmintic effective against threadworm; turns stools red.

py·uria (pī-ū′-rē-à) *n* pus in the urine (more than three leukocytes per high-power field)—**pyuric** *adj.*

PZI *abbr* protamine zinc insulin.

Q

Q fever a febrile disease caused by *Coxiella burnetti*. Human infection transmitted from sheep and cattle in which the organism does not produce symptoms. Pasteurization of milk kills *Coxiella burnetti*.

Quaalude (kwa′-lūd) *n* proprietary name for methaqualone.*

quadri·ceps (kwod′-ri-seps) *n* the quadriceps extensor femoris muscle of the thigh which possesses four heads and is composed of four parts (⇒ Figure 4).

quadri·plegia (kwo-dri-plē′-jē-à) *n* ⇒ tetraplegia—**quadriplegic** *adj.*

quad·ruple vaccine (kwod-rōō′-pl vaksēn′) a vaccine for immunization against diphtheria, pertussis, poliomyelitis and tetanus.

quali·tative (kwal′-i-tā-tiv) *adj* pertaining to quality.

quanti·tative (kwan′-ti-tā-tiv) *adj* pertaining to quantity.

quaran·tine (kwawr′-an-tēn) *n* a period of isolation* of infected or suspected people with the objective of preventing spread to others. For contacts it is usually the same period as the longest incubation period for the specific disease.

quar·tan (kwar′-tan) *adj* the word applied to intermittent fever with paroxysms occurring every 72 h (fourth day).

Quecken·stedt's test (kwek′-en-stets) performed during lumbar puncture. Compression on the internal jugular vein produces a rise in CSF pressure if there is no obstruction to circulation of fluid in the spinal region.

quelling react·ion (kwel′-ing) swelling of the capsule of a bacterium when exposed to specific antisera. The test identifies the genera, species or subspecies of bacteria causing a disease.

Questran (kwes′-tran) *n* proprietary name for lemon-flavored cholestyramine*.

quicken·ing (kwik′-en-ing) *n* the first perceptible fetal movements felt by the mother, usually at 16–18 weeks gestation.

quick·silver (kwik sil′-ver) *n* mercury.

quiesc·ent (kwē-es′-ent) *adj* becoming quiet. Used especially of a skin disease which is settling under treatment.

quinacrine (kwin′-à-krēn) *n* synthetic antimalarial substance, more effective than quinine, and better tolerated. (Atabrine.)

quin·estrol (kwin-es′-trol) *n* a synthetic female sex hormone which suppresses lactation. (Estrovis.)

quinethazone (kwin-eth′-à-zōn) *n* a thiazide diuretic.

quini·dine (kwin′-i-dēn) *n* an alkaloid similar to quinine*, but with a specific effect on the atrial muscle of the heart. Sometimes used in early atrial fibrillation, but only about 50% of patients respond. Therapy should not be continued for more than 10 days unless adequate response has been obtained. (Cardioquin.)

quin·ine (kwī′-nīn) *n* the chief alkaloid of cinchona, once the standard treatment for malaria. For routine use and prophylaxis, synthetic antimalarials are now preferred, but with the increasing risk of drug-resistant malaria, quinine is coming back into use in some areas. The drug also has some oxytocic action and has been employed as a uterine stimulant in labor. The main use is in management of 'night cramps' where it is given as 300–600 mg of bisulfate.

quinin·ism (kwīn′-in-izm) *n* headache, noises in the ears and partial deafness, disturbed vision and nausea arising from an idiosyncratic reaction to, or long-continued use of quinine.

quinsy (kwin′-sē) *n* ⇒ peritonsillar* abscess.

quo·tient (kwō′-shent) *n* a number obtained by division. *intelligence quotient* ⇒ intelligence. *respiratory quotient* the ratio between inspired oxygen and expired carbon dioxide during a specified time.

R

RA latex test for rheumatoid arthritis; discerns the presence in the blood of rheumatoid factor.

rabid (ra'-bid) *adj* infected with rabies.

rabies (rā'-bēz) *n* (*syn* hydrophobia) fatal infection in man caused by a virus; infection follows the bite of a rabid animal, e.g. dog, cat, fox, vampire bat. It is of worldwide distribution; vaccines are available—**rabid** *adj*.

racem·ose (ras'-i-mōs) *adj* resembling a bunch of grapes.

radial artery (rā'-dē-al) ⇒ Figure 9.

radial vein (rā'-dē-al) ⇒ Figure 10.

rad·ical (rad'-i-kal) *adj* pertaining to the root of a thing. *radical operation* usually extensive so that it is curative, not palliative.

radicul·ography (rad-i-kū-lo'-grà-fē) *n* X-ray of the spinal nerve roots after rendering them radiopaque to locate the site and size of a prolapsed intervertebral disc—**radiculogram** *n*.

radio·active (rā-dē-ō-ak'-tiv) *adj* emitting radiation due to instability of the atomic nuclei. *radioactive gold* used for investigation of liver disease. *radioactive iodine ([181]I)* a dose concentrates in the thyroid gland which is subsequently measured. An overactive gland concentrates 45% of the dose in 4 h. an underactive gland less than 20% in 48 h. *radioactive technetium* used for investigation of visceral lesions.

radio·biology (rā-dē-ō-bī-ol'-o-jē) *n* the study of the effects of radiation on living tissue—**radiobiological** *adj*, **radiobiologically** *adv*.

radio·caesium (rā-dē-ō-kē'-zē-um) *n* a radioactive form of the element caesium used in radiation treatment of disease.

radio·carbon (rā-dē-ō-kàr'-bon) *n* a radioactive form of the element carbon used for research into metabolism etc.

radio·graph (rā'-dē-ō-graf) *n* a photographic image formed by exposure to X-rays; the correct term for an 'X-ray'—**radiographic** *adj*.

radiogra·pher (rā-dē-og'-raf-èr) *n* a person qualified in the techniques of diagnostic or therapeutic radiography.

radiogra·phy (rā-dē-og'-raf-ē) *n* the use of X-radiation (a) to create images of the body from which medical diagnosis can be made (diagnostic radiography); or (b) to treat a person suffering from a (malignant) disease, according to a medically prescribed regime (therapeutic radiography).

radio·iodinated human serum albumin (RIHSA) (rā'-dē-ō-ī'-ō-din-āt-ed hū'-man sē'-rum al-bū'min) used for detection and localization of brain lesions, determination of blood and plasma volumes, circulation time and cardiac output.

radio·iodine uptake test (rā'-dē-ō-ī'-ō-dīn up'-tāk) ⇒ radioactive (iodine).

radio·isotope (rā'-dē-ō-īs'-ō-tōp) *n* (*syn* radionuclide) forms of an element which have the same atomic number but different mass numbers, exhibiting the property of spontaneous nuclear disintegration. When taken orally or by injection, can be traced by a Geigercounter. *radioisotope scan* pictorial representation of the amount and distribution of radioactive isotope present in a particular organ.

radiol·ogist (rā-dē-ol'-o-jist) a medical specialist in diagnosis by using X-rays and other allied imaging techniques.

radi·ology (rā-dē-ol'-o-jē) *n* the study of the diagnosis of disease by using X-rays and other allied imaging techniques—**radiological** *adj*, **radiologically** *adv*.

radio·mimetic (rā'-dē-ō-mim-et'-ik) *adj* produces effects similar to those of radiotherapy.

radio·nuclide (rā'-dē-ō-nū'-klīd) *n* ⇒ radioisotope.

radiopaque (rā-dē-ō-pāk') *adj* having the property of significantly absorbing X-rays, thus becoming visible on a radiograph. Barium and iodine compounds are used, as contrast media, to produce artificial radiopacity—**radiopacity** *n*.

radio·sensitive (rā-dē-ō-sen'-si-tiv) *adj* affected by X-rays. Applied to tumors curable by X-rays.

radio·therapist (rā-dē-ō-thèr'-à-pist) *n* a medical specialist in the treatment of disease by X-rays and other forms of radiation.

radio·therapy (rā-dē-ō-thèr'-à-pē) *n* the treatment of proliferative disease, especially cancer, by X-rays and other forms of radiation.

radium (rā'-dē-um) *n* a radioactive element occurring in nature, and still occasionally used in radiotherapy.

radius (rā'-dē-us) ⇒ Figures 2, 3.

radon seeds (rā'-don) capsules containing radon—a radioactive gas produced by the breaking up of radium atoms. Used in radiotherapy.

rale (rāl) *n* abnormal sound heard on auscultation of lungs when fluid is present in bronchi.

Ramsay Hunt syn·drome (ram'-zē hunt)

241

herpes zoster of the ear lobe with facial paralysis and loss of taste.

Ramstedt's oper·ation (ram'-stets) ⇒ pyloromyotomy.

ramus (rā'-mus) *n* a branch, as of a blood vessel or nerve–**rami,** *pl.*

rani·tidine (ra-ni'-tid-īn) *n* an antiulcer drug. It is a histamine H_2 receptor antagonist which decreases gastric acid secretion. (Zantac.)

ran·ula (ran'-ū-là) *n* a cystic swelling beneath the tongue due to blockage of a duct—**ranular** *adj.*

raphe (raf'-ē) *n* a seam, suture, ridge or crease; the median furrow on the dorsal surface of the tongue.

rarefac·tion (rār-e-fak'-shun) *n* becoming less dense, as applied to diseased bone—**rarefied** *adj.*

rash (rash) *n* skin eruption. *nettle rash* ⇒ urticaria.

Rashkind's sept·ostomy (rash'-kīnds sep-tos'-to-mē) when the pulmonary and systemic circulations do not communicate, an artificial atrial septal communication is produced by passing an inflatable balloon-ended catheter through the foramen ovale, filling the balloon with contrast media and pulling it back into the right atrium.

RAST *abbr* radioallergosorbent test. It is an allergen-specific IgE measurement.

rat-bite fever (rat'-bīt fē'-ver) a relapsing fever caused by *Spirillum minus* or by *Streptobacillus moniliformis.* The blood Wassermann* test is positive in the spirillary infection.

rational·ization (rash-on-al-ī-zā'-shun) *n* a mental process whereby a person justifies his or her behavior after the event, so that it appears more rational or socially acceptable.

rauwolfia (raw-wol'-fē-à) *n* dried root contains several alkaloids including reserpine*. It used to be prescribed as a tranquilizer but it has been replaced by more effective drugs. It is still sometimes used to lower blood pressure.

Rauzide (raw'-zīd) *n* proprietary name for bendroflumethazide*.

Raynaud's dis·ease (rā'-nōz) idiopathic trophoneurosis. Paroxysmal spasm of the digital arteries producing pallor and cyanosis of fingers or toes, and occasionally resulting in gangrene. Disease of young women.

Raynaud's pheno·menon (rā'-nōz) ⇒ vibration syndrome.

RBC *abbr* red blood cell or corpuscle. ⇒ blood.

RDS *abbr* respiratory* distress syndrome.

reac·tion (rē-ak'-shun) **1** response to a stimulus. **2** a chemical change, e.g. acid or alkaline reaction to litmus paper. *allergic reaction* ⇒ allergy.

re·agent (rē-ā'-jent) *n* an agent capable of participating in a chemical reaction, so as to detect, measure, or produce other substances.

reagin (rē'-à-jin) *n* IgE antibody.

re·ality orient·ation (RO) (rē-al'-i-tē ōr-ē-en-tā'-shun) *n* a form of therapy useful for withdrawn, confused and depressed patients; they are frequently reminded of their name, the time, place, date and so on. Reinforcement is provided by clocks, calendars and signs prominently displayed in the environment.

rebore (rē'-bōr) *n* ⇒ disobliteration.

recal·citrant (rē-kal'-si-trant) *adj* refractory. Describes medical conditions which are resistant to treatment.

recall (rē'-kawl) *n* part of the process of memory. Memory consists of memorizing, retention and recall.

recannul·ation (rē-kan-ū-lā'-shun) *n* re-establishment of the patency of a vessel.

recept·aculum (rē-sept-ak'-ū-lum) *n* receptacle, often acting as a reservoir. *receptaculum chyli* the pear-shaped commencement of the thoracic duct in front of the first lumbar vertebra. It receives digested fat from the intestine.

recep·tive sens·ory aphasia (rē-sep'-tiv sen'-sor-ē ā-fā'-zē-à) a type of aphasia* in which the patient is unable to put any meaning to the words he hears though he may well be able to understand other forms of communication such as miming, drawing and writing.

recep·tor (rē-sep'-tor) *n* sensory afferent nerve ending capable of receiving and transmitting stimuli.

recess·ive (rē-ses'-iv) *adj* receding; having a tendency to disappear. *recessive trait* a genetically controlled character or trait which is expressed when the specific allele* which determines it is present at both paired chromosomal loci (i.e. 'in double dose'). When the specific allele is present in single dose the characteristic is not manifest as its presence is concealed by the dominant allele at the partner locus. The exception is for X-linked genes in males, in which the single recessive allele on the X-chromosome will express itself so that the character is manifest. ⇒ Mendel's law.

recipi·ent (rē-sip'-ē-ent) *n* a person who receives something from a donor such as blood, bone marrow or an organ. ⇒ blood groups.

Recklinghausen's dis·ease (rek'-ling-howz-enz) a name given to two conditions: (a) osteitis fibrosa cystica—the result of overactivity of the parathyroid glands (hyperparathyroidism) resulting in decalcification of bones and formation of cysts; (b) multiple neurofibromatosis* the tumors can be felt beneath the skin along the course of nerves. There may be pigmented spots (café au lait) on the skin and there may also be pheochromocytoma.

re·cliner's reflux syn·drome (rē-klīn'-erz rē'-fluks) this is due to severe disturbance of the antireflux mechanism which allows stomach contents to leak at any time whatever position the patient is in, although it is most likely to happen when the patient lies down or slumps in a low chair.

recom·binant DNA (rē-kom'-bi-nant) DNA which is produced by deliberately piecing together (recombining chemically) the genic DNA of two different organisms. It is used for the study of the structure and function of both normal and abnormal genes and so, for example, of the molecular basis of human genetic disorders. Its practical applications are in diagnosis (including prenatal diagnosis) and in the manufacture of special gene products used in treatment, such as insulin.

Recombivax-HB (rē-kom'-bi-vaks) *n* proprietary name for hepatitis* B vaccine produced from yeast cultures.

recrud·escence (rē-krōō-des'-ens) *n* the return of symptoms.

rec·tal bladder a term used when the ureters are transplanted into the rectum, which is closed with the establishment of a proximal colostomy, in cases of severe disease of the urinary bladder.

rec·tal varices (rek'-tal vār'-i-sēz) hemorrhoids*.

recto·cele (rek'-tō-sēl) *n* prolapse* of the rectum, so that it lies outside the anus. Usually reserved for herniation of anterior rectal wall into posterior vaginal wall caused by injury to the levator muscles at childbirth. Repaired by a posterior colporrhaphy. ⇒ procidentia.

recto·scope (rek'-tō-skōp) *n* an instrument for examining the rectum. ⇒ endoscope—**rectoscopic** *adj*.

recto·sigmoid (rek-tō-sig'-moyd) *adj* pertaining to the rectum and sigmoid portion of colon.

recto·sigmoidectomy (rek-tō-sig-moyd-ek'-tō-mē) *n* surgical removal of the rectum and sigmoid colon.

recto·uterine (rek-tō-ū'-tèr-īn) *adj* pertaining to the rectum and uterus.

recto·vaginal (rek-tō-vaj'-in-al) *adj* pertaining to the rectum and vagina.

recto·vesical (rek-tō-ves'-ik-al) *adj* pertaining to the rectum and bladder.

rectum (rek'-tum) *n* the lower part of the large intestine between the sigmoid* flexure and anal canal (⇒ Figure 18)—**rectal** *adj*, **rectally** *adv*.

rectus abdominis (rek'-tus ab-dom'-in-is) ⇒ Figure 4.

rectus femoris (rek'-tus fem-ōr'-is) ⇒ Figure 4.

recum·bent (rē-kum'-bent) *adj* lying or reclining—**recumbency** *n*. *recumbent position* lying on the back with the head supported on a pillow; the knees are flexed and parted to facilitate inspection of the perineum.

recur·rent abortion (rē-kur'-ent ab-ōr'-shun) ⇒ abortion.

red lotion an old product containing zinc sulfate which acts as an astringent and assists granulation. Now replaced by zinc* sulfate lotion.

Re·doxon (re-doks'-on) *n* a proprietary preparation of ascorbic* acid.

re·ferred pain pain occurring at a distance from its source, e.g. pain felt in the upper limbs from angina pectoris; that from the gall bladder felt in the scapular region.

re·flex (rē'-fleks) **1** *adj* literally, reflected or thrown back; involuntary, not able to be controlled by the will. *reflex action* an involuntary motor or secretory response by tissue to a sensory stimulus, e.g. sneezing, blinking, coughing. The testing of various reflexes provides valuable information in the localization and diagnosis of diseases involving the nervous system. *reflex zone therapy* treatment of the feet for disorders in other parts of the body whether or not these disorders have resulted in signs and symptoms. **2** *n* a reflex action. *accommodation reflex* constriction of the pupils and convergence of the eyes for near vision. *conditioned reflex* a reaction acquired by repetition or practice. *corneal reflex* a reaction of blinking when the cornea is touched (often absent in hysterical conditions).

re·flux (rē'-fluks) *n* backward flow.

refrac·tion (rē-frak'-shun) *n* the bending of light rays as they pass through media of different densities. In normal vision, the light rays are so bent that they meet on the retina—**refractive** *adj*.

refrac·tory (rē-frak'-tōr-ē) *adj* resistant to treatment; stubborn, unmanageable; rebellious.

regener·ation (rē-jen-ėr-ā'-shun) *n* renewal of tissue.

re·gional ile·itis (rē'-jun-al-il-ē-ī'-tis) (*syn* Crohn's disease) a non-specific chronic recurrent granulomatous disease affecting mainly young adults and characterized by a necrotizing, ulcerating inflammatory process, there usually being an abrupt demarcation between it and healthy bowel. There can be healthy bowel ('skip' area) intervening between two diseased segments. The colon, rectum and anus may also be involved.

Regitine (re'-ji-tēn) *n* proprietary name for phentolamine*.

Reglan (reg'-lan) *n* proprietary name for metoclopramide*.

regres·sion (rē-gresh'-un) *n* in psychiatry, reversion to an earlier stage of development, becoming more childish. Occurs in dementia, especially senile dementia, and, more normally, in a young child following the birth of a sibling.

regurgi·tation (rē-gur-ji-tā'-shun) *n* backward flow, e.g. of stomach contents into, or through, the mouth.

rehabili·tation (rē-hab-il-it-ā'-shun) *n* a planned program in which the convalescent or disabled person progresses towards, or maintains, the maximum degree of physical and psychological independence of which he is capable.

Reiter protein complement fixation (RPCF) test (ri'-ter prō'-tē-en) a test for syphilis; uses an extract prepared from cultivatable treponemata.

Reiter's syn·drome (ri'-terz) a condition in which arthritis occurs together with conjunctivitis and urethritis (or cervicitis in women). It is commonly, but not always, a sexually transmitted infection and should be considered as a cause of knee effusion in young men when trauma has not occurred.

rejec·tion (rē-jek'-shun) *n* **1** the act of excluding or denying affection to another

person. **2** the process which leads to the destruction of grafted tissues.

relaps·ing fever (rē'-lap-sing fē'-ver) louse-borne or tick-borne infection caused by spirochetes of the genus *Borrelia*. Prevalent in many parts of the world. Characterized by a febrile period of a week or so, with apparent recovery, followed by a further bout of fever.

rela·tive humid·ity (rel'-a-tiv hū-mid'-i-tē) ⇒ humidity.

relax·ant (rē-laks'-ant) *n* that which reduces tension. ⇒ muscle.

relaxin (rē-laks'-in) *n* polypeptides secreted by the ovaries to soften the cervix and loosen the ligaments in preparation for birth.

REM sleep *abbr* ⇒ paradoxical sleep.

re·mission (rē-mish'-un) *n* the period of abatement of a fever or other disease.

re·mittent (rē-mit'-ent) *adj* increasing and decreasing at periodic intervals.

re·nal (rē'-nal) *adj* pertaining to the kidney. *renal adenocarcinoma* cancer of the kidney. *renal artery* ⇒ Figures 9, 19, 20. *renal asthma* hyperventilation of lungs occurring in uremia as a result of acidosis. *renal calculus** stone in the kidney. *renal capsule* ⇒ Figure 20. *renal erythropoietic factor* an enzyme released in response to renal (and therefore systemic) hypoxia. Once secreted into the blood, it reacts with a plasma globulin to produce erythropoietin. *renal failure* can only be described within the context of whether it is acute or chronic. Acute renal failure (ARF) occurs when previously healthy kidneys suddenly fail because of a variety of problems affecting the kidney and its circulation. This condition is potentially reversible. Chronic renal failure (CRF) occurs when irreversible and progressive pathological destruction of the kidney leads to terminal or end stage renal disease (ESRD). This process usually takes several years but once ESRD is reached, death will follow unless the patient is treated with some type of dialysis or renal transplant. ⇒ crush syndrome, tubular necrosis, uremia, *renal function tests* ⇒ kidney function tests. *renal glycosuria* occurs in patients with a normal blood sugar and a lowered renal threshold for sugar. *renal edema* inefficient kidney filtration disturbing the electrolyte balance and resulting in edema*. *renal rickets* ⇒ rickets. *renal transplant* kidney* transplant. *renal uremia* uremia* following kidney disease itself, in contrast to uremia from

Renese (ren′-ēs) *n* proprietary name for polythiazide*.

failure of the circulation of the blood (extrarenal uremia). *renal vein* ⇒ Figures 19, 20.

re·nin (ren′-in) *n* an enzyme released into the blood from the kidney cortex in response to sodium loss. It reacts with angiotensinogen (a plasma protein fraction) to produce angiotensin I, which in turn is converted into angiotensin II by an enzyme in the lungs. Excessive production of renin results in hypertensive kidney disease.

ren·nin (ren′-in) *n* milk curdling enzyme found in the gastric juice of human infants and ruminants. It converts caseinogen into casein, which in the presence of calcium ions is converted to an insoluble curd.

renogram (rē′-nō-gram) *n* X-ray of renal shadow following injection of opaque medium, demonstrated in aortograph series—**renographical,** *adj,* **renographically,** *adv.*

reo·virus (rē′-ō-vī-rus) *n* previously called respiratory enteric orphan virus* one of a group of RNA-containing viruses which can infect the respiratory and intestinal tracts without causing serious disease.

repetition strain injuries (re-pe-ti′-shun strān) includes back pain, pain in one or both arms, or legs, and maybe pins and needles. These seem to be caused by inappropriate movements, static muscle position and uncomfortable posture at work.

rep·ression (rē-presh′-un) *n* according to Freud*, the process whereby unacceptable and threatening thoughts and impulses are banished to the unconscious. Freud claimed that repressed thoughts and impulses still influenced behavior and experience, for example in dreams and also in neurotic symptoms.

repro·ductive system (rē-pro-duk′-tiv) the organs and tissues necessary for reproduction. In the male it includes the testes, vas deferens, prostate gland, seminal vesicles, urethra and penis (⇒ Figure 16). In the female it includes the ovaries, fallopian tubes, uterus, vagina and vulva (⇒ Figure 17).

RES *abbr* reticuloendothelial* system.

resec·tion (rē-sek′-shun) *n* surgical excision. *submucous resection (of nasal septum)* incision of nasal mucosa, removal of deflected nasal septum, replacement of mucosa.

resecto·scope (rē-sek′-to-skōp) *n* an instrument passed along the urethra; it permits resection of tissue from the base of the bladder and prostate under direct vision. ⇒ prostatectomy.

resecto·tome (rē-sek′-to-tōm) *n* an instrument used for resection.

reser·pine (rē-sėr′-pin) *n* the chief alkaloid of rauwolfia*. Used mainly in hypertension, sometimes with other drugs. Severe depression has occurred after full and prolonged therapy. Interferes with transmission in sympathetic adrenergic nerves, especially sympathetically mediated vascular reflexes and thus can lead to postural and exercise hypotension. (Serpasil.)

reser·voirs of infection (re′-zer-vwarz) the human ones are the hands, nose, skin and bowel; they have a natural flora which under certain circumstances can become pathogenic.

re·sidual (rē-zid′-ū-al) *adj* remaining. *residual air* the air remaining in the lung after forced expiration. *residual urine* urine remaining in the bladder after micturition.

resins (rez′-ins) *npl* water-insoluble solid or semi-solid amorphous organic polymers that can occur naturally or be manufactured synthetically. *ion exchange resins* ⇒ ion.

resist·ance (rē-zis′-tans) *n* power of resisting. In psychology the name given to the force which prevents repressed thoughts from re-entering the conscious mind from the unconscious. *resistance to infection* the capacity to withstand infection. ⇒ immunity *peripheral resistance* ⇒ peripheral.

resol·ution (rez-ō-lū′-shun) *n* the subsidence of inflammation; describes the earliest indications of a return to normal, as when, in lobar pneumonia, the consolidation begins to liquefy.

reson·ance (rez′-on-ans) *n* the musical quality elicited on percussing a cavity which contains air. *vocal resonance* is the reverberating note heard through the stethoscope when the patient is asked to say 'one, one, one' or '99'.

resor·cinol (rē-sōr′-sin-ol) *n* a drug which acts as a skin abrasive. Useful in a cream for acne and in a lotion for dandruff.

resorp·tion (rē-sōrp′-shun) *n* the act of absorbing again, e.g. absorption of (a) callus following bone fracture (b) roots of the deciduous teeth (c) blood from a hematoma.

245

respir·ation (res-pi-rā'-shun) *n* the process whereby there is gaseous exchange between a cell and its environment—**respiratory** *adj*. *external respiration* involves the absorption of oxygen from the air in the alveoli into the lung capillaries, and excretion of carbon dioxide from the blood in the lung capillaries into the air in the lungs. *internal* or *tissue respiration* is the reverse process—blood vessels supplying the cells carry oxygen which passes from the blood into the tissue cells, and carbon dioxide from the cells passes into the blood in vessels draining the cells. *paradoxical respiration* occurs when the ribs on one side are fractured in two places. During inspiration air is drawn into the unaffected lung via the normal route and also from the lung on the affected side. During expiration air is forced from the lung on the unaffected side, some of which enters the lung on the affected side, resulting in inadequate oxygenation of blood. ⇒ abdominal breathing, anaerobic respiration. Cheyne Stokes respiration, resuscitation.

respir·ator (res'-pi-rā-tor) *n* **1** an apparatus worn over the nose and mouth and designed to purify the air breathed through it. **2** an apparatus which artificially and rhythmically inflates and deflates the lungs when the natural nervous or muscular control of respiration is impaired, as in anterior poliomyelitis. The apparatus works by creation of low pressure around the thorax (tank respirators).

respir·atory dis·tress syn·drome (res'-pir-a-tōr-ē dis-tres') **(RDS)** *neonatal respiratory distress syndrome (NRDS)* dyspnea in the newly born. Due to failure of secretion of protein-lipid complex (pulmonary surfactant) by type II pneumocytes in the tiny air spaces of the lung on first entry of air. Causes atelectasis. Formerly called hyaline membrane disease. Environmental temperature of 32–34° C (90–94° F), oxygen and infusion of sodium bicarbonate are used in treatment. Clinical features include severe retraction of chest wall with every breath, cyanosis, an increased respiratory rate and an expiratory grunt. ⇒ lecithin-sphingomyelin ratio. *adult respiratory distress syndrome* (ARDS) acute respiratory failure due to non-cardiogenic pulmonary edema.

respir·atory fail·ure (res'-pir-a-tōr-ē fāl'-ūr) a term used to denote failure of the lungs to oxygenate the blood adequately. *acute respiratory failure* denotes respiratory insufficiency secondary to an acute insult to the lung; hypoxemia develops, frequently terminating in bronchopneumonia. *acute on chronic respiratory failure* hypoxemia resulting from chronic obstructive airways disease such as chronic bronchitis and emphysema.

respir·atory func·tion tests numerous tests are available for assessing respiratory function. These include measurements of the vital capacity (VC), forced* vital capacity (FVC), forced expiratory volume (FEV) (which is the volume of air that can be expired in 1 s) and the maximal breathing capacity (MBC) which is that quantity of air that can be shifted in 1 min.

respir·atory syn·cytial virus (RSV) (res'-pir-a-tōr-ē sin-sit'-ē-al) causes severe respiratory infection with occasional fatalities in very young children. Infections are less severe in older children.

respir·atory system deals with gaseous exchange. Comprises the nose, nasopharynx, larnyx, trachea, bronchi and lungs (Figures 6, 7).

respir·atory quo·tient (res'-pir-a-tōr-ē kwō'-shent) ⇒ quotient.

respon·aut (res'-pō-nut) *n* a person with permanent severe respiratory paralysis needing mechanical assistance for breathing.

rest·less leg syn·drome restless legs characterized by paresthesiae like creeping, crawling, itching and prickling.

resusci·tation (rē-sus-i-tā'-shun) *n* restoration to life of one who is apparently dead (collapsed or shocked). External massage is carried out for cardiac arrest by placing the patient on his back on a firm surface. The lower portion of the sternum is depressed 35–50 mm each second. To carry out artificial respiration the exhaled breath of the operator inflates the patient's lungs via one of three routes (a) mouth to mouth (b) mouth to nose (c) mouth to nose and mouth—**resuscitative** *adj*.

retar·dation (rē-tàr-dā'-shun) **1** the slowing of a process which has already been carried out at a quicker rate or higher level. **2** arrested growth or function from any cause.

retch·ing (rech'-ing) *n* straining at vomiting.

reten·tion (rē-ten'-shun) *n* **1** retaining of facts in the mind. **2** accumulation of that which is normally excreted. *retention cyst* a cyst* caused by the blocking of a duct. ⇒ ranula. *retention of urine* accumulation of urine within the bladder due to interference of nerve supply, obstruction or psychological factors.

reticu·lar (re-tik'-ū-lar) *adj* resembling a net.

reticulo·cyte (re-tik'-ū-lō-sīt) *n* a young circulating red blood cell which still contains traces of the nucleus which was present in the cell when developing in the bone marrow.

reticulo·cytoma (re-tik-ū-lō-sī-tō'-mà) *n* ⇒ Ewing's tumor.

reticulo·cytosis (re-tik-ū-lō-sī-tō'-sis) *n* an increase in the number of reticulocytes in the blood indicating active red blood cell formation in the marrow.

reticulo·endothelial system (re-tik'-ū-lō-en-dō-thē'-lē-al) **(RES)** a widely scattered system of cells, of common ancestry and fulfilling many vital functions, e.g. defense against infection, antibody, blood cell and bile pigment formation and disposal of cell breakdown products. Main sites of reticuloendothelial cells are bone marrow, spleen, liver and lymphoid tissue.

reticulo·endotheliosis (re-tik'-ū-lō-en-dō-thē-lē-ōs'-is) *n* term loosely used to describe conditions in which there is a reaction of reticuloendothelial cells.

retina (ret'-i-nà) *n* the light-sensitive internal coat of the eyeball, consisting of eight superimposed layers, seven of which are nervous and one pigmented (⇒ Figure 15). It is fragile, translucent and of a pinkish color—**retinal** *adj*.

retin·itis (ret-in-ī'-tis) *n* inflammation of the retina. *retinitis pigmentosa* a noninflammatory familial, degenerative condition which progresses to blindness, for which the word retinopathy is becoming more widely used.

retino·blastoma (ret'-in-ō-blas-tō'-mà) *n* a malignant tumor of the neuroglial element of the retina, occurring exclusively in children. Current research favors a chromosomal abnormality which may be indicated by low blood levels of an enzyme—esterase D.

retin·opathy (ret-in-op'-à-thē) *n* any noninflammatory disease of the retina. ⇒ retinitis.

re·tinoscope (ret'-in-ō-skōp) *n* instrument for detection of refractive errors by illumination of retina using a mirror.

retino·toxic (ret-in-ō-toks'-ik) *adj* toxic to the retina.

retrac·tile (rē-trak'-tīl) *adj* capable of being drawn back, i.e. retracted.

retrac·tor (re-trak'-tor) *n* a surgical instrument for holding apart the edges of a wound to reveal underlying structures.

retro·bulbar (ret-rō-bul'-bar) *adj* pertaining to the back of the eyeball. *retrobulbar neuritis* inflammation of that portion of the optic nerve behind the eyeball.

retro·cecal (ret-rō-sē'-kal) *adj* behind the cecum, e.g. a retrocecal appendix.

retro·flexion (ret-rō-flek'-shun) *n* the state of being bent backwards. ⇒ anteflexion *opp.*

retro·grade (ret'-rō-grād) *adj* going backward. *retrograde pyelography* ⇒ pyelography.

retro·lental fibro·plasia (re-trō-len'-tal fī-brō-plā'-zē-à) ⇒ fibroplasia.

retro·ocular (ret-rō-ok'-ū-lar) *adj* behind the eye.

retro·peritoneal (ret-rō-pėr-it-on-ē'-al) *adj* behind the peritoneum.

retro·pharyngeal (re-trō-fār-in-jē'-al) *adj* behind the pharynx.

retro·placental (ret-rō-plà-sent'-al) *adj* behind the placenta.

retro·pubic (ret-rō-pu'-bik) *adj* behind the pubis.

retro·spection (ret-rō-spek'-shun) *n* morbid dwelling on the past.

retro·sternal (ret-rō-stėrn'-al) *adj* behind the breast bone.

retro·tracheal (ret-rō-trāk'-ē-al) *adj* behind the trachea.

retro·version (ret-rō-vėr'-zhun) *n* turning backward. ⇒ anteversion *opp. retroversion of the uterus* tilting of the whole of the uterus backward with the cervix pointing forward—**retroverted** *adj*.

revascular·ization (rē-vas'-kū-lar-ī-zā'-shun) *n* the regrowth of blood vessel into a tissue or organ after deprivation of its normal blood supply.

re·verse bar·rier nurs·ing ⇒ barrier nursing.

Reye's syn·drome (rīz) 'wet brain and fatty liver' as described in 1963. There is cerebral edema without cellular infiltration, and diffuse fatty infiltration of liver and other organs, including the kidney. The age range of recorded cases is 2 months–15 years. Presents with vomiting, hypoglycemia and disturbed consciousness, jaundice being conspicuous. There is an association with salicylate administration and chicken pox.

Rh *abbr* Rhesus factor. ⇒ blood groups.

rhabdo·myolisis (rab-dō-mī-ol′-is-is) *n* sporadic myoglobinurea; a group of disorders characterized by muscle injury leading to degenerative changes. *non-traumatic rhabdomyolisis* ⇒ crush syndrome.

rhagades (rag′-a-dēz) *npl* superficial elongated scars radiating from the nostrils or angles of the mouth and which are found in congenital syphilis. ⇒ stigmata.

Rheo·macrodex (rē′-ō-mak′-rō-deks) *n* a proprietary low molecular weight dextran*. Antithrombotic. Used to prevent clots in grafted vein.

Rhe·sus factor (rē′-sus) ⇒ blood groups.

Rhe·sus incom·patability, iso·im·munization this problem arises when a Rhesus negative mother carries a Rhesus positive fetus. During the birth there is mixing of fetal and maternal bloods. The mother's body then develops antibodies against the rhesus positive blood. If a subsequent fetus is also Rhesus positive then mother's antibodies will attack the fetal blood supply causing severe hemolysis.

rheu·matic (rōō-mat′-ik) *adj* pertaining to rheumatism.

rheu·matic fever ⇒ rheumatism.

rheu·matism (rōō′-ma-tizm) *n* a non-specific term embracing a diverse group of diseases and syndromes which have in common, disorder or diseases of connective tissue and hence usually present with pain, or stiffness, or swelling of muscles and joints. The main groups are rheumatic fever, rheumatoid arthritis, ankylosing spondylitis, non-articular rheumatism, osteoarthritis and gout. *acute rheumatism* (*syn* rheumatic fever), a disorder, tending to recur but initially commonest in childhood, classically presenting as fleeting polyarthritis of the larger joints, pyrexia and carditis within three weeks following a streptococcal throat infection. Atypically, but not infrequently, the symptoms are trivial and ignored, but carditis may be severe and result in permanent cardiac damage. *non-articular rheumatism* involves the soft tissues and includes fibrositis, lumbago etc.

rheum·atoid (rōō′-ma-toyd) *adj* resembling rheumatism. *rheumatoid arthritis* a disease of unknown etiology, characterized by a chronic polyarthritis mainly affecting the smaller peripheral joints, accompanied by general ill health and resulting eventually in varying degrees of crippling joint deformities and associated muscle wasting. It is not just a disease of joints. Every system may be involved in some way. Many rheumatologists therefore prefer the term 'rheumatoid disease'. There is some question of it being an autoimmune process. *rheumatoid factors* macro gammaglobulins found in most people with severe rheumatoid arthritis. They affect not only joints but lung and nerve tissues and small arteries. It is not yet known whether they are the cause of, or the result of, arthritis. ⇒ pneumoconiosis, Still's disease.

rheuma·tology (rōō-ma-tol′-o-jē) *n* the science or the study of the rheumatic diseases.

rhin·itis (rī-nī′-tis) *n* inflammation of the nasal mucous membrane.

rhin·ology (rī-nol′-o-jē) *n* the study of diseases affecting the nose—**rhinologist** *n*.

rhi·nophyma (rī-nō-fī′-ma) *n* nodular enlargement of the skin of the nose.

rhino·plasty (rī′-nō-plas-tē) *n* plastic surgery of the nasal framework.

rhinor·rhea (rī-nōr-ē′-a) *n* nasal discharge.

rhi·noscopy (rī-nos′-ko-pē) *n* inspection of the nose using a nasal speculum or other instrument—**rhinoscopic** *adj*.

rhino·sporidosis (rī-nō-spōr-i-dō′-sis) *n* a fungal condition affecting the mucosa of the nose, eyes, ears, larynx and occasionally the genitalia.

Rhino·sporidium (rī-nō-spōr-id′-ē-um) *n* a genus of fungi parasitic to man.

rhino·virus (rī′-nō-vī′-rus) *n* there are about 100 different varieties which can cause the common cold.

rhi·zotomy (rī-zot′-o-mē) *n* surgical division of a root; usually the posterior root of a spinal nerve. *chemical rhizotomy* accomplished by injection of a chemical, often phenol*.

rho·dopsin (rō-dop′-sin) *n* the visual purple contained in the retinal rods. Its color is preserved in darkness; bleached by daylight. Its formation is dependent on vitamin* A.

RhoGam (rō′-gam) ⇒ anti-Rhesus* (Rh) serum.

rhom·boid (rom′-boyd) *adj* diamond shaped. *rhomboid muscles* ⇒ Figure 5.

rhon·chus (rong′-kus) *n* an adventitious sound heard on auscultation of the lung. Passage of air through bronchi obstructed by edema or exudate produces a musical note.

rhu·barb (rōō'-barb) *n* the dried root of Chinese *Rheum officinale*. It is purgative in large doses, astringent in small doses.

rhythm (rith'-um) *n* **1** a measured or regular period of time or movement. **2** a means of birth control consisting of calculating the intermenstrual periods of fertility in the female and avoiding coitus during that time.

ribo·flavin (rī'-bō-flā-vin) *n* a constituent of the vitamin* B group. Given in Ménière's disease, angular stomatitis and a variety of other conditions.

ribo·nuclease (rī-bō-nū'-klē-ās) *n* an enzyme that catalyzes the depolymerization of ribonucleic acid. Can be made synthetically.

ribo·nucleic acid (rī-bō-nū-klē'-ik) **(RNA)** nucleic acids found in all living cells. On hydrolysis they yield adenine, guanine, cytosine, uracil, ribose and phosphoric acid. They play an important part in protein synthesis.

ribo·somes (rī'-bō-sōms) *npl* submicroscopic protein-making agents inside all cells.

ribs (ribs) *n* the twelve pairs of bones which articulate with the twelve dorsal vertebrae posteriorly and form the walls of the thorax ($\Rightarrow$ Figure 6). The upper seven pairs are *true ribs* and are attached to the sternum anteriorly by costal cartilage. The remaining five pairs are the *false ribs* the first three pairs of these do not have an attachment to the sternum but are bound to each other by costal cartilage. The lower two pairs are the *floating ribs* which have no anterior articulation. *cervical ribs* are formed by an extension of the transverse process of the 7th cervical vertebra in the form of bone or a fibrous tissue band; this causes an upward displacement of the subclavian artery. A congenital abnormality.

rise-water stool (rīs'-wå-ter) the stool of cholera*. The 'rice grains' are small pieces of desquamated epithelium from the intestine.

rick·ets (rik'-ets) *n* a disorder of calcium and phosphorus metabolism associated with a deficiency of vitamin D, and beginning most often in infancy and early childhood between the ages of 6 months and 2 years. There is proliferation and deficient ossification of the growing epiphyses of bones, producing 'bossing', softening and bending of the long weight-bearing bones, muscular hypotonia, head sweating and, if the blood calcium falls sufficiently, tetany, *fetal rickets* achondroplasia*. *renal rickets* a condition of decalcification (osteoporosis) of bones associated with chronic kidney disease and clinically simulating rickets, occurs in later age groups and is characterized by excessive urinary calcium loss. *vitamin D resistant rickets* due to disease of the lower extremities producing short legs. Genetic illness. No deficiency of vitamin D. Serum levels of phosphorus low. No associated renal disease. Thought to be due to a defect in the tubular reabsorption of phosphorus and a lowered calcium absorption from the gut causing secondary hyperthyroidism and a vitamin D abnormality.

Rickett·sia (rik-et'-sē-å) *n* small pleomorphic parasitic microorganisms which have their natural habitat in the cells of the gut of arthropods. Some are pathogenic to mammals and man, in whom they cause the typhus group of fevers. They are smaller in size than bacteria and larger than the viruses. Many of their physiological characters resemble the bacteria, but like the viruses they are obligate intracellular parasites.

rick·ety ro·sary (rik'-e-tē rōz'-a-rē) a series of protuberances (bossing) at junction of ribs and costal cartilages in children suffering from rickets*.

rider's bone (rī'-derz bōn) a bony mass in the origin of the adductor muscles of the thigh, from repeated minor trauma in horseback-riding.

Riedel's thyroid·itis (re'-delz thī-royd-ī'-tis) a chronic fibrosis of the thyroid gland; ligneous goiter.

Ri·fadin (rif'-å-din) *n* proprietary name for rifampin*.

ri·fampin (rif-am'-pin) *n* an antibiotic. Main indication is in treating tuberculosis in association with other antitubercular drugs. Also useful in leprosy. It colors the urine, sputum and tears red and this can be used as proof of continuing treatment. (Rifadin, Rimactane.)

rifamycin (ri-få-mī'-sin) *n* antibiotic from Streptomyces group of organisms. Useful in resistant tuberculosis, and in Staphylococcal infections.

Rift val·ley fever one of the mosquito*-transmitted hemorrhagic fevers.

rigor (rig'-or) *n* a sudden chill, accompanied by severe shivering. The body temperature rises rapidly and remains high until perspiration ensues and causes a gradual fall in temperature. *rigor mortis* the stiffening of the body after death.

249

RIHSA *abbr* ⇒ radioiodinated* human serum albumin.

Ri·mactane (rī-mak'-tān) *n* proprietary name for rifampin*.

Ri·mifon (rim'-i-fon) *n* proprietary name for isoniazid*.

Ringer's lactate (ring'-erz lak'-tāt) Hartmann's solution.

ring·worm (ring'-werm) *n* (*syn* tinea) generic term used to describe contagious infection of the skin by a fungus, because the common manifestations are circular (circinate) scaly patches. ⇒ dermatophytes.

Rinne's test (rin'-nēz) testing of air conduction and bone conduction hearing, by tuning fork.

RIST *abbr* (radioimmunosorbent test) measures total serum IgE.

risus sardon·icus (ris'-us sàr-don'-i-kus) the spastic grin of tetanus*.

Ritalin (rit'-à-lin) *n* proprietary name for methylphenidate*.

river blind·ness a form of onchocerciasis*.

RN *abbr* registered nurse.

RNA *abbr* ribonucleic* acid.

RO reality* orientation.

Roba·xin (rō-baks'-in) *n* proprietary name for methocarbamol*.

Robinul (rob'-in-ul) *n* proprietary name for glycopyrrolate*.

Rocephin (rō-seph'-in) *n* proprietary name for ceftriaxone*.

Rocky mountain spotted fever a tickborne typhus fever caused by the parasite Rickettsia rickettsii.

rodent ulcer (rō'-dent) a basal cell carcinoma on the face or scalp which, although locally invasive, does not give rise to metastases.

Rogitine (rō'-ji-tēn) *n* proprietary name for phentolamine*. *Rogitine test* if hypertension is permanent an adrenalytic substance, Rogitine (phentolamine) 5 mg, is injected intravenously. A fall in excess of 35 mmHg in the systolic, and 25 mmHg in the diastolic pressure, occurring within 2 min of injection, is highly suggestive of pheochromocytoma.

rolfing (rolf'-ing) *n* massage of tissues around muscle to increase activity of the muscles.

ROM *abbr* range of motion.

Rom·berg's sign (rom'-bergz) a sign of ataxia*. Inability to stand erect (without swaying) when the eyes are closed and the feet together. Also called 'Rombergism'.

Rorschach test (rōr'-shak) a psychological test in which ten ink blots are shown to a person for interpretation.

ro·sacea (rō-zā'-sē-à) *n* a skin disease which shows on flush areas of the face. In areas affected there is chronic dilation of superficial capillaries and hypertrophy of sebaceous follicles, often complicated by an papulopustular eruption.

rose bengal (rōz ben'-gal) a staining agent used to detect diseased corneal and conjunctival epithelium.

ro·seola (rō-zē-ōl'-à) *n* a faint, pink spot, widespread in distribution except for the skin over the hands and face.

rota·viruses (rō-tà-vī'-rus-es) *npl* viruses associated with gastroenteritis in children and infants. Related to, but easily distinguished from, reoviruses*.

ro·tator (rō'-tà-tor) *n* a muscle having the action of turning a part.

Roth spots (roth) round white spots in the retina in some cases of bacterial endocarditis, thought to be of embolic origin.

rough·age (ruf'-aj) *n* ⇒ dietary fiber, bran.

rou·leaux (rōō'-lō) *n* a row of red blood cells, resembling a roll of coins.

round ligament of the uterus (round lig'-a-ment) ⇒ Figure 17.

round·worm (round'-werm) *n* (*Ascaris lumbricoides*) look like earth worms. Worldwide distribution. Parasitic to man. Eggs passed in stools; ingested, hatch in bowel, migrate through tissues, lungs and bronchi before returning to the bowel as mature worms. During migration worms can be coughed up—which is unpleasant and frightening. Heavy infections can produce pneumonia. A tangled mass can cause intestinal obstruction or appendicitis. The best drug for treatment is piperazine. Round-worm of the cat and dog is called *Toxocara*.

Rous sarcomavirus (RSV) (rous sàr-kō'-ma-vī'-rus) a virus of chickens which can cause tumors (sarcomas). A typical member of the RNA tumor virus group; despite much research no viruses belonging to this group have as yet been isolated from human tumors.

Roux·en·Y oper·ation (rōō-an-wī) originally the distal end of divided jejundum was anastomosed to the stomach, and the proximal jejunum containing the duodenal and pancreatic juices was anastomosed to the jejunum about 75 mm below the first anastomosis. The term is now used to include joining of the distal jejunum to a divided bile duct, esophagus or pancreas, in major surgery of these structures.

Rovsing's sign (rov′-sings) pressure in the left iliac fossa causes pain in the right iliac fossa in appendicitis.

RPCF *abbr* Reiter protein complement fixation.

RSI *abbr* repetition* strain injuries.

RSV *abbr* **1** respiratory* syncytial virus **2** Rous* sarcoma virus.

ru·befacients (rū-be-fāsh′-ents) *npl* substances which, when applied to the skin, cause redness (hyperemia).

ru·bella (rū-bel′-à) *n* (*syn* German measles) an acute, infectious, eruptive fever (exanthema) caused by a virus and spread by droplet infection. There is mild fever, a scaly, pink, macular rash and enlarged occipital and posterior cervical glands. Complications are rare, except when contracted in the early months of pregnancy, when it may produce fetal deformities. It is occasionally followed by a painful arthritis.

rubella titer blood test to determine immunity to rubella.

Ruben·stein-Taybi syn·drome a constellation of abnormal findings first described in 1963. It includes mental and motor retardation, broad thumbs and toes, growth retardation, susceptibility to infection in the early years and characteristic facial features.

rubor (rū′-bor) *n* redness; usually used in the context of being one of the four classical signs of inflammation—the others being calor*, dolor*, tumor*.

S

Sabin vaccine (sa′-bin) living attenuated polio virus which can be given orally. Produces active immunity against poliomyelitis.

sac *n* a small pouch or cyst-like cavity—**saccular, sacculated,** *adj*.

sacchar·ides (sak′-à-rīdz) *npl* one of the three main classes of carbohydrates (i.e. sugars).

sac·charin (sak′-à-rin) *n* a well-known sugar substitute. The soluble form is sometimes given intravenously as a test for circulation time, the end point being the perception of a sweet taste in the mouth.

saccharo·lytic (sak-à-rō-lit′-ik) *adj* having the capacity to ferment or disintegrate carbohydrates*—**saccharolysis** *n*.

Saccharo·myces (sak-à-rō-mī′-sēz) *n* a genus of yeasts which includes baker's and brewer's yeast.

sac·charose (sak′-à-rōs) *n* cane sugar; sucrose*.

saccu·lation (sak-ū-lā′-shun) *n* appearance of several saccules.

sac·cule (sak′-ūl) *n* a minute sac (⇒ Figure 13)—**saccular, sacculated** *adj*.

sacral (sā′-kral) *adj* pertaining to the sacrum. *sacral nerve* ⇒ Figure 11.

sacro·anterior (sā-krō-an-tēr′-ē-or) *adj* describes a breech presentation in obstetrics. The fetal sacrum is directed to one or other acetabulum of the mother—**sacroanteriorly** *adv*.

sacro·coccygeal (sā-krō-koks-i-jē′-al) *adj* pertaining to the sacrum* and the coccyx*.

sacro·iliac (sak-rō-il′-ē-ak) *adj* pertaining to the sacrum* and the ilium*.

sacro·ilitis (sak-rō-il-ē-ī′-tis) *n* inflammation of a sacroiliac joint. Involvement of both joints characterizes such conditions as ankylosing spondylitis. Reiter's syndrom and psoriatic arthritis.

sacro·lumbar (sāk-rō-lum′-bàr) *adj* pertaining to the sacrum* and the loins*.

sacro·posterior (sak-rō-pos-tēr′-ē-or) *adj* describes a breech presentation in obstetrics. The fetal sacrum is directed to one or other sacroiliac joint of the mother—**sacroposteriorly** *adv*.

sacro·spinalis muscle (sāk-rō-spin-al′-is) ⇒ Figure 5.

sacrum (sāk′-rum) *n* the triangular bone lying between the fifth lumbar vertebra and the coccyx (⇒ Figures 2, 3). It consists of five vertebrae fused together, and it articulates on each side with the innominate bones of the pelvis, forming the sacroiliac joints—**sacral** *adj*.

saddle nose (sad′-dl nōz) *n* one with a flattened bridge, often a sign of congenital syphilis*.

sadism (sā′-dizm) *n* the obtaining of pleasure from inflicting pain, violence or degradation on another preson, or on the sexual partner. ⇒ masochism *opp*.

sagit·tal (saj′-it-al) *adj* resembling an arrow. In the anteroposterior plane of the body. *sagittal suture* the immovable joint formed by the union of the two parietal bones.

Salazo·pyrin (sal-a-zō-pī′-rin) *n* proprietary name for sulfasalazine*.

SALICYLAMIDE

sali·cylamide (sal-i-sil'-à-mīd) *n* a mild analgesic similar in action to the salicylates, but less likely to cause gastric disturbance.

sali·cylic acid (sal-i-sil'-ik) has fungicidal and bacteriostatic properties, and is used in a variety of skin conditions. It is a constituent of Whitfield's ointment. The plaster is used to remove corns and warts.

saline (sā'-lēn) *n* a solution of salt and water. Normal or physiological saline is a 0.9% solution with the same osmotic pressure as that of blood. ⇒ hypertonic, isotonic.

sal·iva (sà-lī'-và) *n* the secretion of the salivary glands (spittle). It contains water, mucus and ptyalin*—**salivary** *adj.*

sal·ivary (sal'-i-vār-ē) *adj* pertaining to saliva. *salivary calculus* a stone formed in the salivary ducts. *salivary glands* the glands which secrete saliva, i.e. the parotid, submaxillary and sublingual glands.

sali·vation (sal-iv-ā'-shun) *n* an increased secretion of saliva.

Salk vac·cine (solk vak'-sēn) a preparation of killed poliomyelitis virus used as an antigen to produce active artificial immunity to poliomyelitis. It is given by injection.

Salmon·ella (sal-mon-el'-à) *n* a genus of bacteria. Gram-negative rods. Parasitic in many animals and man in whom they are often pathogenic. Some species, such as *Salmonella typhi*, are host-specific, infecting only man, in whom they cause typhoid fever. Others, such as *Salmonella typhimurium*, may infect a wide range of host species, usually through contaminated foods. *Salmonella enteritidis* a motile Gram-negative rod, widely distributed in domestic and wild animals, particularly in rodents, and sporadic in man as a cause of food poisoning.

salpin·gectomy (sal-pin-jek'-to-mē) *n* excision of a fallopian tube.

salpin·gitis (sal-pin-jī'-tis) *n* acute or chronic inflammation of the fallopian tubes. ⇒ hydrosalpinx, pyosalpinx.

salpingo·gram (sal-ping'-ō-gram) *n* radiological examination of tubal patency by retrograde introduction of opaque medium into the uterus and along the tubes—**salpingographic** *adj,* **salpingography** *n,* **salpingographically** *adv.*

salpingo-oophorectomy (sal-ping-ō-ō-ō-fōr-ek'-to-mē) *n* excision of a fallopian tube and ovary.

salpin·gostomy (sal-ping-os'-to-mē) *n* the operation performed to restore tubal patency.

sal·pinx (sal'-pingks) *n* a tube, especially the fallopian tube or the eustachian tube.

sal·salate (sal'-sà-lāt) *n* a non-steroidal anti-inflammatory drug. It is an ester of salicylic* acid which is insoluble in gastric juice, therefore it is less likely than aspirin* to cause gastric irritation and erosion. (Disalcid.)

salve (sav) *n* an ointment.

sal vol·atile (sal vol'-à-til) aromatic solution of ammonia. A household analeptic.

sand·fly (sand'-flī) *n* an insect (*Phlebotomus*) responsible for short, sharp, pyrexial fever called 'sandfly fever' of the tropics. Likewise transmits leishmaniasis.

Sandimmune (sand'-im-ūn) *n* proprietary name for cyclosporin*.

sanguin·eous (sang-gwin'-ē-us) *adj* pertaining to or containing blood.

Sanorex (san'-ōr-eks) *n* proprietary name for mazindol*.

Sansert (san'-sèrt) *n* proprietary name for methysergide*.

santo·nin (san'-tō-nin) *n* an anthelmintic once used for roundworm, but less toxic and more reliable drugs such as piperazine* are now preferred.

sa·phenous (sà-fē'-nus) *adj* apparent; manifest. The name given to the two main veins in the leg, the internal and the external (⇒ Figure 10), and to the nerves (⇒ Figure 11) accompanying them.

sapon·ification (sà-pon'-if-i-kā'-shun) *n* conversion into soaps and glycerol by heating with alkalis. Hydrolysis of an ester by an alkali.

sap·remia (sa-prē'-mē-à) *n* a general bodily reaction to circulating toxins and breakdown products of saprophytic (non-pathogenic) organisms, derived from one or more foci in the body.

sapro·phyte (sap'-rō-fīt) *n* free-living microorganisms obtaining food from dead and decaying animal or plant tissue—**saprophytic** *adj.*

sar·coid (sàr'-koyd) *adj* a term applied to a group of lesions in skin, lungs or other organs, which resemble tuberculous foci in structure, but the true nature of which is still uncertain.

sarcoid·osis (sàr-koyd-ōs'-is) *n* a granulomatous disease of unknown etiology in which histological appearances resemble tuberculosis. May affect any organ of the body, but most commonly presents as a condition of the skin, lymphatic glands or the bones of the hand.

sarcolemma (sàr-kō-lem′-mà) *n* the delicate outer membranous covering of the muscle fibrils.

sar·coma (sàr-kō′-mà) *n* malignant growth of mesodermal tissue (e.g. connective tissue, muscle, bone)—**sarcomata** *pl*, **sarcomatous** *adj*.

sarcoma·tosis (sàr-kō-mà-tō′-sis) *n* a condition in which sarcomata are widely spread throughout the body.

Sar·coptes (sàr-kop′-tēz) *n* a genus of Acerina. *Sarcoptes scabiei* is the itch mite which causes scabies*.

sar·torius (sàr-tō′-rē-us) *n* the 'tailor's muscle' of the thigh, since it flexes one leg over the other (⇒ Figures 4, 5).

scab (skab) *n* a dried crust forming over an open wound.

scabies (skā′-bēz) *n* a parasitic skin disease caused by the itch mite. Highly contagious.

scald (skold) *n* an injury caused by moist heat.

sca·lenus syn·drome (ska-lē′-nus) pain in arm and fingers often with wasting, because of compression of the lower trunk of the brachial plexus behind scalenus anterior muscle at the thoracic outlet.

scalp (skalp) *n* the hair-bearing skin which covers the cranium. *scalp cooling* the application of a cap made of coils through which flows cold water; research shows that it prevents doxorubicin-induced alopecia.

scal·pel (skal′-pl) *n* a surgeon's knife, which may or may not have detachable blades.

scan (skan) *n* an image built up by movement along or across the object scanned, either of the detector or of the imaging agent, to achieve complete coverage, e.g. ultrasound* scan.

scan·ning speech (skan′-ing) a form of dysarthria occurring in disseminated sclerosis. The speech is jumpy or staccato or slow.

scaph·oid (skaf′-oyd) *n* boat-shaped, as a bone of the tarsus and carpus. *scaphoid abdomen* concavity of the anterior abdominal wall, often associated with emaciation.

scap·ula (skap′-ū-là) *n* the shoulderblade—a large, flat triangular bone (⇒ Figures 2, 3)—**scapular** *adj*.

scar (skar) *n* (*syn* cicatrix) the dense, avascular white fibrous tissue, formed as the end-result of healing, especially in the skin.

scarifi·cation (skar-if-i-kā′-shun) *n* the making of a series of small, superficial incisions or punctures in the skin.

scarla·tina (skar-là-tē′-nà) *n* (*syn* scarlet fever) infection by Group A β-hemolytic streptococcus. Occurs mainly in children. Begins commonly iwth a throat infection, leading to fever and the outbreak of a punctuate erythematous rash on the skin of the trunk. Characteristically the area around the mouth escapes (circumoral pallor)—**scarlatinal** *adj*.

scar·let fever (skar′-let) ⇒ scarlatina.

scar·let red a dye once used as a stimulating ointment (2–5%) for clean but slow-healing ulcers, wounds and pressure sores.

SCAT *abbr* sheep cell agglutination test. Rheumatoid factor in the blood is detected by the sheep cell agglutination titer.

Scheuer·mann's dis·ease (shoy′-ermanz) osteochondritis* of the spine affecting the ring epiphyses of the vertebral bodies. Occurs in adolescents.

Schick test (shik) a test used to determine a person's susceptibility or immunity to diphtheria. It consists of the injection of 2 or 3 minims of freshly prepared toxin beneath the skin of the left arm. A similar test is made into the right arm, but in this the serum is heated to 75° C for 10 min, in order to destroy the toxin but not the protein. A positive reaction is recognized by the appearance of a round red area on the left arm within 24–48 h reaching its maximum intensity on the fourth day, then gradually fading with slight pigmentation and desquamation. This reaction indicates susceptibility or absence of immunity. No reaction indicates that the subject is immune to diphtheria. Occasionally a pseudoreaction occurs, caused by the protein of the toxin; in this case the redness appears on both arms, hence the value of the control.

Schilder's dis·ease (shil′-dèrs) a genetically determined degenerative disease associated with mental subnormality.

Schil·ling test (shil′-ing) estimation of absorption of radioactive vitamin B_{12} for confirmation of pernicious anemia.

Schisto·soma (skis-tō-sō′-mà) *n* (*syn Bilharzia*) a genus of blood flukes which require fresh water snails as an intermediate host before infesting humans. *Schistosoma haematobium* is found mainly in Africa and the Middle East. *Schistosoma japonicum* is found in Japan, the Philippines and Eastern Asia. *Schistosoma mansoni* is indigenous to Africa, the Middle East, the Caribbean and South America.

schisto·somiasis (skis-tō-sō-mī'-a-sis) *n* (*syn* bilharziasis) infestation of the human body by *Schistosoma* which enter via the skin or mucous membrane. A single fluke can live in one part of the body, depositing eggs frequently for many years. Prevention is by chlorination of drinking water, proper disposal of human waste and eradication of fresh water snails. Schistosomiasis is a serious problem in the tropics and the Orient. The eggs are irritating to the mucous membranes which thicken and bleed causing anemia, together with pain and dysfunction of the afflicted organ; fibrosis of mucous membranes can cause obstruction.

schisto·somicide (skis-tō-sō'-mi-sīd) *n* any agent lethal to *Schistosoma*—**schistosomicidal** *adj.*

schizo·phrenia (skiz-ō-frē'-nē-a) *n* a group of psychotic mental illnesses characterized by disorganization of the patient's personality. Their course can be at times chronic, at times marked by intermittent attacks which may stop or become retrograde at any stage. Once affected a complete return to the premorbid personality is, however, unlikely. There are three elements common to all cases: a shallowness of emotional life; an inappropriateness of emotion; unrealistic thinking. *catatonic schizophrenia* type of schizophrenia characterized by episodes of immobility with muscular rigidity or stupor, interspersed with periods of acute excitability. *simple schizophrenia* the least disorganized form of schizophrenia characterized by apathy and withdrawal. Onset is usually at an early age but hallucinations and delusions are absent. Increasingly, simple schizophrenics are being cared for in the community.

schizo·phrenic (skiz-ō-fren'-ik) *adj* pertaining to schizophrenia. *schizophrenic syndrome in childhood* considered to be the best diagnostic label, rather than 'autism' or 'psychosis in childhood'.

Schlatter's dis·ease (shlat'-ėrz) (*syn* Osgood-Schlatter's disease) osteochondritis* of the tibial tubercle.

Schlemm's canal (shlems) a lymphati-covenous canal in the inner part of the sclera, close to its junction with the cornea, which it encircles.

Scholz's dis·ease (shōlz) a genetically determined degenerative disease associated with mental subnormality.

Schönlein's dis·ease (shān'-līnz) Henoch*-Schönlein purpura.

Schultz-Charlton test (shultz-chårl'-ton) a blanching produced in the skin of a patient showing scarlatinal rash, around an injection of serum from a convalescent case, indicating neutralization of toxin by antitoxin.

Schwartze's oper·ation (shwårtz) opening of the mastoid process for the excision of infected bone and drainage of cellular suppuration.

sciatica (sī-at'-i-ka) *n* pain in the line of distribution of the sciatic nerve (buttock, back of thigh, calf and foot).

scintillography (sin-til-og'-raf-ē) *n* (*syn* scintiscanning) visual recording of radioactivity over selected areas after administration of suitable radioisotope.

scir·rhous (skir'-rus) *adj* hard; resembling a scirrhus.

scir·rhus (skir'-us) *adj* a carcinoma which provokes a considerable growth of hard, connective tissue; a hard carcinoma of the breast.

scissor leg deform·ity (siz'-or leg) the legs are crossed in walking—following double hip-joint disease, or as a manifestation of Little's disease (spastic cerebral diplegia).

scis·sors gait (siz'-ors) ⇒ gait.

sclera (skle'-ra) *n* the 'white' of the eye (⇒ Figure 15); the opaque bluish-white fibrous outer coat of the eyeball covering the posterior five-sixths; it merges into the cornea at the front—**sclerae** *pl*, **scleral** *adj.*

scler·ema (skler-ē'-ma) *n* a rare disease in which hardening of the skin results from the deposition of mucinous material.

scler·itis (skler-ī'-tis) *n* inflammation of the sclera*.

sclero·corneal (skler-ō-kŏr'-nē-al) *adj* pertaining to the sclera* and the cornea*, as the circular junction of these two structures.

sclero·derma (skler-ō-der'-ma) *n* a disease in which localized edema of the skin is followed by hardening, atrophy, deformity and ulceration. Occasionally it becomes generalized, producing immobility of the face, contraction of the fingers; diffuse fibrosis of the myocardium, kidneys, digestive tract and lungs. When confined to the skin it is termed morphea. ⇒ collagen, dermatomyositis.

scler·osis (skler-ōs'-is) *n* a word used in pathology to describe abnormal hardening or fibrosis of a tissue. ⇒ multiple sclerosis, tuberous sclerosis—**sclerotic** *adj*.

sclero·therapy (skler-ō-thėr'-a-pē) *n* injection of a sclerosing agent for the treatment of varicose veins. When, after the injection, rubber pads are bandaged over the site to increase localized compression, the term *compression sclerotherapy* is used. Sclerotherapy for esophageal varices involves the use of an esophagoscope, either rigid or flexible—**sclerotherapeutic** *adj*, **sclerotherapeutically** *adv*.

scler·otic (skler-ot'-ik) *adj* pertaining to or exhibiting the symptoms of sclerosis.

scler·otomy (skler-ot'-o-mē) *n* incision of sclera for relief of acute glaucoma, prior to doing a decompression operation.

scolex (skō'-leks) *n* the head of the tapeworm by which it attaches itself to the intestinal wall, and from which the segments (proglottides) develop.

scoli·osis (skō-lē-ōs'-is) *n* lateral curvature of the spine, which can be congenital or acquired and is due to abnormality of the vertebrae, muscles and nerves. *idiopathic scoliosis* is characterized by a lateral curvature together with rotation and associated rib hump or flank recession. The treatment is by spinal brace or traction or internal fixation with accompanying spinal fusion. ⇒ Milwaukee brace, halopelvic traction, Harrington rod—**scoliotic** *adj*.

scopol·amine (skōp-ol'-à-mēn) *n* ⇒ hyoscine.

scor·butic (skōr-bū'-tik) *adj* pertaining to scorbutus, the old name for scurvy*.

scot·oma (skō-tō'-mà) *n* a blind spot in the field of vision. May be normal or abnormal—**scotomata** *pl*. *scotopic vision* the ability to see well in poor light.

'screen·ing' (skrēn'-ing) *n* fluoroscopy*.

scrapie (skrā'-pē) *n* a virus disease of sheep and goats.

Scriver test (skrī'-vėr) remarkably efficient in detecting, by a single procedure, 22 aminoacidopathies.

scrof·ula (skrof-ū-là) *n* tuberculosis of bone or lymph gland—**scrofulous** *adj*.

scrofulo·derma (skrof-ū-lō-dėr'-mà) *n* an exudative and crusted skin lesion, often with sinuses, resulting from a tuberculous lesion, underneath, as in bone or lymph glands. Rare in Europe but common in the tropics.

scro·tum (skrō'-tum) *n* the pouch in the male which contains the testes (⇒ Figure 16)—**scrotal** *adj*.

SCU *abbr* special care unit.

scurf (skurf) *n* a popular term for dandruff*.

scurvy (skur'-vē) *n* a deficiency disease caused by lack of vitamin* C (ascorbic acid). Clinical features include fatigue and hemorrhage. Latter may take the form of oozing at the gums or large ecchymoses. Tiny bleeding spots on the skin around hair follicles are characteristic. In children painful subperiosteal hemorrhage (rather than other types of bleeding) is pathognomonic.

scybala (sib'-à-là) *n* rounded, hard, fecal lumps—**scybalum** *sing*.

Sea Legs proprietary name for meclizine*.

seb·aceous (seb-ā'-shus) *adj* literally, pertaining to fat; usually refers to sebum*. *sebaceous cyst* (*syn* wen) a retention cyst in a sebaceous (oil-secreting) gland in the skin. Such cysts are most commonly found on the scalp, scrotum and vulva. *sebaceous glands* the cutaneous glands which secrete an oily substance called 'sebum.' The ducts of these glands are short and straight and open into the hair follicles (⇒ Figure 12).

sebor·rhea (seb-ōr-ē'-à) *n* greasy condition of the scalp, face, sternal region and elsewhere due to overactivity of sebaceous* glands. The seborrheic type of skin is especially liable to conditions such as alopecia, seborrheic dermatitis, acne etc.

sebum (sē'-bum) *n* the normal secretion of the sebaceous* glands; it contains fatty acids, cholesterol and dead cells.

secobarbital (sek-ō-bàrb'-i-tol) *n* a short-acting barbiturate with the general properties of the group, used in mild insomnia and anxiety conditions.

Se·conal (sek'-on-al) *n* proprietary name for secobarbital.

se·cretin (sē-krē'-tin) *n* a hormone produced in the duodenal mucosa, which causes a copious secretion of pancreatic juice.

se·cretion (sē-krē'-shun) *n* a fluid or substance formed or concentrated in a gland and passed into the alimentary tract, the blood or to the exterior.

se·cretory (sē'-krē-tōr-ē) *adj* involved in the process of secretion; describes a gland which secretes.

Sec·tral (sek'-tral) *n* proprietary name for acebutolol*.

sed·ation (sed-ā'-shun) *n* the production of a state of lessened functional activity.

seda·tive (sed'-ȧ-tiv) *n* an agent which lessens functional activity.

sedimentation rate (*abbr*, ESR) ⇒ erythrocyte sedimentation rate.

seg·ment (seg'-ment) *n* a small section; a part—**segmental** *adj*, **segmentation** *n*.

segre·gation (seg-reg-ā'-shun) *n* in genetics, the separation from one another of two alleles, each carried on one of a pair of chromosomes; this happens at meiosis* when the haploid, mature germ cells (the egg and the sperm) are made.

Seid·litz pow·der (sīd'-litz) a once popular aperient. It is dispensed as two powders, one containing sodium potassium tartrate and sodium bicarbonate, the other containing tartaric acid. Both powders are dissolved in water and taken as an effervescent draught.

Seldinger cath·eter (sel'-ding-ėr) a special catheter and guide wire for insertion into an artery, along which it is passed to, for example, the heart.

Selec·tron (sel-ek'-tron) *n* a proprietary device which stores sealed radioactive sources of cesium in a shielded container in readiness for intracavitary treatment of cesium in uterus, cervix or vagina.

seleno·methionine (sel-en-ō-meth-ī'-o-nēn) *n* an injection in which the sulfur atom present in the amino acid methionine is replaced by radioactive selenium. Taken up selectively by the pancreas; valuable in diagnosis of pancreatic disease.

self catheter·ization (self kath-e-ter-ī-zā'-shun) both male and female patients can be taught to pass a catheter into the urinary bladder to evacuate urine intermittently.

self infec·tion (self in-fek'-shun) the unwitting transfer of microorganisms from one part of the body to another in which it produces an infection.

self-monitoring of blood glucose (SMBG) (self mon'-i-tor-ing) blood from a finger prick is applied to a reagent strip to give the hemoglobin A_{lc} ($H6A_{lc}$) level which reflects the blood glucose level.

sella turcica (sel'-lȧ-tur'-si-kȧ) pituitary* fossa.

semen (sē'-men) *n* the secretion from the testicles and accessory male organs, e.g. prostate. It contains spermatozoa*.

semi·circular canals (sem-i-sir'-kū-lar kȧ-nalz') three membranous semicircular tubes contained within the bony labyrinth of the internal ear (⇒ Figure 13). They are concerned with appreciation of the body's position in space.

semi·comatose (sem-i-kō'-mȧ-tōs) *adj* describes a condition bordering on the unconscious.

semi·lunar (sem-i-lū'-nar) *adj* shaped like a crescent or half moon. *semilunar cartilages* the crescentic interarticular cartilages of the knee joint (menisci).

semi·membranosus muscle (sem-i-mem-bran-ōs'-us) ⇒ Figure 5.

semi·nal (sem'-i-nal) *adj* pertaining to semen. *seminal vesicle* ⇒ Figure 16.

semin·iferous (sem-in-if'-ėr-us) *adj* carrying or producing semen.

semin·oma (sem-in-ō'-mȧ) *n* a malignant tumor of the testis—**seminomata** *pl*, **seminomatous** *adj*.

semi·permeable (sem-i-pėr'-mē-ȧ-bl) *adj* describes a membrane which is permeable to some substances in solutions, but not to others.

semi·spinalis muscle (sem-i-spin-al'-is) ⇒ Figure 5.

semi·tendinosus muscle (sem-i-ten-din-ōs'-us) ⇒ Figure 5.

sen·escence (sē-nes'-ens) *n* normal changes of mind and body in increasing age—**senescent** *adj*.

Seng·staken tube (sengz'-tā-ken) incorporates a balloon which after being positioned in the lower esophagus is inflated to apply pressure to bleeding esophageal varices.

senile (sē'-nīl) *adj* suffering from senescence* complicated by morbid processes commonly called degeneration—**senility** *n*.

senna (sen'-nȧ) *n* leaves and pods of a purgative plant from Egypt and India. Once used extensively as 'black draught' or compound senna mixture. (Senokot.)

Sen·okot (sen'-o-kot) *n* proprietary name for standardized senna*.

sen·sible (sen'-sib-l) *n* **1** endowed with the sense of feeling. **2** detectable by the senses.

sensi·tization (sen-si-tī-zā'-shun) *n* rendering sensitive. Persons may become sensitive to a variety of substances which may be food (e.g. shellfish), bacteria, plants, chemical substances, drugs, sera, etc. Liability is much greater in some persons than others. ⇒ allergy, anaphylaxis.

sensori·neural (sen-sor-i-nūr′-al) *adj* pertaining to sensory neurons. *sensorineural deafness* a discriminating term for nerve deafness*.

sen·sory (sen′-sor-ē) *adj* pertaining to sensation. *sensory nerves* those which convey impulses to the brain and spinal cord (⇒ Figure 1).

senti·ment (sen′-ti-ment) *n* a group of emotionally charged tendencies centered on some person or object. Sentiments increase with experience of the environment.

sep·sis (sep′-sis) *n* the state of being infected with pus-producing organisms—**septic** *adj*.

sep·tic abor·tion ⇒ abortion.

septi·cemia (sep-ti-sēm′-ē-à) *n* the persistence and mutliplication of living bacteria in the blood stream—**septicemic** *adj*.

Sep·tra (sep′-trà) *n* a proprietary name for co-trimoxazole*.

sep·tum (sep′-tum) *n* a partition between two cavities, e.g. between the nasal cavities—**septa** *pl*. **septal, septate** *adj*.

se·quela (sē-kwē′-là) *n* pathological consequences of a disease, e.g. pock-marks of smallpox—**sequelae** *pl*.

seques·trectomy (sē-kwes-trek′-to-mē) *n* excision of a sequestrum*.

seques·trum (sē-kwes′-trum) *n* a piece of dead bone which separates from the healthy bone but remains within the tissues—**sequestra** *pl*.

Serax (sēr′-aks) *n* proprietary name for oxazepam*.

serol·ogy (sē-rol′-o-jē) *n* the branch of science dealing with the study of sera—**serological** *adj*, **serologically** *adv*.

sero·purulent (sē-rō-pūr′-ū-lent) *adj* containing serum* and pus*.

ser·osa (sē-rōz′-à) *n* a serous membrane*, e.g. the peritoneal covering of the abdominal viscera—**serosal** *adj*.

sero·sitis (sē-rō-sī′-tis) *n* inflammation of a serous membrane*.

sero·tonin (sē-rō-tōn′-in) *n* a product of tryptophan metabolism. Liberated by blood platelets after injury and found in high concentrations in many body tissues including the CNS. It is a vasoconstrictor, inhibits gastric secretion, stimulates smooth muscle. Serves as a central neurotransmitter and is a precursor of melatonin. Together with histamine it may be concerned in allergic reactions. Called also 5-hydroxytryptamine and 5-HT.

ser·ous (sē′-rus) *adj* pertaining to serum*. *serous membrane* ⇒ membrane.

Ser·pasil (sėr′-pà-sil) *n* proprietary name for reserpine*.

serpigin·ous (sėr-pij′-in-us) *adj* snakelike, coiled, irregular; used to describe the margins of skin lesions, especially ulcers and ringworm.

Ser·ratia (sėr-ā′-shē-à) *n* a genus of Gram-negative bacilli capable of causing infection in humans. It is an endemic hospital resident. ⇒ infection.

ser·ration (sėr-ā′-shun) *n* a saw-like notch—**serrated** *adj*.

serratus muscles (sėr′-a-tus) ⇒ Figures 4, 5.

serum (sē′-rum) *n* supernatant fluid which forms when blood clots—**sera** *pl*. *serum glutamic oxaloacetic transaminase (SGOT)* enzyme normally present in serum and also found in heart, liver and muscle tissue. It is released into the serum as a result of tissue damage and hence its increased presence may be due to myocardial infarction or actue liver disease. *serum sickness* ⇒ anaphylaxis.

serum gonadotropin (sē′-rum gō-nad-ō-trō′-pin) an ovarian stimulating hormone obtained from the blood serum of pregnant mares. It is used in amenorrhea, often in association with estrogens.

SES *abbr* socioeconomic status.

sex-linked refers to genes which are located on the sex chromosomes or, more especially, on the X chromosome. To avoid confusion it is now customary to refer to the latter genes (and the characters determined by them) as X-linked.

sex·ual abuse (seks′-ū-al a-būs′) ⇒ incest.

sex·ual inter·course (seks′-ū-al in′-ter-kōrs) coitus*.

sexually trans·mitted dis·ease (seks′-ū-al-ē tranz-mit′-ed) previously called venereal disease.

SGA *abbr* small for gestational age.

SGOT *abbr* ⇒ serum glutamine oxaloacetic transaminase.

SGPT *abbr* serum* glutamic pyruvic transaminase.

sham feed·ing (sham) enteral* feeding.

shear·ing force (shēr′-ing fōrs) when any part of the supported body is on a gradient, the deeper tissues near the bone 'slide' towards the lower gradient while the skin remains at its point of contact with the supporting surface because of friction which is increased in the presence of moisture. The deep blood vessels are stretched and angulated, thus the deeper tissues become ischemic with consequent necrosis. ⇒ pressure sores.

sheep·skin (shēp'-skin) *n* natural or synthetic fleeces are used to prevent pressure sores. They are placed to distribute pressure over pressure bearing areas whether the patient is confined to bed or chair.

shelf oper·ation an operation to deepen the acetabulum in congenital dislocation of the hip joint, involving the use of a bone graft. Performed at 7–8 years, after failure of conservative treatment.

shia·tsu (shē-àt'-sū) *n* a form of manipulation by thumbs, fingers and palms, without the use of instruments, mechanical or otherwise, to apply pressure to the human skin to correct internal malfunctioning, promote and maintain health and treat specific diseases.

Shigella (shig-el'-là) *n* a genus of bacteria containing some of the organisms causing dysentery. *Shigella flexueri* a pathogenic, Gram-negative rod, which is the most common cause of bacillary dysentery epidemics, and sometimes infantile gastroenteritis. It is found in the feces of cases of dysentery and carriers, whence it may pollute food and water supplies.

shin bone (shin'-bōn) the tibia, the medial bone of the foreleg.

shingles (shing'-ls) *n* a condition arising when the infecting agent (herpes zoster virus) attacks sensory nerves causing severe pain and the appearance of vesicles along the nerve's distribution (usually unilateral). ⇒ herpes zoster virus.

Shirod·kar's oper·ation (shir-od'-kàrs) placing of a purse-string suture around an incompetent cervix during pregnancy. It is removed when labor starts.

shock (shok) *n* the circulatory disturbance produced by severe injury or illness and due in large part to reduction in blood volume. There is discrepancy between the circulating blood volume and the capacity of the vascular bed. Initial cause is reduction in circulating blood volume; perpetuation is due to vasoconstriction, therefore vasoconstrictor drugs are not given. Its features includes a fall in blood pressure, rapid pulse, pallor, restlessness, thirst and a cold clammy skin.

short-circuit oper·ation (shōr ser'-kit) an anastomosis designed to bypass an obstruction in a conducting channel, e.g. gastrojejunostomy.

shortsighted·ness *n* ⇒ Myopia.

shoulder girdle (shōl'-der ger'-dl) formed by the clavicle and scapula on either side.

shoulder lift ⇒ Australian lift.

'show' *n* a popular term for the blood-stained vaginal discharge at the commencement of labor.

shunt (shunt) *n* a term applied to the passage of blood through other than the usual channel.

sialagogue (sī-al'-à-gog) *n* an agent which increases the flow of saliva.

sialo·gram (sī-al'-ō-gram) *n* radiographic image of the salivary glands and ducts, after injection of an opaque medium— **sialography** *n,* **sialographic** *adj,* **sialographically** *adv.*

sialo·lith (sī-al'-ō-lith) *n* a stone in a salivary gland or duct.

sib·ling (sib'-ling) *n* one of a family of children having the same parents.

sickle-cell anemia *n* ⇒ anemia.

side effect any physiological change other than the desired one from drug administration, e.g. the antispasmodic drug propantheline causes the side effect of dry mouth in some patients. The term also covers undesirable drug reactions. Some are predictable, being the result of a known metabolic action of the drug, e.g. yellowing of skin and eyes with mepacrine; thinning of skin and bone and formation of striae with corticosteroids; loss of hair with cyclophosphamide. Unpredictable reactions can be: (a) immediate: anaphylactic shock, angioneurotic edema (b) erythematous: all forms of erythema, including nodosum and multiforme and purpuric rashes (c) cellular eczematous rashes and contact dermatitis (d) specific e.g. light-sensitive eruptions with ledermycin and griseofulvin.

siderosis (sid-ėr-ōs'-is) *n* excess of iron in the blood or tissues. Inhalation of iron oxide into the lungs can cause one form of pneumoconiosis*.

SIDS *abbr* sudden infant death syndrome ⇒ crib death.

sig·moid (sig'-moyd) *adj* shaped like the letter S. *sigmoid colon* ⇒ Figure 18. *sigmoid flexure* ⇒ flexure.

sigmoid·oscope (sig-moyd'-o-skōp) *n* an instrument for visualizing the rectum and sigmoid flexure of the colon. ⇒ endoscope—**sigmoidoscopic** *adj*, **sigmoidoscopy** *n*.

sigmoid·ostomy (sig-moyd-os'-to-mē) *n* the formation of a colostomy in the sigmoid* colon.

sign (sīn) *n* any objective evidence of disease.

Si·lastic (sī-las'-tik) *n* proprietary name for polymeric silicone substances which have the properties of rubber. They are biologically inert and are used in surgical prostheses and implants.

sili·cone (sil'-i-kōn) *n* an organic compound which is water-repellant. *silicone foam dressing* a soft durable substance fits exactly the contours of an open granulating wound in which it encourages healing.

sili·cosis (sil-i-kō'-sis) *n* a form of pneumoconiosis* or 'industrial dust disease' found in metal grinders, stone-workers etc.

sil·ver ni·trate (sil'-ver nī'-trāt) in the form of small sticks, is used as a caustic for warts. Occasionally used as antiseptic eye drops (1%), and as an application to ulcers. Now being used in 0.5% solution for burns to control bacterial infection in postburn period. Causes sodium and chloride loss from wound surface. Sodium chloride given orally or intravenously. Urine tested for chlorides.

silver sulfadiazine silver derivative of sulfadiazine. Topical bacteriostatic agent, which can play a vital role in reducing morbidity. A burn area cannot be sterilized, but the use of silver sulfadiazine means that the bacteria are merely picnicking on the burns rather than getting a deep-seated hold.

Silver·man score (sil'-ver-man) a method of rating respiratory distress by assessing movement of accessory muscles and degree of expiratory grunt.

simian crease (sim'-ē-àn) a fused crease on the palm of the hand associated with congenital abnormalities including Down syndrome.

Simmond's disease (sim'-onds) patient becomes emaciated, suffers from early senility, face wrinkles, hair becomes gray and sparse, blood pressure lowers, pulse slows, bones become frail. Previously called hypopituitary cachexia.

simple frac·ture (sim'-pl frak'-tur) ⇒ fracture.

Sim's pos·ition (simz) an exaggerated left lateral position with the right knee well flexed and the left arm drawn back over the edge of the bed.

Sim's specu·lum (*syn* duck bill speculum) a hinged two-bladed instrument which can be inserted into the vagina; as the blades are separated the cervix and upper vaginal walls are visible.

sinciput (sin'-si-put) *n* the upper half of the skull, including the forehead.

Sine·met (sin'-e-met) *n* a proprietary preparation of levodopa* combined with carbidopa* in 10:1 ratio.

Sine·quan (sin'-e-kwan) *n* proprietary name for doxepin*.

sinew (sin'-oo) *n* a ligament or tendon.

sino·atrial node (sī-nō-ā'-trē-al) ⇒ node.

sinus (sī'-nus) *n* **1** a hollow or cavity, especially the nasal sinuses (⇒ Figure 14). **2** a channel containing blood, especially venous blood, e.g. the sinuses of the brain. **3** a recess or cavity within a bone. **4** any suppurating tract or channel. *sinus arrhythmia* an increase of the pulse rate on inspiration, decrease on expiration. Appears to be normal in some children. ⇒ cavernous, pilonidal.

sinus·itis (sī-nus-ī'-tis) *n* inflammation of a sinus, used exclusively for the paranasal sinuses.

sinus·oid (sī'-nus-oyd) *n* a dilated channel into which arterioles or veins open in some organs and which take the place of the usual capillaries.

sitz-bath (sits bath) *n* a hip bath.

Sjögren-Larsson syn·drome (shō'-gren-Lär'-son) genetically determined congenital ectodermosis. Associated with mental subnormality.

Sjögren syn·drome (shō'-gren) deficient secretion from lacrimal, salivary and other glands, mostly in postmenopausal women. There is keratoconjunctivitis, dry tongue and hoarse voice. Thought to be due to an autoimmune process. Also called kerato-conjunctivitis sicca.

skel·eton (skel'-e-ton) *n* the bony framework of the body, supporting and protecting the soft tissues and organs (⇒ Figures 2, 3)—**skeletal** *adj*. *appendicular skeleton* the bones forming the upper and lower extremeities. *axial skeleton* the bones forming the head and trunk.

Skene's glands (skēnz) two small glands at the entrance to the female urethra; the paraurethral glands.

skin *n* the tissue which forms the outer covering of the body; it consists of two main layers: (a) the epidermis, or cuticle, forming the outer coat (b) the dermis, or cutis vera, the inner or true skin, lying beneath the epidermis. ⇒ Figure 12. *skin shedding* skin is continually shedding its outer keratinized cells as scales. As the skin has a natural bacterial flora, the scales are a potential source of infection for susceptible patients. ⇒ psoriasis.

skull (skul) *n* the bony framework of the head (⇒ Figure 2). ⇒ cranium.

sleep (slēp) *n* a naturally altered state of consciousness occurring in humans in a 24 h biological rhythm. A *sleep cycle* consists of orthodox* sleep and paradoxical* sleep; each cycle lasts approximately 60–90 min, and needs to be completed for the person to gain benefit. *sleep apnea* ⇒ apnea. *sleep deprivation* a cumulative condition arising when there is interference with a person's established rhythm of paradoxical* sleep. It can result in slurred rambling speech, irritability, disorientation, slowed reaction time, malaise, progressing to illusions, delusions, paranoia and hyperactivity.

sleep·sick·ness (slēp'-ing sik'-nes) a disease endemic in Africa, characterized by increasing somnolence caused by infection of the brain by trypanosomes. ⇒ trypanosomiasis.

sleep-walk·ing (slēp'-wok-ing) ⇒ somnambulism.

sling (sling) *n* a bandage used for support.

slipped disc (slipd disk) *n* prolapsed intervertebral disc. ⇒ prolapse.

slipped epiphysis (slipd ē-pif'-i-sis) displacement of an epiphysis, especially the upper femoral one. ⇒ epiphysis.

slough (sluf) *n* septic tissue which becomes necrosed and separates from the healthy tissue.

Slow K a proprietary slow-release potassium chloride product.

slow re·lease drugs *n* drug formulations which do not dissolve in the stomach but in the small intestine where the drug is slowly released and absorbed. Some drugs are now incorporated into a skin patch, which after application permits slow release.

slow virus *n* an infective agent which only produces infection after a long latent period and many cases may never develop overt symptoms but may still be a link in the chain of infectivity. ⇒ Creutzfeldt-Jakob disease.

small-for-dates ⇒ low birthweight.

small·pox (smawl'-poks) *n* (*syn* variola)

caused by a virus eradicated following WHO world-wide campaign. Prophylaxis against the disease is by vaccination. ⇒ vaccinia.

SMBG *abbr* self-monitoring* of blood glucose.

smear (smēr) *n* a film of material spread out on a glass slide for microscopic examination. *cervical smear* microscopic examination of cells scraped from the cervix to detect carcinoma-in-situ. ⇒ carcinoma.

smegma (smeg'-mà) *n* the sebaceous secretion which accumulates beneath the prepuce and clitoris.

smell·ing salts a mixture of compounds usually containing some form of ammonia, which acts as a stimulant, when inhaled.

Smith-Petersen nail (smith pē'-ter-son) a trifin, cannulated metal nail used to provide internal fixation for intracapsular fractures of the femoral neck.

smokers' blind·ness (*syn* tobacco amblyopia) absorption of cyanide in the nicotine of smoke. The sight gets worse, color vision goes, the victim can go blind. Cyanide prevents absorption of vitamin B_{12}. Injection of hydroxycobalamin is therapeutic.

snare (snār) *n* a surgical instrument with a wire loop at the end; used for removal of polypi.

Snellen's test types (snel'-enz) a chart for testing visual acuity.

snow *n* solid carbon dioxide. Used for local freezing of the tissues in minor surgery.

snuf·fles (snuf'-lz) *n* a snorting inspiration due to congestion of nasal mucous membrane. It is a sign of early congenital (prenatal) syphilis when the nasal discharge may be purulent or blood-stained.

S.O.A.P. notes method of recording nursing notes using subjective and objective data, assessment and plan.

SOB *abbr* shortness of breath.

social isolation a term which can be applied to one person, a family or a group of people. Those 'isolated' do not interact with other human beings in the usual pattern, for any one of a number of reasons.

socio·cultural (sō-sē-ō-kul'-tūr-al) *adj* pertaining to culture in its sociological setting.

soci·ology (sō-sē-ol'-o-jē) *n* the scientific

study of interpersonal and intergroup social relationships—**sociological** *adj*.

socio·medical (sō-sē-ō-med'-i-kal) *adj* pertaining to the problems of medicine as affected by sociology.

so·dium acid phos·phate (sō'-dē-um as'-id fos'-fāt) saline purgative and diuretic. It increases the acidity of the urine, and is given with hexamine as a urinary antiseptic.

so·dium amy·tal (sō'-dē-um am'-i-tol) amobarbital.

so·dium bi·carbonate (sō-dē-um bī-kàr'-bon-āt) a domestic antacid, given for heartburn, etc. For prolonged therapy alkalis that cause less rebound acidity are preferred.

so·dium chlor·ide (sō'-dē-um klōr'-īd) Salt, present in body tissues. Used extensively in shock and dehydration as intravenous normal saline, or as dextrosesaline in patients unable to take fluids by mouth. Used orally as replacement therapy in Addison's disease, in which salt loss is high. When salt is lost from the body, there is compensating production of renin.

so·dium ci·trate (sō'-dē-um sī'-trat) an alkaline diuretic very similar to potassium citrate. Used also as an anticoagulant for stored blood, and as an addition to milk feeds to reduce curdling.

sodium flouride ((sō'-dē-um flōr'-īd) white powder used in drinking water and solutions for preventing dental caries.

so·dium iodide (sō'-dē-um ī'-ō-dīd) used occasionally as an expectorant, and as a contrast agent in retrograde pyelography.

so·dium per·borate (sō'-dē-um pėr'-bōr-āt) aqueous solutions have antiseptic properties similar to those of hydrogen peroxide, and are used as mouthwashes, etc.

sodium peroxide (sō'-dē-um pėr'oks'-īd) used for bleaching.

so·dium pro·pionate (sō'-dē-um prō'-pi-on-āt) used as an antimycotic in fungal infections as gel, ointment, lotion and pessaries.

so·dium salicyl·ate (sō'-dē-um sal-is'-il-āt) has the analgesic action of salicylates in general, and formerly used in rheumatic fever. Large doses are essential. Chronic rheumatoid conditions do not respond so well.

so·dium sulf·ate (so'-dē-um sul'-fāt) a popular domestic purgative. A 25% solution is used as a wound dressing. Given intravenously as a 4.3% solution in anuria.

so·dium tetra·decyl sulf·ate (sō'-dē-um tet'-rà-dek'-l sul'-fāt) a sclerosant liquid for injection into veins to obliterate them and shrink varicosities.

soft palate ⇒ Figure 14.

soft sore the primary ulcer of the genitalia occurring in the venereal disease chancroid.

solar plexus (sō'-lar pleks'-us) a large network of sympathetic (autonomic) nerve ganglia and fibers, extending from one adrenal gland to the other. It supplies the abdominal organs.

soleus muscle (sō'-lē-us) ⇒ Figures 4, 5.

Solu-Cortef (sol'-ū-kōr'-tef) *n* hydrocortisone sodium succinate, used for severe asthma.

sol·ute (sol'-ūt) *n* that which is dissolved in a solvent.

sol·ution (sol-oo'-shun) *n* a fluid which contains a dissolved substance or substances. *saturated solution* one in which the maximum possible quantity of a particular substance is dissolved. Therefore further additions of the substance remain undissolved.

sol·vent (sol'-vent) *n* an agent which is capable of dissolving other substances (solutes). The component of a solution which is present in excess.

so·matic (som-at'-ik) *adj* pertaining to the body. *somatic cells* body cells, as distinct from germ cells*. *somatic nerves* nerves controlling the activity of striated, skeletal muscle.

somato·statin (som-at'-ō-sta'-tin) *n* growth hormone release-inhibiting hormone (GH-RIH).

somato·trophin (som-at-ō-trō'-fin) *n* ⇒ growth hormone.

Sombulex (som'-bū-leks) *n* proprietary name for hexobarbital*.

somnam·bulism (som-nam'-bū-lizm) *n* (*syn* sleepwalking) a state of dissociated consciousness in which sleeping and waking states are combined. Considered normal in children but as an illness having a hysterical basis in adults.

Sonne dys·entery (son'-nē dis'-en-tėr-ē) bacillary dysentery caused by infection with *Shigella sonnei* (Sonne bacillus). The organism is excreted by cases and carriers in their feces, and contaminates hands, food and water, from which new hosts are infected.

sono·graph (son'-ō-graf) *n* graphic record of sound waves. **sonogram**, *n*.

sopor·ific (sop-ōr-if'-ik) *adj, n* describes an agent which induces profound sleep.

Sor·bitol (sōr'-bi-tōl) *n* proprietary liquid for parenteral feeding.

sordes (sōr'-dēz) *npl* dried, brown crusts which form in the mouth, especially on the lips and teeth, in illness.

sot·alol (sot'-à-lol) *n* an antihypertensive of the beta-adrenoceptor blocking type exemplified by propanolol.

souf·fle (sōō'-fl) *n* puffing or blowing sound. *funic souffle* auscultatory murmur of pregnancy. Synchronizes with the fetal heartbeat and is caused by pressure on the umbilical cord. *uterine souffle* soft, blowing murmur which can be auscultated over the uterus after the fourth month of pregnancy.

sound *n* an instrument to be introduced into a hollow organ or duct to detect a stone or to dilate a stricture.

source isol·ation is for patients who are sources of microorganisms which may spread from them to infect others. *strict source isolation* is for highly transmissible and dangerous diseases. *standard source isolation* is for other communicable diseases.

soya bean (soy'-à-bēn) a highly nutritious legume* used in Asiatic countries in place of meat. It contains high-quality protein and little starch. Is useful in diabetic preparations. Soya protein is a constituent of soya milk used as a substitute for cow's milk by strict vegetarians (vegans) and by persons with cow's milk allergy.

span·sules (span'-sūls) *n* a chemically prepared formulation for drugs designed to obtain controlled release via oral route.

Spar·ine (spār'-ēn) *n* proprietary name for promazine*.

spasm (spazm) *n* convulsive, involuntary muscular contraction.

spas·modic colon (spaz-mod'-ik kō'-lon) megacolon*.

spas·modic dysmenor·rhea (spaz-mod'-ik dis'-men-ōr-ē'-a) ⇒ dysmenorrhea.

spas·molytic (spaz-mō-lit'-ik) *adj, n* current term for antispasmodic drugs—spasmolysis *n*.

spas·tic (spas'-tik) *adj* in a condition of muscular rigidity or spasm, e.g. spastic diplegia (Little's disease). *spastic dystonic syndrome* abnormality of gait and foot posture usually due to brain damage at birth. Difficult to treat because imbalance in various opposing muscles has developed over a long period. *spastic gait* ⇒ gait. *spastic paralysis* results mainly from upper motor neuron lesions. There are exaggerated tendon reflexes.

spas·ticity (spas-tis'-it-ē) *n* condition of rigidity or spasm of muscle.

spat·ula (spat'-ū-là) *n* a flat flexible knife with blunt edges for making poultices and spreading ointment. *tongue spatula* a rigid, blade-shaped instrument for depressing the tongue.

species (spē'-shēz) *n* a systematic category, subdivision of genus. Natural groups of organisms actually or potentially interbreeding but biologically different so that they are reproductively isolated from one another. The individuals within a species group have common characteristics and differ generally fairly clearly from those of a related species.

specific (spes-if'-ik) *adj* special; characteristic; peculiar to. *specific disease* one that is always caused by a specified organism. *specific dynamic action* ⇒ action. *specific gravity* the weight of a substance, as compared with that of an equal volume of water, the latter being represented by 1000.

spectino·mycin (spek-tin'-ō-mī'-sin) *n* an antibiotic which is useful for resistant microorganisms. It is the drug of choice in the treatment of gonorrhea.

spectro·photometer (spek-trō-fō-to'-me-tèr) a spectroscope combined with a photometer for quantitatively measuring the relative intensity of different parts of a light spectrum—**spectrophotometric** *adj.*

spectro·scope (spek'-trō-skōp) *n* an instrument for observing spectra of light.

specu·lum (spek'-ū-lum) *n* an instrument used to hold the walls of a cavity apart, so that the interior of the cavity can be examined—**specula** *pl.*

speech mechan·ism (spēch mek'-an-izm) involves the processes of breathing, phonation, articulation, resonance and prosody. It is disturbed in various combinations in dysarthria* and dysphasia*.

speech ther·apy (spēch thèr'-à-pē) a paramedical specialty. It aims to maximize the many essential skills concerned with language ability in those people born with mental or physical handicap; or in those who have lost these skills because of disease.

sperm (spèrm) *n* an abbreviated form of the word spermatozoon* or spermatozoa. *sperm count* an infertility test. If there are less than 60 million sperms in an ejaculation of semen there is accompanying sterility; between 300 and 500 million is normal.

sper·matic (sperm-at'-ik) *adj* pertaining to or conveying semen. *spermatic cord* suspends the testicle in the scrotum and contains the spermatic artery and vein and the vas deferens ($\Rightarrow$ Figure 16).

spermaticidal (sperm-at-is-ī'-dal) *adj* lethal to spermatozoa*.

spermato·genesis (sperm-at-ō-jen'-es-is) *n* the formation and development of spermatozoa—**spermatogenetic** *adj*.

spermator·rhea (sperm-at-ōr-ē'-à) *n* involuntary discharge of semen without orgasm.

spermato·zoon (sperm-at-ō-zō'-on) *n* a mature, male reproductive cell—**spermatozoa** *pl*.

spermi·cide, spermato·cide (sperm'-i-sīd) *n* an agent that kills spermatozoa—**spermicidal** *adj*.

sphe·noid (sfē'-nóyd) *n* a wedge-shaped bone at the base of the skull containing a cavity, the sphenoidal sinus—**sphenoidal** *adj*.

sphero·cyte (sfēr'-ō-sīt) *n* round red blood cell, as opposed to biconcave—**spherocytic** *adj*.

sphero·cytosis (sfēr-ō-sī-tō'-sis) *n* (*syn* acholuric jaundice) a heredofamilial genetic disorder transmitted as a dominant gene, i.e. with a one in two chance of transmission. It exists from birth but can remain in abeyance throughout life; sometimes discovered by 'accidental' examination of the blood. $\Rightarrow$ jaundice.

sphinc·ter (sfink'-tèr) *n* a circular muscle, contraction of which serves to close an orifice ($\Rightarrow$ Figure 19).

sphincter·otomy (sfink-tèr-ot'-o-mē) *n* surgical division of a muscular sphincter.

sphingo·myelinase (sfing-ō-mī'-el-in-ās) *n* an essential enzyme in lipid metabolism and storage.

sphygmo·cardio·graph (sfig-mō-kàr'-dē-ō-graf) *n* an apparatus for simultaneous graphic recording of the radial pulse and heart-beats—**sphygmocardiographic** *adj*, **sphygmocardiographically** *adv*.

sphygmo·graph (sfig'-mō-graf) *n* an apparatus attached to the wrist, over the radial artery, which records the movements of the pulse beat—**sphygmographic** *adj*.

sphygmo·manometer (sfig-mō-man-om'-e-tèr) *n* an instrument used for measuring the blood pressure.

spica (spī'-kà) *n* a bandage applied in a figure-of-eight pattern.

spic·ule (spī'-kūl) *n* a small, spike-like fragment, especially of bone.

spigot (spig'-ot) *n* glass, wooden or plastic peg used to close a tube.

spina bifida (spī'-nà-bif'-id-à) a congenital defect in which there is incomplete closure of the neural canal, usually in the lumbo-sacral region. *spina bifida occulta* the defect does not affect the spinal cord or meninges. It is often marked externally by pigmentation, a hemangioma, a tuft of hair or a lipoma which may extend into the spinal canal. *spina bifida cystica* an externally protruding spinal lesion. It may vary in severity from meningocele to myelomeningocele. The condition can be detected in utero in mid-pregnancy by an increased concentration of alphafetoprotein in the amniotic fluid or by ultrasonography.

spinal (spī'-nal) *n* pertaining to the spine. *spinal anesthetic* a local anesthetic solution is injected into the subarachnoid space, so that it renders the area supplied by the selected spinal nerves insensitive. *spinal canal* $\Rightarrow$ vertebral canal. *spinal caries* disease of the vertebral bones. *spinal column* $\Rightarrow$ vertebral column. *spinal cord* the continuation of nervous tissue of the brain down the spinal canal to the level of the first or second lumbar vertebra ($\Rightarrow$ Figures 1, 11). *spinal nerves* 31 pairs leave the spinal cord and pass out of the spinal canal to supply the periphery.

spine (spīn) *n* 1 a popular term for the bony spinal or vertebral column. 2 a sharp process of bone—**spinous, spinal** *adj*.

spinnbarkheit (spin'-bàr-kīt) *n* viscosity of cervical mucus, useful in estimating time of ovulation.

Spir·illum (spī-ril'-um) *n* a bacterial genus. Cells are rigid screws or portions of a turn. Common in water and organic matter. *Spirillum minus* is found in rodents and may infect man, in whom it causes one form of rat*-bite fever—**spirilla** *pl*, **spirillary** *adj*.

spiro·chete (spī'-rō-kēt) *n* bacterium having a spiral shape—**spirochetal** *adj*.

spiro·chetemia (spī-rō-kēt-ēm'-ē-à) *n* spirochetes in the blood stream. This kind of bacteremia occurs in the secondary stage of syphilis and in the syphilitic fetus—**spirochetemic** *adj*.

spiro·graph (spī'-rō-graf) *n* an apparatus which records the movement of the lungs—**spirographic** *adj*, **spirography** *n*, **spirographically** *adv*.

spi·rometer (spī-ro'-met-ėr) *n* an instrument for measuring the capacity of the lungs—**spirometric** *adj*, **spirometry** *n*.

spirono·lactone (spī-ron-ol-ak'-tōn) *n* a potassium-sparing antialdosterone preparation. It acts on the complex biochemical processes involved in edematous accumulation and causes renal excretion of sodium and water. (Aldactone.)

spittle (spit'-tl) *n* (*syn* sputum) matter which is expectorated from the lungs.

Spitz·Holter valve (spits hōl'-ter) a special valve used to drain hydrocephalus.

splanch·nic (splangk'-nik) *adj* pertaining to or supplying the viscera.

splanchni·cectomy (splangk-knik-ek'-to-mē) *n* surgical removal of the splanchnic nerves, whereby the viscera are deprived of sympathetic impulses; occasionally performed in the treatment of hypertension or for the relief of certain kinds of visceral pain.

splanch·nology (splangk-nol'-o-jē) *n* the study of the structure and function of the viscera.

spleen (splēn) *n* a lymphoid, vascular organ immediately below the diaphragm, at the tail of the pancreas, behind the stomach. It can be enlarged in reactive and neoplastic conditions affecting the reticuloendothelial system.

splen·ectomy (splen-ek'-to-mē) *n* surgical removal of the spleen.

splenic anemia (splen'-ik a-nē'-mē-a) *n* ⇒ anemia.

splen·itis (splen-ī'-tis) *n* inflammation of the spleen*.

splenius capitis muscle (splen'-ē-us kap'-i-tus) ⇒ Figure 5.

spleno·caval (splen-ō-kā'-val) *adj* pertaining to the spleen and inferior vena cava, usually referring to anastomosis of the splenic vein to the latter.

splenogram (splen'-ō-gram) *n* radiographic picture of the spleen after the injection of radio-opaque medium—**splenograph, splenography,** *n*, **splenographical,** *adj*.

spleno·megaly (splen-ō-meg'-à-lē) *n* enlargement of the spleen.

spleno·portal (splen-ō-pōr'-tal) *adj* pertaining to the spleen and portal vein.

spleno·portogram (splen-ō-port'-ō-gram) *n* radiographic demonstration of the spleen and portal vein after injection of radio-opaque medium—**splenoportographical** *adj*, **splenoportograph, splenoportography** *n*, **splenoportographically** *adv*.

spleno·renal (splen-ō-rē'-nàl) *adj* pertaining to the spleen and kidney, as anastomosis of the splenic vein to the renal vein; a procedure carried out in some cases of portal hypertension.

splint (splint) *n* a mechanism for immobilizing a joint.

spon·dyl(e) (spon'-dil) *n* a vertebra*.

spondyl·itis (spon-dil-ī'-tis) *n* inflammation of one or more vertebrae—**spondylitic** *adj*. ankylosing spondylitis a condition characterized by ossification of the spinal ligaments and ankylosis of sacroiliac joints. It occurs chiefly in young men.

spondyl·ography (spon-dil-og'-raf-ē) *n* a method of measuring and studying the degree of kyphosis by directly tracing the line of the back.

spondylo·listhesis (spon-dil-ō-lis-thē'-sis) *n* forward displacement of lumbar vertebra(e)—**spondylolisthetic** *adj*.

spondyl·osis deformans (spon-dil-ōs'-is dē-fōr'-mans) degeneration of the whole intervertebral disc, with new bone formation at the periphery of the disc. Commonly called 'osteoarthritis of spine'.

spongio·blastoma multi·forme (spon-jē-ō-blas-tō'-mà mul'-ti-fōrm) a highly malignant rapidly growing brain tumor.

spon·taneous frac·ture ⇒ fracture.

spor·adic (spōr-ad'-ik) *adj* scattered; occurring in isolated cases; not epidemic—**sporadically** *adv*.

spore (spōr) *n* a phrase in the life-cycle of a limited number of bacterial genera where the vegetative cell becomes encapsulated and metabolism almost ceases. These spores are highly resistant to environmental conditions such as heat and desiccation. The spores of important species such as *Clostridium tetani* and *Clostridium botulinum* are ubiquitous so that sterilization procedures must ensure their removal or death.

spori·cidal (spōr-i-sīd'-al) *adj* lethal to spores—**sporicide** *n*.

sporo·trichosis (spōr-ō-trik-ōs'-is) *n* infection of a wound by a fungus (*Sporotrichum schenkii*). There results a primary sore with lymphangitis and subcutaneous painless granulomata. Occurs amongst agricultural workers.

sporu·lation (spōr-ū-lā′-shun) *n* the formation of spores by bacteria.

spotted fever (spot′-ed fē′-ver) 1 cerebrospinal fever. Organism responsible is *Neisseria meningitides,* transferred by droplet infection. Occurs in epidemics ⇒ meningitis. 2 *Rocky Mountain spotted fever* is a tick borne typhus* fever.

sprain (sprān) *n* injury to the soft tissues surrounding a joint, resulting in discoloration, swelling and pain.

Sprengel's shoulder deform·ity (spreng′-elz) congenital high scapula, a permanent elevation of the shoulder, often associated with other congenital deformities, e.g. the presence of a cervical rib or the absence of vertebrae.

sprue (sprōō) *n* a chronic malabsorption disorder associated with glossitis, indigestion, weakness, anemia and steatorrhea.

spuri·ous diar·rhea (spū′-rē-us dī′-á-rē′-á) the leakage of fluid feces past a solid impacted mass of feces. More likely to occur in children and the elderly.

spu·tum (spū′-tum) *n* ⇒ spittle.

squamous (skwā′-mus) *adj* scaly. *squamous epithelium* the non-glandular epithelial covering of the external body, surfaces. *squamous carcinoma* carcinoma arising in squamous epithelium; epithelioma.

squills (skwilz) *n* dried bulbs of Mediterranean plant, used in Gee's linctus and other cough preparations as an expectorant.

squint (skwint) *n* (*syn* strabismus) incoordinated action of the muscles of the eyeball, such that the visual axes of the two eyes fail to meet at the objective point. *convergent squint* when the eyes turn towards the medial line. *divergent squint* when the eyes turn outwards.

SR *abbr* sedimentation rate.

SSE *abbr* soap suds enema.

stac·cato speech (stá-kát′-ō) with interruptions between words or syllables. The scanning speech of disseminated sclerosis and cerebellar disease.

stag·nant loop syn·drome (stag′-nant lōop) stagnation of contents of any surgically created 'loop' of intestine with consequent increase in bacterial population and interference with absorption of food.

St Anthony's fire (sānt an′-thon-ēz) a disease characterized by either (a) a burning sensation and later gangrene of the ex-tremities or (b) convulsions. It is due to a mixture of mycotoxins*.

staped·ectomy (stă-ped-ek′-to-mē) *n* surgical removal of stapes for otosclerosis. After stapedectomy, stapes can be replaced by a prosthesis. Normal hearing is restored in 90% of patients.

stapedial mobilization, stapediolysis (stă-ped-ē′-al) release of a stapes rendered immobile by otosclerosis.

stapes (stā′-pēz) *n* the stirrup-shaped medial bone of the middle ear. *mobilization of stapes* forcible pressure on stapes to restore its mobility. Gain in hearing not permanent, but a stapedectomy can be done later—**stapedial** *adj.*

Staphcillin (staf-sil′-in) *n* proprietary name for methicillin*.

Staphylococcus (staf-il-ō-kok′-us) *n* a genus of bacteria. Gram-positive cocci occurring in clusters. May be saprophytes or parasites. Common commensals of man, in whom they are responsible for much minor pyogenic infection, and a lesser amount of more serious infection. Produce several exotoxins. These include leukocidins which kill white blood cells and hemolysins which destroy red blood cells. A common cause of hospital cross infection—**staphylococcal** *adj. Staphylococcus epidermis* one of the most common microorganisms causing bacteremia in patients who have had bone marrow transplant. In addition to an overall 8% fatality rate, the following conditions—protracted illness, extensive soft tissue infections, endocarditis, pneumonia and infected emboli have occurred. The organism is frequently resistant to all antimicrobials except vancomycin.

staphyloma (staf-il-ōm′-á) *n* a protrusion of the cornea or sclera of the eye—**staphylomata** *pl.*

starch (stárch) *n* the carbohydrate present in potatoes, rice, maize, etc. Widely used as an absorbent dusting powder.

stasis (stā′-sis) *n* stagnation; cessation of motion. *intestinal stasis* sluggish bowel contractions resulting in constipation.

status (stat′-us) *n* state; condition. *status asthmaticus* repeated attacks of asthma* without any period of freedom between spasms. *status epilepticus* describes epileptic attacks following each other almost continuously. *status lymphaticus* is a condition found postmortem in patients who have died without apparent cause. The thymus may be found hypertrophied with increase in lymphatic tissue elsewhere.

STD *abbr* sexually* transmitted diseases.

steapsin (stē-ap′-sin) *n* the lipase* of the pancreatic juice which splits fat into fatty acids and glycerine.

steathorrea (stē-at-ōr-ē′-à) *n* a syndrome of varied etiology associated with multiple defects of absorption from the gut and characterized by the passage of pale, bulky, greasy, foul-smelling stools.

stegomyia (steg-ō-mī′-ē-à) *n* a genus of mosquitoes, some of which transmit the malaria* parasite. Found in most tropical and subtropical countries.

Stein-Leventhal syndrome (stīn lev′-en-thal) secondary amenorrhea, infertility, bilateral polycystic ovaries and hirsutism occurring in the second or third decades of life. Sometimes treated by wedge resection of ovary.

Steinmann's pin (stīn′-manz) an alternative to the use of a Kirschner wire of applying skeletal traction to a limb. It has its own introducer and stirrup.

Stelazine (stel′-à-zēn) *n* proprietary name for trifluoperazine*.

stellate (stel′-āt) *adj* star-shaped. *stellate ganglion* a large collection of nerve cells (ganglion) on the sympathetic chain in the root of the neck. *stellate ganglionectomy* surgical removal of the stellate ganglion; sometimes performed for Meniere's disease when the attacks of vertigo are crippling and are unrelieved by conventional treatment.

Stellwag's sign (stel′-wags) occurs in exophthalmic goiter (thyrotoxicosis). Patient does not blink as often as usual, and the eyelids close only imperfectly when he does so.

stenosis (sten-ō′-sis) *n* a narrowing—**stenosis** *pl*, **stenotic** *adj*. *pyloric stenosis* **1** narrowing of the pylorus due to scar tissue formed during the healing of a duodenal ulcer. **2** congenital hypertrophic pyloric stenosis due to a thickened pyloric sphincter muscle. ⇒ Ramstedt's operation.

stercobilin (ster-kō-bī′-lin) *n* the brown pigment of feces; it is derived from the bile pigments.

stercobilinogen (ster-kō-bil-in′-ō-jen) *n* ⇒ urobilinogen.

stercoraceous (ster-kōr-ash′-ē-us) *adj* pertaining to or resembling feces—**stercoral** *adj*.

stereotactic surgery (stē-rē-ō-tak′-tik) electrodes and cannulae are passed to a

predetermined point in the brain for physiological observation or destruction of tissue in diseases such as paralysis agitans, multiple sclerosis and epilepsy. Intractible pain can be relieved by this method—**stereotaxy** *n*.

sterile (ster′il) *adj* free from microorganisms—**sterility** *n*.

steriliz·ation (ster-il-ī-zā′-shun) *n* **1** treatment which achieves the killing or removal of all types of microorganisms including spores. It is accompanied by using heat, radiation, chemicals or filtration. **2** rendering incapable of reproduction.

Steri-Strip (ster′-ē strip) *n* proprietary sterile skin closure strips; wound edges are brought within 3 mm (to allow for drainage); strips of adhesive are placed across the wound with space between. Lastly a strip is placed on either side, parallel to the wound.

sternal puncture (ster′nal punk′-tūr) insertion of a special guarded hollow needle with a stylet, into the body of the sternum for aspiration of a bone marrow sample.

sterno·clavicular (ster-nō-clav-ik′-ū-lar) *adj* pertaining to the sternum* and the clavicle*.

sterno·cleidomastoid muscle (ster-nō-klī-dō-mas′-toyd) a strap-like neck muscle arising from the sternum and clavicle, and inserting into the mastoid process of temporal bone. ⇒ torticollis.

sterno·costal (ster-nō-kos′-tal) *adj* pertaining to the sternum* and ribs.

stern·otomy (ster-not′-o-mē) *n* surgical division of the sternum*.

sternum (ster′-num) *n* the breast bone—**sternal** *adj*.

Sterogyl 15 (ster′-ō-jil) proprietary name for calciferol*.

steroids (ster′-oyds) *npl* a term embracing a naturally occurring group of chemicals allied to cholesterol and including sex-hormones, adrenal cortical hormones, bile acids etc. By custom it often now implies the natural adrenal glucocorticoids, i.e. hydrocortisone and cortisone, or synthetic analogues such as prednisolone and prednisone.

sterol (ster′-ol) *n* a solid alcohol. Cholesterol and many hormones secreted by the adrenal cortex and the gonads are examples. They all contain the same basic ring structure.

stertor (ster′-tor) *n* loud snoring; sonorous breathing—**stertorous** *adj*.

stetho·scope (steth'-ō-skōp) *n* an instrument used for listening to the various body sounds, especially those of the heart and chest. **stethoscopic** *adj*, **stethoscopically** *adv*.

Stevens-Johnson syndrome (stē'-venz jon'-son) severe variant of the allergic response—erythema multiforme. It is an acute hypersensitivity state and can follow a viral or bacterial infection, drugs—such as long-acting sulfonamides, some anticonvulsants and some antibiotics. In some cases no cause can be found. Lung complications during the acute phase can be fatal. Mostly it is a benign condition, and there is complete recovery.

stibo·phen (stī'-bō-fen) *n* a complex antimony compound used in the treatment of schistosomiasis.

stig·mata (stig-mà'-tà) *n* marks of disease, or congenital abnormalities, e.g. facies of congenital syphilis—**stigma** *sing*.

stil·bestrol (stil-bes'-trol) *n* an orally active synthetic estrogen, indicated in all conditions calling for estrogen therapy. Large doses are given in prostatic carcinoma. ⇒ diethylstilbestrol.

stil·ette (stil-et') *n* a wire or metal rod for maintaining patency of hollow instruments.

still·born (stil'-bōrn) *n* born dead.

Still's disease (stilz) a form of rheumatoid polyarthritis, involving enlargement of the spleen, lymphatic nodes and glands, occurring in infants and young children. Sufferers are often retarded. Also called 'arthritis deformans juvenilis'.

stimulant (stim'-ū-lant) *n* stimulating. An agent which excites or increases function.

stimulus (stim'-ū-lus) *n* anything which excites functional activity in an organ or part.

stitch (stich) *n* **1** a sudden, sharp, darting pain. **2** a suture.

Stockholm technique (stok'-hōlm) a method of treating carcinoma of the cervix by radium on three successive occasions at weekly intervals.

Stokes-Adams syn·drome (stōks-ad'-amz) a fainting (syncopal) attack, commonly transient, which occurs in patients with heart block. If severe, may take the form of a convulsion, or patient may become unconscious.

stoma (stō'-mà) *n* the mouth; any opening—**stomata** *pl*, **stomal** *adj*.

stomach (stum'-ak) *n* the most dilated part of the digestive tube, situated between the esophagus (cardiac orifice) and the beginning of the small intestine (pyloric orifice); it lies in the epigastric, umbilical and left hypochrondriac regions of the abdomen. The wall is composed of four coats: serous, muscular, submucous and mucous. **stomach pH electrode** an apparatus used to measure gastric contents in situ.

stomachics (stum-ak'-iks) *npl* agents which increase the appetite, especially bitters.

stoma·titis (stō-mà-tī'-tis) *n* inflammation of the mouth. *angular stomatitis* fissuring in the corners of the mouth consequent upon riboflavin deficiency. Sometimes misapplied to: (a) the superficial maceration and fissuring at the labial commisures in perlèche and (b) the chronic fissuring at the site in elderly persons with sagging lower lip or malapposition of artificial dentures. *aphthous stomatitis* recurring crops of small ulcers in the mouth. Relationship to herpes simplex suspected, but not proven ⇒ aphthac. *gangrenous stomatitis* ⇒ cancrum oris.

stone (stōn) *n* calculus; a hardened mass of mineral matter.

stool (stool) *n* the feces. An evacuation of the bowels.

stove-in chest there may be multiple anterior or posterior fractures of the ribs (causing paradoxical breathing) and fractures of sternum, or a mixture of such fractures.

strabismus (stà-bis'-mus) *n* ⇒ squint.

strain (strān) *n* the damage, usually muscular that results from excessive physical effort.

stramonium (strà-mō'-nē-um) *n* a plant resembling belladonna* in its properties, and used as an antispasmodic in bronchitis and parkinsonism.

strangu·lated her·nia (strāng'-ū-lā-ted hér'-nē-à) ⇒ hernia.

strangu·lation (strāng-ū-lā'-shun) *n* constriction which impedes the circulation—**strangulated** *adj*.

strangury (strang'-gū-rē) *n* a painful urge to micturate with slow voiding of small amounts of urine.

Strassman oper·ation (stras'-man) a plastic operation to make a bicornuate uterus a near normal shape.

stratified (strat'-i-fīd) *adj* arranged in layers.

stratum (strat'-um) *n* a layer or lamina, e.g. the various layers of the epithelium of the skin, i.e. stratum granulosum, stratum lucidum.

straw·berry tongue (straw'-bėr-ē) the tongue is thickly furred with projecting red papillae. As the fur disappears the tongue is vividly red like an overripe strawberry. A characteristic of scarlet* fever.

Strepto·bacillus (strep-tō-ba-sil'-us) *n* pleomorphic bacterium which may be Gram-positive in young cultures.

Strepto·coccus (strep-tō-kok'-us) *n* a genus of bacteria. Gram-positive cocci, often occuring in chains of varying length. Require enriched media for growth and the colonies are small. Saprophytic and parasitic species. Pathogenic species produce powerful exotoxins include leukocidins which kill white blood cells and hemolysins which kill red blood cells. In man streptotocci are responsible for numerous infections such as scarlatina, tonsillitis, erysipelas, endocarditis and wound infections in hospital, with rheumatic fever and glomerulonephritis as possible sequelae—**streptococcal** *adj*.

strepto·dornase (strep-tō-dōr'-nās) *n* an enzyme used with streptokinase* in liquefying pus and blood clots.

strepto·kinase (strep-tō-kī'-nās) *n* an enzyme derived from cultures of certain hemolytic streptococci. Plasminogen activator. Used with streptodornase*. Its fibrinolytic effect has been used as thrombolytic therapy to speed removal of intravascular fibrin.

strepto·lysins (strep-tō-lī'-sins) *npl* exotoxins produced by streptococci. Antibody produced in the tissues against streptolysin may be measured and taken as an indicator of recent streptococcal infection.

strepto·mycin (strep-tō-mī'-sin) *n* an antibiotic effective against many organisms, but used mainly in tuberculosis. Treatment must be combined with other drugs to reduce drug resistance. It is not absorbed when given orally, hence used in some intestinal infections.

Strepto·thrix (strep'-to-thriks) *n* a filamentous bacterium which shows true branching. ⇒ Streptobacillus.

stress (stres) *n* the wear and tear on the body in response to stressful agents. Selye called such agents stressors and said that they could be physical, physiological, psychological or sociocultural.

stress test (*syn* oxytocin challenge test) the administration of low doses of Pi-

tocin, I.V., to a pregnant woman while the fetal heart and uterine contractions are recorded via external fetal monitor. Used to evaluate for placental insufficiency in women with low estriol values or suspected of postmaturity.

striae (strī'-ē) *npl* streaks; stripes; narrow bands. *striae gravidarum* lines which appear, especially on the abdomen, as a result of stretching of the skin in pregnancy; due to rupture of the lower layers of the dermis. They are red at first and then become silvery-white—**stria** *sing*, **striated** *adj*.

stric·ture (strik'-tūr) *n* a narrowing, especially of a tube or canal, due to scar tissue or tumor.

stri·dor (strī'-dor) *n* a harsh sound in breathing, caused by air passing through constricted air passages—**stridulous** *adj*.

stroke (strōk) *n* a popular term for apoplexy resulting from a vascular accident in the brain, which can result in hemiplegia. ⇒ cerebrovascular accident.

stroma (strō'-mà) *n* the interstitial or foundation substance of a structure.

Strongyl·oides (strong'-i-loyds) *n* a genus of intestinal worms that can infest man.

strongyl·oidiasis (strong-i-loyd-ī'-à-sis) *n* infestation with *Strongyloides stercoralis*, usually acquired through the skin from contaminated soil, but can be through mucous membrane. At the site of larval penetration there may be an itchy rash. As the larvae migrate through the lungs there may be pulmonary symptoms with larvae in sputum. There may be varying abdominal symptoms. Because of autoinfective life cycle, treatment aims at complete elimination of the parasite. Thiabendazole 25 mg per kg twice daily for 2 days; given either as a suspension or tablets which should be chewed. Driving a car is inadvisable during therapy.

stron·tium (stron'-tē-um) *n* a metallic element chemically similar to calcium and present in bone. Isotopes of strontium are used in radioisotope scanning of bone to detect abnormalities.

stron·tium-90 (stron'-tē-um nīn'-tē) a radioactive isotope with a relatively long half-life (28 years). It is incorporated into bone tissue where turnover is slow. It is the most dangerous constituent of atomic fall-out.

strophan·thus (strō-fan'-thus) *n* African plant with cardiac properties similar to digitalis, but of more rapid action. The active principle, strophanthin, is sometimes given by intravenous injection.

strophu·lus (strof'-ū-lus) *n* ⇒ miliaria.

strych·nine (strik'-nēn) *n* a bitter alkaloid obtained from nux vomica. Has been used as a tonic in association with other bitter drugs.

Stryker bed (strī'-kėr) constructed so that a patient can be rotated as required to the prone or supine position. Used mainly for spinal conditions and burns.

STS *abbr* serological test for syphilis.

student's elbow (stoo'-dents el'-bō) olecranon bursitis*.

stupe (stūp) *n* a medical fomentation. Opium may be added to relieve pain. Turpentine may be added to produce counterirritation.

stu·por (stū'-por) *n* a state of marked impairment of, but not complete loss of consciousness. The victim shows gross lack of responsiveness, usually reacting only to noxious stimuli. In psychiatry there are three main varieties of stupor: depressive, schizophrenic and hysterical—**stuporous** *adj.*

Sturge-Weber syn·drome (sturj web'-er) (*syn* nevoid amentia) a genetically determined congenital ectodermosis, i.e. a capillary hemangioma above the eye may be accompanied by similar changes in vessels inside the skull giving rise to epilepsy and other cerebral manifestations.

St Vitus' dance (sānt vī'-tus dans) ⇒ chorea.

sty (stī) *n* (*syn* hordeolum) an abscess in the follicle of an eyelash.

styl·oid (stī'-loyd) *adj* long and pointed; resembling a pen or stylus.

styp·tic (stip'-tik) *n* an astringent applied to stop bleeding. A hemostatic.

sub·acute (sub-à-kūt') *adj* moderately severe. Often the stage between the acute and chronic phases of disease. *subacute bacterial endocarditis* septicemia due to bacterial infection of a heart valve. Petechiae of the skin and embolic phenomena are characteristic. The term infective endocarditis is now preferred, since other microorganisms may be involved. *subacute combined degeneration of the spinal cord* a complication of untreated pernicious anemia (PA) and affects the posterior and lateral columns. *subacute sclerosing panencephalitis (SSPE)* a slow* virus infection caused by the measles virus; characterized by diffuse inflammation of brain tissue.

subarach·noid hemor·rhage (sub-à-rak'-noyd hem'-ōr-aj) bleeding, usually from a ruptured berry aneurysm into the subarachnoid space accompanied by headache and a stiff neck. Blood is present in the CSF. Cerebral angiography reveals the site of bleeding and treatment depends on this.

subarach·noid space (sub-à-rak'-noyd spās) the space beneath the arachnoid membrane, between it and the pia mater. It contains cerebrospinal fluid.

sub·carinal (sub-kar-ī'-nal) *adj* below acarina, usually referring to the carina tracheae.

sub·clavian (sub-klā'-vē-an) *adj* beneath the clavicle. *subclavian artery* ⇒ Figure 9. *subclavian vein* ⇒ Figure 10.

sub·clinical (sub-klin'-i-kal) *adj* insufficient to cause the classical identifiable disease.

sub·conjunctival (sub-kon-jungk-tī'-val) *adj* below the conjunctiva—**subconjunctivally** *adj.*

subcon·scious (sub-kon'-shus) *adj n* that portion of the mind outside the range of clear consciousness, but capable of affecting conscious mental or physical reactions.

sub·costal (sub-kos'-tal) *adj* beneath the rib.

sub·cutaneous (sub-kū-tā'-nē-us) *adj.* beneath the skin—**subcutaneously** *adv. subcutaneous edema* is demonstrable by the 'pitting' produced by pressure of the finger. *subcutaneous tissue* ⇒ Figure 12.

sub·cuticular (sub-kū-tik'-ū-lar) *adj* beneath the cuticle, as a subcuticular abscess.

sub·dural (sub-dūr'-al) *adj* beneath the dura mater; between the dura and arachnoid membranes. *subdural hematoma* the bleeding comes from a small vein or veins lying between the dura and brain. It develops slowly and may present as a space-occupying lesion with vomiting, papilledema, fluctuating level of consciousness, weakness, usually a hemiplegia on the opposite side to the clot. Finally there is a rise in blood pressure and a fall in pulse rate.

sub·endocardial (sub-en-dō-kàr'-dē-al) *adj* immediately beneath the endocardium.

sub·hepatic (sub-hep-at'-ik) *adj* beneath the liver.

sub·involution (sub-in-vol-ū'-shun) *adj* failure of the gravid uterus to return to its normal size within a normal time after childbirth. ⇒ involution.

subjec·tive (sub-jek'-tiv) *adj* internal; personal; arising from the senses and not perceptible to others. ⇒ objective *opp*.

subli·mate (sub'-lim-āt) 1 *n* a solid deposit resulting from the condensation of a vapor. 2 *vt* in psychiatry, to redirect a primitive desire into some more socially acceptable channel, e.g. a strong tendency to agressiveness subliminated into sporting activity—**sublimation** *n*.

Subli·maze (sub'-li-māz) *n* proprietary name for fentanyl*.

sublim·inal (sub-lim'-in-al) *adj* inadequate for perceptible response. Below the threshold of consciousness. ⇒ liminal.

sub·lingual (sub-ling'-gwal) *adj* beneath the tongue.

sublux·ation (sub-luks-ā'-shun) incomplete dislocation of a joint.

submandib·ular (sub-man-dib'-ū-lar) *adj* below the mandible.

submax·illary (sub-maks'-il-ār-ē) *adj* beneath the lower jaw.

sub·mucosa (sub-mū-kō'-sà) *n* the layer of connective tissue beneath a mucous membrane—**submucous, submucosal** *adj*.

sub·mucous (sub-mū'-kus) *adj* beneath a mucous membrane. *submucous resection* removal of a deflected nasal septum.

subnor·mality (sub-nōr-mal'-it-ē) *n* a state of arrested or incomplete development of mind (not amounting to severe subnormality) which includes subnormality of intelligence and is of a nature or degree which requires or is susceptible to medical treatment or other special care or training of the patient. *severe subnormality* a state of arrested or incomplete development of mind which includes subnormality of intelligence and is of such a nature or degree that the patient is incapable of living an independent life or of guarding himself against serious exploitation, or will be so incapable when of an age to do so.

sub·occipital (sub-ok-sip'-it-al) *adj* beneath the occiput; in the nape of the neck.

sub·periosteal (sub-per-ē-os'-tē-al) *adj* beneath the periosteum of bone.

sub·phrenic (sub-fren'-ik) *adj* beneath the diaphragm.

subscapularis muscle (sub-skap-ū-lār'-is) ⇒ Figure 4.

sub·sultus (sub-sul'-tus) *adj* muscular tremor. *subsultus tendinum* twitching of tendons and muscles particularly around the wrist in severe fever, such as typhoid.

succinyl·choline (sucks-in-il-kōl'-ēn) *n* a short-acting muscle relaxant.

succinyl·sulfa·thiazole (sucks-in-il-sul-fà-thī'-à-zōl) *n* a sulfonamide* formerly used in gastrointestinal infections and in bowel surgery. It is poorly absorbed and is not effective against systemic infections.

succus (suk'-us) *n* a juice, especially that secreted by the intestinal glands and called *succus entericus*.

suc·cussion (suk-ush'-un) *n* splashing sound produced by fluid in a hollow cavity on shaking the patient, e.g. liquid content of dilated stomach in pyloric stenosis. *hippocratic succussion* the splashing sound, on shaking, when fluid accompanies a pneumothorax.

su·crose (sū'-krōs) *n* a disaccharide obtained from sugar cane, sugar beet and maple syrup. It is normally hydrolyzed into dextrose and fructose in the body.

sucro·suria (sū-krōs-ū'-rē-à) *n* the presence of sucrose in the urine.

suction abortion (suk'-shun) abortion performed by using an instrument that sucks the contents of the uterus.

su·damina (sū-dam'-in-à) *n* sweat rash.

Sudan blind·ness a form of onchocerciasis*.

sud·den infant death syn·drome ⇒ crib death.

sudor (sū'-dor) *n* sweat—**sudoriferous** *adj*.

sudor·ific (sū-dor-if'-ik) *adj, n* (*syn* diaphoretic) describes an agent which induces sweating.

suggest·ibility (sug-jest-i-bil'-i-tē) *n* may be heightened in hospital patients, in the dependence on others that illness brings, in children, in the mentally subnormal and in those with a tendency to hysteria.

sugges·tion (sug-jest'-chun) *n* the implanting in a person's mind of an idea which he accepts fully without logical reason. Suggestion is utilized when the idea of recovery is given to, and accepted by, a patient. In psychiatric practice suggestion is used as a therapeutic measure sometimes under hypnosis or narcoanalysis.

Sulamyd (sul'-à-mid) *n* proprietary name for sulfacetamide*.

sul·cus (sul'-kus) *n* a furrow or groove, particularly those separating the gyri or convolutions of the cortex of the brain—**sulci** *pl*.

sulfa·cetamide (sul-fà-sēt'-à-mīd) *n* a sulfonamide* used mainly as eye drops, and systemically for urinary tract infections. (Sulamyd.)

sulfa·diazine (sul-fà-dī'-à-zīn) *n* a powerful sulfonamide* compound for systemic use in many infections. Often the drug of choice in meningococcal infections as its penetration into cerebrospinal fluid is greater than the other sulfonamides. It is less effective against staphylococcal infections.

sulfa·dimeth·oxine (sul-fà-dī-meth-oks'-īn) *n* a sulfonamide, useful as a prophylactic of urinary infection as resistance does not occur. (Madribon.)

sulfa·dimidine (sul-fà-dī'-mi-dīn) *n* one of the most effective and least toxic of the sulfonamides*, and the reduced incidence of side effects increases its value in pediatrics. The sodium salt may be given by injection.

sulf·hemo·globin (sulf-hē-mō-glo'-bin) *n* ⇒ sulfmethemoglobin.

sulfa·salazine (sulf-a-sal'-à-zēn) *n* a sulfonamide compound which, after ingestion, is said to be distributed largely in connective tissue. It is used in the treatment of ulcerative colitis. (Salazopyrin, Azulfidine.)

sulfhemo·globinemia (sulf-hē-mō-glō'-bin-ēm'-ē-à) *n* a condition of circulating sulfmethemoglobin* in the blood.

sulfa·methoxazole (sulf-meth-oks'-à-zōl) *n* sulfonamide that has a pattern of absorption and excretion very similar to trimethoprim, and so used in mixed products.

sulfin·pyrazone (sulf-in-pī'-rà-zōn) *n* uricosuric* agent. It is now being tried out as a prophylactic after myocardial infarction. (Anturam.)

sulfmethemo·globin (sulf-meth-hē-mō-glō'-bin) *n* (*syn* sulfemoglobin) a sulfide oxidation product of hemoglobin*, produced in vivo by certain drugs. This compound cannot transport oxygen or carbon dioxide and, not being reversible in the body, is an indirect poison.

sulfona·mides (sul-fon'-à-mīds) *npl* a group of bacteriostatic agents, effective orally, but must be maintained in a definite concentration in the blood. They are antimetabolites; they inhibit formation of folic acid, which for many organisms is an essential metabolite.

sulfonamidopyrimidines (sul-fon-à-mīd'-ō-pi-rim'-id-ēnz) *npl* oral blood-sugar lowering agents.

sul·fones (sul'-fōnz) *npl* a group of synthetic drugs, represented by dapsone*, useful for leprosy.

sulfony·lureas (sul-fon-il-ū'-rē-as) *npl* sulfonamide* derivatives that are oral hypoglycemic agents. They increase insulin output from a functioning pancreas so that injections of insulin may be unnecessary. Of chief value in 'middle-age onset' diabetes.

sul·fur (sul'-fur) *n* an insoluble yellow powder once used extensively as sulfur ointment for scabies. Still used in lotions and baths for acne and other skin disorders.

sul·furic acid (sul-fūr'-ik) the concentrated acid is widely employed in industry, and is very corrosive. The dilute acid (10%) has been given for its astringent action, but is now rarely used.

sun·stroke (sun'-strōk) *n* ⇒ heat-stroke.

super·cilium (sū-per-sil'-ē-um) *n* the eyebrow—**superciliary** *adj.*

superego (sū-per-ē'-gō) *n* part of the mind concerned with morality and self criticism; it operates at a partly conscious, partly unconscious level. Corresponds roughly to the long term 'conscience'.

Superinone (sū-per'-in-ōn) *n* proprietary name for tyloxapol*.

su·perior (sū-pē'-rē-or) *adj* in anatomy, the upper of two parts—**superiorly** *adj.*

super·numerary (sū-per-nū'-mer-ār-ē) *n* in excess of the normal number; additional.

supin·ate (sū'-pin-āt) *vt* turn or lay face or palm upward ⇒ pronate *opp.*

supin·ator (sū'-pin-āt-or) *n* that which suppinates, usually applied to a muscle ⇒ pronator *opp.*

su·pine (sū'-pīn) *adj* 1 lying on the back with face upwards. 2 of the hand, with the palm upwards. ⇒ prone *opp.*

supposi·tory (sup-oz'-i-tōr-ē) *n* medicament in a base that melts at body temperature. Inserted into the rectum.

sup·pression (sup-resh'-un) *n* 1 cessation of a secretion (e.g. urine) or a normal process (e.g. menstruation). 2 in psychology, the voluntary forcing out of the mind of painful thoughts. This often results in the precipitation of a neurosis.

suppu·ration (sup-ūr-ā'-shun) *n* the formation of pus—**suppurative** *adj,* **suppurate** *vi.*

supra·clavicular (sū-prà-klà-vik'-ū-lar) *adj* above the collar bone (clavicle).

supra·condylar (sū-prà-kon'-dil-ar) *adj* above a condyle*.

supra·orbital (sū-prà-ŏr'-bit-al) *adj* above the orbits. *supraorbital ridge* the ridge covered by the eyebrows.

supra·pubic (sū-prà-pū'-bik) *adj* above the pubis.

supra·renal (sū-prà-rē'-nal) *adj* above the kidney. ⇒ adrenal.

supra·spinatus muscle (sū-per-spin-ā'-tus) ⇒ Figure 5.

supra·sternal (sū-prà-ster'-nal) *adj* above the breast bone (sternum).

sur·amin (sūr'-à-min) *n* a drug which is used intravenously in the early stages of trypanosomiasis, filariasis and onchocerciasis. Contraindications are renal disease or adrenal insufficiency. (Antrypol.)

surface muscles (sur'-fas) ⇒ Figures 4, 5.

sur·factant (sur-fak'-tant) *n* a mixture of phospholipids, chiefly lecithin* and sphingomyelin secreted into the pulmonary alveoli; it reduces the surface tension of pulmonary fluids, contributing to the elastic properties of pulmonary tissues. Can be instilled via a tracheal catheter for respiratory distress syndrome. ⇒ pneumocytes, zinc.

sur·gery (sur'-je-rē) *n* that branch of medicine which treats diseases, deformities and injuries, wholly or in part, by manual or operative procedures.

sur·gical dres·sings (sur'-ji-kal) ⇒ wound dressings.

sur·gical emphy·sema (sur'-ji-kal em-fis-ēm'-à) air in the subcutaneous tissueplanes following the trauma of surgery or injury.

Sur·montil (sur-mon'-til) *n* proprietary name for trimipramine*.

suscepti·bility (sus-sept-ib-il'-it-ē) *n* the opposite of resistance. Includes a state of reduced capacity to deal with infection.

sus·pensory band·age (sus-pen'-sor-ē) applied so that it supports and suspends the scrotum*.

suspensory ligaments (sus-pen'-sor-ē lig'-à-ments) ⇒ Figure 15.

suture (sū'-tūr) *n* **1** the junction of cranial bones. **2** in surgery, a ligature*.

swab (swàb) *n* **1** a small piece of cotton wool or gauze. **2** a small piece of sterile cotton wool, or similar material, on the end of a shaft of wire or wood, enclosed in a protecting tube. It is used to collect material for bacteriological examination.

sweat (swet) *n* the secretion from the sudoriferous glands. *sweat gland* ⇒ Figure 12.

sweat test a petri dish prepared with agar, silver nitrate and potassium chromate. With palm of hand pressed to this, excessive chorides in sweat gives distinctive white print, as in cystic fibrosis.

Swenson's oper·ation (swen'-sonz) for congenital intestinal aganglionosis (Hirschsprung's disease).

swimmer's ear otitis externa, caused by water remaining in the ear canal after swimming.

sy·cosis barbae (sī-kŏ'-sis bar'-bā) (*syn* barber's itch) a pustulal folliculitis of the beard area in men. Now rare due to antibiotics and improved hygiene.

sy·cosis nuchae (sī-kŏ'-sis noōk'-ā) a folliculitis at the nape of the neck which leads to keloid thickening (acne keloid).

Sydenham's chorea (sid'-en-hamz kŏr-ē'-à) St. Vitus Dance ⇒ chorea.

sym·biosis (sim-bī-ŏ'-sis) *n* a relationship between two or more organisms in which the participants are of mutual aid and benefit to one another. ⇒ antibiosis *opp.*—**symbiotic** *adj.*

sym·blepharon (sim-blef'-a-ron) *n* adhesion of the lid to the eyeball.

Syme's ampu·tation (simz) amputation just above the ankle joint. Provides an end-bearing stump. Especially useful in primitive conditions where elaborate artificial limbs are not available.

Symmetrel (sim'-e-trel) *n* proprietary name for amantadine*.

sympath·ectomy (sim-pà-thek'-tō-mē) *n* surgical excision of part of the sympathetic nervous system.

sympath·etic ner·vous sys·tem (sim-pà-thet'-ik) a portion of the autonomic nervous system. It is composed of a chain of ganglia on either side of the vertebral column in the thora-columbar region and sends fibers to all plain muscle tissue.

sympatho·lytic (sim-pà-thō-lit'-ik) *n* a drug which opposes the effects of the sympathetic nervous system.

sympatho·mimetic (sim-pà-thō-mim-et'-ik) *adj* capable of producing changes similar to those produced by stimulation of the sympathetic nerves.

symphy·sis (sim'-fis-is) *n* a fibrocartilaginous union of bones—**symphyseal** *adj.*

symp·tom (sim'-tum) *n* a subjective phenomenon or manifestation of disease—**symptomatic** *adj. symptom complex* a group of symptoms which, occuring together, typify a particular disease or syndrome.

symptoma·tology (sim-tum-à-tol′-o-jē) *n* 1 the branch of medicine concerned with symptoms. 2 the combined symptoms typical of a particular disease.

Syn·lalar (sin′-là-lar) *n* proprietary name for fluocinolone*.

syn·apse, synapsis (sin′-aps, sin-ap′-sis) *n* the point of communication between two adjacent neurons.

syn·chysis (sin′-kis-is) *n* degenerative condition of the vitreous humor of the eye, rendering it fluid. *synchysis scintillans* fine opacities in the vitreous.

Syncillin (sin-sil′-lin) *n* proprietary name for phenethicillin*.

syn·cope (sin′-ko-pē) *n* (*syn* faint) literally, sudden loss of strength. Caused by reduced cerebral circulation often following a fright, when vasodilation is responsible. May be symptomatic of cardiac arrhythmia, e.g. heart block.

syncytium (sin-sit′-ē-um) *n* a mass of protoplasm that is multinucleated.

syn·dactyly, syndactylism, syndactylia (sin-dak′-til-ē) *n* webbed fingers or toes—**syndactylous** *adj.*

syn·drome (sin′-drōm) *n* a group of symptoms and/or signs which, occurring together, produce a pattern or symptom complex, typical of a particular disease.

syn·echia (sin-ek′-ē-a) *n* abnormal union of parts, especially adhesion of the iris to the cornea in front, or the lens capsule behind—**synechiae** *pl.*

syner·gism, synergy (sin′-er-jizm, sin′-er-jē) *n* the harmonious working together of two agents, such as drugs, microorganisms, muscles, etc—**synergic** *adj.*

syner·gist (sin′-er-jist) *n* an agent co-operating with another. One partner in a synergic action.

syner·gistic action (sin-er-jist′-ik) ⇒ action.

Syn·kavite (sin′-kà-vīt) *n* proprietary name for menadiol*.

syn·kinesis (sin-kin-ē′-sis) *n* the ability to carry out precision movements.

syno·vectomy (sin-ō-vek′-to-mē) *n* excision of synovial membrane.

syn·ovial fluid (sin-ō′-vē-al) the fluid secreted by the membrane lining a joint cavity.

syn·ovial mem·brane (sin-ō′-vē-al) ⇒ membrane.

syn·ovioma (sin-ō-vē-ōm′-à) *n* a tumor of synovial membrane—benign or malignant.

syno·vitis (sī-nō-vī′-tis) *n* inflammation of a synovial membrane.

syn·thesis (sin′-the-sis) *n* the process of building complex substances from simpler substances by chemical reactions—**synthetic** *adj.*

Synthroid (sin′-throyd) *n* proprietary name for levothyroxine*.

Syn·tocinon (sin-tō′-sin-on) *n* a proprietary brand of synthetic oxytocin*.

syph·ilide (sif′-il-īd) *n* a syphilitic skin lesion.

syph·ilis (sif′-il-is) *n* a venereal disease caused by *Treponema pallidum*. Infection is acquired or it may be congenital—when it is prenatal. *Acquired syphilis* manifests in: (a) the primary stage, appears 4–5 weeks (or later) after infection when a primary chancre associated with swelling of local lymph glands appears (b) the secondary stage in which the skin eruption (syphilide) appears (c) the third stage occurs 15–30 years after initial infection. Gummata appear, or neurosyphilis* and cardiovascular syphilis supervene. The commonest types of nervous system involvement are general paralysis of the insane and tabes dorsalis (locomotor ataxia). Cardiovascular involvement produces aortic aneurysm and impairment or destruction of the aortic valve—**syphilitic** *adj. congenital syphilis* is acquired by the fetus from the infected mother.

syr·inge (si-rinj′) *n* a device for injecting, instilling or withdrawing fluids. The principal components are a cylindrical barrel to one end of which a hollow needle is attached, and a close-fitting plunger.

syringo·myelia (si-ring′-ō-mī-ēl′-ē-à) *n* an uncommon, progressive disease of the nervous system of unknown cause, beginning mainly in early adult life. Cavitation and surrounding fibrous tissue reaction, in the upper spinal cord and brain stem, interfere with sensation of pain and temperature, and sometimes with the motor pathways. The characteristic symptom is painless injury, particularly of the exposed hands. Touch sensation is intact. ⇒ Charcot's joint.

syringo·myelocele (si-ring-gō-mī′-el-ō-sēl) *n* the most severe form of meningeal hernia (spina* bifida). The central canal is dilated and the thinned-out posterior part of the spinal cord is in the hernia.

system for identifying motivated abilities (SIMA) a self-explanatory term. The tests are especially useful in diagnosing the level of mental deterioration.

sys·temic circul·ation (sis-tem′-ik sir-kū-lā′-shun) oxygenated blood leaves the left ventricle and after flowing throughout the body, returns deoxygenated to the right atrium.

sys·tole (sis′-tol-ē) *n* the contraction phase of the cardiac cycle, as opposed to diastole*—**systolic** *adj*.

sys·tolic mur·mur (sis-tol′-ik mur′-mur) a cardiac murmur occurring between the first and second heart sounds due to valvular disease, e.g. mitral systolic murmur.

T

TAB *abbr* a vaccine containing killed *Salmonella typhi, Salmonella paratyphi A* and *S. paratyphi B*; and used to produce active artificial immunity in man, against typhoid* and paratyphoid* fever.

tabes (tā′-bēz) *n* wasting away—**tabetic** *adj*. *tabes dorsalis* is a variety of neurosyphilis in which the posterior (sensory) columns of the spinal cord and the sensory nerve roots are diseased. ⇒ Charcot's joint, locomotor ataxia. *tabes mesenterica* is tuberculous enlargement of peritoneal glands found in children.

tab·etic gait (ta-bet′-ik gāt) ⇒ gait.

tabo·paresis (tā-bō-par-ēs′-is) *n* a condition of general paralysis of the insane in which the spinal cord shows the same lesions as in tabes* dorsalis.

Tace (tās) *n* proprietary name for chlorotrianisene*.

tachisto·scope (tak-is′-tō-skōp) *n* enables words and patterns to be presented for predetermined periods in the right or left visual field. Used in centers for training 'word blind' people.

tachy·cardia (tak-i-kàr′-dē-à) *n* excessively rapid action of the heart. *paroxysmal tachycardia* a temporary but sudden marked increase in frequency of heartbeats, because the conducting stimulus is originating in an abnormal focus.

tachy·phasia (tak-i-fā′-zē-à) *n* extreme rapidity of flow of speech occurring in some mental disorders.

tachyp·nea (tak-ip′-nē-à) *n* abnormal frequency of respiration—**tachypneic** *adj*.

tac·tile (tak′-tīl) *adj* pertaining to the sense of touch.

Taenia (tē′-nē-à) *n* a genus of flat, parasitic worms; cestodes or tapeworms. *Taenia echinococcus* the adult worm lives in the dog's intestine (the definitive host) and man (the intermediate host) is infested by swallowing eggs from the dog's excrement. These become embryos in the human small intestine, pass via the blood stream to organs, particularly the liver, and develop into hydatid cysts. *Taenia saginata* larvae present in infested, undercooked beef; the commonest species in Britain. In man's (the definitive host) intestinal lumen they develop into the adult tapeworm, which by its four suckers attaches itself to the gut wall. *Taenia solium* resembles *Taenia saginata*, but has hooklets as well as suckers. Commonest species in Eastern Europe. The larvae are ingested in infested, undercooked pork; man can also be the intermediate host for this worm by ingesting eggs which, developing into larvae in his stomach, pass via the bowel wall to reach organs, and there develop into cysts. In the brain these may give rise to epilepsy.

taenia (tē′-nē-à) *n* a flat band. *taenia coli* three flat bands running the length of the large intestine and consisting of the longitudinal muscle fibers.

taeniacide (tē′-nē-à-sīd) *n* an agent that destroys tapeworms—**taeniacidal** *adj*.

taenia·fuge (tē′-nē-à-fūj) *n* an agent that expels tapeworms.

Tagamet (tag′-à-met) *n* proprietary name for cimetidine.

talc (talk) *n* a naturally occurring soft white powder consisting of magnesium silicate. Used extensively as a dusting powder, prior to the donning of surgical gloves.

talipes (tal′-i-pēz) *n* any of a number of deformities of foot and ankle.

talus (tāl′-us) *n* the astragalus; situated between the tibia proximally and the calcaneus* distally, thus directly bearing the weight of the body. It is the second largest bone of the ankle.

Talwin (tol′-win) *n* proprietary name for pentazocine*.

tamox·ifen (ta-moks′-i-fen) *n* a synthetic anti-estrogenic compound. Now the drug of choice for postmenopausal metastatic breast cancer.

tampon·ade (tam-pon-ad') *n* insertion of a tampon. ⇒ cardiac.

Tan·dearil (tan'-dĕr-il) *n* proprietary name for oxyphenbutazone*.

tan·nic acid (tan'-ik as'-id) a brown powder obtained from oak galls. It has astringent properties, and is used as suppositories for hemorrhoids.

tanta·lum (tan'-tà-lum) *n* a rare metal sometimes used in the form of wire or gauze to reinforce weak areas of the body, as in the repair of a large hernia.

tape·worm (tāp'-worm) *n* ⇒ taenia.

tapote·ment (tap-ōt-mon') *n* (*syn* tapping) percussion in massage. It includes *beating* with the clenched hand; *clapping* with the palm of the hand; *hacking* with the little finger side of the hand, and *punctuation* with the tips of the fingers.

tap·ping (tap'-ing) *n* 1 ⇒ aspiration. 2 ⇒ tapotement.

Tar·actan (tar-ak'-tan) *n* proprietary name for chlorprothixene*.

tar·salgia (tar-sal'-jē-à) *n* pain in the foot.

tarso·metatarsal (tar-sō-met-à-tar'-sal) *adj* pertaining to the tarsal and metatarsal region.

tarso·plasty (tar'-sō-plas-tē) *n* any plastic operation to the eyelid.

tarsor·rhaphy (tar-sōr'-à-fē) *n* suturing of the lids together in order to protect the cornea when it is anesthetic, or to allow healing.

tar·sus (tar'-sus) *n* 1 the seven small bones of the foot (⇒ Figure 2). 2 the thin elongated plates of dense connective tissue found in each eyelid, contributing to its form and support—**tarsal** *adj*.

tar·tar (tar'-tar) *n* the deposit, calculus, which forms on the teeth. *tartar emetic* ⇒ antimony and potassium tartrate.

Tay-Sachs' dis·ease (tā'-saks) the primary defect appears to be a deficiency of the enzyme β-D-N-acetylhexosamidase which leads to a massive accumulation of a specific lipid substance called GM₂, or Tay-Sachs ganglioside—hence the alternative name, gangliosidosis.

Tay's choroid·itis (tāz kōr-oyd-ī'-tis) ⇒ choroiditis.

T-bandage used to hold a dressing on the perineum in position.

TBI *abbr* ⇒ total body irradiation.

team nursing a method of giving nursing care in which two or more members of the nursing staff, one of whom is the team leader, are assigned to work together to provide care for a group of patients.

tears (tērz) *npl* the secretion formed by the lacrimal gland. They contain the enzyme lysozyme* which acts as an antiseptic.

tease (tēz) *vt* to draw or pull out into fine threads, as in separating the fibers of a particle of muscle tissue.

teat (tēt) *n* a nipple.

Tebrazid (teb'-rà-zid) *n* proprietary name for pyrazinamide*.

teeth (tēth) *npl* the structures used for mastication. The deciduous, milk or primary set, 20 in number, is shed by the age of 7 years, and is normally replaced by the permanent or secondary teeth. The permanent set, 32 in number, is usually complete in the late teens.—**tooth** *sing. bicuspid teeth* ⇒ bicuspid. *canine or eye teeth* have sharp fang-like edge for tearing food. ⇒ canine. *Hutchinson's teeth* have a notched edge and are characteristic of congenital syphilis. *incisor teeth* have knife-like edge for biting food. *premolar and molar teeth* have a squarish termination for chewing and grinding food. *teething* discomfort, often associated with the signs of inflammation, during the eruption of teeth in infants. *wisdom teeth* are the last molar teeth, one at either side of each jaw.

Teg·retol (teg'-re-tol) *n* proprietary name for carbamazepine*.

tegu·ment (teg'-ū-ment) *n* the skin or covering of the animal body.

telangiec·tasis (tel-an-jē-ek'-ta-sis) *n* dilatation of the capillaries on a body surface.

tel·emetry (tel-em'-et-rē) *n* the graphing of measurements at a distance from the subject by using radio signals.

Tele·paque (tel-ē-pāk') *n* proprietary name for iopanoic* acid.

tele·therapy (tel-ē-thēr'-à-pē) *n* treatment with cobalt or caesium beams—**teletherapeutic** *adj,* **teletherapeutically** *adv*.

Temaril (tem'-à-ril) *n* proprietary name for trimeprazine*.

tem·azepam (tem-az'-e-pam) *n* short-acting benzodiazepine*.

Temovate (tem'-ō-vāt) *n* proprietary name for clobetasol* proprionate.

tempera·ment (tem'-per-à-ment) *n* the habitual mental attitude of the individual.

temple (tem'-pl) *n* that part of the head lying between the outer angle of the eye and the top of the earflap.

tem·poral (tem'-por-al) *adj* relating to the temple. *temporal bones* one on each side of the head below the parietal bone, containing the middle ear.

temporo·mandibular (tem-por-ō-man-dib'-ū-lar) *adj* pertaining to the temporal region or bone, and the lower jaw.

temporo·mandibular joint syn·drome (TMJ) pain in the region of the temporomandibular joint frequently caused by malocclusion of the teeth, resulting in malposition of the condylar heads in the joint and abnormal muscle activity, and by bruxism.

Tempra (tem'-prà) *n* proprietary name for acetaminophen*.

TEN *abbr* toxic* epidermal necrolysis.

tenaculum (ten-ak'-ū-lum) *n* an instrument with a hook on the end for holding parts, as in an operation.

Tenckhoff cath·eter (ten'-kof) a Silastic* tube with spaced perforations in the last 7 cm of the tube, suitable for continuous ambulatory peritoneal dialysis.

ten·don (ten'-don) *n* a firm, white, fibrous inelastic cord which attaches muscle to bone—**tendinous** *adj*.

tendon·itis (ten-don-ī'-tis) *n* inflammation of a tendon.

tenes·mus (ten-es'-mus) *n* painful, ineffectual straining to empty the bowel or bladder.

ten·oplasty (ten'-ō-plas-tē) *n* a reconstructive operation on a tendon—**tenoplastic** *adj*.

Ten·ormin (ten'-ōr-min) *n* proprietary name for atenolol*.

tenor·rhaphy (ten-ōr'-à-fē) *n* the suturing of a tendon.

tenosyno·vitis (ten-ō-sī-nō-vī'-tis) *n* inflammation of the thin synovial lining of a tendon sheath, as distinct from its outer fibrous sheath. It may be caused by mechanical irritation or by bacterial infection.

ten·otomy (ten-ot'-o-mē) *n* division of a tendon.

Ten·uate (ten'-ū-āt) *n* proprietary name for diethylpropion*.

tera·togen (ter-at'-ō-jen) *n* anything capable of disrupting fetal growth and producing malformation. Classified as drugs, poisons, radiations, physical agents such as ECT, infections, e.g. rubella and rhesus and thyroid antibodies. ⇒ dysmorphogenic—**teratogenic, teratogenetic** *adj*, **teratogenicity, teratogenesis** *n*.

tera·tology (ter-à-tol'-o-jē) *n* the scientific study of teratogens and their mode of action—**teratological** *adj*, **teratologist** *n*, **teratologically** *adv*.

tera·toma (ter-à-tō'-mà) *n* a tumor of embryonic origin and composed of various structures, including both epithelial and connective tissues; most commonly found in the ovaries and testes, the majority being malignant—**teratomata** *pl*, **teratomatous** *adj*.

ter·butaline (ter-bū'-tà-lēn) *n* a bronchodilator useful in acute exacerbations of asthma. (Bricanyl.)

teres muscles (tē'-rēz) ⇒ Figure 5.

Terra·mycin (ter-à-mī'-sin) *n* proprietary name for oxytetracycline*.

ter·tiary (ter'-shē-à-rē) *adj* third in order.

tes·ticle (tes'-tik-l) *n* ⇒ testis—**testicular** *adj*.

tes·tis (tes'-tis) *n* one of the two glandular bodies contained in the scrotum of the male (⇒ Figure 16); they form spermatozoa and also the male sex hormones. *undescended testis* the organ remains within the bony pelvis or inguinal canal. ⇒ cryptorchism—**testes** *pl*.

testos·terone (tes-tos'-ter-ōn) *n* the hormone derived from the testes and responsible for the development of the secondary male characteristics. Used in carcinoma of the breast, to control uterine bleeding and in male underdevelopment.

test-tube baby one produced by in* vitro fertilization.

teta·nus (tet'-à-nus) *n* (*syn* lockjaw) disease caused by *Clostridium tetani*, an anaerobe commonly found in ruminants and manure. Affected patients develop a fear of water and muscle spasms. Tetanus toxoid injections produce active immunity. ATS injection produces passive immunity—**tetanic** *adj*.

tet·any (tet'-à-nē) *n* condition of muscular hyperexcitability in which mild stimuli produce cramps and spasms. Found in parathyroid deficiency and alkalosis. Associated in infants with gastrointestinal upset and rickets.

tetracaine (tet'-rà-kān) *n* ophthalmic anesthetic. (Pontocaine.)

tetra·chloro·ethylene (tet-rà-klōr-ō-eth'-il-ēn) *n* an anthelmintic given in hookworm. A single dose is used.

tetra·coccus (tet-rà-kok'-us) *n* coccal bacteria arranged in cubical packets of four.

tetra·cycline (tet-rȧ-sī'-klin) *n* a broad spectrum antibiotic related to both chlortetracycline* and oxytetracycline* and used for similar purposes. As a rule it causes less gastrointestinal disturbances. There is less absorption of oral tetracycline when the stomach is full, or contains aluminium, calcium and magnesium. Causes fluorescence in body cells. This disappears rapidly from normal cells when the drug is discontinued and is retained by cancerous cells for 24–30 h after dosage ceases. (Achromycin.)

tetra·dacytlous (tet-rȧ-dak'-til-us) *adj* having four digits on each limb.

tetradeca·peptide (tet-rȧ-dek-ȧ-pep'-tīd) *n* a peptide containing 14 amino acids.

tetral·ogy of Fallot (tet-ral'-o-jē ov fal-lō') a form of congenital heart defect which comprises cyanosis, a septal defect between the ventricles, hypertrophy of the right ventricle, with narrowing of the outlet, and displacement of the aorta to the right. It is amenable to corrective surgery.

tetra·plegia (tet-rȧ-plē'-jē-ȧ) *n* (*syn* quadriplegia) paralysis of all four limbs—**tetraplegic** *adj*.

thala·motomy (thal-ȧ-mot'-o-mē) *n* usually operative (sterotaxic) destruction of a portion of thalamus. Can be done for intractable pain.

thala·mus (thal'-ȧ-mus) *n* a collection of grey matter at the base of the cerebrum (⇒ Figure 1). Sensory impulses from the whole body pass through on their way to the cerebral cortex—**thalami** *pl*, **thalamic** *adj*.

thalass·emia (thal-ȧ-sēm'-ē-ȧ) *n* a hemolytic anemia which is inherited in an autosomal recessive pattern. There are three classifications: (a) *minor*, denotes the carrier and he/she is asymptomatic (b) *intermediate*, a very mild form which may require an occasional blood transfusion (c) *major*, a severe form in which the affected bone marrow produces fetal type hemoglobin. The breakdown of hemoglobin and recurrent blood transfusions leads to iron overload which is treated with chelating agents such as desferrioxamine.

THAM *abbr* tris*-hydroxylmethyl aminomethane. Proprietary name for tromethamine*.

thanat·ology (than-ȧ-tol'-o-jē) *n* the scientific study of death, including its etiology and diagnosis.

theca (thē'-kȧ) *n* an enveloping sheath, especially of a tendon—**thecal** *adj. theca*

vertebralis the membranes enclosing the spinal cord.

the·nar (thē'-nȧr) *adj* pertaining to the palm of the hand and the sole of the foot. *thenar eminence* the palmar eminence below the thumb.

theo·bromine (thē-ō-brō'-mēn) *n* a drug allied to caffeine*, but with a less stimulating and more powerful diuretic action. It has been given with phenobarbitbone to reduce frequency and severity of anginal attacks.

theo·phylline (thē-of'-i-lin) *n* a diuretic related to caffeine* but more powerful. It is used mainly as its derivative aminophylline* in the treatment of congestive heart failure, dyspnea and asthma.

thera·peutic abor·tion (thèr-ȧ-pū'-tik) ⇒ abortion.

thera·peutic embol·ization (thèr-ȧ-pū'-tik em-bol-ī-zā'-shun) the deliberate infarction of a tumor to reduce its size and vascularity before removal by surgery.

thera·peutics (thèr-ȧ-pū'-tiks) *n* the branch of medical science dealing with the treatment of disease—**therapeutic** *adj*, **therapeutically** *adv*.

ther·apy (thèr'-ȧ-pē) *n* treatment.

ther·mal (ther'-mal) *adj* pertaining to heat.

thermo·genesis (ther-mō-jen'-es-is) *n* the production of heat—**thermogenetic** *adj*.

thermo·labile (ther-mō-lā'-bīl) *adj* capable of being easily altered or discomposed by heat.

thermoly·sis (ther-mol'-is-is) *n* heat-induced chemical dissociation. Dissipation of body heat—**thermolytic** *adj*.

ther·mometer (ther-mom'-et-er) *n* an instrument containing a substance, the volume of which is altered by temperature. The low reading clinical thermometer is marked so that it registers hypothermic body temperatures—**thermometric** *adj*.

thermo·phil (thèr'-mō-fil) *n* a microorganism accustomed to growing at a high temperature—**thermophilic** *adj*.

Thermo·scan (thèr'-mō-skan) *n* a proprietary apparatus capable of scanning the distribution of heat over an area. Sufficiently sensitive to record temperature differentials down to 0° C. Among the many conditions which can be studied are blood flow disorders, viability of skin grafts, onset of malignant breast tumors and the extent of varicose veins.

thermo·stable (thèr-mō-stā'-bl) *adj* unaffected by heat. Remaining unaltered at a high temperature, which is usually specified—**thermostability** *n*.

thermo·therapy (thĕr-mŏ-ther'-à-pē) *n* heat treatment. ⇒ hyperthermia.

thesaur·osis (thē-sawr-ō'-sis) *n* a term currently used with reference to hair sprays. Macromolecules are taken up by cells of the reticuloendothelial system with a consequent inflammatory reaction. Similar to sarcoidosis*.

thiabenda·zole (thī-à-ben'-dà-zōl) *n* best available treatment for *Strongyloides* infestation. No starvation or purgation necessary. Stated to clear the infection in about 50% of patients with trichuriasis. Effective orally for larva migrans caused by some species of Ancylostoma. Has been used as a second-line drug for threadworms in three doses of 50 mg/kg at weekly intervals. (Mintezol.)

thia·mine (thī'-à-min) *n* (*syn* vitamin B₁) concerned in carbohydrate metabolism; indicated therapeutically in thiamine deficiency disorders, such as beri-beri, and some forms of neuritis; also as adjunct to oral antibiotic therapy; deficiency may cause mental confusion or cardiomyopathy.

thia·zides (thī'-à-zīdz) *npl* saluretic diuretic group of drugs ⇒ diuretics.

Thiersch skin graft (tērsh'-ēz) a thin sheet of split skin graft which is applied to a raw surface.

thiethyl·perazine (thī-eth-il-pér'-à-zēn) *n* a phenothiazine* tranquilizer which is useful for nausea, vomiting and vertigo. (Torecan.)

Thimerosal (thī-mèr'-o-sol) *n* organic iodine solution, useful for preparation of skin prior to surgery. (Merthiolate.)

thio·guanine (thī-ō-gwan'-ēn) *n* an antimetabolite. Interferes with synthesis of nucleoprotein, thus useful in acute leukemia.

thio·pental (thī-ō-pen'-tal) *n* a barbiturate given by intravenous injection as a short-acting basal anesthetic. The effect can be extended by additional doses, and in combination with curare compounds adequate relaxation for major surgery can be achieved. (Pentothal.) ⇒ barbiturates.

thio·ridazine (thī-ō-rid'-a-zēn) *n* sedative, tranquilizer. Closely resembles chlorpromazine*. (Mellaril.)

thiothixene (thī-ō-thiks'-ēn) *n* antipsychotic used in schizophrenia.

thiouracil (thī-ō-ū'-ras-il) *n* an antithyroid drug, now rarely used.

thora·centesis (thŏr-à-sen-tē'-sis) *n* aspiration of the pleural cavity.

tho·racic (thŏr-as'-ik) *adj* pertaining to the thorax. *thoracic aorta* ⇒ Figure 9. *thoracic nerve* ⇒ Figure 11. *thoracic duct* a channel conveying lymph (chyle) from the receptaculum chyli in the abdomen to the left subclavian vein. *thoracic inlet syndrome* ⇒ cervical rib.

thoraco·plasty (thŏr'-à-kō-plas-tē) *n* an operation on the thorax in which the ribs are resected to allow the chest wall to collapse and the lung to rest; used in the treatment of tuberculosis. Since the advent of antituberculous drugs it is rarely necessary.

thoraco·scope (thŏr'-à-kō-skōp) *n* an instrument which can be inserted into the pleural cavity through a small incision in the chest wall, to permit inspection of the pleural surfaces and division of adhesions by electric diathermy—**thoracoscopic** *adj,* **thoracospy** *n*.

thora·cotomy (thŏr-à-kot'-o-mē) *n* surgical exposure of the thoracic cavity.

tho·rax (thŏr'-aks) *n* the chest cavity—**thoracic** *adj*.

Thorazine (thŏr'-à-zēn) *n* proprietary name for chlorpromazine*.

thread·worm (thred'-werm) *n* Enterobius vermicularis. Tiny threadlike worms that infest man's intestine. Females migrate to anus to lay eggs, thus spread of, and reinfestation is easy. The whole family should be treated simultaneously using piperazine over a week, together with hygiene measures to prevent reinfestation. A further course after a 10 day interval is advisable to deal with worms that have since hatched, as the eggs are not affected by the drug.

threat·ened abor·tion (thret'-end) ⇒ abortion.

thre·onine (thrē'-on-ēn) *n* an essential amino* acid.

thrill *n* vibration as perceived by the sense of touch.

throm·bectomy (throm-bek'-to-mē) *n* surgical removal of a thrombus from within a blood vessel.

thrombin (throm'-bin) *n* not normally present in circulating blood; generated from prothrombin (Factor II). The extrinsic and intrinsic pathways lead to production of thrombin. The extrinsic pathway is tested by the prothrombin time (PT). The intrinsic pathway involves principally Factors IX and VIII among others. The partial thromboplastin time (PTT) or a modification called the partial thromboplastin time with kaolin (PTTK) detects abnormalities in this pathway ⇒ blood, Christmas disease, hemophilia.

thrombo·angiitis (throm-bō-an-jē-īt'-is) *n* clot formation within an inflamed vessel. *thromboangiitis obliterans* ⇒ Buerger's disease.

thrombo·arteritis (throm-bō-ȧr-ter-īt'-is) *n* inflammation of an artery with clot formation.

thrombo·cyte (throm'-bō-sīt) *n* (*syn* platelet) plays a part in the clotting of blood ⇒ blood.

thrombo·cythemia (throm-bō-sī-thē'-mē-à) *n* a condition in which there is an increase in circulating blood platelets which can encourage clotting within blood vessels. ⇒ thrombocytosis.

thrombo·cytopenia (throm-bō-sī-tō-pē'-nē-à) *n* a reduction in the number of platelets in the blood which can result in spontaneous bruising and prolonged bleeding after injury—**thrombocytopenic** *adj.*

thrombo·cytopenic pur·pura (throm-bō-sī-tō-pē'-nik pur'-pur-à) a syndrome characterized by a low blood platelet count, intermittent mucosal bleeding and purpura. It can be symptomatic, i.e. secondary to known disease or to certain drugs; or idiopathic, a rare condition of unknown cause (purpura hemorrhagica) occurring principally in children and young adults. In both forms the bleeding time is prolonged.

thrombo·cytosis (throm-bō-sī-tō'-sis) *n* an increase in the number of platelets in the blood. It can arise in the course of chronic infections and cancers. It is likely to cause the complication of thrombosis.

thrombo·embolic (throm-bō-em'-bol-ik) *adj* a word which is used to describe the phenomenon whereby a thrombus or clot detaches itself and is carried to another part of the body in the bloodstream to block a blood vessel there.

thrombo·endarter·ectomy (throm-bō-end-ȧr-ter-ek'-to-mē) *n* removal of a thrombus and atheromatous plaques from an artery.

thrombo·endarter·itis (throm-bō-end-ȧr-ter-īt'-is) *n* inflammation of the inner lining of an artery with clot formation.

thrombo·gen (throm'-bō-jen) *n* a precursor of thrombin.

thrombo·genic (throm-bō-jen'-ik) *adj* capable of clotting blood—**thrombogenesis, thrombogenicity** *n,* **thrombogenically** *adv.*

thrombo·kinase (throm-bō-kī'-nās) *n* ⇒ thromboplastin.

thrombo·lytic (throm-bō-lit'-ik) *adj* pertaining to disintegration of a blood clot—**thrombolysis** *n. thrombolytic therapy* the attempted removal of preformed intravascular fibrin occlusions using fibrinolytic agents.

thrombo·phlebitis (throm-bō-fle-bī'-tis) *n* inflammation of the wall of a vein with secondary thrombosis within the involved segment—**thrombophlebitic** *adj. thrombophlebitis migrans* recurrent episodes of thrombophlebitis affecting short lengths of superficial veins; deep vein thrombosis is uncommon and pulmonary embolism rare.

thrombo·plastin (throm'-bō-plas-tin) *n* (*syn* thrombokinase) an enzyme which converts prothrombin into thrombin. *intrinsic thromboplastin* produced by the interaction of several factors during the clotting of blood. Much more active than tissue thromboplastin. *tissue thromboplastin* thromboplastic enzymes are present in many tissues, and tissue extracts are used in clotting experiments and in the estimation of prothrombin time.

throm·bosis (throm-bō'-sis) *n* the intravascular formation of a blood clot—**thromboses** *pl,* **thrombotic** *adj.*

throm·bus (throm'-bus) *n* an intravascular blood clot—**thrombi** *pl.*

thrush (thrush) *n* ⇒ candidiasis.

thymec·tomy (thī-mek'-to-mē) *n* surgical excision of the thymus.

thymo·cytes (thī'-mō-sīts) *n* cells found in the dense lymphoid tissue in the lobular cortex of the thymus gland—**thymocytic** *adj.*

thy·mol (thī'-mol) *n* the chief antiseptic constituent of oil of thyme. Widely employed in mouthwashes and dental preparations, and has been given as an anthelmintic in hookworm.

thymo·leptic (thī-mō-lep'-tik) *n* a term for drugs primarily exerting their effect on the brain, thus influencing 'feeling' and behavior.

thy·moma (thī-mō'-mà) *n* a tumor arising in the thymus—**thymomata** *pl.*

thy·mosin (thī-mō'-sin) *n* hormone secreted by the epithelial cells of the thymus gland. Provides the stimulus for lymphocyte production within the thymus; confers on lymphocytes elsewhere in the body the capacity to respond to antigenic stimulation.

thy·mus (thī'-mus) *n* a gland lying behind the breast bone and extending upward as far as the thyroid gland. It is well developed in infancy and attains its greatest size towards puberty; and then the lymphatic tissue is replaced by fatty tissue. It has an immunological role. Autoimmunity is thought to result from pathological activity of this gland—**thymic** *adj*.

thyro·calcitonin (thī-rō-kal-si-tō'-nin) *n* ⇒ calcitonin.

thyro·glossal (thī-rō-glos'-al) *adj* pertaining to the thyroid gland and the tongue. *thyroglossal cyst* a retention*cyst caused by blockage of the thyroglossal duct; it appears on one or other side of the neck. *thyroglossal duct* the fetal passage from the thyroid gland to the back of the tongue where its vestigial end remains as the foramen cecum. In this area thyroglossal cyst or fistula can occur.

thy·roid (thī'-royd) *n* the ductless gland found on both sides of the trachea. It secretes thyroxine, which controls the rate of metabolism. The commercial material is prepared from the thyroid gland of the ox, sheep or pig, dried and reduced to powder and adjusted in strength to contain 0.1% of iodine as thyroxine. Used in myxedema and cretinism. *thyroid cartilage* ⇒ Figure 6. *thyroid antibody test* the presence and severity of autoimmune thyroid disease is diagnosed by the levels of thyroid antibody in the blood. *thyroid-stimulating hormone test (TSH)* radioimmunoassay of the level of thyroid-stimulating hormone in the serum. Useful in diagnosing mild hypothyroidism.

thyroid·ectomy (thī-royd-ek'-to-mē) *n* surgical removal of the thyroid gland.

thyroid·itis (thī-royd-īt'-is) *n* inflammation of the thyroid gland. *Autoimmune thyroiditis* or Hashimoto's disease is a firm goiter ultimately resulting in hypothyroidism. *Riedel's thyroiditis* ⇒ Riedel's*.

thyro·toxicosis (thī-rō-toks-ik-ōs'-is) *n* one of the autoimmune thyroid diseases. A condition due to excessive production of the thyroid gland hormone (thyroxine*), usually due to a thyroid stimulating immunoglobulin, and resulting classically in anxiety, tachycardia, sweating, increased appetite with weight loss, and a fine tremor of the out-stretched hands, and prominence of the eyes (Graves' dis-

ease). It is much more common in women than in men. In older patients cardiac irregularities may be a prominent feature. Thyrotoxicosis may also be due to increased thyroxine production by a single thyroid nodule or a multinodular goiter—**thyrotoxic** *adj*.

thyro·toxic crisis (thī-rō-toks'-ik krī'-sis) the sudden worsening of symptoms in a patient with thyrotoxicosis; may occur immediately after thyroidectomy if the patient is not properly prepared.

thyro·trophic (thī-rō-trō'-fik) *adj* describes a substance which stimulates the thyroid gland, e.g. thyrotrophin (thyroid stimulating hormone, TSH) secreted by the anterior pituitary gland.

thyrox·ine (thī-roks'-ēn) *n* the principal hormone of the thyroid gland. It raises the basal metabolic rate. Thyroxine is used in the treatment of hypothyroidism. (Eltroxin.)

TIA *abbr* transient* ischemic attacks.

tibia (tib'-ē-à) *n* the shin-bone; the larger of the two bones in the lower part of the leg; it articulates with the femur*, fibula* and talus*—**tibial** *adj*.

tibial artery (tib'-ē-al ar'-ter-ē) ⇒ Figure 9.

tibial vein (tib'-ē-al vān) ⇒ Figure 10.

tibiofibular (tib-ē-ō-fib'-ū-lar) *adj* pertaining to the tibia and the fibula.

tic (tik) *n* purposeless involuntary, spasmodic muscular movements and twitchings, due partly to habit, but often associated with a psychological factor.

tic douloureux (tik doo'-loor-er) (trigeminal neuralgia) spasms of excruciating pain in the distribution of the trigeminal nerve.

tick (tik) *n* a blood-sucking parasite, larger than a mite. Some of them are concerned in the transmission of relapsing fever, typhus, etc.

tidal air (tī'-dal èr) the volume of air which passes in and out of the lungs in normal breathing.

Tietze syn·drome (tēt'-sēz) costochondritis which is self-limiting and of unknown etiology. There is no specific treatment. Different diagnosis is myocardial infarction.

timolol maleate (tim'-ol-ol mal'-ē-āt) a hypotensive beta-blocking agent. (Blocadren.)

tinc·ture (tink'-tūr) *n* the solution of a drug in alcohol.

tine test (tīn) a multiple puncture test using disposable equipment. The plastic holder has four small tines coated with undiluted tuberculin. The reaction is read in 48–72 h.

tinea (tin'-ē-à) *n* ⇒ ringworm. *tinea barbae* sycosis* barbae. *tinea capitis* ringworm of the head. *tinea corporis* (*syn* circinata) ringworm of the body. *tinea cruris* (*syn* dhobie itch) ringworm of the crutch area. *tinea incognita* unrecognized ringworm to which topical corticosteroids have been inappropriately applied, obscuring the usual signs of ringworm. *tinea pedis* ringworm of the foot.

tin·nitus (tin-ī'-tus) *n* a buzzing, thumping or ringing sound in the ears.

tint·ometer (tin-tom'-et-ėr) *n* an apparatus for measuring the degree of redness in the skin, an early sign of hyperemia which may progress to inflammation.

tis·sue (tish'-ū) *n* a collection of cells or fibers of similar function, forming a structure. *tissue respiration* ⇒ respiration.

ti·tration (tī-trā'-shun) *n* volumetric analysis by aid of standard solutions.

titer (tī'-ter) *n* a standard of concentration per volume, as determined by titration.

TLC *abbr* tender loving care.

TMJ *abbr* temporomandibular* joint syndrome.

TNM system a method of staging the extent of the malignant process. The initial letters indicate Tumor, Nodes (lymph) and Metastases (distant). Each category has four main divisions—T1–4, N and M0–3. The combined score permits allocation to Stages 1–4.

tobacco ambly·opia (tō-bak'-ō am-blī-ōp'-ē-à) ⇒ smokers' blindness.

tobra·mycin (tō-brà-mī'-sin) *n* an antibiotic similar to gentamicin* but said to be less toxic. (Nebcin.)

toc·ography (tok-og'-raf-ē) *n* process of recording uterine contractions using a tocograph or a parturiometer.

toc·opherol (tok-of'-er-ol) *n* synthetic vitamin E, similar to that found in wheatgerm oil. It has been used in habitual abortion, and empirically in many other conditions with varying success.

Tof·ranil (tof'-ran-il) *n* proprietary name for imipramine*.

tolaz·amide (tol-az'-à-mīd) *n* one of the sulfonylureas*. (Tolinase.)

tolaz·oline (tol-az'-ol-ēn) *n* a peripheral vasodilator, used in circulatory disorders such as Raynaud's disease and re-

lated conditions. Has also been used in ophthalmic conditions such as keratitis. (Priscoline.)

tolbut·amide (tol-bū'-tà-mīd) *n* a sulfonamide* derivative which stimulates functioning islets of Langerhans to pour out more insulin. Has been used with success in the oral treatment of diabetes, so that insulin injections may be reduced or withdrawn. Of no value in juvenile diabetes. (Orinase.) *tolbutamide test* after blood is withdrawn for estimation of its fasting sugar content, an intravenous injection of tolbutamide is given. Blood is taken for glucose levels 20 and 30 min later. Differentiates diabetes which can be controlled by oral antidiabetic drugs (non-insulin dependent) from diabetes which cannot be so controlled (insulin dependent).

toler·ance (tol'-ėr-ans) *n* ability to endure the application or administratiion of a substance, usually a drug. One may have to increase the dose of the drug as tolerance develops, e.g. nitrites. *exercise tolerance* exercise accomplished without pain or marked breathlessness. American Heart Association's classification of functional capacity: Class I—no symptoms on ordinary effort; Class II—slight disability on ordinary effort; Class III—marked disability on ordinary effort which prevents any attempt at housework; Class IV—symptoms at rest or heart failure.

Tolinase (tol'-i-nās) *n* proprietary name for tolazamide*.

tol·naftate (tol-naf'-tāt) *n* an antifungal agent, useful for athlete's foot. (Tinactin.)

tomo·graphy (to-mo'-graf-ē) *n* a technique of using X-rays to create an image of a specific, thin layer through the body (rather than the whole body)—**tomographic** *adj*, **tomogram** *n*, **tomograph** *n*, **tomographically** *adv*.

tone (tōn) *n* the normal, healthy state of tension.

tongue (tung) *n* the mobile muscular organ contained in the mouth; it is concerned with speech, mastication, swallowing and taste. ⇒ strawberry tongue.

tonic (ton'-ik) *adj* used to describe a state of continuous muscular contraction, as opposed to intermittent contraction.

ton·ography (ton-og'-raf-ē) *n* continuous measurement of blood, or intraocular, pressure. *carotid compression tonography* normally occlusion of one common carotid artery causes an ipsilateral fall of

281

intraocular pressure. Used as a screening test for carotid insufficiency.

tonom·eter (ton-om'-et-er) *n* an instrument for measuring intraocular pressure.

tonsil·lectomy (ton-sil-lek'-to-mē) *n* removal of the tonsils. *tonsillectomy position* the three quarters prone position to prevent inhalation (aspiration) pneumonia and asphyxiation.

tonsil·litis (ton-sil-lī'-tis) *n* inflammation of the tonsils.

tonsil·loliths (ton-sil'-lō-liths) *npl* concretions arising in the body of the tonsil.

tonsillo·pharyngeal (ton-sil-lō-fär-in-jē'-al) *adj* pertaining to the tonsils* and pharynx*.

tonsil·lotome (ton-sil'-lō-tōm) *n* instrument for excision of tonsils.

ton·sils (ton'-sils) *npl* the small bodies, one on each side, covered by mucous membrane, embedded in the fauces between the palatine arch; composed of about 10–18 lymph follicles—**tonsillar** *adj*.

tooth (tōōth) ⇒ Figure 14, teeth.

top·ectomy (top-ek'-to-mē) *n* modified frontal lobotomy. Small incisions made in thalamofrontal tracts.

tophus (tō'-fus) *n* a small, hard concretion forming on the ear-lobe, on the joints of the phalanges, etc. in gout—**tophi** *pl*.

top·ical (top'-i-kal) *adj* describes the local application of such things as anesthetics, drugs, powders and ointments to skin and mucous membrane—**topically** *adv*.

top·ography (top-og'-raf-ē) *n* a description of the regions of the body—**topographical** *adj*, **topographically** *adv*.

TOPV *abbr* trivalent oral polio vaccine.

TORCH infections infectious diseases which may be transmitted to the fetus through the placenta. Includes toxoplasmosis, rubella, cytomegalo virus and herpes simplex.

Tore·can (tōr'-e-kan) *n* proprietary name for thiethylperazine*.

tor·sion (tōr'-shun) *n* twisting.

torti·collis (tōr-ti-kol'-is) *n* (*syn* wryneck) a painless contraction of one sternocleidomastoid* muscle. The head is slightly flexed and drawn towards the contracted side, with the face rotated over the other shoulder.

total body ir·radiation (TBI) a treatment used in the early treatment of some cancers.

total co·lonic lav·age (*syn* whole gut irrigation) a preoperative procedure before extensive bowel surgery. A large amount of fluid, e.g. 1 l per half hour, is introduced into the stomach via a nasogastric tube while the patient sits on a padded commode. The infusion is continued until the effluent is clear, usually 4–6 h. Has been used for fecal impaction.

total par·enteral nu·trition (TPN) solutions containing all essential nutrients administered by a central venous line; only liquids and low density solutions are administered. ⇒ parenteral feeding.

Toti's oper·ation (tō'-tēz) ⇒ dacryocystorhinostomy.

tourni·quet (turn'-i-ket) *n* an apparatus for the compression of the blood vessels of a limb. Designed for compression of a main artery to control bleeding. It is also used to obstruct the venous return from a limb and so facilitate the withdrawal of blood from a vein. Tourniquets vary from a simple rubber band to a pneumatic cuff.

tox·emia (toks-ē'-mē-à) *n* a generalized poisoning of the body by the products of bacteria or damaged tissue—**toxemic** *adj*.

toxic (toks'-ik) *adj* poisonous, caused by a poison. *toxic epidermal necrolysis (TEN)* a syndrome in which the appearance is of scalded skin. It can occur in response to drug reaction, staphylococcal infection, systemic illness, and it can be idiopathic. *toxic shock syndrome* (*syn* tampon shock syndrome) a recently recognized cluster of signs and symptoms which occur in some women who use tampons. There is high temperature, vomiting and diarrhea. *Staphylococcus aureus* is present in the vagina of about 5% of women; it produces a toxin and the victim develops blood poisoning. Tampons are thought to encourage production of toxin by acting as a plug. The condition is sometimes fatal.

tox·icity (toks-is'-i-tē) *n* the quality or degree of being poisonous.

toxi·cology (toks-i-kol'-o-jē) *n* the science dealing with poisons, their mechanisms of action and antidotes to them—**toxicological** *adj*, **toxicologically** *adv*.

toxico·mania (toks-i-kō-mā'-nē-à) *n* WHO definition: Periodic or chronic state of intoxication produced by repeated consumption of a drug harmful to the individual or society. Characteristics are: (a) uncontrollable desire or necessity to continue consuming the drug and to try to get it by all means (b) tendency to increase the dose (c) psychic and physical dependency as a result.

toxin (toks'-in) *n* a product of bacteria that damages or kills cells.

Toxo·cara (toks-ō-kār'-à) *n* genus of roundworm of the cat and dog. Man can be infested (toxocariasis) by eating with hands soiled from these pets. The worms cannot become adult in man (incorrect host) so the larval worms wander through the body, attacking mainly the liver and the eye. Treatment is unsatisfactory, but the condition usually clears after several months.

tox·oid (toks'-oyd) *adj* a toxin altered in such a way that it has lost its poisonous properties but retained its antigenic properties. *toxoid antitoxin* a mixture of toxoid and homologous antitoxin in floccule form, used as a vaccine, e.g. in immunization against diphtheria.

Toxo·plasma (toks-ō-plaz'-mà) *n* a protozoon whose natural host in the US is the domestic cat. Cats' feces are allegedly the source of most human infections in this country and, like another possible source, undercooked meat, should be avoided by pregnant women.

toxo·plasmosis (toks-ō-plaz-mō'-sis) *n* *Toxoplasma* parasites which, commonly occurring in mammals and birds, may infect man. Intrauterine fetal and infant infections are often severe, producing encephalitis, convulsions hydrocephalus and eye diseases, resulting in death or, in those who recover, mental retardation and impaired sight. Infection in older children and adults may result in pneumonia, nephritis or skin rashes. Skull X-ray reveals flecks of cerebral calcification. Skin and antibody tests confirm the diagnosis.

TPI test *Treponema pallidum* immobilization test; a modern, highly specific test for syphilis in which syphilitic serum immobilizes and kills spirochetes grown in pure culture.

TPN *abbr* total* parenteral nutrition.

trabec·ulae (tràb-ek'-ū-lē) *npl* the fibrous bands or septa projecting into the interior of an organ, e.g. the spleen; they are extensions from the capsule surrounding the organ—**trabecula** *sing,* **trabecular** *adj.*

trabec·ulotomy (trab-ek-ū-lot'-o-mē) *n* operation for glaucoma. It aims at creating a channel through the trabecular meshwork from the canal of Schlemm to the angle of the anterior chamber.

trace elements (trās el'-e-ments) metals and other elements that are regularly present in very small amounts in the tissues and known to be essential for normal metabolism (e.g. copper, cobalt, manganese, fluorine etc).

tracer (trās'-er) *n* a substance or instrument used to gain information. Radioactive tracers have extended knowledge in physiology; some are used in diagnosis.

tra·chea (trā'-kē-à) *n* (*syn* windpipe) the fibrocartilaginous tube lined with mucous membrane passing from the larynx* to the bronchi* ($\Rightarrow$ Figure 6). It is about 115 mm long and about 25 mm wide—**tracheal** *adj.*

tra·cheitis (trā-kē-ī'-tis) *n* inflammation of the trachea; most commonly the result of a viral infection such as the common cold.

trachelor·rhaphy (trā-kel-ōr'-à-fē) *n* operative repair of a uterine cervical laceration.

tracheo·bronchial (trā-kē-ō-brongk'-ē-al) *adj* pertaining to the trachea* and the bronchi*.

tracheo·bronchitis (trā'-kē-ō-brongk-ī'-tis) *n* inflammation of the trachea and bronchi $\Rightarrow$ acute bronchitis.

tracheo·esophageal (trā'-kē-ō-ē-sof-à-jē'-al) *adj* pertaining to the trachea* and the esophagus*. *tracheo-esophageal fistula* usually occurs in conjunction with esophageal atresia. The fistula usually connects the distal esophagus to the trachea.

tracheost·omy (trā-kē-os'-to-mē) *n* fenestration in the anterior wall of the trachea by removal of a circular piece of cartilage from the third and fourth rings, for establishment of a safe airway and reduction of 'dead space'—**tracheostome** *n.*

tracheot·omy (trā-kē-ot'-o-mē) *n* vertical slit in the anterior wall of the trachea at the level of the third and fourth cartilaginous rings.

tra·choma (trà-kō'-mà) *n* contagious inflammation affecting conjunctiva, cornea and eyelids. It is due to *Chlamydia trachomatis* which resembles a virus, which behaves like a bacterium, though it multiplies intracellularly; it is sensitive to sulfonamides and antibiotics. If untreated, trachoma leads to blindness.

Tracrium (trak'-rē-um) *n* proprietary name for atracurium*.

trac·tion (trak'-shun) *n* a drawing or pulling on the patient's body to overcome muscle spasm and to reduce or prevent deformity. A steady pulling exerted on some part (limb or head) by means of weights and pulleys. ⇒ Balkan beam, Braun's frame, Bryant's traction, halopelvic traction, Milwaukee brace, Russell traction.

trac·totomy (trak-tot'-o-mē) *n* incision of a nerve tract. Surgical relief of intractable pain. Using stereotactic measures this operation is now being done for some forms of mental illness.

tragus (trā'-gus) *n* the projection in front of the external auditory meatus—**tragi** *pl*.

trait (trāt) *n* an individual characteristic forming part of the whole personality.

trance (trans) *n* a term used for hypnotic sleep and for certain self-induced hysterical stuporous states.

tranquil·izers (tran'-kwi-lī-zerz) *npl* drugs used to relieve tension or combat psychotic symptoms without significant sedation. These drugs do not affect a basic disease, but reduce symptoms so that the patent feels more comfortable and is more accessible to help from psychotherapy. Greatly exaggerate the effects of alcohol.

trans·abdominal (trans-ab-dom'-in-al) *adj* through the abdomen, as the transabdominal approach for nephrectomy—**transabdominally** *adv*.

trans·amniotic (trans-am-nē-ot'-ik) *adj* through the amniotic membrane and fluid, as a transamniotic transfusion of the fetus for hemolytic disease.

trans·cutaneous (trans-kū-tā'-nē-us) *adj* through the skin, for example absorption of applied drugs; or the monitoring of the oxygen and carbon dioxide content of blood in skin vessels. *transcutaneous electrical nerve supply* four pads are placed on either side of the spine from a battery-operated apparatus which can be controlled by the patient for relief of pain.

tran·section (trans-sek'-shun) *n* the cutting across or mechanical severance of a structure.

trans·frontal (trans-front'-al) *adj* through the frontal bone; an approach used for hypophysectomy.

trans·fusion (trans-fū'-zhun) *n* the introduction of fluid into the tissue or into a blood vessel. *blood transfusion* the intravenous replacement of lost or destroyed blood by compatible citrated human blood. Also used for severe anemia with deficient blood production.

Fresh blood from a donor or stored blood from a blood bank may be used. It can be given 'whole', or with some plasma removed ('packed-cell' transfusion). If incompatible blood is given severe reaction follows. ⇒ blood groups. *intrauterine transfusion* of the fetus endangered by Rhesus incompatibility. Red cells are transfused directly into the abdominal cavity of the fetus, on one or more occasions. This enables the induction of labor to be postponed until a time more favorable to fetal welfare.

Trans·derm·Nitro (trans'-dėrm nī'-trō) a proprietary preparation of glyceryl trinitrate which facilitates controlled absorption via the skin so that a constant blood level can be maintained.

trans·sient is·chemic attacks (TIA) (tranz'-ē-ent ish-ēm'-ik) ⇒ drop attacks, vertebrobasilar insufficiency.

trans·illumination (trans-il-ū-min-ā'-shun) *n* the transmission of light through the sinuses for diagnostic purposes.

trans·irrigation (trans-ir-i-gā'-shun) *n* diagnostic puncture and lavage, as performed in maxillary sinusitis.

trans·location (trans-lō-kā'-shun) *n* transfer of a segment of a chromosome to a different site on the same chromosome (shift) or to a different one. Can be a direct or indirect cause of congenital abnormality.

trans·lucent (trans-lū'-sent) *adj* intermediate between opaque and transparent.

trans·lumbar (trans-lum'-bar) *adj* through the lumbar region. Route used for injecting aorta prior to aortography.

trans·methylation (trans-meth-il-ā'-shun) *n* a process in the metabolism of amino acids in which a methyl group is transferred from one compound to another.

trans·migration (trans-mī-grā'-shun) *n* the transit of a cell across a membrane from one side of a vessel to the other.

trans·mural (trans-mū'-ral) *adj* through the wall, e.g. of a cyst, organ or vessel—**transmurally** *adv*.

trans·nasal (trans-nā'-sal) *adj* through the nose—**transnasally** *adv*.

tran·sonic (trans-on'-ik) *adj* allowing the passage of ultrasound.

trans·peritoneal *adj* (trans-pār-it-on-ē'-al) across or through the peritoneal cavity. ⇒ dialysis.

trans·placental (trans-plas-en'-tal) *adj* through the placenta—**transplacentally** *adv*.

trans·plant (trans'-plant) *n* customarily

refers to the surgical operation of grafting an organ, which has been removed from a cadaver that has been declared brain dead, or from a living relative. If the recipient's malfunctioning organ is removed and the transplant is placed in its bed it is referred to as an *orthotopic transplant* (e.g. liver and heart). If the transplanted organ is not placed in its normal anatomical site the term *heterotopic transplant* is used—**transplantation** *n*, **transplant** *vt*.

transplant·ation (trans-plant-ā'-shun) *n* commonly refers to the transplantation of healthy bone marrow to treat inborn errors such as: immune deficiency; the deficiency anemias such as thalassemia and aplastic anemia; and mucopolysaccharidoses, a group of diseases in which the enzyme that breaks down body mucus is absent.

trans·rectal (trans-rek'-tal) *adj* through the rectum, as a transrectal injection into a tumor—**transrectally** *adv*.

trans·sphenoidal (trans-sfen-oyd'-al) *adj* through the sphenoid bone; an approach used for hypophysectomy.

trans·thoracic (trans-thōr-as'-ik) *adj* across or through the chest, as in transthoracic needle biopsy of a lung mass.

transu·date (trans'-ū-dāt) *n* a fluid that has passed out of the cells either into a body cavity (e.g. ascitic fluid in the peritoneal cavity) or to the exterior (e.g. serum from the surface of a burn).

trans·urethral (trans-ūr-ēth'-ral) *adj* by way of the urethra.

trans·vaginal (trans-vaj'-in-al) *adj* through the vagina, as an incision to drain the uterorectal pouch, transvaginal injection into a tumor, pudendal block or culdoscopy—**transvaginally** *adv*.

trans·ventricular (trans-ven-trik'-ū-lar) *adj* through a ventricle. Term used mainly in cardiac surgery—**transventricularly** *adv*.

transverse colon (trans'-vėrs kō'-lon) ⇒ Figure 18.

trans·vesical (trans-ves'-ik-al) *adj* through the bladder, by custom referring to the urinary bladder—**transvesically** *adv*.

tranyl·cypromine (tra-nl-sī'-prō-mēn) *n* a monamine* oxidase inhibitor. (Parnate.)

tra·pezius muscles (trà-pē'-zē-us) ⇒ Figures 4, 5.

Trasi·cor (tras'-i-kōr) *n* proprietary name for oxprenolol*.

trauma (traw'-mà) *n* **1** bodily injury. **2** emotional shock—**traumatic** *adj*.

traumatol·ogist (traw-mà-tol'-o-jist) *n* a surgeon who specializes in traumatology.

trauma·tology (traw-mà-tol'-o-jē) *n* the branch of surgery dealing with injury caused by accident—**traumatological** *adj*, **traumatologically** *adv*.

Trecator (trē-kā'-tor) *n* proprietary name for ethionamide*.

Trema·toda (trem-à-tō'-dà) *n* a class of parasitic worms which include many pathogens of man such as the *Schistosoma* of schistosomiasis.

tremor (trem'-or) *n* involuntary trembling. *intention tremor* an involuntary tremor which only occurs on attempting voluntary movement; a characteristic of multiple sclerosis.

trench foot (trench-foot) (*syn* immersion foot) occurs in frostbite* or other conditions of exposure where there is 'deprivation' of local blood supply and secondary bacterial infection.

trench mouth infection of tonsils by Vincent's bacillus.

Trendelen·burg's oper·ation (tren-del'-en-burgs) ligation of the long saphenous vein in the groin at its junction with the femoral vein. Used in cases of varicose veins.

Trendelen·burg's pos·ition lying on an operating or examination table, with the head lowermost and the legs raised.

Trendelen·burg's sign a test of the stability of the hip, and particularly of the ability of the hip abductors (gluteus medius and minimus) to steady the pelvis upon the femur. Principle: normally, when one leg is raised from the ground the pelvis tilts upwards on that side, through the hip abductors of the standing limb. If the abductors are inefficient (e.g. in poliomyelitis, severe coxa vara and congenital dislocation of the hip), they are unable to sustain the pelvis against the body weight and it tilts downwards instead of rising.

tre·phine (trē-fīn') *n* an instrument with sawlike edges for removing a circular piece of tissue, such as the cornea or skull.

Trepon·ema (trep-on-ēm'-à) *n* a genus of slender spiral-shaped bacteria which are actively motile. Best visualized with dark-ground illumination. Cultivated in the laboratory with great difficulty. *Treponema pallidum* is the causative organism of syphilis; *Treponema pertenue* the spirochete that causes yaws. *Treponema carateum;* the spirochete that causes pinta.

treponema·tosis (trep-on-ĕm-à-tōs'-is) *n* the term applied to the treponemal diseases.

treponemi·cide (trep-on-ĕm'-i-sīd) *n* lethal to *Treponema*—**treponemicidal** *adj*.

tri·age (trĕ-azh) *n* a system of priority classification of patients in any emergency situation.

trial of labor where there is a question of cephalopelvic disproportion, the pregnant woman is allowed to labor under supervision to determine whether the delivery can proceed vaginally.

triam·cinolone (trī-am-sin'-o-lōn) *n* a steroid with good anti-inflammatory effect and very little electrolyte retaining activity. Because of stimulation of protein breakdown it can cause muscle wasting. (Aristocort, Kenalog.)

triam·terene (trī-am'-ter-ēn) *n* a diuretic that increases excretion of sodium chloride but lessens potassium loss at distal kidney tubule.

tri·angular band·age (trī-ang'-ū-lar) useful for arm slings, for securing splints, in first aid work and for inclusive dressings of a part, as a whole hand or foot.

TRIC *abbr* trachoma inclusion conjunctivitis. Agent responsible for infections of eye, genital tract and urethritis. ⇒ conjunctivitis.

tri·ceps (trī'-seps) *n* the three-headed muscle on the back of the upper arm (⇒ Figures 4, 5).

trich·iasis (trik-ī'-à-sis) *n* abnormal ingrowing eyelashes causing irritation from friction on the eyeball.

trichi·nosis (trik-i-nō'-sis)*n* a disease caused by eating undercooked pig meat infected with *Trichinella spiralis* (the trichina worm). The female worms living in the small bowel produce larvae which invade the body and, in particular, form cysts in skeletal muscles; the usual symptoms are diarrhea, nausea, colic, fever, facial edema, muscular pains and stiffness.

trichlor·acetic acid (trī-klōr-à-sē'-tik as'-id) a powerful caustic and astringent. Used as a crystal for application to warts and ulcers.

trichloro·ethylene (trī-klōr-ō-eth'-il-ēn) *n* volatile liquid whose vapor is a good analgesic but poor general anesthetic. Inhaled in small doses, it is useful in relieving the pain of trigeminal neuralgia and in self-administered obstetric anaesthesia. (Trilene.)

tricho·monacide (trik-ō-mōn'-à-sīd) *n* lethal to the protozoa belonging to the genus *Trichomonas*.

Tricho·monas (trik-ō-mōn'-às) *n* a protozoan parasite of man. *Trichomonas vaginalis* produces infection of the urethra and vagina often associated with profuse discharge (leukorrhea). The organism is best recognized by microscopic examination of the discharge. ⇒ amoeba protozoa.

tricho·moniasis (trik-ō-mō-nī'-à-sis) *n* inflammation of the vagina (urethra in males) caused by *Trichomonas vaginalis*.

tricho·phytosis (trik-ō-fī-tō'-sis) *n* infection with a species of the fungus *Trichophyton,* e.g. ringworm* of the hair or skin.

trichuri·asis (tri-kū-rī'-à-sis) *n* infestation with *Trichuris trichiura*.

Tri·churis (tri-kū'-ris) *n* a genus of nematodes. *Trichuris trichiura* the whipworm.

triclo·fos (trī'-klō-fōs) *n* derivative of chloral* hydrate causing less gastric irriation. (Triclos.)

Triclos (trī'-klos) *n* proprietary name for triclofos*.

tri·cuspid (trī'-kus'-pid) *adj* having three cusps. *tricuspid valve* that between the right atrium and ventricle of the heart.

tri·fluoper·azine (trī-flū-ō-pėr'-à-zēn) *n* a tranquilizer and antiemetic. More potent and less sedative than chlorpromazine*. (Stelazine.)

trigem·inal (trī-jem'-in-al) *adj* triple; separating into three sections, e.g. the trigeminal nerve, the fifth cranial nerve, which has three branches, supplying the skin of the face, the tongue and teeth. *trigeminal neuralgia* ⇒ tic douloureux.

trig·ger fin·ger (trig'-ger fing'-er) a condition in which the finger can be actively bent but cannot be straightened without help; usually due to a thickening on the tendon which prevents free gliding.

tri·gone (trī'-gōn) *n* a triangular area, especially applied to the bladder base, bounded by the ureteral openings at the back and the urethral opening at the front—**trigonal** *adj*.

trihexyphenidyl (trī-heks-ē-fen'-i-dl) *n* antispasmodic used mainly for rigidity of parkinsonism. Side effects include dryness of mouth, nausea and vertigo. (Artane.)

tri·iodo·thyronine (trī-ī-ō-dō-thī'-ron-ēn) *n* a thyroid hormone that plays a part in maintaining the body's metabolic process.

Tri·lene (trī'-lēn) *n* proprietary name for trichloroethylene.

trime·prazine (trī-mep'-rā-zēn) *n* an antihistamine with sedative action. A phenothiazine* derivative. Used in the treatment of pruritis, urticaria and preoperatively for children. (Temaril.)

tri·mester (trī-mes'-ter) *n* a period of 3 months.

tri·methaphan (trī-meth'-ā-fan) *n* a brief-acting blocking agent used by intravenous injection to produce a fall in blood pressure during bloodless field surgery. (Arfonad.)

tri·methoprim (trī-meth'-ō-prim) *n* an antibacterial agent. Has selective inhibiting action on the enzyme that converts folic acid into folinic acid, needed by many bacteria. When used with sulfonamides* the ensuing action is bactericidal. The sulfonamide must have a similar pattern of absorption and excretion. ⇒ co-trimoxazole.

tri·mipramine (trī-mip'-rā-mēn) *n* an antidepressant similar to imipramine*. (Surmontil.)

tripelennamine (trī-pel-en'-ā-mēn) *n* an antihistamine, useful in the treatment of allergies.

triple antigen (*syn*, DPT) contains diphtheria, whooping-cough and tetanus antigens.

triple test (tri'-pl) a Dreiling tube is passed through the mouth into the duodenum and pancreatic function tests are carried out. In these, the enzymes secretin and pancreozymin are given to stimulate the pancreas and the juice is aspirated as it flows into the duodenum. It is possible to recognize a tumor in the pancreas from analysis of the volume and chemistry of this juice. Some of the juice is then examined by the pathologist using Papanicolaou's method to show cancer cells and thirdly, the radiologist performs a hypotonic duodenogram which, unlike the conventional barium meal, frequently demonstrates tumors of the pancreas or ampulla. The test takes 2 h to complete.

triple vac·cine ⇒ vaccines.

trip·loid (trip'-loyd) *adj* possessing three chromosomal sets. ⇒ genome, haploid.

trismus (triz'-mus) *n* spasm in the muscles of mastication.

tri·somy (trī'-sō-mē) *n* the presence in triplicate of a chromosome that should normally be present only in duplicate. This increases the chromosome number by one (single trisomy), e.g. to 47 in man. *trisomy 18* ⇒ Edward syndrome. *trisomy 21* ⇒ Down syndrome.

tro·car (trō'-kar) *n* a pointed rod which fits inside a cannula*.

trochan·ters (trō-kan'-ters) *npl* two processes, the larger one (*trochanters major*) on the outer, the other (*trichanters minor*) on the inner side of the femur between the shaft and neck; they serve for the attachment of muscles—**trochanteric** *adj*.

troch·lea (trō'-klē-à) *n* any part which is like a pulley in structure or function—**trochlear** *adj*.

tromethamine (trō-meth'-ā-mēn) *n* an alkali used to treat acidosis. (THAM.)

tro·phic (trō'-fik) *adj* pertaining to nutrition.

tropho·blastic tissue (trof-ō-blas'-tik) cells, covering the embedding ovum and concerned with the nutrition of the ovum.

tropic·amide (tro-pik'-à-mīd) *n* a synthetic drug which has mydriatic and cyclophegic actions. (Mydracil.)

Trouseau's sign (trōō-sōz') ⇒ carpopedal spasm.

Trypano·soma (trī-pan-ō-sō'-mà) *n* a genus of parasitic protozoa. Their life cycle alternates between blood-sucking arthropods and vertebrate hosts, and in the latter they appear frequently in the blood stream as fusiform, actively motile structures some 10–40 μm in length. A limited number of species are pathogenic to man.

trypano·somiasis (trī-pan-ō-sō-mī'-à-sis) *n* disease produced by infestation with *Trypanosoma*. In man this may be with *Trypanosoma rhodesiense* in East Africa or *Trypanosoma gambiense* in West Africa, both transmitted by the tsetse fly, and with *Trypanosoma cruzii*, transmitted by bugs, in South Africa. In West Africa infection of the brain commonly produces the symptomatology of 'sleeping sickness'.

tryparsamide (trī-pàr'-sà-mīd) *n* an organic arsenic compound of value in the treatment of trypanosomiasis. It is usually given by intravenous injection, as it is more irritant and less effective orally.

tryp·sin (trip'-sin) *n* a proteolytic enzyme present in pancreatic juice. Given in digestive disorders. Specially purified forms are used to liquefy clotted blood and other secretions, and in ophthalmology to facilitate removal of cataracts.

tryp·tophan (trip'-tō-fan) *n* one of the essential amino* acids necessary for growth. It is a precursor of serotonin*. Adequate levels of tryptophan may compensate deficiencies of niacin and thus mitigate pellagra.

tsetse fly (tsĕt'-sē) a fly of the genus *Glossina*, the vector of *Trypanosoma* in Africa. The *Trypanosoma* live part of their life cycle in the flies and are transferred to new hosts, including man, in the salivary juices when the fly bites for a blood meal.

tubal (tū'-bal) *adj* pertaining to a tube. *tubal abortion* ⇒ abortion. *tubal ligation* tying of both fallopian tubes as a means of sterilization. *tubal pregnancy* ⇒ ectopic pregnancy.

Tub·arine (tū'-bàr-ēn) *n* proprietary name for tubocurarine*.

tubercle (tū'-ber-kl) *n* **1** a small rounded prominence, usually on bone. **2** the specific lesion produced by *Mycobacterium tuberculosis*.

tuberculide, tuberculid (tū-ber'-kū-līd) *n* a small lump. Metastatic manifestation of tuberculosis*, producing a skin lesion, e.g. papulonecrotic tuberculide, rosacea-like tuberculide.

tubercu·lin (tū-ber'-kū-lin) *n* a sterile extract of either the crude (old tuberculin) or refined (PPD) complex protein constituents of the tubercle bacillus. Its commonest use is in determining whether a person has or has not previously been infected with the tubercle bacillus, by injecting a small amount into the skin and reading the reaction, if any, in 48–72 h; negative reactors have escaped previous infection. ⇒ Mantoux reaction.

tubercu·loid (tū-ber'-kū-loyd) *adj* resembling tuberculosis*. Describes one of the two types of leprosy.

tubercu·loma (tū-ber-kū-lō'-mà) *n* a caseous tubercle, usually large, its size suggesting a tumor.

tubercu·losis (tū-ber-kū-lō'-sis) *n* a specific infective disease caused by *Mycobacterium tuberculosis* (Koch's tubercle bacillus)—**tubercular, tuberculous** *adj*. *avian tuberculosis* endemic in birds and rarely seen in man. **bovine tuberculosis** endemic in cattle and transmitted to man via infected cow's milk. ⇒ bovine. *human tuberculosis* endemic in man and the usual cause of pulmonary and other forms of tuberculosis. *miliary tuberculosis* a generalized acute form in which, as a result of bloodstream dissemination, minute, multiple tuberculous foci are scattered throughout many organs of the body.

tuberculo·static (tū-ber-kū-lō-stat'-ik) *adj* inhibiting the growth of *Myobacterium tuberculosis*.

tuber·ous scler·osis (tū'-ber-us skler-ōs'-is) (*syn* epiloia) an inherited sclerosis of brain tissue resulting in mental defect. It may be associated with epilepsy.

tuber·osity (tū-ber-os'-it-ē) *n* a bony prominence.

tubo·curarine (tū-bō-kūr-àr'-ēn) *n* the muscle-relaxing drug derived from the South American arrow poison curare. Action reversed by neostigmine given intravenously together with atropine*, which depresses the vagus nerve and so quickens the heart beat. Causes hypertension and histamine release and is now often replaced by pancuronium*, alcuronium* or vecuronium*. (Tubarine.)

tubo·ovarian (tū-bō-ō-vėr'-ē-an) *adj* pertaining to or involving both tube and ovary, e.g. tubo-ovarian abscess.

tubu·lar necro·sis (tū'-bū-lar nek-rō'-sis) acute necrosis of the renal tubules which may follow the crush syndrome, severe burns, hypotension, intrauterine hemorrhage and dehydration. The urine flow is greatly reduced and acute renal* failure develops.

tu·bule (tū'-būl) *n* a small tube. *collecting tubule* straight tube in the kidney medulla conveying urine to the kidney pelvis. *convoluted tubule* coiled tube in the kidney cortex. *seminiferous tubule* coiled tube in the testis. *uriniferous tubule* nephron*.

Tuinal (tū'-in-al) *n* a proprietary mixture of amobarbital* and secobarbital*.

tula·remia (tū-là-rē'-mē-à) *n* (*syn* deer-fly fever, rabbit fever, tick fever) an endemic disease of rodents, caused by *Pasteurella tularensis*; transmitted by biting insects and acquired by man either in handling infected animal carcases or by the bite of an infected insect. Suppuration at the inoculation site is followed by inflammation of the draining lymph glands and by severe constitutional upset—**tularemic** *adj*.

tulle gras (tūl'-grà) a non-adhesive dressing for wounds. Gauze impregnated with soft paraffin and sterilized.

tu·mescence (tū-mes'-ens) *n* a state of swelling; turgidity.

tu·mor (tū'-mor) *n* a swelling. A mass of abnormal tissue which resembles the normal tissues in structure, but which fulfils no useful function and which grows at the expense of the body. Benign, simple or innocent tumors are encapsulated, do not infiltrate adjacent tissue or cause metastases and are unlikely to recur if removed—**tumorous** *adj. malignant tumor* not encapsulated, infiltrates adjacent tissue and causes metastases. ⇒ cancer.

tunica (tōō'-ni-ka) *n* a lining membrane; a coat. *tunica adventitia* the outer coat of an artery. *tunica intima* the lining of an artery. *tunica media* the middle muscular coat of an artery.

tun·nel reimplant·ation oper·ation a surgical procedure used to reimplant the ureter.

tur·binate (tur'-bin-āt) *adj* shaped like a top or inverted cone. *turbinate bone* three on either side forming the lateral nasal walls.

tur·binated (tur'-bin-ā-ted) *adj* scroll-shaped, as the three turbinate processes which project from the lateral nasal walls.

turbin·ectomy (tur-bin-ek'-to-mē) *n* removal of turbinate bones.

tur·gid (tur'-jid) *adj* swollen; firmly distended, as with blood by congestion—**turgescence** *n*, **turgidity** *n*.

Turner syn·drome (tur'-ner) a condition of multiple congenital abnormalities in females, with infantile genital development, webbed neck, cubitus valgus and, often, aortic coarctation. The ovaries are almost completely devoid of germ cells and there is failure of pubertal development. Most subjects with Turner syndrome have a single sex chromosome, the X, and thus only 45 chromosomes in their body cells.

tussis (tus'-sis) *n* a cough.

Tylenol (tī'-len-ol) *n* proprietary name for acetaminophen*.

ty·losis (tī-lō'-sis) *n* ⇒ keratosis.

tylox·apol (tī-loks'-à-pol) *n* a drug which increases the volume and decreases the viscosity of bronchial mucus. (Superinone.)

tym·panic (tim·pan'-ik) *adj* pertaining to the tympanum*. *tympanic membrane* ⇒ membrane.

tym·panites, tympanism (tim-pan-i'-tēz, tim'-pan-izm) *n* (*syn* meteorism) abdominal distension due to accumulation of gas in the intestine.

tym·panitis (tim-pan-ī'-tis) *n* inflammation of the tympanum.

tympano·plasty (tim'-pan-ō-plas-tē) *n* any reconstructive operation on the middle ear designed to improve hearing. Normally carried out in ears damaged by chronic suppurative otitis media with associated conductive deafness—**tympanoplastic** *adj*.

tym·panum (tim'-pan-um) *n* the cavity of the middle ear.

ty·phoid fever (tī'-foyd fē'-ver) an infectious fever usually spread by contamination of food, milk or water supplies with *Salmonella typhi,* either directly by sewage, indirectly by flies or by faulty personal hygiene. Symptomless carriers harboring the germ in the gallbladder and excreting it in their stools are the main source of outbreaks of disease in this country. The average incubation period is 10–14 days. A progressive febrile illness marks the onset of the disease, which develops as the germ invades lymphoid tissue, including that of the small intestine (Peyer's patches) to profuse diarrheal (pea soup) stools which may become frankly hemorrhagic; ultimate recovery usually begins at the end of the third week. A rose-colored rash may appear on the upper abdomen and back at the end of the first week. ⇒ TAB.

ty·phus (tī'-fus) *n* an acute infectious disease characterized by high fever, a skin eruption and severe headache. It is a disease of war, famine or catastrophe, being spread by lice, ticks or fleas. Infecting organism is *Ricketisia prowazekii,* sensitive to sufonamides and antibiotics.

tyr·amine (tī'-rà-mēn) *n* an amine present in several foodstuffs, especially cheese. It has a similar effect in the body to epinephrine*, consequently patients taking drugs in the monoamine oxidase inhibitor (MAOI) group should not eat cheese, otherwise a dangerously high blood pressure may result.

tyro·sine (tī'-rō-sēn) *n* an amino acid essential for growth. Combines with iodine to form thyroxine.

tyrosin·osis (tī-rō-sin-ō'-sis) *n* due to abnormal metabolism of tyrosine; excess parahydroxyphenylpyruvic acid is excreted in the urine.

tyroth·ricin (tī-roth'-ri-sin) *n* a mixture of gramicidin* and other antibiotics. It is too toxic for systemic therapy, but is valuable in a number of infected skin conditions.

U

UAO *abbr* upper airway obstruction.

UHBI *abbr* upper hemi-body irradiation*.

ul·cer (ul'-ser) *n* destruction of either mucous membrane or skin from whatever cause, producing a crater or indentation. An inflammatory reaction occurs and if it penetrates a blood vessel bleeding ensues. If the ulcer is in the lining of a hollow organ it can perforate through the wall.

ulcer·ative (ul'-ser-à-tiv) *adj* pertaining to or of the nature of an ulcer. ⇒ colitis.

ulcero·genic (ul-ser-ō-jen'-ik) *adj* capable of producing an ulcer.

Ull·rich syn·drome (ul'-rik) ⇒ Noonan syndrome.

ulna (ul'-nà) *n* the inner bone of the forearm. ⇒ Figures 2, 3.

ulnar artery (ul'-nar) ⇒ Figure 9.

ultra·sonography (ul-trà-son-og'-raf-ē) *n* production of a visible image from the use of ultrasound. A controlled beam is directed into the body. The echoes of reflected ultrasound are used to build up an electronic image of the various structures of the body. *realtime ultrasonography* an ultrasound imaging technique involving rapid pulsing to enable continuously viewing of movement to be obtained, rather than stationary images—**ultrasonograph** *n*, **ultrasonographically** *adv*.

ultra·sound (ul'-tra-sownd) *n* sound waves with a frequency of over 20 000 Hz and inaudible to the human ear.

ultraviolet (ul-trà-vī'-ō-let) *adj* referring to rays beyond the visible spectrum at the violet end.

umbili·cal cord (um-bil'-i-kal) the navel string attaching the fetus to the placenta.

umbili·cal hernia ⇒ hernia.

umbili·cated (um-bil'-i-kāt-ed) *adj* having a central depression, e.g. a smallpox vesicle.

umbili·cus (um-bil'-i-kus) *n* (*syn* navel) the abdominal scar left by the separation of the umbilical cord after birth—**umbilical** *adj*.

uncinate (un'-sin-āt) *adj* hook-shaped, unciform.

uncon·sciousness (un-kon'-shus-nes) *n* state of being unconscious; insensible.

'under·arm, pill' six small capsules containing levonorgestrel* are inserted under the skin of a woman's forearm; the implants release small amounts of the drug; the effect is achieved in 24 h and lasts for 5 years.

un·dine (un'-dēn) *n* a small, thin glass flask used for irrigating the eyes.

undu·lant fever (un'-dū-lant) brucellosis*.

unguen·tum (un-gwen'-tum) *n* ointment.

uni·cellular (ū-ni-sel'-ū-lar) *adj* consisting of only one cell.

uni·lateral (ū-ni-lat'-er-al) *adj* relating to or on one side only—**unilaterally** *adv*.

uni·ocular (ūn-i-ok'-ū-lar) *adj* pertaining to, or affecting one eye.

uni·ovular (ū-ni-ō'-vū-lar) *adj* (*syn* monovular) pertaining to one ovum, as uniovular twins (identical). ⇒ binovular *opp*.

uni·para (ū-nip'-à-rà) *n* a woman who has borne only one child. ⇒ primipara—**uniparous** *adj*.

Unna's paste (ōo'-naz pāst) a glycogelatin and zinc oxide preparation once used in the treatment of varicose ulcers in association with supportive bandaging.

up·per respir·atory tract infec·tions (URTI) the upper respiratory tract is the commonest site of infection in all age groups. The infections include rhinitis—usually viral—sinusitis, tonsillitis, adenoiditis, pharyngitis, otitis media and croup (laryngitis), often involving the tonsils and posterior cervical lymph glands. Such infections seldom require hospital treatment, but epiglottitis can be rapidly fatal.

ura·chus (ū'-rak-us) *n* the stemlike structure connecting the bladder with the umbilicus in the fetus; in postnatal life it is represented by a fibrous cord situated between the apex of the bladder and the umbilicus, known as the median umbilical ligament—**urachal** *adj*.

urate (ū'-rāt) *n* any salt of uric acid; such compounds are present in the blood, urine and tophi or calcareous concretions.

ura·turia (ū-rà-tūr'-ē-à) *n* excess of urates in the urine—**uraturic** *adj*.

urea (ū-rē'-à) *n* the chief nitrogenous end-product of protein metabolism; it is excreted in the urine of which it is the main nitrogenous constituent. Can be given as an osmotic diuretic by intravenous infusion to reduce intracranial and intraocular pressure and topically to moisturize, soften and smooth dry, rough skin. *urea clearance test, urea concentration test* urine is collected under specified conditions after administration of an oral dose of urea. The speed and the concentration at which the urea appears in the urine is a measure of the level at which the kidneys are functioning.

Urea·phil (ū-rē′-à-fil) *n* a proprietary urea preparation used to produce dehydration in cerebral edema, raised intraocular pressure and as a diuretic in resistant cases. Has a low potential for sodium retention, thus increases urinary output.

uremia (ūr-ēm′-ē-à) *n* a clinical syndrome due to renal failure resulting from either disease of the kidneys themselves, or from disorder or disease elsewhere in the body which induces kidney dysfunction and which results in gross biochemical disturbance in the body, including retention of urea and other nitrogenous substances in the blood (azotemia). Depending on the cause it may or may not be reversible. The fully developed syndrome is characterized by nausea, vomiting, headache, hiccough, weakness, dimness of vision, convulsions and coma. ⇒ renal—**uremic** *adj.*

uremic snow (ūr-ēm′-ik snō) ⇒ uridrosis.

ureter (ūr′-e-ter) *n* the tube passing from each kidney to the bladder for the conveyance of urine (⇒ Figures 19, 20); its average length is from 25–30 cm—**ureteric, ureteral** *adj.*

ureter·ectomy (ūr′-et-er-ek′-to-mē) *n* excision of a ureter.

ureter·itis (ūr-et-er-ī′-tis) *n* inflammation of a ureter.

uretero·colic (ūr-et-er-kol′-ik) *adj* pertaining to the ureter* and colon*, usually indicating anastomosis of the two structures.

uretero·colostomy (ūr′-et-er-ō-kol-os′-to-mē) *n* (*syn* utero-colic anastomosis) surgical transplantation of the ureters from the bladder to the colon so that urine is passed by the bowel; sometimes carried out to relieve strangury in tuberculosis of the bladder, or prior to cystectomy for bladder tumors.

uretero·ileal (ūr-et-er-ō-il′-ē-al) *adj* pertaining to the ureters* and ileum* as the anastomosis necessary in ureteroileostomy (ileal conduit).

uretero·ileostomy (ūr′-et-er-ō-il-ē-os′-to-mē) *n* ⇒ ileoureterostomy.

uretero·lith (ū-rē′-ter-ō-lith) *n* a calculus* in the ureter.

uretero·lithotomy (ūr-et-er-ō-lith-ot′-o-mē) *n* surgical removal of a stone from a ureter.

uretero·sigmoidostomy (ū-rē′-ter-ō-sig-moyd-os′-to-mē) *n* ureterocolostomy*.

ureter·ostomy (ūr-et-er-os′-to-mē) *n* the formation of a permanent fistula through which the ureter discharges urine. ⇒ cutaneous, ileoureterostomy, rectal bladder.

uretero·vaginal (ūr-et-er-ō-vaj′-in-al) *adj* pertaining to the ureter* and vagina*.

uretero·vesical (ūr-et-er-ō-ves′-i-kal) *adj* pertaining to the ureter* and urinary bladder*.

urethra (ūr-ēth′-rà) *n* the passage from the bladder through which urine is excreted (⇒ Figure 19); in the female it measures 25–40 mm; in the male 250 cm—**urethral** *adj.*

urethral syn·drome (ūr-ēth′-ral) symptoms of urinary infection although the urine is sterile when withdrawn by catheter. Suggests that infection is confined to the urethra and adjoining glands.

ureth·ritis (ūr-ēth-rī′-tis) *n* inflammation of the urethra. *non-specific urethritis* ⇒ non-gonococcal urethritis.

urethro·cele (ūr-ēth′-rō-sēl) *n* prolapse of the urethra, usually into the anterior vaginal wall.

ureth·rography (ūr-ēth-rog′-raf-ē) *n* radiological examination of the urethra. Can be an inclusion with cystography either retrograde (ascending) or during micturition—**urethrographic** *adj*, **urethrogram** *n*, **urethrograph** *n*, **urethrographically** *adv.*

ureth·rometry (ūr-ēth-rom′-et-rē) *n* measurement of the urethral lumen using a urethrometer—**urethrometric** *adj*, **urethrometrically** *adv.*

urethro·plasty (ūr-ēth′-rō-plas-tē) *n* any plastic operation on the urethra—**urethroplastic** *adj.*

urethro·scope (ūr-ēth′-rō-skōp) *n* an instrument designed to allow visualization of the interior of the urethra—**urethroscopic** *adj*, **urethroscopy** *n*, **urethroscopically** *adv.*

urethro·stenosis (ūr-ēth-rō-sten-ōs′-is) *n* urethral stricture*.

ureth·rotomy (ūr-ēth-rot′-o-mē) *n* incision into the urethra; usually part of an operation for stricture.

urethro·trigonitis (ūr-ēth-rō-trig-on-ī′-tis) *n* inflammation of the urinary bladder. ⇒ trigone.

URI *abbr* upper respiratory infection.

uric acid (ūr′-ik as′-id) an acid formed in the breakdown of nucleoproteins in the tissues, the end-product of purine metabolism, and excreted in the urine. It is relatively insoluble and excessive amounts are liable to give rise to stones. Present in excess in the blood in gout and a gout-like syndrome occurring in male infants, manifesting as early as 4 months with self-destructive behavior, cerebral palsy and mental retardation.

uricosuric (ū-rik-ō-sū′-rik) *adj* enhances renal excretion of uric acid due to impairment of tubular reabsorption. Such substances are used in chronic gout.

uri·drosis (ūr-id-rō′-sis) *n* (*syn* uremic snow) excess of urea in the sweat; it may be deposited on the skin as fine white crystals.

urin·alysis (ūr-in-al′-is-is) *n* examination of the urine.

uri·nary (ūr′-in-ār-ē) *adj* pertaining to urine. *urinary bladder* a muscular distensible bag situated in the pelvis (⇒ Figures 16, 19). It receives urine from the kidneys via two ureters and stores it until the volume causes reflex evacuation through the urethra. *urinary system* comprises two kidneys, two ureters, one urinary bladder and one urethra. The kidneys filter the urine from the blood; the ureters convey the urine to the bladder, which stores it until there is sufficient volume to elicit the desire to pass urine and it is then conveyed to the exterior by the urethra. ⇒ Figures 19, 20. *urinary tract infection (URI)* the second most prevalent infection in hospitals, but the most common hospital-acquired infection. It occurs most frequently in the presence of an indwelling catheter. The most common infecting agent is *Escherichia coli*, suggesting that autogenous infection via the periurethral route is the commonest pathway.

uri·nation (ūr-in-ā′-shun) *n* ⇒ micturition.

urine (ūr′-in) *n* the amber-colored fluid which is excreted from the kidneys at the rate of about 1500 ml every 24 h in the adult; it is slightly acid and has a specific gravity of 1005–1030.

urini·ferous (ūr-in-if′-er-us) *adj* conveying urine*.

urino·genital (ūr-in-ō-jen′-i-tal) *n* ⇒ urogenital.

uri·nometer (ūr-in-om′-et-er) *n* an instrument for estimating the specific gravity of urine.

Urispas (ūr′-is-pas) *n* proprietary name for flavoxate*.

urobilin (ūr-ō-bil′-in) *n* a brownish pigment formed by the oxidation of urobilinogen and excreted in the feces and sometimes found in urine left standing in contact with air.

urobilino·gen (ūr-ō-bil-in′-ō-jen) *n* (*syn* stercobilinogen) a pigment formed from bilirubin* in the intestine by the action of bacteria. It may be reabsorbed into the circulation and converted back to bilirubin in the liver and re-excreted in the bile or urine.

urobilin·uria (ūr-ō-bil-in-ūr′-ē-à) *n* the presence of increased amounts of urobilin in the urine. Evidence of increased production of bilirubin in the liver, e.g. after hemolysis.

uro·chrome (ūr′-ō-krōm) *n* the yellow pigment which gives urine its normal color.

uro·dynamics (ūr-ō-dī-nam′-iks) *n* the use of sophisticated equipment to measure bladder function. Particularly useful in diagnosing the cause of urinary incontinence.

uro·genital (ūr-ō-jen′-i-tal) *adj* (*syn* urinogenital) pertaining to the urinary and the genital organs.

Uro·grafin (ūr′-ō-graf-in) *n* a proprietary contrast medium suitable for urography.

urog·raphy (ūr-og′-raf-ē) *n* (*syn* pyelography) radiographic visualization of the renal pelvis and ureter by injection of a radioopaque liquid. The liquid may be injected into the blood stream whence it is excreted by the kidney (intravenous urography) or it may be injected directly into the renal pelvis or ureter by way of a fine catheter introduced through a cystoscope (retrograde or ascending urography)—**urographic** *adj*, **urogram** *n*, **urographically** *adv*. *intravenous urography (IVU)* demonstration of the urinary tract following an intravenous injection of an opaque medium.

uro·kinase (ūr-ō-kī′-nās) *n* an enzyme which dissolves fibrin clot. Used for traumatic and postoperative hyphema. It has been tried in hyaline membrane disease.

urol·ogist (ūr-ol′-o-jist) *n* a person who specializes in disorders of the female urinary tract and the male genitourinary tract.

urol·ogy (ūr-ol′-o-jē) *n* that branch of science which deals with disorders of the female urinary tract and the male genitourinary tract—**urological** *adj*, **urologically** *adv*.

uropathy (ūr-op′-à-thē) *n* disease in any part of the urinary system.

urostomy (ūr-os′-to-mē) *n* a word sometimes used to encompass conditions described by complex but specific words such as cutaneous ureterostomy, ileoureterostomy, rectal bladder, ureterocolostomy.

URTI *abbr* upper* respiratory tract infection.

urti·caria (ur-ti-kār′-ē-à) *n* (*syn* nettlerash, hives) an allergic skin eruption characterized by multiple, circumscribed, smooth, raised, pinkish, itchy weals, developing very suddenly, usually lasting a few days and leaving no visible trace. Common provocative agents in susceptible subjects are ingested foods such as shellfish, injected sera and contact with, or injection of, antibiotics such as penicillin and streptomycin. ⇒ angioedema. *factitial urticaria* ⇒ dermographia.

uter·ine tubes (ū′-ter-in) ⇒ fallopian tubes. ⇒ Figure 17.

utero·placental (ū-ter-ō-pla-sent′-al) *adj* pertaining to the uterus* and placenta*.

utero·rectal (ū-ter-ō-rek′-tal) *adj* pertaining to the uterus* and the rectum*.

utero·sacral (ū-ter-ō-sā′-kral) *adj* pertaining to the uterus* and sacrum*.

utero·salpingography (ū-ter-ō-sal-ping-og′-raf-ē) *n* (*syn* hysterosalpingography) radiological examination of the uterus and uterine tubes involving retrograde introduction of an opaque medium during fluoroscopy. Used to investigate patency of fallopian tubes.

utero·vaginal (ū-ter-ō-vaj′-in-al) *adj* pertaining to the uterus* and the vagina*.

utero·vesical (ū-ter-ō-ves′-ik-al) *adj* pertaining to the uterus* and the urinary bladder*.

uterus (ū′-ter-us) *n* the womb (⇒ Figure 17; a hollow muscular organ into which the ovum is received through the fallopian tubes and where it is retained during development, and from which the fetus is expelled through the vagina. ⇒ bicornuate—**uteri** *pl*, **uterine** *adj*.

UTI *abbr* urinary* tract infection.

utricle (ū′-tri-kl) *n* a little sac or pocket (⇒ Figure 13).

uvea (ū′-vē-à) *n* the pigmented part of the eye, including the iris, ciliary body and choroid—**uveal** *adj*.

uveitis (ū-vē-ī′-tis) *n* inflammation of the uvea*.

uvula (ū′-vū-là) *n* the central, tag-like structure hanging down from the free edge of the soft palate (⇒ Figure 14).

uvu·lectomy (ū-vū-lek′-to-mē) *n* excision of the uvula.

uvu·litis (ū-vū-lī′-tis) *n* inflammation of the uvula.

V

vacci·nation (vak-sin-ā′-shun) *n* originally described the process of inoculating persons with discharge from cowpox to protect them from smallpox. Now applied to the inoculation of any antigenic material for the purpose of producing active artificial immunity.

vac·cines (vak′-sēnz) *npl* suspensions or products of infectious agents, used chiefly for producing active immunity. *triple vaccine* protects against diphtheria, tetanus and whooping-cough. In addition to these, *quadruple vaccine* protects against polio-myelitis ⇒ Sabin, Salk, TOPV, BCG.

vac·cinia (vak-sin′-ē-à) *n* virus used to confer immunity against smallpox. Its origins are obscure but it is probably a cowpox-smallpox hybrid—**vaccinial** *adj*.

vac·uum extrac·tor (vak′-ūm eks-trak′-tor) **1** an instrument used to assist delivery of the fetus. **2** an instrument used as a method of abortion.

VADAS *abbr* voice* activated domestic appliance system.

vagal (vā′-gal) *adj* pertaining to the vagus* nerve.

vag·ina (và-jī′-nà) *n* literally, a sheath; the musculomembranous passage extending from the cervix uteri to the vulva (⇒ Figure 17); it measures 75 mm along the anterior wall and 90 mm along the posterior wall—**vaginal** *adj*.

vagin·ismus (vaj-in-is′-mus) *n* painful muscular spasm of the vaginal walls resulting in dyspareunia or painful coitis.

vagin·itis (vaj-in-ī′-tis) *n* inflammation of the vagina. *senile vaginitis* can cause adhesions which may obliterate the vaginal canal. *Trichomonas vaginitis* characterized by an intensely irritating discharge; due to a ciliated protozoon which normally inhabits the bowel ⇒ Trichomonas.

vago·lytic (vā-gō-lit′-ik) *adj* that which neutralizes the effect of a stimulated vagus nerve.

vagot·omy (vā-got′-o-mē) *n* surgical division of the vagus nerves; done in conjunction with gastroenterostomy in the treatment of peptic ulcer or pyloroplasty.

vagus nerve (vă′-gus) the parasympathetic pneumogastric nerve; the 10th cranial nerve, composed of both motor and sensory fibers, with a wide distribution in the neck, thorax and abdomen, sending important branches to the heart, lungs, stomach etc—**vagi** *pl*, **vagal** *adj*.

valgus, valga, valgum (val′-gus) *adj* exhibiting angulation away from the midline of the body, e.g. hallux valgus.

val·ine (vă′-lēn) *n* one of the essential amino* acids, α-aminoisovalerianic acid.

Val·ium (val′-ē-um) proprietary name for diazepam*.

Val·salva ma·neuver (val-sal′-và man-ōō′-ver) the maximum intrathoracic pressure achieved by forced expiration against a closed glottis; occurs in such activities as lifting heavy objects or straining at stool; the glottis narrows simultaneously with contraction of the abdominal muscles.

valve (valv) *n* a fold of membrane in a passage or tube permitting the flow of contents in one direction only—**valvular** *adj*.

valvo·plasty (val′-vō-plas-tē) *n* a plastic operation on a valve, usually reserved for the heart; to be distinguished from valve replacement or valvotomy—**valvoplastic** *adj*.

val·votomy, valvulotomy (val-vot′-o-mē) *n* incision of a stenotic valve, by custom referring to the heart, to restore normal function.

valvu·litis (val-vū-lī′-tis) *n* inflammation of a valve, particularly in the heart.

valvu·lotomy (val-vū-lo′-to-mē) *n* ⇒ valvotomy.

Vanceril (van′-ser-il) *n* proprietary name for beclomethasone.

Vancocin (van′-kō-sin) *n* proprietary name for vancomycin*.

vanco·mycin (van-kō-mī′-sin) *n* an antibiotic for overwhelming staphylococcal infections. Natural resistance to vancomycin is rare. Has to be given intravenously. (Vancocin.)

Van den Bergh's test (van′-den bergs) estimation of serum bilirubin*. Direct positive reaction (conjugated) occurs in obstructive and hepatic jaundice. Indirect positive reaction (unconjugated) occurs in hemolytic jaundice.

vanillylmandelic acid (van-il′-l man-del′-ik) *n* a metabolite of epinephrine* which is excreted in the urine.

Vaquez's dis·ease (va-kăz′) polycythemia* vera.

var·icella (văr-i-sel′-à) *n* ⇒ chickenpox—**varicelliform** *adj*.

varicella zoster hyperimmune globulin (VZIG) a blood product which when injected produces immunity to varicella and zoster.

var·ices (văr′-i-sēz) *n* dilated, tortuous (or varicose) veins. ⇒ varicose veins—**varix** *sing*.

varico·cele (văr′-i-kō-sēl) *n* varicosity of the veins of the spermatic cord.

var·icose ulcer (văr′-i-kōs) (*syn* gravitational ulcer) an indolent type of ulcer* which occurs in the lower third of a leg afflicted with varicose* veins.

var·icose veins dilated veins, the valves of which become incompetent so that blood flow may be reversed. Most commonly found in the lower limbs where they can result in a gravitational ulcer; in the rectum, when the term 'rectal varices' (hemorrhoids) is used; and in the lower esophagus, when they are called esophageal varices.

va·riola (văr-ē-ō′-là) *n* ⇒ smallpox.

vario·loid (văr′-ē-ō-loyd) *n* attack of smallpox modified by previous vaccination.

varix (văr′-iks) *n* ⇒ varices.

varus, vara, varum (văr′-us) *adj* displaying displacement or angulation towards the midline of the body, e.g. coxa vara.

vas (vas) *n* a vessel—**vasa** *pl*, *vas deferens* the excretory duct of the testis. *vasa vasorum* the minute nutrient vessels of the artery and vein walls.

vas·cular (vas′-kū-lar) *adj* supplied with vessels, especially referring to blood vessels.

vascular·ization (vas′-kū-lar-īz-ā′-shun) *n* the acquisition of a blood supply; the process of becoming vascular.

vascul·itis (vas-kū-lī′-tis) *n* (*syn* angiitis) inflammation of a blood vessel.

vasculo·toxic (vas′-kū-lō-toks′-ik) *adj* any substance which brings about harmful changes in blood vessels.

vasec·tomy (vas-ek′-to-mē) *n* surgical excision of part of the vas deferens usually for sterilization.

vaso·constrictor (văs-ō-kon-strik′-tor) *adj* any agent which causes a narrowing of the lumen of blood vessels.

Vasodilan (vă-sō-dī′-lan) *n* proprietary name for isoxuprine*.

vasodilator (văs-ō-dī'-lă-tor) *adj* any agent which causes a widening of the lumen of blood vessels.

vaso·epididy·mostomy (văs'-ō-ep-id-id-ē-mos'-to-mē) *n* anastomosis of the vas deferens to the epididymis.

vaso·motor nerves (vă-sō-mō'-tor) nerves which cause changes in the caliber of the blood vessels, usually constriction.

vaso·pressin (vă-sō-pres'-in) *n* formed in the hypothalamus. Passes down the nerves in the pituitary stalk to be stored in the posterior lobe of the pituitary gland. It is the anti-diuretic hormone (ADH). A synthetic preparation is available—pitressin, which can be given intranasally or by injection in diabetes insipidus.

vaso·pressor (vă-sō-pres'-or) *n* a drug which increases blood pressure usually, but not always, by vasoconstriction of arterioles.

vaso·spasm (vă'-sō-spazm) *n* constructing spasm vessel walls—**vasospastic** *adj.*

vaso·vagal attack (vă-sō-vā'-gal) faintness, pallor, sweating, feeling of fullness in epigastrium. When part of the pastgastrectomy syndrome it occurs a few minutes after a meal.

Vas·oxyl (văz-oks'-l) *n* proprietary name for methoxamine*.

vastus muscles (vas'-tus) ⇒ Figure 4.

VBI *abbr* vertebrobasilar* insufficiency.

vec·tor (vek'-tor) *n* a carrier of disease.

veg·etations (vej-e-tā'-shuns) *npl* growths or accretions composed of fibrin and platelets occurring on the edge of the cardiac valves in endocarditis.

vegetat·ive (vej'-e-tā-tiv) *adj* pertaining to the non-sporing stage of a bacterium.

ve·hicle (vē'-hi-kl) *n* an inert substance in which a drug is administered, e.g. water in mixtures.

vein (vān) *n* a vessel conveying blood from the capillaries back to the heart. It has the same three coats as an artery, the inner one being fitted with valves—**venous** *adj.*

Velban (vel'-ban) *n* proprietary name for vinblastine*.

Vel·osef (vel'-ō-sef) *n* proprietary name for cephradine*.

Vel·peau's band·age (vel'-pōz) an arm to chest bandage for a fractured clavicle.

vena cava (vē'-nả kā'-vả) ⇒ Figure 8.

vene·puncture (vē'-ne-pungk'-tūr) *n* insertion of a needle into a vein.

ve·nereal (ve-nē'-rē-al) *adj* pertaining to or caused by sexual intercourse. *venereal disease* ⇒ sexually-transmitted disease.

venereol·ogy (ve-nē-rē-ol'-o-jē) *n* the study and treatment of sexually-transmitted disease.

venesec·tion (vē'-ne-sek'-shun) *n* (*syn* phlebotomy) a clinical procedure, formerly by opening the cubital vein with a scalpel (now usually by venepuncture), whereby blood volume is reduced in congestive heart failure.

venoclysis (vē-nō-klī'-sis) *n* the introduction of nutrient or medicinal fluids into a vein.

ven·ography (vē-nog'-raf-ē) *n* (*syn* phlebography) radiological examination of the venous system involving injection of an opaque medium—**venographic** *adj,* **venogram** *n,* **venograph** *n,* **venographically** *adv.*

venom (ven'-um) *n* a poisonous fluid produced by some scorpions, snakes and spiders.

ven·otomy (vē-not'-o-mē) *n* incision of a vein. ⇒ venesection.

ve·nous (vē'-nus) *adj* pertaining to the veins.

venti·lators (ven'-ti-lă-tors) *npl* apparatuses for providing assisted ventilation. They have built-in controls which can change the assistance from intermittent positive pressure to intermittent mandatory ventilation or even to continuous positive airways pressure.

Ven·tolin (ven'-tō-lin) *n* proprietary name for albuterol*.

ven·tral (ven'-tral) *adj* pertaining to the abdomen or the anterior surface of the body—**ventrally** *adv.*

ven·tricle (ven'-tri-kl) *n* a small belly-like cavity—**ventricular** *adj ventricle of the brain* four cavities filled with cerebrospinal fluid within the brain. *ventricle of the heart* the two lower muscular chambers of the heart (⇒ Figure 8).

ven·tricular punc·ture (ven-trik'-ū-lar) a highly skilled method of puncturing a cerebral ventricle for a sample of cerebrospinal fluid.

ventriculo·cystern·ostomy (ven-tri'-kū-lō-sis-tern-os'-to-mē) *n* artificial communication between cerebral ventricles and subarachnoid space. One of the drainage operations for hydrocephalus.

ventriculo·scope (ven-trik′-ū-lō-skōp) *n* an instrument via which the cerebral ventricles can be examined—**ventriculoscopic** *adj*, **ventriculoscopically** *adv*.

ventricul·ostomy (ven-trik′-ū-los′-to-mē) *n* an artificial opening into a ventricle. Usually refers to a drainage operation for hydrocephalus.

ventro·suspension (ven-trō-sus-pen′-shun) *n* fixation of a displaced uterus to the anterior abdominal wall.

Ven·turi (ven-tū′-rē) *n* a device used in e.g. oxygen therapy masks incorporating an injector*.

ven·ule (ven′-ūl) *n* 1 a small vein. 2 a syringe-like apparatus for collecting blood from a vein.

ver·apamil (ver-à-pam′-il) *n* a synthetic drug which appears to have a quinidine*-like action on the myocardium. Useful for angina of effort. (Calan, Isoptin.)

vermi·cide (ver′-mi-sīd) *n* an agent which kills intestinal worms—**vermicidal** *adj*.

vermi·form (ver′-mi-fôrm) *adj* wormlike. *vermiform appendix* the vestigial, hollow, wormlike structure attached to the cecum.

vermi·fuge (ver′-mi-fūj) *n* an agent which expels intestinal worms.

Vermox (ver′-moks) *n* proprietary name for mebendazole*.

vernix caseosa (ver′-niks kās-ē-ōs′-à) the fatty substance which covers the skin of the fetus at birth and keeps it from becoming sodden by the liquor amnii.

ver·ruca (ve-roo′-kà) *n* wart. ⇒ condyloma—**verrucae**, *pl*, **verrucous**, **verrucose** *adj*, *verruca necrogenica* (postmortem wart) develops as result of accidental inoculation with tuberculosis while carrying out a postmortem. *verruca plana* the common multiple, flat, tiny warts often seen on children's hands, knees and face. *verruca plantaris* a flat wart on the sole of the foot. Highly contagious. *verruca seborrheica* (*syn* basal cell papilloma) the brown, greasy wart seen in seborrheic subjects, commonly on the chest or back, which increase with aging. *verruca vulgaris* the common wart of the hands or feet, of brownish color and rough pitted surface, caused by the human papillomavirus.

ver·sion (ver′-zhun) *n* turning—applied to the maneuver to alter the position of the fetus *in utero*. *cephalic version* turning the child so that the head presents. *external cephalic version (ECV)* the conversion of a transverse into a head presentation to facilitate labor. The technique is safer with the use of ultrasound and tachographic monitoring. *internal version* is turning the child by one hand in the uterus, and the other on the patient's abdomen. *podalic version* turning the child to a breech presentation. This version may be external or internal.

ver·tebra (ver′-te-brà) *n* one of the irregular bones making up the spinal column—**vertebrae** *pl*, **vertebral** *adj*.

ver·tebral column (ver′-te-bral) (*syn* spinal column) made up of 33 vertebrae, articulating with the skull above and the pelvic girdle below. The vertebrae are so shaped that they enclose a cavity (spinal* canal, neural canal) which houses the spinal* cord. There is more low back pain and sciatica in people who have a narrow spinal canal.

vertebro·basilar insuf·ficiency (VBI) (ver′-te-brō-bās′-i-lar) a syndrome caused by lack of blood to the hindbrain. May be progressive, episodic or both. Clinical manifestations include giddiness and vertigo, nausea, ataxia, drop* attacks and signs of cerebellar disorder such as nystagmus.

ver·tex (ver′-teks) *n* the top of the head.

ver·tigo (ver′-ti-gō) *n* giddiness, dizziness—**vertiginous** *adj*.

vesi·cal (ves′-i-kal) *adj* pertaining to the urinary bladder.

vesi·cant (ves′-i-kant) *n* a blistering substance.

ves·icle (ves′-i-kl) *n* 1 a small bladder, cell or hollow structure. 2 a skin blister—**vesicular** *adj*, **vesiculation** *n*.

vesi·costomy (ves-i-kos′-to-mē) ⇒ cystostomy.

vesico·ureteric (ves′-i-kō-ū-rē-ter′-ik) *adj* pertaining to the urinary bladder* and ureter*. Vesicoureteric reflux can cause pyelonephritis.

vesico·vaginal (ves-i-kō-va′-ji-nal) *adj* pertaining to the urinary bladder* and vagina*.

vesicu·litis (ves-i-kū-lī′-tis) *n* inflammation of a vesicle, particularly the seminal vesicles.

vesiculo·papular (ves-i-kū-lō-pap′-ū-lar) *adj* pertaining to or exhibiting both vesicles and papules.

vessel (ves′-el) *n* a tube, duct or canal, holding or conveying fluid, especially blood and lymph.

vesti·bule (ves′-ti-būl) *n* 1 the middle part of the internal ear, lying between the semicircular canals and the cochlea (⇒ Figure 13). 2 the triangular area between the labia minora—**vestibular** *adj.*

ves·tigial (ves-ti'-jē-al) *adj* rudimentary; indicating a remnant of something formerly present.

vi·able (vī'-à-bl) *adj* capable of living a separate existence—**viability** *n.*

Vibramycin (vī-brà-mī'-sin) *n* proprietary name for doxycycline*.

vi·bration syn·drome (vī-brā'-shun) (*syn* Raynaud's phenomenon) impotency and paralysis of the arm and hands in workers using vibrating machines.

Vibrio (vib'-rē-ō) *n* a genus of curved, motile microorganisms. *Vibrio cholerae,* or the *comma vibrio,* causes cholera.

vicari·ous (vī-kār'-ē-us) *adj* substituting the function of one organ for another. *vicarious menstruation* bleeding from the nose or other part of the body when menstruation is abnormally suppressed.

vil·lus (vil'-us) *n* a microscopic fingerlike projection; found in the mucous membrane of the small intestine or on the outside of the chorion of the embryonic sac—**villi** *pl,* **villous** *adj.*

vin·blastine (vin-blas'-tēn) *n* an alkaloid from periwinkle. An antimitotic used mainly in Hodgkin's disease and choriocarcinoma resistant to other therapy. Given intravenously. (Velan.)

Vincent's angina (vin'-sents an-jī'-na) infection of the mouth or throat by spirochete and a bacillus in synergism. To be differentiated from Ludwig's angina.

vin·cristine (vin-kris'-tēn) *n* an antileukemic drug. Derived from an extract of the periwinkle plant. Given intravenously. (Oncovin.)

vinyl ether an inhalation anesthetic similar to ether, but more rapid and less sustained in effect. Rarely used due to its flammability when used in dosage adquate to cause anesthesia.

viomycin (vī-ō-mī'-sin) *n* an antibiotic used in the treatment of tuberculosis when the disease is resistant to other drugs.

viral hemor·rhagic fevers (vī'-ral hem-ōr-aj'-ik) fevers which occur mainly in the tropics: they are often transmitted by mosquitoes or ticks; they may have a petechial skin rash. Examples are chikungunya, Ebola, denque, Lassa fever, Marburg disease, Rift valley fever and yellow fever.

viral hepa·titis (vī'-ral hep-à-tī'-tis) ⇒ hepatitis.

viremia (vī-rē'-mē-à) *n* the presence of virus in the blood—**viremic,** *adj. maternal viremia* can cause fetal damage.

viri·cidal (vī-ri-sī'-dal) *adj* lethal to a virus—**viricide** *n.*

viril·ism (vī'-ril-ism) *n* the appearance of secondary male characteristics in the female.

vi·rology (vī-rol'-o-jē) *n* the study of viruses and the diseases caused by them—**virological** *adj.*

viru·lence (vī'-rū-lens) *n* infectiousness; the disease-producing power of a microorganism: the power of a microorganism to overcome host resistance—**virulent** *adj.*

vi·rus (vī'-rus) *n* very small microorganisms parasitic within living cells. They differ from bacteria in having only one kind of nucleic acid, either DNA or RNA; in lacking the apparatus necessary for energy production and protein synthesis; and by not reproducing by binary fission but by independent synthesis of their component parts which are then assembled. They cause many kinds of acute and chronic diseases in man, and can cause tumors in animals. Some of the more important groups are: (a) *poxviruses,* e.g. smallpox, molluscum contagiosum (b) *herpesviruses,* e.g. herpes simplex virus, cytomegalovirus, varicella-zoster virus, Epstein-Barr virus (c) *adenoviruses,* (d) *papovaviruses,* e.g. polyoma virus, which can cause tumors in laboratory animals (e) *reoviruses,* e.g. rotaviruses (f) *togaviruses,* e.g. yellow fever virus (g) *picornaviruses* (h) *myxoviruses* (i) *paramyxoviruses* (j) *rhabdoviruses,* e.g. rabies virus (k) *coronaviruses,* e.g. some common cold viruses (l) *arenaviruses,* e.g. Lassa fever virus. Groups a–d are DNA viruses, groups e–l are RNA viruses. Those viruses which are spread by arthropods—insects and ticks—are known as arboviruses, these include reoviruses, togaviruses and rhabdoviruses.

vis·cera (vis'-èr-à) *npl* the internal organs—**viscus** *sing,* **visceral** *adj.*

viscer·optosis (vis-er-op-tō'-sis) *n* downward displacement or falling of the abdominal organs.

vis·cid (vis'-kid) *adj* sticky, glutinous, mainly used to describe sputum.

Vistaril (vis'-tà-ril) *n* proprietary name for hydroxyzine* hydrochloride.

vis·ual (viz'-ū-al) *adj* pertaining to vision. *visual acuity* ⇒ acuity. *visual field* the area within which objects can be seen.

visual purple the purple pigment in the retina of the eye, which is called rhodopsin.

vi·tal capac·ity (vī'-tal kap-as'-i-tē) the amount of air expelled from the lungs after a deep inspiration. ⇒ forced vital capacity.

vital·lium (vī-tal'-ē-um) *n* an alloy which can be left in the tissues in the form of nails, plates, tubes etc.

vitalo·graph (vī-tal'-ō-graf) *n* apparatus for measuring the forced* vital capacity.

vit·amin (vī'-tà-min) *n* essential food factor, chemical in nature, present in certain foodstuffs. Some vitamins can now be synthesized commercially. Their absence causes deficiency diseases.

vit·amin A (vī'-tà-min ā) (*syn* retinol) a fat-soluble anti-infective substance present in all animal fats. In its provitamin form, β carotene, it is present in carrots, cabbage, lettuce, tomatoes and other fruits and vegetables; in the body it is converted into retinol. It is essential for healthy skin and mucous membranes; it aids night vision. Deficiency can result in stunted growth, night blindness and xerophthalmia and is an important cause of blindness in certain parts of the world, e.g. India.

vit·amin B (vī'-tà-min bē) refers to any one of a group of water-soluble vitamins— the vitamin B complex, all chemically related and often occurring in the same foods ⇒ biotin, cyanocobalamin, folic acid, nicotinic acid, pantothenic acid, pyridoxine, riboflavine, thiamine.

vit·amin B₁ (vī'-tà-min bē-wun') thiamine*.

vit·amin B₂ (vī'-tà-min bē-too͞o) riboflavine*.

vit·amin B₆ (vī'-tà-min bē-siks) pyridoxine*.

vit·amin B₁₂ (vī'-tà-min bē-twelv) cyanocobalamin*.

vit·amin C (vī'-tà-min sē) ascorbic* acid.

vit·amin D (vī'-tà-min dē) a fat-soluble vitamin which has two main forms: ergocalciterol (vitamin D_2, calciferol*) and cholecalciferol (vitamin D_3); the production of both is dependent on UVR acting on two different sterols. Good sources are oily fish and dairy produce. *vitamin D resistant rickets* ⇒ rickets.

vit·amin E (vī'-tà-min ē) a group of chemically related compounds known as tocopherols*. It is an intracellular fat-soluble antioxidant and maintains the stability of polyunsaturated fatty acids and other fatlike substances. It is thought that deficiency results in muscle degeneration, a hemolytic blood disease, and is associated with the aging process. *vitamin E deficiency syndrome* occurs in small infants, less than 2 kg and under 35 weeks gestation. Diagnosis at between 6 and 11 weeks reveals low hemoglobin and reticulocytosis; there is good response to vitamin E including a rise in haemoglobin and loss of edema. The condition is aggravated by giving iron. Deficiency in older children results in cerebellar* ataxia and is associated with abetalipoproteinemia.

vit·amin K (vī'-tà-min kā) menadiol*, phytomenadione*. *vitamin K test* after injection of vitamin K, the serum prothrombin rises in obstructive jaundice, but remains depressed in toxic jaundice.

viti·ligo (vit-il-i'-gō) *n* a skin disease of probable autoimmune origin characterized by areas of complete loss of pigment.

vitrec·tomy (vit-rek'-to-mē) *n* surgical removal of the vitreous humor from the vitreous chamber.

vit·reous (vit'-rē-us) *adj* resembling jelly. *vitreous chamber* the cavity inside the eyeball and behind the lens. *vitreous humor* the jelly-like substance contained in the vitreous chamber (⇒ Figure 15).

Vivactil (vī-vak'-til) *n* proprietary name for protriptyline*.

VNA *abbr* visiting nurse association.

vocal cords (vō'-kal kōrds) membranous folds stretched anteroposteriorly across the larynx. Sound is produced by their vibration as air from the lungs passes between them.

voice activated domestic appliance system (VADAS) a microprocessor and voice input system to enhance the lives of disabled people by allowing them to control their environment.

vol·atile (vol'-à-tīl) *adj* evaporating rapidly.

vol·ition (vol-i'-shun) *n* the will to act— **volitional** *adj*.

Volk·mann's ischemic contrac·ture (vōlk'-manz) a flexion deformity of the wrist and fingers from fixed contracture of the flexor muscles in the forearm. The cause is ischemia of the muscles by injury or obstruction to the brachial artery, near the elbow.

volun·tary (vol'-un-tār-ē) *adj* under the control of the will; free and unrestricted; as opposed to reflex or involuntary.

volvu·lus (vol'-vū-lus) *n* a twisting of a section of bowel, so as to occlude the lumen a cause of intestinal obstruction.

vomit (vom'-it) *n* ejection of the stomach contents through the mouth: sickness.

vomit·ing of preg·nancy (vom'-it-ing uv preg'-nans-ē) ⇒ hyperemesis.

vomi·tus (vom'-it-us) *n* vomited matter.

von Reckling·hausen's dis·ease (von-rek'-ling-how-zenz) Recklinghausen's disease.

von Wille·brand's dis·ease (von-vil'-e-brandz) an inherited bleeding disease due to deficiencies relating to the factor VIII proteins in plasma. The inheritance is autosomal dominant, affecting both sexes, and is essentially a disorder of the primary hemostatic mechanism with deranged platelet-endothelial cell interaction. In severe cases von Willebrand's disease results in a clotting defect resembling hemophilia*.

Voss oper·ation (vos) described in 1956 for relief of pain in early degenerative disease of the hip joint. Division of surrounding main muscles allows healing of articulating surfaces and increases the joint space.

vulva —(vul'-và) *n* the external genitalia of the female—**vulval** *adj.*

vul·vectomy (vul-vek'-to-mē) *n* excision of the vulva.

vulvitis (vul-vī'-tis) *n* inflammation of the vulva.

vulvo·vaginal (vul-vō-vaj'-in-al) *adj* pertaining to the vulva* and the vagina*.

vulvo·vaginitis (vul-vō-vaj-in-ī'-tis) *n* inflammation of the vulva and vagina.

vulvo·vaginoplasty (vul-vō-vaj'-in-ō-plas'-tē) *n* recently devised operation for congenital absence of the vagina, or acquired disabling stenosis—**vulvovagino-plastic** *adj.*

VZIG *abbr* varicella* zoster hyperimmune immunoglobulin.

W

Waldeyer's ring (val'-dī-erz) a lymphatic circle surrounding the pharynx.

Wängensteen tube (wang'-en-stēn) has radio-opaque tip. Used for gastrointestinal aspiration.

war·farin (wawr'-fär-in) *n* the oral anticoagulant of choice. Coumarin derivative.

wart (wawrt) *n* ⇒ verruca.

wash·ing soda (wosh'-ing sō'-da) sodium carbonate.

Wasser·man test (wos'-er-man) carried out in the diagnosis of syphilis. It is a complement-fixation test and is not entirely specific ⇒ TPI test.

water·brash (wot'er brash) ⇒ pyrosis.

Water·house-Friderichsen syn·drome (wot'-er-hows frid-er-ik'-sen) shock with widespread skin hemorrhages occurring in meningitis, especially meningococcal. There is bleeding in the adrenal glands.

Waterston's oper·ation (wot'-er-stons) anastomosis of the right pulmonary artery to the ascending aorta. Used as a palliative measure in the treatment of Fallot's tetralogy in the young child.

WBC *abbr* white blood cell or corpuscle. ⇒ blood.

weal (wēl) *n* a superficial swelling, characteristic of urticaria, nettle-stings, etc.

Weber's test (web'-erz) a tuning fork test for the diagnosis of deafness.

Weil-Felix test (wel fē'-liks) an agglutination reaction used in the diagnosis of the typhus group of fevers. Patient's serum is titrated against a heterologous antigen.

Weil's dis·ease (vīlz) spirochetosis icterohemorrhagica, a type of jaundice with fever caused by a leptospire voided in the urine of rats. A disease of miners, sewer workers etc who work in dirty water.

wen (wen) *n* ⇒ sebaceous.

Wertheim's hyster·ectomy (vert'-hīmz) an extensive operation for removal of carcinoma of the cervix, where the uterus, cervix, upper vagina, tubes, ovaries and regional lymph glands are removed.

Wharton's jelly (war'-tunz) a jelly-like substance contained in the umbilical cord.

Wheel·house's oper·ation (whēl'-hows-ez) external urethrotomy for impassable stricture.

whip·worm (whip'-werm) *n* *Trichuris trichiura*, a round-worm which infests the intestine of man in the humid tropics. Eggs are excreted in the stools. The worms do not normally produce symptoms, but heavy infestations of over 1000 worms cause blood diarrhea, anemia and prolapse of the rectum. Treatment unsatisfactory but recently thiabendazole has cleared the infestation in about 50% of patients treated.

White·head's var·nish (whīt'-heds var-nish) a solution of iodoform, benzoin, storax and tolu in ether, used as an antiseptic and protective application to wounds.

white fluids emulsions of tar acids and phenols in water, widely used for general disinfectant purposes.

white leg thrombophlebitis* occurring in women after childbirth.

'whites' *npl* a popular term for leukorrhea*.

White's tar paste zinc paste with the addition of about 6% coal tar. Valuable in infantile eczema.

Whit·field's oint·ment (whit'-fēlds) an antifungal preparation (ung, acid benz. co.) containing salicylic and benzoic acids.

whit·low (wit'-lō) *n* ⇒ paronychia.

WHO *abbr* World Health Organization.

whole gut irrigation ⇒ total colonic lavage.

whoop·ing cough (hōop'-ing kof) ⇒ pertussis.

Widal test (vē-dal') an agglutination reaction for typhoid fever. The patient's serum is put in contact with *Salmonella typhi*. The result is positive if agglutination occurs, proving the presence of antibodies in the serum.

wife/woman batter·ing physical assault on a woman by her husband/partner. Believed to be a frequently unreported crime.

Wilms tumor (vilmz) the commonest abdominal tumor of childhood, and one which usually affects the kidneys. Usually diagnosed during the pre-school period. Prognosis is uncertain and depends on the stage of the tumor and child's age at onset of diagnosis and treatment.

Wilson's dis·ease (wil'-sunz) hepaticolenticular degeneration with choreic movements. Due to disturbance of copper metabolism. No urinary catecholamine excretion. Associated with mental subnormality. Can be treated with BAL and penicillamine. Asymptomatic relatives can be given prophylactic penicillamine.

window (oval and round) (win'-dō) ⇒ Figure 13.

wind·pipe (wind'-pīp) *n* ⇒ trachea.

winter·green (win'-ter-grēn) ⇒ methylsalicylate.

winter vomit·ing dis·ease caused by a ubiquitous, yet still unidentified virus. Syndrome simulates food poisoning.

witch hazel (wich hā'-zel) *n* ⇒ hamamelis.

womb (wōōm) *n* the uterus.

Wood's light special ultraviolet light used for the detection of ringworm.

wool·sorters' disease (wool'-sōr-terz) ⇒ anthrax.

wool test a test for detecting color blindness. The person is asked to select skeins of wool of matching colors.

worms (wermz) *n* ⇒ ascarides, taenia, *Trichuris*.

wound (wōōnd) *n* most commonly used when referring to injury to the skin or underlying tissues of organs by a blow, cut, missile or stable. It also includes injury to the skin caused by chemicals, cold, friction, heat, pressure and rays; and manifestation in the skin of internal conditions, e.g. pressure sores and ulcers.

wound drains (wōōnd drānz) most commonly used in abdominal wounds. They may be inserted as a therapeutic measure, e.g. to drain an abscess, or to prevent complications (prophylaxis) e.g. due to the escape of bile. Drainage may be active where the drain is attached to suction apparatus producing a 'closed wound suction'. A passive drain provides a path of least resistance to the skin and any exudate seeps into a surgical dressing; this system provides a route for bacteria to enter the body ⇒ healing.

wound dress·ings (*syn* surgical dressings) previously they absorbed exudate from the wound which dried, so that when separated from the wound, some of the newly formed tissue was removed. It has been demonstrated conclusively that wounds heal more quickly in a moist environment than in a dry one. Modern dressings aim to be permeable to water vapor and gases but not to bacteria or liquids; this retains serous exudate which is actively bactericidal. They do not adhere to the wound surface and on removal do not damage new tissue ⇒ Debrisan, OpSite.

wound heal·ing ⇒ healing, moist wound healing.

wrist (rist) *n* the carpus (⇒ Figure 3). *wrist drop* paralysis of the muscles which raise the wrist because of damage to the radial nerve.

wry·neck (rī'-nek) *n* ⇒ torticollis.

Wycillin (wī-sil'-in) *n* proprietary name for penicillin G.

Wydase (wī'-dās) *n* proprietary name for hyaluronidase*.

X

Xanax (zan'-aks) *n* proprietary name for alprazolam*.

xanthel·asma (zan-thel-az'-mà) *n* a variety of xanthoma. *xanthelasma palpebrarum* small yellowish plaques appear on the eyelids.

xan·thine (zan'-thēn) *n* 2.6-dioxypurine found in liver, muscle, pancreas and urine. Some derivatives are diuretic. Present in some renal calculi and possesses stimulant properties to muscle tissue, especially the heart.

xanthin·uria (zan-thēn-ūr'-ē-à) *n* rare hereditary disorder in man in which xanthine oxidase enzyme is lacking, resulting in excessive urinary xanthine and hypoxanthine in place of uric acid.

xan·thoma (zan-thō'-mà) *n* a collection of cholesterol under the skin producing a yellow discoloration—**xanthomata** *pl*.

xenon (zen'-on) *n* a rare gas that is chemically inert, but which can produce general anesthesia. Has never been used clinically.

Xen·opsylla (zen-op-sil'-à) *n* a genus of fleas. *Xenopsylla cheopis* is the rat flea that transmits bubonic plague.

xero·derma, xerodermia (zē-rō-dèr'-mà) *n* dryness of the skin ⇒ ichthyosis. *xeroderma pigmentosum* (*syn* Kaposi's disease) a familial dermatosis probably caused by failure of normal skin repair following ultraviolet damage. Pathological freckle formation (ephelides*) may give rise to keratosis, neoplastic growth and a fatal termination.

xeroph·thalmia (zē-rōf-thal'-mē-à) *n* dryness and ulceration of the cornea which may lead to blindness. Associated with lack of vitamin A.

xe·rosis (zē-rō'-sis) *n* dryness. *xerosis conjunctivae* ⇒ Bitot's spots.

xe·rostomia (zē-rō-stō'-mē-à) *n* dry mouth.

xiphoid process (zī'-foyd pro'-ses) the lower tip of the sternum.

X-rays *npl* short wavelength, penetrating rays of electromagnetic spectrum, produced by electrical equipment. The word is popularly used to mean radiographs*.

xy·lene (zī'-lēn) *n* a clear inflammable liquid resembling benzene. Has been used as an ointment in pediculosis. (Xylol.)

Xylo·caine (zī'-lō-kān) *n* proprietary name for lidocaine*.

Xylol (zī'-lol) *n* proprietary name for xylene*.

xylo·metazoline (zī-lō-met-a-zōl'-ēn) *n* a nasal vasoconstrictor; gives quick relief but the action is short; there is a danger of rebound congestion after repeated use.

xy·lose (zī'-lōs) *n* wood sugar.

xy·lose test more convenient than fat balance and equally accurate. Xylose is given orally and its urinary excretion is measured. Normally 25% of loading dose is excreted. Less than this indicates malabsorption syndrome.

XXY syn·drome Klinefelter* syndrome.

Y

yaws (yawz) *n* a tropical disease which resembles syphilis so closely that they may be one and the same disease but modified by differences of climate, social habit and hygiene. Pinta (S. America) and bejel (Transjordan) may be similar variants. All these diseases are caused by an identical spirochete and produce a positive Wassermann test in the blood. Only syphilis is a sexually-transmitted disease. The general term for the group is 'treponematosis'.

yeast (yēst) *n* saccharomyces. A unicellular fungus which will cause fermentation and which reproduces by budding only. Said to be rich in vitamin B complex.

yel·low fever (yel'-ō fē'-ver) an acute febrile illness of tropical areas, caused by a group B arbovirus and spread by a mosquito (*Aedes aegypti*). Characteristic features are jaundice, black vomit and anuria. An attenuated virus variant known as 17D is prepared as vaccine for immunization.

Yersinia (yer-sin'-ē-à) *n* current name for Pasteurella.

Yomesan (yom'-e-san) *n* proprietary name for niclosamide*.

yttrium 90 (**Y**) (i'-trē-um) *n* a substance emitting beta particles with a half-life of 64 h. Implantations of this in bone wax are left in the pituitary fossa after hypophysectomy for breast cancer.

Z

Zan·tac (zan'-tak) *n* proprietary name for ranitidine*.

Zar·ontin (zar-on'-tin) *n* proprietary name for ethosuximide*.

Zinacef (zin'-à-sef) *n* proprietary preparation of cefuroxime*.

zinc (zingk) *n* a trace element which forms an essential part of many enzymes and plays an important role in protein synthesis and cell multiplication. Zinc absorption is reduced by alcohol and the contraceptive pill. In animal trials it has been shown to affect the production of lung surfactant. Deficiency in zinc is associated with anemia, short stature, hypogonadism, impaired wound healing and geophagia*. Zinc salts have many topical applications (e.g. astringents, antiseptics and deodorants) but when absorbed by the system they are often poisonous and cause chronic symptoms resembling those produced by lead. *zinc oxide* a widely used mild astringent, present in calamine lotion and cream. Lassar's paste, Unna's paste and many other dermatological applications. *zinc peroxide* a white powder with an antiseptic action similar to that of hydrogen* peroxide, but much slower and prolonged in action. Used as ointment, lotion and mouthwash. *zinc stearate* a mild astringent used as a dusting powder in eczematous conditions. *zinc sulfate* a constituent of red lotion and other stimulating lotions for the treatment of ulcers. Occasionally used as an emetic.

Zollin·ger-Ellison syn·drome (zol'-in-ger el'-i-son) the presence of ulcerogenic tumor of the pancreatic islets of Langerhans, hypersecretion of gastric acid, fulminating ulceration of esophagus, stomach, duodenum and jejunum. Frequently accompanied by diarrhea. Diagnosed by gastric secretion and blood gastrin studies.

zona (zō'-nà) *n* a zone; a girdle; herpes zoster. *zona pellucida* the vitelline membrane surrounding the ovum.

zonula ciliaris (zō'-nū-là-sil-ē-ār'-is) suspensory ligament attaching the periphery of the lens of the eye to ciliary body. Zonula.

zonule (zō'-nūl) *n* small zone, belt or girdle. Zonula.

zonulo·lysis (zō-nū-lō-lī'-sis) *n* breaking down the zonula ciliaris—sometimes necessary before intracapsular extraction of the lens—**zonulolytic** *adj*.

zo·onosis (zō-on-ōs'-is) *n* disease in man transmitted from animal. Farm workers are at risk—**zoonoses** *pl*.

zoster (zos'-ter) *n* herpes* zoster.

zy·goma (zī-gō'-mà) *n* the cheekbone—**zygomatic** *adj*.

zy·gote (zī'-gōt) *n* the fertilized ovum. The diploid* cell derived from the fusion after fertilization of two gametes, ova and sperm, each of which carries the basic, haploid*, chromosome complement.

Zyloprim (zī'-lō-prim) *n* proprietary name for allopurinal*.

zymo·gen (zī'-mō-jen) *n* an inactive precursor of an active enzyme which is converted to the active form by the action of acid, another enzyme or by other means.

APPENDICES

Appendix 1 Illustrations of major body systems

Acknowledgments

Figures 1, 2, 3, 4, 5, 8, 11, 13, 14, 15,
18, 19 and 20 from the Royal Society
of Medicine Family Medical Guide, Longman

Figures 6, 7, 9, 10, 12, 16 and 17 from
Wilson KJW: Ross & Wilson's
Foundations of Anatomy and
Physiology, 5th ed Churchill
Livingstone, Edinburgh, 1981.

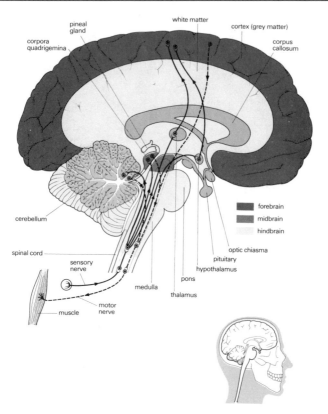

Figure 1 Brain – midline section

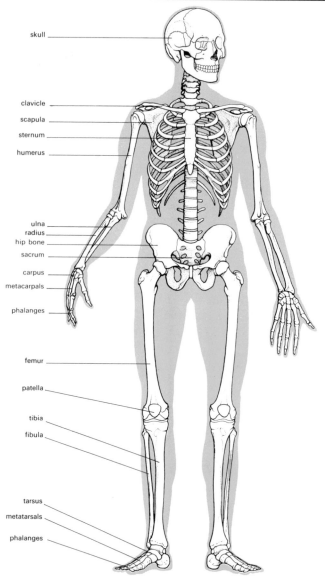

skull

clavicle

scapula

sternum

humerus

ulna
radius
hip bone
sacrum
carpus
metacarpals

phalanges

femur

patella

tibia

fibula

tarsus
metatarsals
phalanges

Figure 2 Skeleton – front view

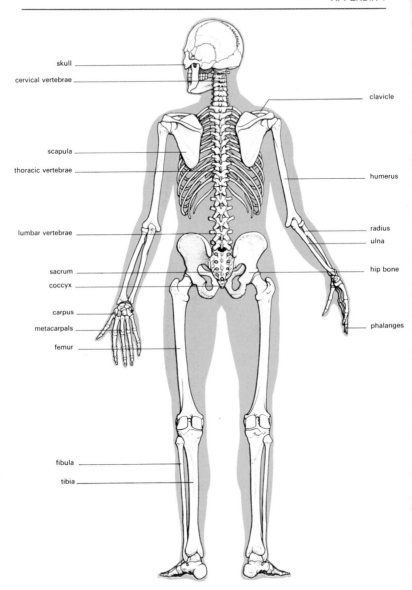

skull

cervical vertebrae

clavicle

scapula

thoracic vertebrae

humerus

lumbar vertebrae

radius

ulna

sacrum

hip bone

coccyx

carpus

metacarpals

phalanges

femur

fibula

tibia

Figure 3   Skeleton – back view

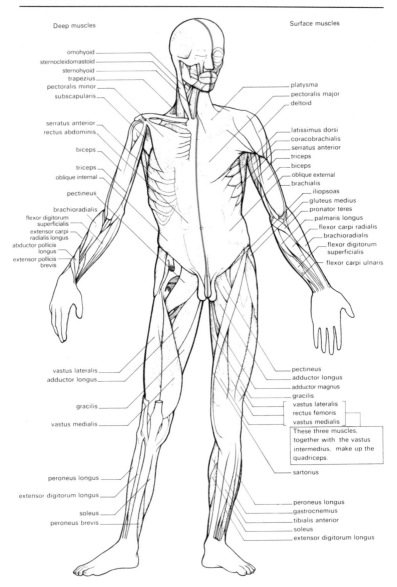

Deep muscles

Surface muscles

omohyoid
sternocleidomastoid
sternohyoid
trapezius
pectoralis minor
subscapularis

platysma
pectoralis major
deltoid

serratus anterior
rectus abdominis

latissimus dorsi
coracobrachialis
serratus anterior
triceps

biceps

biceps
oblique external

triceps
oblique internal

brachialis
iliopsoas
gluteus medius
pronator teres
palmaris longus
flexor carpi radialis
brachioradialis
flexor digitorum
superficialis
flexor carpi ulnaris

pectineus

brachioradialis
flexor digitorum
superficialis
extensor carpi
radialis longus
abductor pollicis
longus
extensor pollicis
brevis

vastus lateralis
adductor longus

pectineus
adductor longus
adductor magnus
gracilis
vastus lateralis
rectus femoris
vastus medialis

gracilis

vastus medialis

These three muscles,
together with the vastus
intermedius, make up the
quadriceps.

sartorius

peroneus longus

extensor digitorum longus

soleus
peroneus brevis

peroneus longus
gastrocnemius
tibialis anterior
soleus
extensor digitorum longus

Figure 4 Muscles – front view

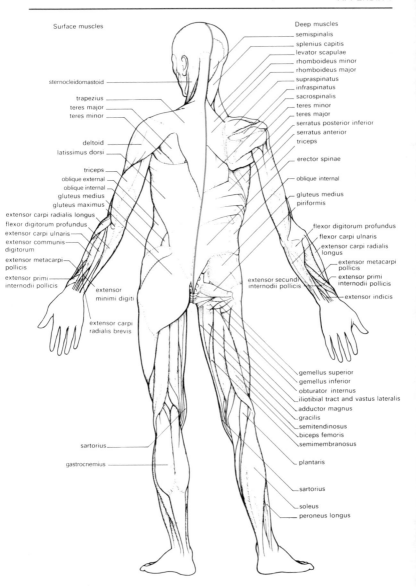

Surface muscles

Deep muscles
semispinalis
splenius capitis
levator scapulae
rhomboideus minor
rhomboideus major
supraspinatus
infraspinatus
sacrospinalis
teres minor
teres major
serratus posterior inferior
serratus anterior
triceps

sternocleidomastoid

trapezius
teres major
teres minor

erector spinae

deltoid
latissimus dorsi

oblique internal

gluteus medius
piriformis

triceps
oblique external
oblique internal
gluteus medius
gluteus maximus

extensor carpi radialis longus
flexor digitorum profundus
extensor carpi ulnaris
extensor communis
digitorum

flexor digitorum profundus
flexor carpi ulnaris
extensor carpi radialis
longus

extensor metacarpi
pollicis

extensor metacarpi
pollicis
extensor primi
internodii pollicis

extensor primi
internodii pollicis

extensor
minimi digiti

extensor secundi
internodii pollicis

extensor indicis

extensor carpi
radialis brevis

gemellus superior
gemellus inferior
obturator internus
iliotibial tract and vastus lateralis
adductor magnus
gracilis
semitendinosus
biceps femoris
semimembranosus

sartorius

plantaris

gastrocnemius

sartorius

soleus
peroneus longus

Figure 5 Muscles – back view

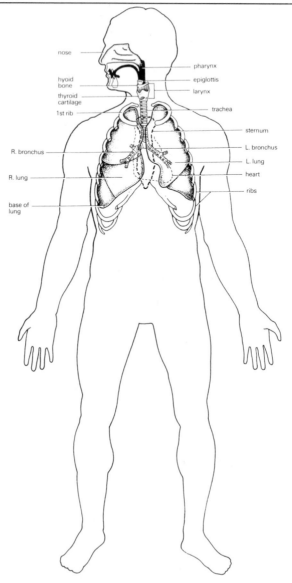

Figure 6 Respiratory system and related structures

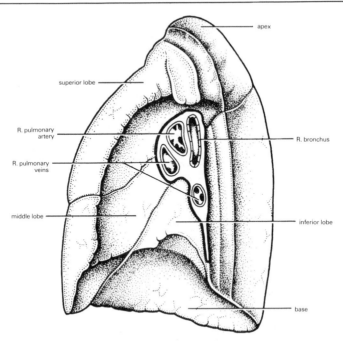

Figure 7 Respiratory system – the right lung

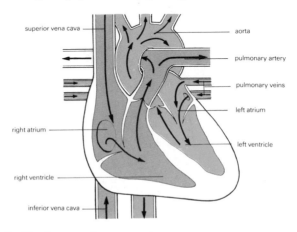

Figure 8 Circulatory system

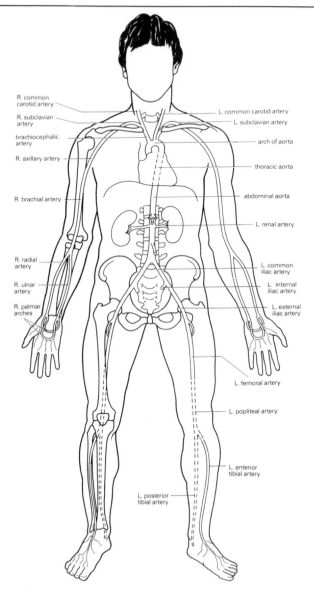

Figure 9 Circulatory system – arteries

R. common carotid artery
R. subclavian artery
brachiocephalic artery
R. axillary artery
R. brachial artery
R. radial artery
R. ulnar artery
R. palmar arches

L. common carotid artery
L. subclavian artery
arch of aorta
thoracic aorta
abdominal aorta
L. renal artery
L. common iliac artery
L. internal iliac artery
L. external iliac artery
L. femoral artery
L. popliteal artery
L. anterior tibial artery
L. posterior tibial artery

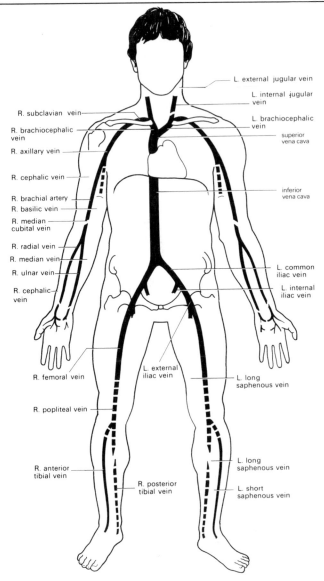

Figure 10 Circulatory system – veins

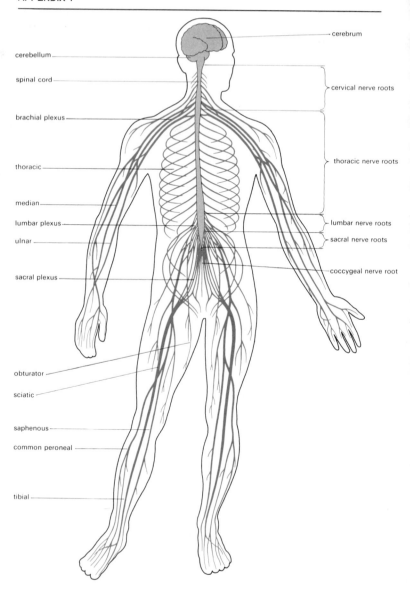

Figure 11 Nervous system

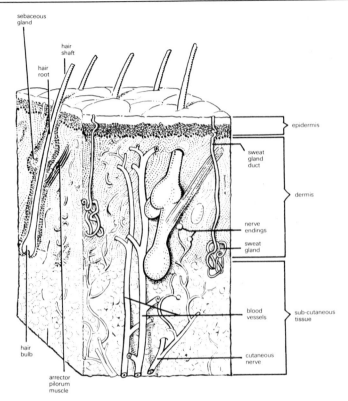

Figure 12 Skin

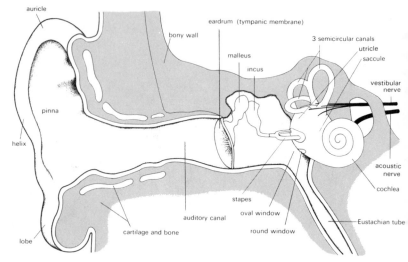

Figure 13 Ear

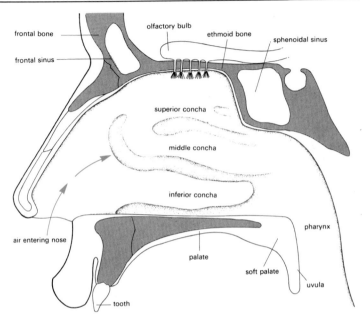

Figure 14 Nose

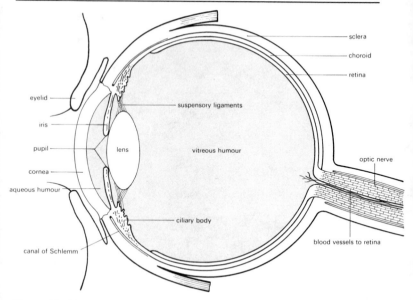

Figure 15 Eye

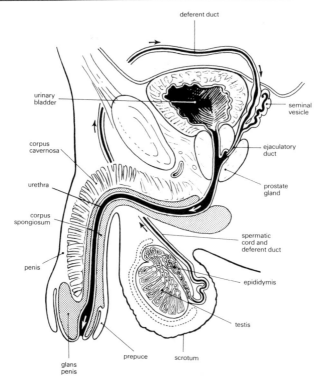

Figure 16 Male reproductive system

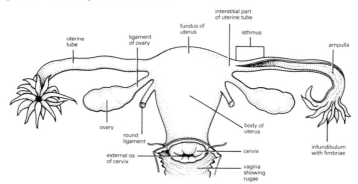

Figure 17 Female reproductive system

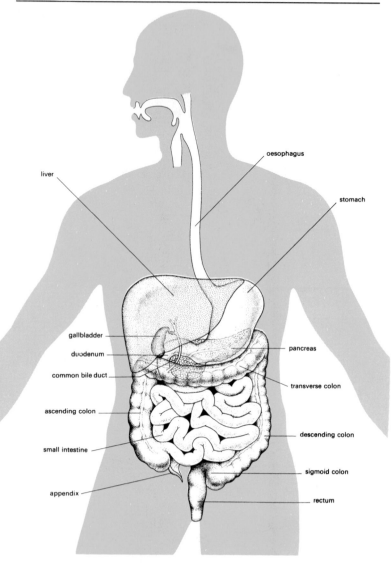

Figure 18 Digestive system

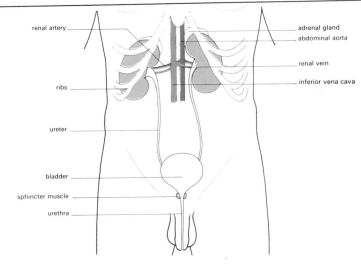

Figure 19 Urinary system

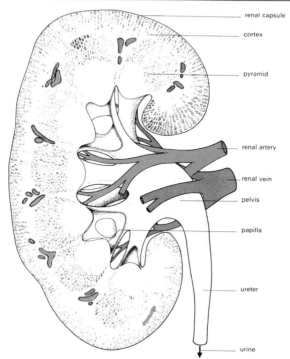

Figure 20 Urinary system – the kidney

Appendix 2 SI units and the metric system

Acknowledgment

Conversion scales are taken from
Goodsell D. Coming to terms with
SI metric. Nursing Mirror 141:55, 1975.

Système International (SI) Units

At an international convention in 1960, the General Conference of Weights
and Measures agreed to promulgate an International System of Units,
frequently described as SI or Système International. This is merely the
name for the current version of the metric system, first introduced in
France at the end of the 18th century.

In any system of measurement, the magnitude of some physical quantities
must be arbitrarily selected and declared to have unit value. These
magnitudes form a set of standards and are called *basic units*. All other
units are *derived units*.

Basic units

The SI has seven basic units.

Name of SI units	Symbol for SI unit	Quantity
meter	m	length
kilogram	kg	mass
second	s	time
mole	mol	amount of substance
ampere	A	electric current
kelvin	°K	thermodynamic temperature
candela	cd	luminous intensity

Derived units

Derived units are obtained by appropriate combinations of
basic units:
– unit area results when unit length is multiplied by unit
  width

– unit density results when unit weight (mass) is divided
by unit volume

Name of SI unit	Symbol for SI unit	Quantity
joule	J	work, energy, quantity of heat
pascal	Pa	pressure
newton	N	force

Decimal multiples and submultiples

The metric system uses multiples of 10 to express number.
Multiples and submultiples of the basic unit are
expressed as decimals and the following prefixes are used:
The most widely used prefixes are kilo, milli and micro
(μ):

$$0.000\ 001\ g = 10^{-6}g = 1\ \mu g$$

Multiples and sub-multiples of units

1 000 000 000 000	10^{12}	tera	T
1 000 000 000	10^{9}	giga	G
1 000 000	10^{6}	mega	M
1 000	10^{3}	kilo	k
100	10^{2}	hecto	h
10	10^{1}	deca	da
0.1	10^{-1}	deci	d
0.01	10^{-2}	centi	c
0.001	10^{-3}	milli	m
0.000 001	10^{-6}	micro	μ
0.000 000 001	10^{-9}	nano	n
0.000 000 000 001	10^{-12}	pico	p
0.000 000 000 000 001	10^{-15}	femto	f
0.000 000 000 000 000 001	10^{-18}	atto	a

Rules for using units

a. The symbol for a unit is unaltered in the plural and
should not be followed by a full stop except at the end
of the sentence:

5 cm *not* 5 cm. or 5 cms.

b. The decimal sign between digits is indicated by a full
stop in typing. No commas are used to divide large
numbers into groups of three, but a half-space (whole
space in typing) is left after every third digit. If the
numerical value of the number is less than 1 unit, a zero
should precede the decimal sign:

0.123 456 *not* .123,456

c. The SI symbol for 'day' (i.e. 24 hours) is 'd', but urine and fecal excretions of substances should preferably be expressed as 'per 24 hours':

g/24 h

d. 'Squared' and 'cubed' are expressed as numerical powers and not by abbreviation:

square centimeter is cm^2 *not* sq cm.

Commonly used measurements

a. Temperature is expressed as degrees Celsius (°C) and the standard thermometer is graded 32–42°C.

1° Celsius = 1° Centigrade

b. The calorie is replaced by the joule:

1 calorie = 4.2 J
1 Calorie (dietetic use) = 4.2 kilojoules = 4.2 kJ

The previous 1000 Calorie reducing diet is expressed (approximately) as a 4000 kJ diet.

1 g of fat provides	38 kJ
1 g of protein provides	17 kJ
1 g of carbohydrate provides	16 kJ

c. Equivalent concentration mEq/l is commonly used for reporting results of monovalent electrolyte measurements (sodium, potassium, chloride and bicarbonate). It is not part of the SI system and should be replaced by molar concentration—in these examples mmol/l.

For these four measurements, the numerical value will not change.

d. The SI unit of pressure is the pascal (Pa). Blood gas measurements should be given in the SI unit kPa instead of mmHg.

1 mmHg = 133.32 Pa
1 kPa = 7.5006 mmHg

Column measurement will be *retained* in clinical practice *as at present*.

blood pressure (in mmHg)
cerebrospinal fluid (in mmH_2O)
central venous pressure (in cmH_2O)

Weights and measures

Metric   Imperial

Linear measure

	1 millimeter	=	0.039	in	1 inch	=	25.4	mm
10 mm	= 1 centimeter	=	0.394	in	1 foot	=	0.305	mm
10 cm	= 1 decimeter	=	3.94	in	1 yard	=	0.914	m
10 dm	= 1 meter	=	39.37	in	1 mile	=	1.61	km
1000 m	= 1 kilometer	=	0.6214	mile				

Square measure

	1 sq centimeter	=	0.155	sq in	1 square inch	=	6.452	cm^2
100 cm^2	= 1 sq meter	=	1.196	sq yd	1 square foot	=	9.29	dm^2
100 m^2	= 1 are	=	119.6	sq yd	1 square yard	=	0.836	m^2
100 ares	= 1 hectare	=	2.471	acres	1 acre	=	4047	m^2
100 ha	= 1 sq kilometer	=	0.386	sq miles	1 square mile	=	259	ha

Cubic measure

	1 cu centimeter	=	0.061	in^3	1 cubic inch	=	16.4	cm^3
1000 cu cm	= 1 cu decimeter	=	0.035	ft^3	1 cubic foot	=	0.0283	m^3
1000 cu dm	= 1 cu meter	=	1.308	yd^3	1 cubic yard	=	0.765	m^3

Capacity measure

	1 milliliter	=	0.002	pt	1 fluid ounce	=	28.4	cm^3
10 ml	= 1 centiliter	=	0.018	pint	1 pint	=	0.568	l
10 cl	= 1 deciliter	=	0.176	pt	1 quart	=	1.136	l
10 dl	= 1 liter	=	1.76	pt	1 gallon	=	4.546	l
1000 l	= 1 kiloliter	=	220.0	gall				

Weight

	1 milligram	=	0.015	grain	1 grain	=	64.8	mg
10 mg	= 1 centigram	=	0.154	grain	1 dram	=	1.772	g
10 cg	= 1 decigram	=	1.543	grain	1 ounce	=	28.35	g
10 dg	= 1 gram	=	15.43	grain	1 pound	=	0.4536	kg
		=	0.035	oz	1 stone	=	6.35	kg
1000 g	= 1 kilogram	=	2.205	lb	1 quarter	=	12.7	kg
1000 kg	= 1 tonne				1 hundred weight	=	50.8	kg
	(metric ton)	=	0.984	(long)	1 ton	=	1.016	tonnes
				ton	1 short ton	=	0.907	tonnes

Temperature

$$°\text{Fahrenheit} = \left(\frac{9}{5} \times x°C\right) + 32$$

$$°\text{Centigrade} = \frac{5}{9} \times \left(x°F - 32\right)$$

where x is the temperature to be converted

Conversion scales for certain chemical pathology tests and units of measurement

Chemical pathology Blood plasma

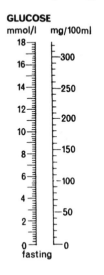

GLUCOSE
mmol/l   mg/100ml

fasting

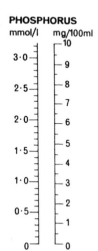

PHOSPHORUS
mmol/l   mg/100ml

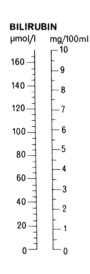

BILIRUBIN
µmol/l   mg/100ml

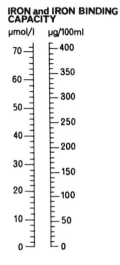

IRON and IRON BINDING CAPACITY
µmol/l   µg/100ml

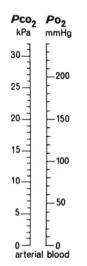

Pco₂   Po₂
kPa   mmHg

arterial blood

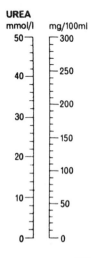

UREA
mmol/l   mg/100ml

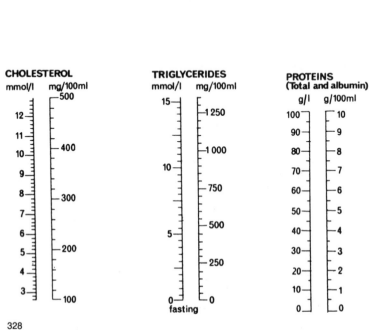

CREATININE

µmol/l	mg/100ml
	10
800	9
700	8
600	7
500	6
400	5
300	4
200	3
100	2
0	1
	0

URATE (Uric acid)

mmol/l	mg/100ml
0·9	15
0·8	14, 13
0·7	12, 11
0·6	10
0·5	9, 8
0·4	7, 6
0·3	5, 4
0·2	3
0·1	2, 1
0	0

CALCIUM

mmol/l	mg/100ml
4	17, 15
3	13, 11
2	9, 7
1	5, 3

CHOLESTEROL

mmol/l	mg/100ml
12	500
11	400
10	
9	
8	300
7	
6	200
5	
4	
3	100

TRIGLYCERIDES

mmol/l	mg/100ml
15	1 250
	1 000
10	750
	500
5	250
0	0

fasting

PROTEINS
(Total and albumin)

g/l	g/100ml
100	10
90	9
80	8
70	7
60	6
50	5
40	4
30	3
20	2
10	1
0	0

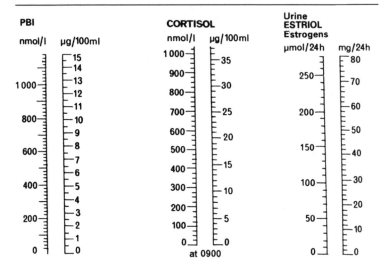

PBI

nmol/l   µg/100ml

CORTISOL

nmol/l   µg/100ml

at 0900

Urine
**ESTRIOL
Estrogens**

µmol/24h   mg/24h

General measurements

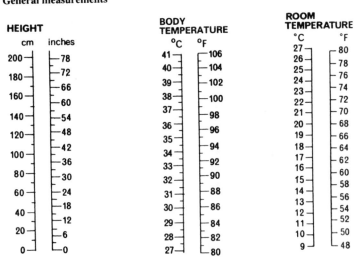

HEIGHT

cm   inches

**BODY
TEMPERATURE**

°C   °F

**ROOM
TEMPERATURE**

°C   °F

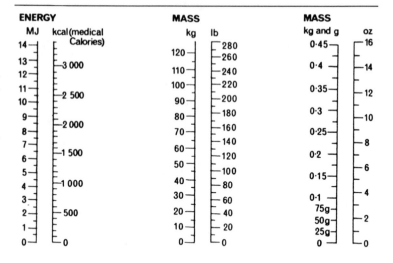

ENERGY

MJ	kcal (medical Calories)
14	
13	3 000
12	
11	2 500
10	
9	2 000
8	
7	1 500
6	
5	
4	1 000
3	
2	500
1	
0	0

MASS

kg	lb
	280
120	260
110	240
100	220
90	200
80	180
70	160
60	140
50	120
40	100
30	80
20	60
10	40
0	20
	0

MASS

kg and g	oz
0·45	16
0·4	14
0·35	12
0·3	10
0·25	8
0·2	
0·15	6
0·1	4
75g	
50g	2
25g	
0	0

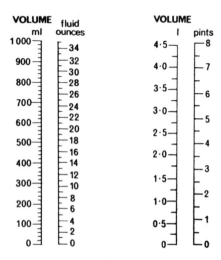

VOLUME

ml	fluid ounces
1 000	34
900	32 / 30
800	28 / 26
700	24 / 22
600	20
500	18 / 16
400	14 / 12
300	10 / 8
200	6 / 4
100	2
0	0

VOLUME

l	pints
4·5	8
4·0	7
3·5	6
3·0	5
2·5	4
2·0	3
1·5	2
1·0	
0·5	1
0	0

PRESSURE

FORCE

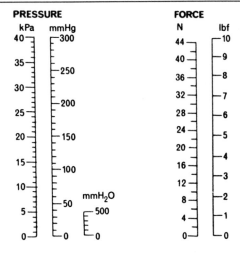

Appendix 3 Normal characteristics

Blood

Normal ranges vary between laboratories. These ranges should be taken as a guide only

Test	Measurement
Albumin *see* Protein	
Alkali reserve	55–70 ml CO_2/100 ml (23.8–34.6 mEq/l)
Amino acid nitrogen	2.5–4.0 mmol/l
Aminotransferases *see* Transaminases	
Ammonia	12–60 μmol/l
Amylase	90–300 iu/l
Antistreptolysin 'O' titer	Up to 200 U/ml
Ascorbic acid	0.7–1.4 mg/100 ml
Bicarbonate	24–30 mmol/l
Bilirubin—total conjugated	0.5–1.7 μmol/l Up to 0.3 μmol/l
Bleeding time	1–6 min
Blood volume	Approx 1/12 or 8% body weight
Bromsulphthalein	Less than 15% after 25 min
Calcium	2.1–2.6 mmol/l
Carbon dioxide (whole blood)	4.5–6.0 kPa
Carbonic acid	1.1–1.4 mmol/l
Carbon monoxide	Less than 0.8 vol %

Test	Measurement
Carotenoids	1.0–5.5 μmol/l
Cephalin-cholesterol reaction	0–1 +
Ceruloplasmin (copper oxidase)	0.3–0.6 g/l
Chloride	95–105 mmol/l
Cholesterol	3.5–7.0 mmol/l
Cholinesterase	2–5 iu/l
Clotting time	4–10 min
Factor V assay (AcG)	75–125%
Factor VIII assay (AHG)	50–200%
Factor IX assay (PTC, Christmas factor)	75–125%
Factor X assay (Stuart factor)	75–125%
Clot retraction	Starts 1h Complete 24h
CO_2 combining power *see* Alkali reserve	
Colloidal gold	0–1 units
Color index	0.85–1.15
Congo red	60–100% retained in bloodstream
Copper	75–140 μg/100ml
Corticosteroids (cortisol)	0.3–0.7 μmol/l
Creatine	15–60 μmol/l
Creatine kinase	4–60 iu/l
Creatinine	60–120 μmol/l
Copper	13–24 μmol/l

Enzymes *see* individual enzymes

Erythrocyte sedimentation rate (ESR) Men	3–5 mm/1 h; 7–15 mm/2h (Westergren)
Women	7–12 mm/l h; 12–17/2h (Westergren)

Test	Measurement
Fasting blood sugar *see* Glucose	
Fatty acids (free)	0.3–0.6 mmol/l
Fibrinogen *see* Protein Flocculation tests *see under* individual tests	
Folic acid	greater than 3 ng/ml
Gammaglobulin *see* Protein	
Gamma-glutamyl-transpeptidase	5–30 iu/l
Globulin *see* Protein	

Glucose (whole blood, fasting)
   venous
   capillary (arterial)
	
	3.0–5.0 mmol/l
	3.3–5.3 mmol/l

Glucose tolerance	max. 180 mg/100 ml returns fasting $1\frac{1}{2}$–2h
Glutamic oxalacetic transaminase (GOT) *see also* Transaminases	5–40 units/ml
Glutamic pyruvic transaminase (GPT) *see also* Transaminases	5–35 units/ml
Glycerol *see* Triglyceride	
Haptoglobins	20–110 μmol/l
Hematocrit *see* PCV	
Hemoglobin	12–18g/dl
Hydrogen ion activity exponent (pH)	7.36–7.42
Hydrogen ion concentration	35–44 nmol/l
Icteric index	4–6U

Iron
   Men
 	
   Women
	
	13–32 μmol/l
	
	Approx 3.25 μmol/l less

Iron-binding capacity (total)	45–70 μmol/l
Kahn	negative
Ketones	0.06–0.2 mmol/l
Lactate	0.75–2.0 mmol/l

Test	Measurement
Lactate dehydrogenase	
total	60–250 iu/l
'heart specific'	50–150 iu/l
Lead (whole blood)	0.5–1.7 μmol/l
LE cells	None
Leucine aminopeptidase	1–3 μmol/h ml
Lipase	18–280 iu/l
Lipids (total)	4.5–10 g/l
β-Lipoproteins	3.5–6.5 g/l
Liver function *see* individual tests	
Magnesium	0.7–1.0 mmol
Methemoglobin	None
5'-Nucleotidase	2.15 iu/l
Osmolality	275–295 mosmol/kg
Oxygen (whole blood)	11–15 kPa
Oxygen capacity	14.4–24.7 ml
Oxygen combining power	
Men	17.8–22.2 ml
Women	16.1–18.9 ml
Paul-Bunnell	Agglutination up to 1:20
CO_2	4.5–6.0 kPa
pH	7.36–7.42
Phosphatase	
Acid-total	3.5–20 iu/l
Acid-prostatic	0–3.5 iu/l
Alkaline-total	20–90 iu/l
Phosphate (inorganic)	0.8–1.4 mmol/l
Phospholipids	
(as fatty acids)	5.0–9.0 mmol/l
(as phosphorus)	1.9–3.2 mmol/l
Phosphorus *see* Phosphate, inorganic	
Platelets	200–500 × 10^9/l

Test	Measurement
PO_2 (whole blood)	11–15 kPa
Potassium	3.8–5.0 mmol/l
Protein	
—Total	62–80 g/l
—Albumin	35–50 g/l
—Globulin (total)	18–32 g/l
—Gammaglobulin	7–15 g/l
—Fibrinogen	2–4 g/l
—A–G ratio	1.5:1–2.5:1
Protein-bound iodine	0.3–0.6 μmol/l
Prothrombin time	11–18 s
Pseudocholinesterase *see also* Cholinesterase	60–90 Warburg units
Pyruvate (fasting)	0.05–0.08 mmol/l
Red cell count	
Total:	$4.0–6.0 \times 10^{12}$/l
Reticulocytes	0.1–2.0/100 RBCs
Packed cell volume (PCV)	
Men:	40–54%
Women:	36–47%
Mean cell volume (MCV)	78–94 μm^3
Mean corpuscular hemoglobin concentration (MCHC)	32–36%
Mean corpuscular hemoglobin (MCH)	27–32 pg
Mean cell diameter	6.7–7.7 μm
Red cell fragility	Hemolysis slight 0.44% NaCl Hemolysis complete 0.3% NaCl
Sodium	136–148 mmol/l
Sulfhemoglobin	None
Thymol	
flocculation	0
turbidity	0–4 units
Thyroxine	0.04–0.85 μmol/l
Transaminase	
alanine (at 25°C)	4–12 iu/l
aspartate (at 25°C)	5–15 iu/l
Transferrin	0.12–0.2 g/l
Triglyceride	0.3–1.8 mmol/l

Test	Measurement
Urea	3.0–6.5 mmol/l
Uric acid	0.1–0.45 mmol/l
Vitamin A	1.0–3.0 μmol/l
Vitamin B_{12}	150–800pg/ml
Vitamin C *see* Ascorbic acid—	
Wasserman reaction (WR)	Negative
White cell count *Total*	4.0–10.0 × 10^9/l
Differential Neutrophils Eosinophils Basophils Lympocytes Monocytes	2 500–7 500 × 10^6/l 200–400 × 10^6/l 0–50 × 10^6/l 1 500 × 3 500 × 10^6/l 400–800 × 10^6/l
Zinc sulfate reaction	2.8 units

Cerebrospinal fluid

Pressure (adult)	50 to 200 mm water
Cells	0 to 5 lymphocytes/mm³
Glucose	3.3–4.4 mmol/l
Protein	100–400 mg/l

Feces

Normal fat content

Daily output on normal diet	less than 7g
Fat (as stearic acid)	11–18 mmol/24h

Urine

Total quantity per 24 hours	1000 to 1500 ml
Specific gravity	1.012 to 1.030
Reaction	pH 4 to 8

Average amounts of inorganic and organic solids in urine each 24 hours

Calcium	2.5–7.5 mmol
Creatinine	9–17 mmol
Estriol	varies widely during pregnancy—μmol
5H1AA	15–75 μmol
HMMA*	10–35 μmol
Hydroxyproline	0.08–0.25 mmol
Magnesium	3.3–5.0 mmol
Phosphate	15–50 mmol
Urea	250–500 mmol

17-ketosteroids:
Men	8 to 15 mg/24 hours
Women	5 to 12 mg/24 hours

* 4-Hydroxy-3-methoxy mandelic acid.

Vitamins

Vitamin & daily intake	Sources	Function	Properties	Deficiencies
Fat-soluble				
A (retinol) 750–1200 μg (retinol equivalents)	Carrots, spinach, apricots, tomatoes, liver, kidney, oily fish, egg yolk, milk, butter, cheese	Normal development of bones and teeth. Antiinfective. Essential for healthy skin and mucous membranes. Aids night vision.	Synthesized in the body from carotene, present in vegetables. Can be stored in liver.	Poor growth. Rough dry skin and mucous membranes encouraging infection. Lessened ability to see in poor light. Xerophthalmia and eventual blindness.
D (Calciferol)	Oily fish, egg yolk, butter, margarine. Ultra-violet rays of sunlight.	Anti-rachitic. Assists absorption and metabolism of calcium and phosphorus.	Produced in the body by action of sunlight on ergosterol in skin.	Rickets in children; osteomalacia and osteoporosis in adults.
E (tocopherol)	Wheat germ, egg yolk, milk, cereals, liver, green vegetables.	Not fully understood in human body, perhaps controls oxidation in body tissues.		
K	Green vegetables, especially cabbage, peas.	Anti-hemorrhagic. Essential for the production of prothrombin.	Only absorbed in the presence of bile.	Delayed clotting time. Liver damage.

Vitamin & daily intake	Sources	Function	Properties	Deficiencies
Water-soluble				
B-complex B1 aneurin (thiamin) 1–1.5 mg	Wholemeal flour and bread, brewers' yeast, cereals, milk, eggs, liver, fish, vegetables.	Anti-neuritic. Anti-beri-beri. Anti-pellagra. Health of nervous system.	Destroyed by excessive heat, e.g. toast and baking soda	Beri-beri. Neuritis. Poor growth in children.
B2 riboflavin 1.5–2.5 mg Nicotinic acid 15–18 mg		Steady and continuous release of energy from carbohydrates.	Can withstand normal cooking and food processing.	Fissures at corner of mouth and tongue. Inflammation. Corneal opacities. Pellagra: dermatitis diarrhea dementia.
B6 (pyridoxine)	As other B-complex foods	Protein metabolism.	Relieves post-radiotherapy nausea and vomiting.	Nervousness and insomnia.
B12 (cobalamin)	Liver, kidney, and other B-complex foods.	Essential for red blood cell formation.	Requires intrinsic factor secreted by gastric cells for absorption.	Pernicious anemia.
Cytamin	Prepared from growth of Streptomyces.	Maintenance therapy for patients with pernicious anemia.		
Folic acid	Liver and green vegetables	Assists production of red blood cells.		Some forms of macrocytic anemia. Premature babies and elderly people on poor diets.
C (ascorbic acid) 30–60 mg	Fresh fruit: oranges, lemons, grapefruit, blackcurrants; green leaf vegetables, potatoes, turnips, rose hip syrup	Formation of bones, connective tissue, teeth and red blood cells.	Destroyed by cooking in the presence of air and by plant enzymes released when cutting and grating raw food. Lost by long storage.	Sore mouth and gums. Capillary bleeding. Scurvy. Delayed wound healing.

Weights and heights

Weight for age, birth to 5 years, sexes combined.

Means for boys are 0.05 to 0.15 kg heavier and for girls 0.05 to 0.15 kg lighter.

Age (months)	Weight (kg) Standard	80% Standard	60% Standard	Age (months)	Weight (kg) Standard	80% Standard	60% Standard
0	3.4	2.7	2.0	31	13.7	11.0	8.2
				32	13.8	11.1	8.3
1	4.3	3.4	2.5	33	14.0	11.2	8.4
2	5.0	4.0	2.9				
3	5.7	4.5	3.4	34	14.2	11.3	8.5
				35	14.4	11.5	8.6
4	6.3	5.0	3.8	36	14.5	11.6	8.7
5	6.9	5.5	4.2				
6	7.4	5.9	4.5	37	14.7	11.8	8.8
				38	14.85	11.9	8.9
7	8.0	6.3	4.9	39	15.0	12.05	9.0
8	8.4	6.7	5.1				
9	8.9	7.1	5.3	40	15.2	12.2	9.1
				41	15.35	12.3	9.2
10	9.3	7.4	5.5	42	15.5	12.4	9.3
11	9.6	7.7	5.8				
12	9.9	7.9	6.0	43	15.7	12.6	9.4
				44	15.85	12.7	9.5
13	10.2	8.1	6.2	45	16.0	12.9	9.6
14	10.4	8.3	6.3				
15	10.6	8.5	6.4	46	16.2	12.95	9.7
				47	16.35	13.1	9.8
16	10.8	8.7	6.6	48	16.5	13.2	9.9
17	11.0	8.9	6.7				
18	11.3	9.0	6.8	49	16.65	13.35	10.0
				50	16.8	13.5	10.1
19	11.5	9.2	7.0	51	16.95	13.65	10.2
20	11.7	9.4	7.1				
21	11.9	9.6	7.2	52	17.1	13.8	10.3
				53	17.25	13.9	10.4
22	12.05	9.7	7.3	54	17.4	14.0	10.5
23	12.2	9.8	7.4				
24	12.4	9.9	7.5	55	17.6	14.2	10.6
				56	17.7	14.3	10.7
25	12.6	10.1	7.6	57	17.9	14.4	10.75
26	12.7	10.3	7.7				
27	12.9	10.5	7.8	58	18.05	14.5	10.8
				59	18.25	14.6	10.9
28	13.1	10.6	7.9	60	18.4	14.7	11.0
29	13.3	10.7	8.0				
30	13.5	10.8	8.1				

Desirable weights for men and women aged 25 years and over according to height and frame, based on measurements made in indoor clothing without shoes.

Height (meters)	Weight in (kg) Small frame	Medium frame	Large frame
Men			
1.550	51–54	54–59	57–64
1.575	52–56	55–60	59–65
1.600	53–57	56–62	60–67
1.625	55–58	58–63	61–69
1.650	56–60	59–65	63–71
1.675	58–62	61–67	64–73
1.700	60–64	63–69	67–75
1.725	62–66	64–71	68–77
1.750	64–68	66–73	70–79
1.775	65–70	68–75	72–81
1.800	67–72	70–77	74–84
1.825	69–74	72–79	76–86
1.850	71–76	74–82	78–88
1.875	73–78	76–84	81–90
1.900	74–79	78–86	83–93
Women			
1.425	42–44	44–49	47–54
1.450	43–46	45–50	48–55
1.475	44–48	46–51	49–57
1.500	45–49	47–53	51–58
1.525	46–50	49–54	52–59
1.550	48–51	50–55	53–61
1.575	49–53	51–57	55–63
1.600	50–54	53–59	57–64
1.625	52–56	54–61	59–66
1.650	54–58	56–63	60–68
1.675	55–59	58–65	62–70
1.700	57–61	60–67	64–72
1.725	59–63	62–69	66–74
1.750	61–65	63–70	68–76
1.775	63–67	65–72	69–79

Appendix 4 Poisons

Acknowledgment
The information about poisons has been updated with the help of S.J. Hopkins PhD FPS, Consultant Pharmacist, Addenbrooke's Hospital, Cambridge.

Basic principles of treatment

In all cases of poisoning, certain general principles should be followed. It is a common misconception that for each poison there is a specific antidote. In practice, a true pharmacological antagonist is available in only 2.0% of poisonings. In the great majority of instances, therefore, the treatment consists primarily in the application of basic principles of supportive treatment. If the poison is a gas, or the vapor of a volatile liquid, the patient must be removed at once to fresh air and given oxygen and artificial respiration if needed. Subsequent treatment is supportive to maintain vital functions. If the poison has been ingested in most cases it is necessary to remove as much as possible of the unabsorbed substance from the stomach. Outside of the hospital this is best achieved by pharyngeal irritation using the finger or by administration of syrup of Ipecac as directed by the local Poison Control Center. In the hospital, gastric aspiration and lavage should be given provided the patient retains an adequate cough and gag reflex, or is sufficiently unconscious to allow the introduction of a cuffed endotracheal tube to protect the airway. These procedures should only be performed with the patient lying on his side with the head dependent. An adequate size of tube must be used, and 300 ml quantities of lukewarm water should be used for lavage until the recovered fluid runs clear. As a general rule nothing should be left in the stomach after lavage for fear of subsequent vomiting and pulmonary aspiration. Emetic drugs have been enthusiastically recommended to avoid the use of gastric aspiration and lavage. Apomorphine, common salt, mustard and copper sulfate have been used as emetics, but are now regarded as dangerous, and should **not** be used. Syrup of ipecac is quite widely used in a dose of 15 ml followed by 200 ml of water, and provided its limitations are recognized is the treatment of choice in children. The onset of its emetic effect is usually delayed for about 18 min and occasionally it may produce undesirable toxic effects after absorption.

Common errors in treatment

1. Analeptic therapy

Bemegride is not a specific barbiturate antagonist and its use in poisonings due to hypnotic drugs is associated with frequent serious side-effects including cardiac arrhythmias, convulsions and even irreversible brain damage. The use of analeptics cannot be justified.

2. Bladder catheterization

This highly dangerous procedure is seldom necessary even in deeply unconscious patients. With adequate nursing care, there should be no undue risk of skin breakdown due to incontinence of urine. Bladder catheterization is justified in prolonged bladder distension and occasionally when forced diuresis therapy is being given.

3. Prophylactic antibiotics

With good nursing care, including frequent turning of the patient and careful attention to mouth hygiene prophylactic administration of antibiotics is unnecessary. These drugs should be given only when there is clear clinical or X-ray evidence of infection.

Guide to poisonous substances and treatment

Substance	Clinical features	Treatment
Acids Strong hydrochloric acid. Spirits of salts. Strong sulfuric acid (oil of vitriol). Strong nitric acid. (See Bleaches (b)) **Alkalis** Caustic soda (sodium hydroxide). Caustic potash (potassium hydroxide). Strong ammonia	Severe burning of mouth and throat, causing dyspnea due to edema of glottis. Severe abdominal pains, thirst, shock, dark and bloodstained vomit, gastroenteritis.	Plenty of water to dilute the poison. *Acids:* Neutralize with milk of magnesia or calcium hydroxide (56 ml to ½ liter of warm water). Carbonates, as chalk, sodium bicarbonate and washing soda also effective, but cause liberation of carbon dioxide. Soap can be used if no other alkali available. *Alkalis:* Neutralize with acetic acid (56 ml to ½ liter), or vinegar (112 ml to ½ liter); lemon juice also effective, if available in sufficient quantity. General measures include morphine for pain, and arachis or olive oil as demulcent.
Amphetamine and related substances	Alertness, tremor, confusion, delirium, hallucinations, panic attacks, lethargy, exhaustion, headache, sweating, cardiac arrhythmias, hypertension or hypotension, dryness of mouth, diarrhea and abdominal colic, ulcers of the lips in addicts, convulsions and deep unconsciousness.	Gastric aspiration and lavage. If markedly excited chlorpromazine i.m. is the most effective treatment. Intensive supportive therapy. Forced acid diuresis if essential. For severe hypertension, phentolamine 5–10 mg i.v.
Anticoagulants Phenindione Warfarin Rodenticides	Hematuria, hemoptysis, bruising and hematemesis; occasionally bleeding elsewhere. Orange yellow urine. Prolonged prothrombin time.	Gastric aspiration and lavage. Vit. K; 20 mg i.v. Blood transfusion if necessary.

Substance	Clinical features	Treatment
Antidepressants Amitriptyline Butriptyline Desipramine Doxepin Imipramine Nortriptyline Protriptyline Trimipramine	Dryness of the mouth, dilated pupils, tachycardia leading to bizarre cardiac arrhythmias, hypotension, cardiac failure or arrest, urinary retention, varying degrees of unconsciousness, pressure of speech, increased limb reflexes, convulsions, torticollis and ataxia. Respiratory failure. Cardiac complications are common and particularly dangerous in children.	Gastric aspiration and lavage. Intensive supportive therapy. In the majority of patients these measures are all that are necessary. The central nervous system effects and some of the cardiac abnormalities can be abolished by the slow i.v. injection of physostigmine salicylate 1–3 mg, which may be repeated once after 10 min. If ineffective, convulsions may be controlled by diazepam 10 mg i.v. or sodium phenobarbital 300 mg i.m. β-Adrenergic blocking drugs may correct difficult cardiac arrhythmias.
Antihistamines	In adults, toxic doses cause deep central depression. In children and infants, the effect is often stimulatory, and confusion and convulsions may result. Hypotension, tachycardia and occasionally cardiac arrhythmias. Respiratory depression. Dryness of the mouth, nausea and constipation. Hyperpyrexia. Agranulocytosis and aplastic anemia may develop.	Intensive supportive therapy. Gastric aspiration and lavage. Sedation may be required in the form of diazepam or sodium phenobarbital i.m. Antibiotics, steroid drugs and blood transfusion may be necessary in severe blood dyscrasia.
Atropine Belladonna Scopolamine Homatropine Propantheline and other anticholinergic drugs. Deadly Nightshade	Blurring of vision, taxia, mental confusion, hallucinations. Tachycardia, hypertension, cardiac arrhythmias. Dryness and burning of the mouth with marked thirst, nausea and vomiting. Urinary urgency and possible acute retention. Hyperpyrexia. Death usually results from respiratory failure.	Intensive supportive therapy. Gastric aspiration and lavage. Peripheral effects may be relieved by subcutaneous injection of neostigmine 0.25 mg. When central nervous stimulation is marked, sedation with a short-acting barbiturate or diazepam may be necessary. Physostigmine salicylate (1–4 mg) i.m. or i.v. will rapidly antagonize the central nervous complications, but repeat doses may be required every 1 to 2 hours.

Substance	Clinical features	Treatment
Barbiturates *Long-acting* Barbital Phenobarbital *Medium-acting* Allobarbital Butobarbital Amylobarbital *Short-acting* Pentobarbital Cyclobarbital Quinalbarbital *Ultra-short-acting* Hexobarbital Thiopental	Impaired level of consciousness. Limb reflexes very variable. Withdrawal fits and delirium during the phase of recovery occur in patients habituated to the drug. Cardiovascular depression with hypotension and 'shock'. Respiratory depression. Hypothermia. Renal failure. Bullous lesions occur in 6% of patients with this condition.	Intensive supportive therapy. Gastric aspiration and lavage. Forced osmotic alkaline diuresis and/or hemodialysis are of value in patients severely poisoned with long-acting barbiturates but are less effective with the other types.
Benzodiazepines Chlordiazepoxide Diazepam Flurazepam Lorazepam Oxazepam Temazepam	Physical dependence may occur when the drug has been taken for some time. Also an additive effect occurs when taken in combination with alcohol, barbiturate, phenothiazine, monoamine oxidase inhibitors and imipramine. Loss of consciousness, bradycardia and hypotension. Respiratory depression.	Intensive supportive therapy. Gastric aspiration and lavage.
Bleaches *a.* Containing sodium hypochlorite	If inhaled: Cough and pulmonary edema. If ingested: Irritation of the mouth and pharynx; edema of pharynx and larynx. Nausea and vomiting.	Gastric aspiration and lavage using 2.5% sodium thiosulfate (if not available milk or milk of magnesia). If severely ill sodium thiosulfate (1%) 250 ml i.v.
b. Containing oxalic acid	Irritation of the mouth and throat. Nausea and vomiting. Muscular twitchings and convulsions. Shock and cardiac arrest. Acute renal failure the onset of which may be delayed.	Intensive supportive therapy. Gastric aspiration and lavage adding 10 g calcium lactate to the lavage fluid. Calcium gluconate 10% 10 ml i.v. and repeat as necessary. Provided the renal output is adequate at least 5 liters of fluid should be given for 3 days.

Substance	Clinical features	Treatment
Carbamates Meprobamate	Impairment of consciousness, muscle weakness and incoordination, nystagmus. Respiratory depression. Hypotension. Hypothermia. Withdrawal fits may occur.	Intensive supportive therapy. Gastric aspiration and lavage. Forced osmotic alkaline diuresis in severely poisoned patients and, if ineffective, hemodialysis.
Carbon monoxide and coal gas	Vertigo and ataxia; acute agitation and confusion; deep coma may develop. Papilledema, increased limb reflexes and possibly extensor plantar responses. Acute myocardial infarction, tachycardia, arrhythmias and hypotension. Respiratory stimulation, which may progress to respiratory failure. Nausea, vomiting, hematemesis and fecal incontinence are common. Bullous lesions may occur. Sequelae include Parkinsonism, hemiparesis and impairment of higher intellectual function.	Urgent. Remove from exposure. Intensive supportive therapy. Give a mixture of 95% O_2 and 5% CO_2 or by hyperbaric oxygen if available. In the presence of cerebral edema 500 ml of 20% mannitol i.v. over 15 min followed by 500 ml 5% dextrose over the next 4 hours.
Contraceptives, oral	Mild nausea or vomiting. Withdrawal bleeding in girls may occur.	Intensive supportive therapy. Gastric aspiration and lavage.
Cresol Phenol Lysol	Strong smell of carbolic acid in patient's breath or vomit. Corrosion of lips and buccal mucosa but little pain. Marked abdominal pain, nausea and vomiting. Hematemesis or gastric perforation. After absorption, initial excitement then impaired consciousness. Hypotension. Dark urine, oliguria and renal failure. Liver failure may occur. Respiratory failure is a common cause of death.	Intensive supportive therapy. Gastric aspiration and lavage with care. Wash ulcers with copious water or 50% alcohol. Medical measures for hepatic and renal failure. Hemodialysis may be required.

Substance	Clinical features	Treatment
Cyanide	Very toxic. *Mild poisoning* Headach, dyspnea, vomiting, ataxia and loss of consciousness occur gradually. *Severe poisoning* The above features develop very rapidly and the patient becomes deeply unconscious. The smell of bitter almonds is not necessarily present. The skin remains pink unless breathing has ceased. Rapid, thready pulse. Hypotension. Limb reflexes are often absent and the pupils are dilated.	Speed is essential. As long as the heart sounds are audible, recovery may be anticipated with appropriate treatment. Treatment includes: (1) If the poisoning is due to inhalation, remove from contaminated atmosphere. (2) Break an ampule of amyl nitrite under the patient's nose whilst applying artificial respiration where this is necessary. (3) Cobalt edetate (Kelocyanor), which is the treatment of choice. Dose 300–600 mg i.v. initially, but a second dose of 300 mg may be given if recovery does not occur within 1–2 minutes, followed by i.v. glucose 5%. (4) Alternatively, give sodium nitrite (3%) in a dose of 10 ml over 3 minutes i.v. (5) Slow i.v. infusion of 50 ml of 25% sodium thiosulfate. (6) If the poison has been ingested, gastric aspiration and lavage, with 300 ml 25% sodium thiosulfate left in the stomach. Hyperbaric oxygen may reduce the cellular anoxia. *Note:* Ketocyanor and the other antidotes should be kept in an emergency kit in all emergency depts. Ketocyanor may cause nausea and vomiting, but recovery is rapid. Remember that Ketocyanor is relatively toxic except in cyanide poisoning, so careful diagnosis is important. If given in error, treat cobalt toxicity with i.v. infusion of sodium calcium edetate.
Detergents	Nausea, vomiting and diarrhea. Most are not very toxic.	Supportive therapy

Substance	Clinical features	Treatment
Digitalis and Digoxin	Nausea and vomiting, diarrhea. Bradycardia. Cardiac arrhythmias. Mental confusion.	Intensive supportive therapy. Gastric aspiration and lavage. In hypokalemic arrhythmia, potassium chloride 1.0 g orally every 20 min; if vomiting occurs 1 g in 200 ml 5% dextrose infused over 30 min. Lidocaine 500 mg in 500 ml saline/dextrose i.v. administered at a rate depending on the clinical response is the best treatment for ventricular ectopics. Atropine sulfate 0.6 mg i.m. repeated as necessary for bradycardia. Cardiac pacing may occasionally be required.
Glutethimide	Similar to barbiturate poisoning, but depth of coma may vary considerably. Sudden apnea may occur, probably due to sudden raised intracranial pressure. Pupils dilated and unresponsive to light. Hypotension may be severe. Myocardial infarction may occur.	Intensive supportive therapy. Gastric aspiration and lavage with a mixture of castor oil and water. Leave 50 ml of castor oil in stomach to reduce absorption. If there is any suspicion of raised intracranial pressure give 500 ml 20% mannitol i.v. over 20 min followed by 500 ml 5% dextrose over next 4 hours.
Iron salts	*Stage 1.* Epigastric pain, nausea and vomiting. Hematemesis. Tachypnea and tachycardia followed by bloody diarrhea and collapse. *Stage 2.* An interval of hours or even several days may elapse during which there are no further signs and symptoms. Then severe headache, confusion, delirium, convulsions and loss of consciousness. Respiratory and circulatory failure. *Stage 3.* If patient survives, liver failure and renal failure may occur.	Intensive supportive therapy. Immediate i.m. injection of desferrioxamine 1–2 g, followed by gastric aspiration and lavage with desferrioxamine 2 g in 1 liter of water. Afterwards 10 g desferrioxamine should be left in the stomach. I.v. infusion of desferrioxamine 15 mg/kg per hour to a maximum dose of 80 mg/kg per 24 hours. Medical measures for hepatic and renal failure may be necessary.

Substance	Clinical features	Treatment
Lead	Severe abdominal pain, vomiting, diarrhea, oliguria, collapse, coma, 'Shock' and hepatic failure may occur. Acute hemolytic anemia.	Intensive supportive therapy. Gastric aspiration and lavage. When colic is severe calcium gluconate (10%) 10 ml i.v. Calcium sodium edetate up to 40 mg/kg twice daily for 5 days by i.v. infusion. Penicillamine orally in doses of 20–40 mg daily following initial therapy. Sodium bicarbonate (5%) or sodium lactate (M/6) by i.v. infusion for acidosis. Peritoneal or hemodialysis in severe poisoning.
Methyl alcohol Methanol Wood alcohol	Headache, blurring of vision which may lead to blindness, dilatation of pupils and papilledema, loss of consciousness. Nausea and vomiting. Hyperventilation.	Intensive supportive therapy. Gastric aspiration and lavage. Ethylalcohol 50% 1 ml per kg stat, then 0.5 ml per kg every 2 hours. Treat acidosis with i.v. infusions of sodium bicarbonate 5% or sodium lactate (M/6), repeated if necessary for some hours.
Methaqualone	Hypertonia, myoclonia, extensor plantar responses, papilledema and impairment of level of consciousness. Tachycardia, acute myocardial infarction. Respiratory depression. Bleeding tendencies may occur.	Intensive supportive therapy. Gastric aspiration and lavage. Hemodialysis in severe poisoning.
Opium alkaloids Heroin Morphine Meperidene Codeine Dipipanone Pentazocine Propoxyphene	Impaired level of consciousness; pinpoint pupils. Convulsions may occur particularly in young children. Respiratory and circulatory depression. Methemoglobinemia may occur.	Intensive supportive therapy. Gastric aspiration and lavage. Naloxone (Narcan) 0.4 mg i.v. and repeated 3 min later is usually sufficient to re-establish normal respiration and conscious level.

Substance	Clinical features	Treatment
Organophosphorous compounds	These insecticides are very toxic. Headache, restlessness, ataxia, muscle weakness, convulsions. Salivation, nausea, vomiting, colic and diarrhea. Bradycardia, hypotension, peripheral circulatory failure. Bronchospasm, cyanosis, acute pulmonary edema. Respiratory failure is the usual cause of death.	Intensive supportive therapy. Gastric aspiration and lavage if ingested. As soon as cyanosis is corrected, atropine sulfate 2 mg i.v. and repeated at 15-min intervals until fully atropinized. Pralidoxime 30 mg per kg i.v. slowly and repeat half-hourly as necessary. If sedation or control of convulsions is required, diazepam 10 mg may be used.
Paracetamol	Pallor, nausea and sweating. Hypotension, tachycardia and other cardiac arrhythmias. Excitement and delirium progressing to CNS depression and stupor. Hypothermia, hypoglycemia and metabolic acidosis. Tachypnea. Hemolysis. Renal failure. Jaundice and hepatic failure, which is the commonest mode of death. Severity of poisoning best assessed on blood levels. If the plasma paracetamol level is above 2000 mmol per liter and especially if the plasma half-life is greater than 4 hours hepatic damage is likely.	Intensive supportive therapy. If the plasma paracetamol half-life is greater than 4 hours give acetylcysteine 150 mg/kg by i.v. infusion in glucose 5% over 15 minutes, followed by 50 mg/kg over 4 hours and 100 mg/kg over 16 hours may protect the liver against paracetamol damage. Methionine 2.5 g orally initially, repeated 4-hourly up to a total of 10 g is also of value. *Note* Acetylcysteine may increase liver damage unless given within 12 hours of poisoning. Intravenous infusions of sodium bicarbonate to correct acidemia, i.v. glucose for hypoglycemia, and if hemolysis is severe corticosteroids and blood transfusion may be necessary. Hemodialysis may be required for renal failure.
Paraquat	Burning sensation in mouth at time of ingestion followed by nausea, vomiting and diarrhea. After a few hours painful buccal ulceration develops. Several days after ingestion a progressive alveolitis and bronchiolitis is probable and is the usual cause of death. Severe renal and hepatic impairment may occur.	Careful gastric aspiration and lavage with 300 ml of Fuller's earth suspension 30% with 15 g of magnesium sulfate. Leave 300 ml of suspension in stomach. Give another 300 ml later to promote excretion of unabsorbed drug by purging. Intensive supportive therapy. Immediate forced diuresis is safe before renal damage occurs.

Substance	Clinical features	Treatment
Petroleum distillates	Nausea, vomiting and diarrhea. If inhaled or aspirated, intense pulmonary congestion and chemical pneumonitis. Depression of consciousness and respiration with occasional convulsions.	*No* gastric aspiration or lavage. 250 ml liquid paraffin orally. If pneumonitis, hydrocortisone 100 mg i.m. 6-hourly for 48 hours with antibiotics as indicated. Mechanical ventilation may be necessary.
Phenothiazines	Impaired level of consciousness, Parkinsonism, torticollis, oculogyric crises, restlessness and convulsions. Hypotension, tachycardia, cardiac arrhythmias. Hypothermia. Respiratory depression in severe poisoning.	Intensive supportive therapy. Gastric aspiration and lavage. Convulsions should be treated with diazepam 10 mg, or orphenadrine 20 mg or procyclidine 10 mg by injection. Cogentin (benztropine mesylate) 2 mg i.v. is effective for Parkinsonism.
Phenytoin	Stimulation and possibly euphoria, vertigo, headache, cerebellar ataxia, nystagmus, tremor, loss of consciousness. Nausea, and vomiting. Respiratory depression.	Intensive supportive therapy. Gastric aspiration and lavage.
Primidone	Similar to phenytoin but loss of consciousness tends to be more marked.	Intensive supportive therapy. Gastric aspiration and lavage. Forced alkaline osmotic diuresis or hemodialysis may be necessary in severe poisoning.
Quinine and quinidine	Tinnitus; blurred vision; headache and dizziness. Impaired consciousness; rapid, shallow breathing. Tachycardia, hypotension, cardiac arrhythmias and arrest may occur. Acute hemolysis and renal failure.	Intensive supportive therapy. Gastric aspiration and lavage. ECG monitoring is required and cardiac arrhythmias treated with appropriate drugs. In marked visual impairment stellate ganglion block may produce dramatic improvement. Forced acid diuresis may be of value in severe poisoning.

Substance	Clinical features	Treatment
Salicylates Aspirin (acetylsalicylic acid) Methyl salicylate Sodium salicylate	Alertness and restlessness, tinnitus, deafness. Hyperventilation. Hyperpyrexia and sweating, nausea and vomiting. Dehydration and oliguria. Unconsciousness may occur in severe poisoning; hypoprothrombinemia occurs in some patients. Hypokalemia may be severe. Metabolic acidemia and hypoglycemia are often marked in children.	Gastric aspiration and lavage in all patients. Forced alkaline diuresis if the plasma salicylate is above 500 mg/liter in adults or 300 mg/liter in children. In very severe poisoning hemodialysis. Intensive supportive therapy.
Snake bite Adder bite (Viper berus)	Local features: Swelling, pain and redness. General features: Agitation, restlessness, abdominal colic, vomiting and diarrhea. Collapse and respiratory failure may result.	Specific antivenom should *not* be used as serious anaphylactic shock may result, unless in the severely ill patient when only the Zagreb antivenom should be given by i.v. infusion. Adrenaline should be available for serum reactions. Cleanse the site and immobilize the bitten part. Hydrocortisone 100 mg i.m. Antibiotics and tetanus antitoxin are of little value. Intensive supportive therapy.
Thiazides	Polyuria, dehydration, hypokalemia, hyponatremia, hypochloremia and alkalemia. Acute renal failure may occur. Also acute hepatic failure is occasionally found and in susceptible patients an acute attack of gout may result.	Intensive supportive therapy. Gastric aspiration and lavage. Potassium chloride 2 g 3-hourly depending on the degree of hypokalemia. Intravenous fluids may be necessary to correct dehydration.

Further information may be obtained from various Poison Control Centers.

Appendix 5 Poison Control Centers*

Alabama	205-832-3194
Alaska	907-465-3100
Arizona	602-626-6016
Arkansas	501-661-2301
California	916-322-4336
Colorado	303-320-8476
Connecticut	203-674-3456
Delaware	302-655-3389
District of Columbia	202-673-6741
Florida	904-487-1566
Georgia	404-894-5170
Hawaii	808-531-7776
Idaho	208-334-4245
Illinois	217-785-2080
Indiana	317-633-0332
Iowa	515-281-4964
Kansas	913-862-9360 ext. 541
Kentucky	502-564-3970
Louisiana	318-425-1524
Maine	207-871-2950
Maryland	301-528-7604
Massachusetts	617-727-2700
Michigan	517-373-1406
Minnesota	612-623-5284
Mississippi	601-354-7660
Missouri	314-751-2713
Montana	406-449-3895

Nebraska	402-471-2122
Nevada	702-885-4750
New Hampshire	603-646-5000
New Jersey	609-292-5666
New Mexico	505-843-2551
New York	518-474-3785
North Carolina	919-684-8111
North Dakota	701-224-2388
Ohio	614-466-5190
Oklahoma	405-271-5454
Oregon	503-225-8968
Pennsylvania	717-787-2307
Rhode Island	401-277-5727
South Carolina	803-758-5654
South Dakota	605-773-3361
Tennessee	615-741-2407
Texas	512-458-7254
Utah	801-533-6161
Vermont	802-658-3456
Virginia	804-786-5188
Washington	206-522-7478
West Virginia	304-348-4211
Wisconsin	608-267-7174
Wyoming	307-777-7955

* These numbers are subject to change. For further listings and updated information, contact the National Clearinghouse for Poison Control Centers, Food and Drug Administration, U.S. Department of Health and Human Services, Bethesda, Md., 20016.

AA	Alcoholics Anonymous
AACCN	American Association of Critical Care Nurses
AACN	American Association of Colleges of Nursing
AAMD	American Association for Mental Deficiency
AANA	American Association of Nurse Anesthetists
AAPA	American Academy of Pediatrics
AARC	American Association for Retired Citizens
AARCA	American Association for Rehabilitation Therapy
AATA	American Art Therapy Association
ACCH	Association for Care of Children in Hospitals
ACHA	American College Health Association
ACLU	American Civil Liberties Union
ACNM	American College of Nurse-Midwives
ACOG	American College of Obstetricians and Gynecologists
ACS	American Cancer Society
AHA	American Hospital Association
AHM	Academy of Holistic Medicine
AMA	American Medical Association
ANA	American Nurses' Association
ANAD	Anorexia Nervosa and Associated Disorders
AOA	Administration on Aging
AORN	Association of Operating Room Nurses
APHA	American Public Health Association
ARC	American Red Cross
ASPO	American Society for Psychoprophylaxis in Obstetrics

BA	Bachelor of Arts
BS	Bachelor of Science
BSN	Bachelor of Science in Nursing

CAL	Computer Assisted Learning
CDC	Centers for Disease Control
CEC	Council for Exceptional Children
CFF	Cystic Fibrosis Foundation
CIH	Children in Hospitals

CNM	Certified Nurse-Midwife
CSPI	Center for Science in the Public Interest

DC	Doctor of Chiropractic
DDS	Doctor of Dental Surgery
DH	Dental Hygienist
DMD	Doctor of Dental Medicine
DMV	Doctor of Veterinary Medicine
DO	Doctor of Osteopathy
DP	Doctor of Pharmacy
DPH	Doctor of Public Health
DPM	Doctor of Podiatric Medicine

EDNA	Emergency Department Nurses' Association
EENT	Eye, Ear, Nose and Throat
EMS	Emergency Medical Services
EMT	Emergency Medical Technician

FACA	Fellow of the American College of Anesthetists
FACC	Fellow of the American College of Cardiology
FACD	Fellow of the American College of Dentists
FACFP	Fellow of the American College of Family Practitioners
FACO	Fellow of the American College of Otolaryngology
FACOG	Fellow of the American College of Obstetricians and Gynecologists
FACP	Fellow of the American College of Physicians
FACR	Fellow of the American College of Radiologists
FACS	Fellow of the American College of Surgeons
FCAP	Fellow of the College of American Pathologists
FCGP	Fellow of the American College of General Practitioners
FCMS	Fellow of the College of Medicine and Surgery
FCOT	Fellow of the College of Occupational Therapists
FCPath	Fellow of the College of Pathologists
FCP	Fellow of the College of Clinical Pharmacology
FCPS	Fellow of the College of Physicians and Surgeons
FDA	Food and Drug Administration
FDS	Fellow in Dental Surgery
FNP	Family Nurse Practitioner
FNS	Frontier Nursing Service

GN	Graduate Nurse
HEW	Health, Education and Welfare
HMO	Health Maintenance Organization
HO	House Officer
ICEA	International Childbirth Education Association
ICN	International Council of Nurses; Intensive Care Nursery
ICNM	International College of Nurse-Midwives
LLL	La Leche League
LPN	Licensed Practical Nurse
MA	Master of Arts
MCA	Maternity Center Association
MD	Medical Doctor
MDA	Muscular Dystrophy Association
MO	Medical Officer
MPH	Master of Public Health
MS	Master of Science
MSN	Master of Science in Nursing
NA	Nurse Anesthetist
NAACOG	Nurses' Association of the American College of Obstetricians and Gynecologists
NAPNAP	National Association of Pediatric Nurse Associates and Practitioners
NAPSAC	National Association of Parents and Professionals for Safe Alternatives in Childbirth
NARC	National Association for Retarded Citizens
NCDAI	National Clearinghouse for Drug Abuse Information
NHI	National Health Insurance
NHS	National Health Service
NIOSH	National Institute for Occupational Safety and Health
NLN	National League of Nursing
NREMT	National Registry of Emergency Medical Technicians
OT	Occupational Therapist

PA	Physician's Assistant; Parents' Anonymous
PhD	Doctor of Philosophy
PHN	Public Health Nurse
PNP	Pediatric Nurse Practitioner
PPFA	Planned Parenthood Federation of America
PSR	Physicians for Social Responsibility
PSRO	Peer Standards Review Organization
PT	Physical Therapist
RN	Registered Nurse
RNA	Registered Nurse Anesthetist
SN	Student Nurse
ST	Speech Therapist
VNA	Visiting Nurse Association
WHO	World Health Organization

a.a.	of each
abd	abdomen
a.c.	before meals
Ac.	acid
ACTH	adrenocorticotropin
ADL	activities of daily living
ADP	adenosine diphosphate
ad lib	as desired
adm	admission
alk.	alkaline
A.M.	morning
a.m.a.	against medical advice
amp	ampule
amt	amount
ANS	autonomic nervous system
ante	before
AP	anteroposterior
AROM	artificial rupture of membranes
ASHD	arteriosclerotic heart disease
ASD	atrial septal defect
ATP	adenosine triphosphate
A-V	atrio-ventricular
A&W	alive and well

BCP	birth control pills
B.E.	barium enema
bene	well
b.i.d.	twice a day
BM	bowel movement
BMR	basal metabolic rate
BP	blood pressure
BRP	bathroom privileges
BS	blood sugar
BSE	breast self exam
BSP	bromosulfophthalein
BT	bleeding time

BUN	blood urea nitrogen
Bx	biopsy

C	centigrade
$\bar{c}$	with
Ca	calcium, cancer
Cal	calorie
cap	capsule
cath	catheter
C.B.C.	complete blood count
C.B.R.	complete bed rest
cc	cubic centimeter
CC	chief complaint
C.C.U.	coronary care unit
CF	cystic fibrosis
CHF	congestive heart failure
CHO	carbohydrate
chol.	cholesterol
cm	centimeter
CMV	cytomegalo virus
CNS	central nervous system
c/o	complains of
C.O.	cardiac output
contra	against
CPD	cephalopelvic disproportion
C&S	culture and sensitivity
CS	cesarean section
CSF	cerebrospinal fluid
CSS	central sterile supply
CST	convulsive shock therapy
CV	cardiovascular
CVA	cerebrovascular accident
CVP	central venous pressure
CVS	clean voided specimen
Cx	cervix

d.c	discontinue
D&C	dilation and curettage
DD	differential diagnosis
dig.	digitalis

dil.	dilute
disch.	discharge
DNA	deoxyribonucleic acid
DOA	dead on arrival
DOB	date of birth
DOE	dyspnea on exertion
DPT	diphtheria, pertussis, tetanus
dr	dram
Dr.	doctor
D.R.	delivery room
drsg.	dressing
DSD	dry sterile dressing
DTs	delirium tremens
DTR	deep tendon reflex
D/W	dextrose and water
Dx	diagnosis
ECG, EKG	electrocardiogram
ECT	electroconvulsive therapy
EDC	estimated date of confinement
EEG	electroencephalogram
e.g.	for example
elix.	elixir
E.R.	emergency room
E.S.P.	extrasensory perception
ESR	erythrocyte sedimentation rate
et al.	and others
ext.	extract
f	frequency; female
F	fahrenheit
F.B.S.	fasting blood sugar
Fe	iron
FEV	forced expiratory volume
FH	family history
FHR	fetal heart rate
fld	fluid
FSH	follicle stimulating hormone
G	gravida
gal	gallon

GC	gonococcus
GH	growth hormone
GI	gastrointestinal
Gm, g	gram
gr	grain
gtt	drops
GTT	glucose tolerance test
GU	genitourinary
h(hr)	hour
Hb(Hgb)	hemoglobin
HCL	hydrochloric
Hct	hematocrit
Hg	mercury
HMD	hyaline membrane disease
h/o	history of
HPI	history of present illness
H.R.	heart rate
h.s.	hour of sleep
ht	height
HT	hypertension
Hx	history
ICF	intracellular fluid
ICU	Intensive Care Unit
ID	Intradermal
I&D	incision and drainage
i.e.	that is
IM	intramuscular
inj	injection
I&O	intake and output
IPPB	intermittent positive pressure breathing
IQ	intelligence quotient
IU	international unit
IUD	intrauterine device
IV	intravenous
IVP	intravenous pyelogram
K	potassium
kg	kilogram

L	left; liter
lap	laparotomy
lb	pound
LE	lupus erythematosis
LGA	large for gestational age
LH	luteinizing hormone
liq	liquid
LLQ	left lower quadrant
LMP	last menstrual period
LOA	left occiput anterior
LOP	left occiput posterior
LOT	left occiput transverse
LP	lumbar puncture
LUQ	left upper quadrant
l&w	living and well
m	meter
mEq	milliequivalent
mg	milligram
MI	myocardial infarction
min	minute; minim
ml	milliliter
mm	millimeter
MS	multiple sclerosis
MSU	midstream urine
multip	multipara
NB	note carefully; newborn
neg	negative
neuro	neurology
N-G	nasogastric
nil	none
no.	number
noct	at night
NPN	non protein nitrogen
NPO	nothing by mouth
NS	normal saline
NSVD	normal spontaneous vaginal delivery
nullip	nullipara
N&V	nausea and vomiting

OA	occiput anterior
OB, Obs	obstetrics
O.C.	oral contraceptive
od	daily
OD	right eye; overdose
OOB	out of bed
OP	occiput posterior
OPD	outpatient department
O.R.	operating room
Ortho	orthopedics
os	opening
OS	left eye
OT	occupational therapy
oz	ounce

$\bar{p}$	after
P	para; pulse
PA	physician's assistant
Pap	Papanicolaou smear
para	number of pregnancies
path	pathology
PBI	protein bound iodine
p.c.	after meals
PE	physical examination
per	by; through
PERLA	pupils equal and reactive to light and accommodation
P.H.	past history
PI	present illness
PID	pelvic inflammatory disease
PKU	phenylketonuria
p.m.	afternoon
P.O.R.	problem oriented record
pos	positive
postop	postoperative
preop	preoperative
prep	preparation
p.r.	per rectum
p.r.n.	when needed
pro time	prothrombin time

PSP	phenolsulfon phthalein
pt	patient, pint
PT	physical therapy
PTA	prior to admission
PVC	premature ventricular contraction
q.	every
q.d.	every day
q.h.	every hour
q.h.s.	at bedtime
q.i.d.	4 times a day
q.o.d.	every other day
qt	quart
R, Rt	right
RBC	red blood cell
RDS	respiratory distress syndrome
REM	rapid eye movement
Rh	Rhesus factor
RHD	rheumatic heart disease
RLQ	right lower quadrant
RNA	ribonucleic acid
R/O	rule out
ROA	right occiput anterior
ROM	range of motion
ROP	right occiput posterior
ROT	right occiput transverse
RR	respiratory rate; recovery room
RUQ	right upper quadrant
Rx	therapy; treatment
$\bar{s}$	without
sc	subcutaneous
SD	standard deviation
sg	specific gravity
SGA	small for gestational age
SIDS	sudden infant death syndrome
sig	label
SOB	shortness of breath
$\overline{ss}$	one half
SSE	soap suds enema

stat	immediately
Sx	symptoms
TB	tuberculosis
Tbsp.; T.	tablespoon
t.i.d.	three times a day
TLC	tender loving care
t.o.	telephone order
TPR	temperature, pulse, respiration
tsp	teaspoon
TUR	transurethral resection
U	unit
U/A	urinalysis
ung	ointment
URI	upper respiratory infection
UTI	urinary tract infection
vag	vaginal
VD	venereal disease
VDRL	venereal disease research laboratory
Vit	vitamin
v.o.	verbal order
vol	volume
VS	vital signs
WBC	white blood cell
WC	wheelchair
WDWN	well developed, well nourished
WNL	within normal limits
wt	weight